ADOLESCENT MEDICINE

ADOLESCENT MEDICINE

Edited by
Adele D. Hofmann

in collaboration with
Donald E. Greydanus

Addison-Wesley Publishing Company
Medical/Nursing Division, Menlo Park, California
Reading, Massachusetts • London • Amsterdam • Don Mills, Ontario • Sydney

Sponsoring Editor: Richard W. Mixter
Production Coordinator: Nancy Sjoberg
Copy Editor: Suzanne Aboulfadl

Library of Congress Cataloging in Publication Data
  Main entry under title:

  Adolescent medicine.

  Includes index.
  1. Adolescent medicine. I. Hofmann, Adele D.
II. Greydanus, Donald E. [DNLM: 1. Adolescent
medicine—Handbooks. WS 460 H236]
RJ550.H3 1983   616   82-16345
ISBN 0-201-11071-7
ABCDEFGHIJ-MA-89876543

The authors and publishers have exerted every effort
to ensure that drug selection and dosage set forth in
this text are in accord with current recommendations
and practice at the time of publication. However, in
view of ongoing research, changes in government
regulations and the constant flow of information
relating to drug therapy and drug reactions, the
reader is urged to check the package insert for each
drug for any change in indications of dosage and for
added warnings and precautions. This is particularly
important where the recommended agent is a new
and/or infrequently employed drug.

Addison-Wesley Publishing Company
Medical/Nursing Division
2725 Sand Hill Road
Menlo Park, California 94025

Contributors

Richard R. Brookman, M.D.
Director, Adolescent Medicine
Associate Professor of Pediatrics
Department of Pediatrics
Medical College of Virginia,
Virginia Commonwealth University
Richmond, Virginia

H. Paul Gabriel, M.D.
Director, Pediatric Psychiatry Consultation-Liason
  Service
New York University Medical Center and
  Bellevue Hospital Center
Professor of Clinical Psychiatry
New York University School of Medicine
New York, New York

Donald E. Greydanus, M.D.
Director, Adolescent Medical Clinic
Department of Pediatrics
Strong Memorial Hospital
Assistant Professor of Pediatrics
University of Rochester School of Medicine and
  Dentistry
Rochester, New York

Adele D. Hofmann, M.D.
Director, Adolescent Medical Unit
Department of Pediatrics
New York University Medical Center and
  Bellevue Hospital Center
Associate Professor of Pediatrics
New York University School of Medicine
New York, New York

Robert L. Johnson, M.D.
Director of Adolescent Medicine
Department of Pediatrics
University Hospital—Newark and Children's Hospital
  of New Jersey—Newark
Assistant Professor of Pediatrics
University of Medicine and Dentistry of New Jersey—
  New Jersey Medical School
Newark, New Jersey

George J. D. Mellendick, M.D.
Chairman, Department of Community Medicine
Perth Amboy General Hospital
Perth Amboy, New Jersey
Assistant Clinical Professor of Pediatrics
New York University School of Medicine
New York, New York

C. Anita Robinson, M.D.
Fellow, Adolescent Medical Unit
New York University Medical Center and
  Bellevue Hospital Center
New York, New York
Director, Adolescent Medicine
D.C. General Hospital
Assistant Professor
Howard University Medical School
Washington, D.C.

Ira M. Sacker, M.D.
Chief, Adolescent Medical Program
Department of Pediatrics
The Brookdale Hospital Medical Center
Assistant Professor of Pediatrics
State University of New York (SUNY) Downstate
Brooklyn, New York

Shepard H. Splain, D.O.
Physician-in-Charge of Sports Medicine
The Brookdale Hospital Medical Center
Brooklyn, New York
Clinical Associate, Department of Surgery
  (Orthopaedics)
New York College of Osteopathic Medicine
New York, New York

Natalia M. Tanner, M.D.
Attending Physician
Children's Hospital of Michigan
Clinical Associate Professor of Pediatrics
School of Medicine, Wayne State University
Detroit, Michigan

Editor's Foreword

Adolescent medicine is comprised of that body of knowledge and set of skills necessary to meet the primary health care needs of young people from the onset of puberty to the acquisition of autonomous adulthood, or approximately from 10-21 years of age. The parameters of this discipline encompass a broad range of issues varying from the biological to the psychosocial and from prevention to remediation of specific health problems.

Many medical problems are directly consequent to certain behaviors that are characteristic of the adolescent years, including sexual experimentation, indiscriminate drug and alcohol consumption, inexperienced automobile driving, and competitive athletics. Additional dimension is added to adolescent health care by the inevitable interplay between illness on the one hand and the intense body image concerns that stem from preoccupation with pubertal changes on the other hand. These factors render the adolescent singularly vulnerable to psychological complications of organic disease.

Another aspect of adolescent health care relates to parental and societal concern about adolescent behavior in general and the frequency with which the process of emancipation, both normal and deviant, is manifest in a distressing manner. The primary care physician will often be the first port of call for school problems, intrafamily conflicts, predelinquent acts, suicidal proclamations or attempts, and the like. In many instances he or she will be therapist as well as diagnostician.

While the behavioral aspects of adolescent medicine are widely recognized today, it is still often suggested that this is a healthy time of life from the biological perspective. It is certainly true that morbidity and mortality are lower in the second decade of life than in either infancy or old age. But it is a serious error to consider that teenagers are entirely immune from health problems. The following indicates the scope of health needs that may be encountered:

1. The 1976 mortality rates for 10-14 year olds and 15-19 year olds were 0.03% (0.3/1000) and 0.1% (1.0/1000), respectively, as compared to 0.07% (0.7/1000) for children less than 5 years and 0.13% (1.3/1000) for 20-25 year olds. Accidents, homicide, suicide, malignant neoplasms, and cardiovascular disease lead the list of causes of adolescent deaths. The incidence of significant morbidity is similar in magnitude to that of any age group between 6-35 years.

2. Seventy-two percent of 12-19 year olds visit a physician at least once a year.

3. Cross-sectional surveys of various adolescent populations have found an incidence of 40%-60% of abnormal findings on physical examination. Significant unremediated disease is particularly prevalent among those who live in poverty. Diseases commonly encountered among all economic groups include dermatologic problems, dental caries and periodontal disease, allergic conditions, epilepsy, cardiac problems, adjustment reactions and other behavioral concerns, deviations in growth and development, and a wide range of gynecologic and sexuality-related problems.

4. Inquiries from adolescents themselves about high-priority health matters find 90% wanting help for one or more of the following: acne, how far to go with sex, depression, obesity, getting along with parents, worries about health, dental care, nervousness, making friends, frequent fatigue, and birth control.

5. Nearly 11 million adolescents are sexually active today. Two out of every three boys and one out of every three girls between 15 and 19 years have had sexual intercourse at least once. One million girls become pregnant each year, with 600,000 actually giving birth; 35,000 of these births are to adolescents less than 16 years old.

6. The rate of gonorrhea among youths 15-19 years of age is second only to that among persons 20-25 years of age. It is the most frequently encountered reportable infectious disease and is virtually epidemic.

7. Increasing numbers of handicapped children are surviving into adolescence and an increasing number of severely and permanently injured youths are being salvaged as a result of advances in medical technology. The problems of chronic disease or disability during the teenage years cause special management considerations, particularly in the psychosocial dimension.

When one examines these trends together, it becomes evident that there are, in fact, many health problems that occur in adolescence and each poses a singular and taxing challenge to the health care professional.

To be effective, health care for young people also needs to be provided in a manner that is responsive to relevant developmental issues, such as puberty, intellectual maturation, and psychosocial advance. Failure to attend to these matters in any care plan risks poor compliance on the patient's part and overlooks important opportunities to help the adolescent accomplish his or her developmental tasks in the best way possible. At no other time in postnatal life does the human being accelerate in the rate of growth or experience such dramatic changes in bodily functions, physical appearance, cognitive capacity, and interpersonal relationships with parents and peers as during adolescence.

The adolescent patient cannot be managed as either a small adult or large child. The former bestows a degree of autonomy for which he or she is not yet ready, while the latter employs an inappropriate level of dependency that is guaranteed to precipitate struggles over control and, possibly, poor compliance with medical regimens. Rather, the health care approach should be one that supports the adolescent's interest in self-determination through *guided* decision-making and a collaborative physician-patient relationship in which the physician is clearly an authority but avoids delivering care in an authoritarian manner.

A final dimension of adolescent medicine requires the reorganization of customary appointment times and fee scales. A primary health care system that looks to high volume and low cost in contending with escalating medical expenses cannot satisfactorily manage many adolescent health problems. Caring for adolescents takes time; time to obtain psychosocial developmental data and time to provide counseling to young people and their parents. These are essential components of care. In the ordinary course of events, a first visit takes a minimum of 45 minutes and follow-up visits frequently require half an hour. Thus, appointment scheduling and fee scales must be adjusted accordingly. Parents are generally understanding of these higher costs when they are explained in advance. Attempting to see young people in lesser circumstances will only result in frustration for the physician and inadequate care for the patient.

Adele D. Hofmann

Preface

Adolescent Medicine is a response to the rapidly growing and widespread interest in the health care of young people between 10 and 21. The purpose of this book is to provide practical information relative to the diagnosis and management of health problems of this age group. It has been carefully coordinated and integrated by selected specialists in adolescent medicine, an orthopedist, and a psychiatrist, all of whom have had extensive direct experience in taking care of adolescents and in teaching adolescent medicine to physicians and other health care professionals.

Adolescent Medicine has been written for primary care physicians (including family physicians, general internists, and pediatricians), medical students, house officers in primary care disciplines, nurse practitioners, and physicians' assistants who want a practical, quick, how-to reference guide. Particular attention has been given to those problems that are relatively common or have singular implications for adolescents. Because this book's approach is that of a pragmatic, ready-to-use handbook, no attempt has been made to be all-inclusive or comprehensive in coverage. The reader who wishes additional information after reading *Adolescent Medicine* is directed to the more extensive texts listed in the bibliographies at the end of each chapter.

However, certain subjects are treated in this book in ways that are not available in other volumes devoted to adolescent medicine. Particularly distinctive sections include those on the emergency management of drug overdose and athletic injuries, the programmed approach to helping both the adolescent and family adjust to the physical and emotional viscissitudes of chronic illness or disability, and the detailed guide to adolescent interviewing and counseling techniques.

Adolescent Medicine is divided into four parts. Part One covers normal adolescence and general health care principles. This includes information on setting the stage for a health visit, the elements of a complete history and physical examination, and an optimal health maintenance plan for adolescents, outlining recommended procedures and the frequency with which they should be performed. Part Two comprises an organ system review, giving special attention to differential diagnoses, management protocols, and potential complications of the various diseases or their management. Rarely seen conditions or, conversely, those that are seen so frequently (for example, the common cold) as to be already sufficiently familiar to health care professionals have been omitted. Part Three focuses on issues of particular significance in adolescence, such as sexuality, nutrition, sports medicine, drug and alcohol abuse, chronic illness, and legal issues. Part Four offers guidance in managing the commonly encountered psychological problems of adolescence, such as psychosomatic illness, parent-adolescent alienation, depression, suicide, and school problems. Appendices give tables of normal values cited by age and, when available, by sexual maturity rating and addresses of organizations that may be helpful in providing additional professional or lay information and/or educational materials.

I wish to express my deep appreciation to each contributor for his or her unflagging interest in and commitment to this book and cheerful willingness in revising manuscript drafts on a number of occasions. A very special thanks to C. Anita Robinson, M.D., who diligently ferreted out the data for the appendix tables during her fellowship year with the editor. I am also grateful to my family, who survived on sparse fare and inattention while wife and mother became a recluse for a good many weekends over the better part of a year. My thanks also to Addison-Wesley for making this book possible and for having the vision to include a handbook on adolescent medicine in their publishing program. Particular appreciation and gratitude goes to all our secretaries who spent untold hours converting our hieroglyphics into manuscript form. In this regard I wish to extend my particular thanks to Mrs. Rita Fox. Lastly, none of us could have written this book were it not for both our patients and our own adolescent children and all they have taught us. Our warm appreciation goes to all those young people we have seen over the years or raised in our homes who so richly contributed to our understanding of the adolescent dimension.

Adele D. Hofmann

Contents

Tables

ADOLESCENT MEDICINE

PART ONE

ORIENTATION TO ADOLESCENT HEALTH CARE

1

Adolescent Growth and Development

Robert L. Johnson, M.D.

Puberty
Maturational events □ Clinical application of pubertal growth principles
Cognitive Maturation
Adolescence

Growth and development of the adolescent can be divided into three closely related maturational phenomena: biologic growth, or puberty; cognitive advance and the arrival of abstract thought; and psychosocial development—the process of adolescence itself (Figure 1-1).

Puberty

Puberty is characterized by sexual maturation and statural growth. Both result from a complex process in which gonadal hormones rapidly rise to a point sufficient to stimulate maturation of end-organ tissues such as those of the reproductive and musculoskeletal systems. In brief, although the amount of sex steroids produced has been slowly increasing since about 6 years of age, children do not reach puberty until some as yet incompletely understood confluence of events triggers hypothalamic production of follicle-stimulating hormone-releasing factor (FSHRF) and luteinizing hormone–releasing factor (LHRF). Current concepts suggest this system is controlled by a highly sensitive negative feedback mechanism that inhibits the synthesis of effective levels of the releasing hormones in early life. With increasing age, the feedback system decreases in sensitivity, allowing the releasing hormones to reach endocrinologically effective levels. The Frisch-Revelle hypothesis suggests this decreasing sensitivity is related to a statistically significant correlation between menarche and the achievement of a "critical" body weight of 47.8 kg. When they later found an even closer correlation between menarche and a

characteristic ratio between total body fat, total body water, and lean mass, Frisch and Revelle modified the critical body weight theory to incorporate a critical body composition concept. Subsequent investigators have not been able to replicate these studies with the same degree of consistency, although the concept based on body composition appears to be more broadly applicable than that based on body weight.

Whatever the triggering mechanisms, FSHRF and LHRF, which consist of short-chain peptides, then travel from a storage site in nerve endings in the median eminence through a capillary network to the anterior pituitary gland. There they stimulate the final states of synthesis and secretion of the gonadotrophic hormones—follicle-stimulating hormone (FSH) and luteinizing hormone (LH). In the female, FSH stimulates growth of the ovarian follicle and elaboration of estrogenic hormones. LH initiates ovulation, the formation of the corpus luteum, and progesterone production. In the male, LH acts on the Leydig cells, thus prompting testicular maturation and testosterone production. FSH, acting with LH, stimulates the final stage of spermatogenesis (Figure 1-2).

MATURATIONAL EVENTS

The first visible signs of puberty are the development of secondary sexual characteristics. As described by Tanner, the male adolescent experiences a gradual increase in the volume of his testes and scrotal size and an increase in the length and diameter of his

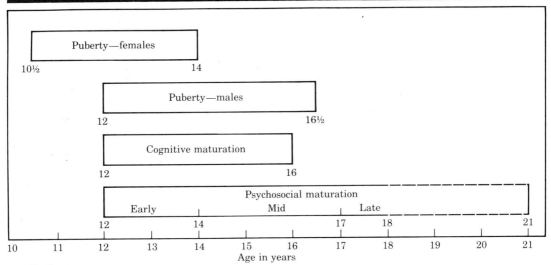

FIGURE 1-1
AVERAGE AGE RELATIONSHIPS OF PUBERTAL, COGNITIVE AND PSYCHOSOCIAL MATURATION
IN ADOLESCENCE

penis. In the female, a breast bud forms and grows, causing enlargement and contour changes of the breast. In both sexes pubic hair begins to grow.

Shortly thereafter, most teenagers experience a rapid increase in linear growth. Initially, the length of the long bones increases, creating a rise in the body's center of gravity. This is followed by growth of the spine, which reestablishes equilibrium in the ratio of upper to lower body segments. Tanner calls this stage of acceleration the growth spurt. During it, the average girl grows at a peak velocity of 8 cm per year; the average boy at a rate of 10 cm per year, adding as much as 20 cm to his height. Although linear growth is a most striking feature of puberty, a similar dimensional increase occurs in every body system except the lymphatic, in which total tissue volume decreases.

CLINICAL APPLICATION OF PUBERTAL GROWTH PRINCIPLES

Anyone who observes a group of adolescents of equal chronologic age quickly becomes aware of the great temporal variability in the physical expression of puberty. In any group of 14-year-olds, some are fully mature; others are in the midst of rapid change; and the remainder have not entered puberty at all—yet all are within the normal range of variation. Indeed, we all have our own biologic time clocks. Clearly, a purely chronologic conception of puberty is of limited value.

To improve the ability to assess the progress of

a particular youth, most individuals have adopted the use of the maturational stages proposed by Tanner in *Growth at Adolescence* (1962). He describes five growth stages based on the progression of breast and pubic hair development in girls and genital and pubic hair development in boys. Chapter 2 explains these stages in detail.

The importance of maturational stages lies in their correlation with other pubertal events. Understanding these relationships, as demonstrated in Figure 1-3, and their standard deviations greatly facilitates evaluation of normal and problematic growth states such as delayed puberty, short stature, or primary amenorrhea. Puberty in females can begin at any time between 8 and 14 years of age, but once initiated usually is completed within 3 years. The growth spurt commonly starts at the onset of stage 2, reaches a peak midway between stages 3 and 4, and ends at stage 5. Menarche occurs approximately 2½ years after the onset of puberty, or during stage 4. At this time the adolescent female has attained 90%–95% of her adult height.

Puberty starts 1½–2 years later in the male than in the female and takes nearly twice as long to complete. The growth spurt usually begins at stage 3, reaches a peak during stage 4, and is all but complete by stage 5. Some males, however, continue to grow up to 2 cm more in the ensuing 5 years. Another characteristic of male puberty is a period of rapid muscle growth at the end of stage 4, often referred to as the strength spurt.

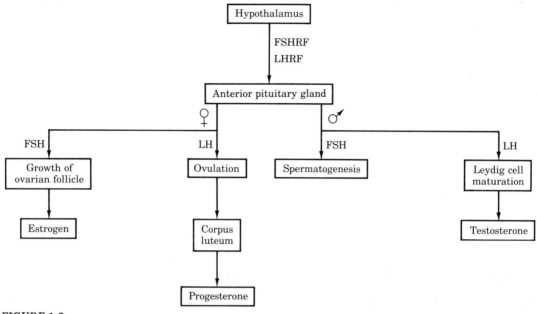

FIGURE 1-2
ENDOCRINE RESPONSE AT PUBERTY

Cognitive Maturation

As defined by Piaget, the early and midteen years are characterized by the movement from concrete to abstract operations in problem solving and directed thinking. Concrete thought is limited to considering things and specific situations in existential terms. The concrete thinker lacks the ability to extract general principles from one experience and apply them to a wholly new experience. The future cannot be appreciated except as a direct projection of clearly visible current options. Moral concepts are limited to coopting existing societal rules.

Abstract thinking permits the conceptualization of possibilities beyond past and present experience. It concerns words, hypotheses, ideas, and epistomologic form—hence the synonym, formal thought. Emerging abstractive competence is evident in the preoccupation of adolescents with fantasy and ideas. It has particular significance for psychosocial development in facilitating the formulation of identity, the achievement of independence, the making of career and life-style choices, and the evolution of a personal value system. Abstractive ability may not be so critical in highly structured cultures where growing up is simply a recapitulation of established tradition, but it becomes more important in a rapidly changing society where options and projected outcomes are measurable only in conjectural rather than predictable terms. These circumstances require the capacity for imaginative and creative thought.

It is important for the primary care physician to take this process into account in adopting any care plan. Teenagers who are capable of formal thought are better able to appreciate the consequences of their acts and to consider delaying immediate gratification for a more worthwhile but later goal. As applied to the medical setting, this means such adolescents are able to perceive treatment benefits and risks in future terms, much as the physician perceives them. But concrete thinkers, or those in whom abstractive process is still developing, need therapeutic recommendations with more immediate benefits. A young adolescent, for example, is unable to comprehend the long-range health implications of smoking; they have no reality and the adolescent cannot project into the future. But he may be able to accept the advantage of avoiding smoking if the physician stresses applications to his present life such as improved exercise tolerance in sports, the economic benefit of diverting money from cigarette purchases to clothing and records, or improved relations with a peer group who no longer views smoking as a status symbol.

On the average, abstractive ability begins to

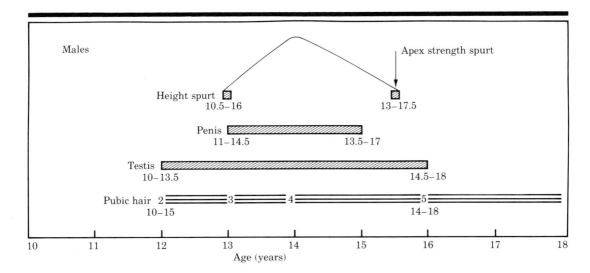

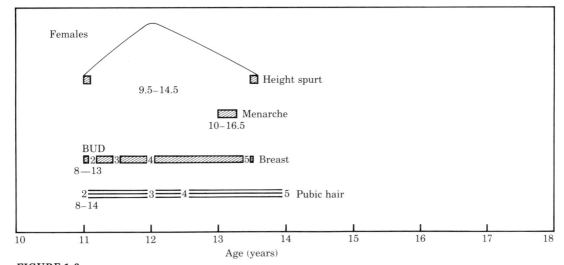

FIGURE 1-3
DIFFERENTIAL MATURATION IN MALES AND FEMALES

Numbers in bar representing pubic hair development refer to Tanner stage; other numbers define the normal age range, in years, for the initiation or completion of any event. From Tanner, J. M. 1962. *Growth at adolescence.* 2nd ed. Oxford: Blackwell.

emerge at about age 12 years and is fully operational by about age 16. Thereafter judgment may be enhanced by experience but not by additional intelligence or reasoning power. Like any other developmental parameter, however, wide variations exist among individuals. A particularly gifted youngster may abstract in the preteen years, whereas slower youths may not reach this point until the last year or two of high school. It also is true that this ability is not universally acquired; 30% of the normal populace never become abstractive thinkers; although if they are going to be, it happens in adolescence.

Even if capable of formal thought, no one uses it all the time. It may not be called for in simple situations. At other times, judgment and rationality may succumb to irrationality stemming from overriding stress and anxiety factors or chronic maladaptive patterns. Thus even an abstracting adolescent

TABLE 1-1
CHARACTERISTICS OF EARLY ADOLESCENCE

GROWTH	1. Secondary sexual characteristics have begun to appear. 2. Growth rapidly accelerating; reaches peak velocity.
COGNITION	1. Concrete thought dominant. 2. Existential orientation. 3. Cannot perceive long-range implications of current decisions and acts.
PSYCHOSOCIAL SELF	1. Preoccupation with rapid body change. 2. Former body image disrupted.
FAMILY	1. Defining independence-dependence boundaries. 2. No major conflicts over parental control.
PEER GROUP	1. Seeks peer affiliation to counter instability generated by rapid change. 2. Compares own normality and acceptance with same-sex age mates.
SEXUALITY	1. Self-exploration and evaluation. 2. Limited dating. 3. Limited intimacy.
AGE RANGE	Initiates between ages 11–13 and merges with midadolescence at 14–15 years.

TABLE 1-2
CHARACTERISTICS OF MID-ADOLESCENCE

GROWTH	1. Secondary sexual characteristics well advanced. 2. Growth decelerating; stature reaches 95% of adult height.
COGNITION	1. Rapidly gaining competence in abstract thought. 2. Capable of perceiving future implications of current acts and decisions but variably applied. 3. Reverts to concrete operations under stress.
PSYCHOSOCIAL SELF	1. Reestablishes body image as growth decelerates and stabilizes. 2. Preoccupation with fantasy and idealism in exploring expanded cognition and future options.
FAMILY	1. Major conflicts over control. 2. Struggle for emancipation.
PEER GROUP	1. Strong need for identification to affirm self-image. 2. Looks to peer group to define behavioral code during emancipation process.
SEXUALITY	1. Multiple plural relationships. 2. Heightened sexual activity. 3. Testing ability to attract and parameters of masculinity or femininity. 4. Preoccupation with romantic fantasy.
AGE RANGE	Begins around 14–15 years and blends into late adolescence about age 17.

may have difficulty seeing a range of options and acting on them with a clear head when the issue at hand is a particularly provocative one. In adolescence such tension is often caused by intrafamily contests over control, insecure peer relationships, important examinations and, last but not least, the ambivalence surrounding sexuality.

Adolescence

The biologic events of puberty have not changed since the time of Caine and Abel. Although evidence suggests that maturation now begins at an earlier age and that adolescents are attaining a larger ultimate size, the events just described are universal in their sequencing and expression. Adolescence is the psychosocial process through which a child becomes an adult. This process, though linked to the more constant features of puberty, is unique for each society. For the young Kunte Kinte of Alex Haley's *Roots*, it was a brief, predetermined 6-week period of training followed by ritual circumcision. There were no variations and no uncertainties. For J. D. Salinger's Holden Caulfield, it was a long tedious process that had no clear beginning or end; it was full of mysteries and pitfalls. For too many teenagers today, it is the 9 months involved in giving birth to a child.

To become adults, teenagers must accomplish two tasks: emancipation (establishing independence within the family) and identity formation in the sexual, intellectual, and functional modes. Adolescents negotiate these tasks against the background of their worlds—family, school, peer group, and self.

As with puberty, adolescence can be divided

TABLE 1-3
CHARACTERISTICS OF LATE ADOLESCENCE

GROWTH	Physically mature; statural and reproductive growth virtually complete.
COGNITION	1. Established abstract thought processes. 2. Future oriented. 3. Capable of perceiving and acting on long-range options.
PSYCHOSOCIAL SELF	1. Emancipation completed. 2. Intellectual and functional identity established. 3. May experience *crisis of 21* when facing societal demands for autonomy.
FAMILY	Transposition of child-parent dependency relationship to the adult-adult model.
PEER GROUP	Recedes in importance in favor of individual friendships.
SEXUALITY	1. Forms stable relationships. 2. Capable of mutuality and reciprocity in caring for another rather than former narcissistic orientation. 3. Plans for future in thinking of marriage, family. 4. Intimacy involves commitment rather than exploration and romanticism.
AGE RANGE	Approximately 17–21 years; upper end particularly variable; dependent on cultural, economic, and educational factors.

into stages that exemplify the characteristics of the psychosocial process. Tables 1-1, 1-2, and 1-3 list the features of early, mid, late adolescence. The rapidly developing physical changes in early adolescents focus their attention on their bodies; they become narcissistic. They test the limits of their independence but create no conflicts over control. In completing 95% of adult growth, midadolescents have established a new body image; abstract thought begins to emerge, and they steep themselves in fantasy and idealism. The major struggle for emancipation develops, and the influence of the peer group attains major proportions. Late adolescents have emancipated themselves and established intellectual and sexual identities. They must still determine their functional identities, and for the first time face major decisions that have long-lasting consequences. The enormity of this insight frequently generates what can be termed the crisis of age 21.

The foregoing is intended as a brief orientation; later chapters detail various elements of growth and development in specific clinical situations.

Bibliography

PUBERTY

Barnes, H. V. 1975. Physical growth and development during puberty. *Med. Clin. North Am.* 59:1305.

Crawford, J. D., and Osler, D. C. 1975. Body composition at menarche: the Frisch-Revelle hypothesis revisited. *Pediatrics* 56:449.

Finkelstein, J. W. 1980. The endocrinology of adolescence. *Pediatr. Clin. North Am.* 27:53.

Katchadourian, H. A. 1977. *Biology of adolescence.* San Francisco: W. H. Freeman.

Kogut, M. D. 1973. Growth and development in adolescence. *Pediatr. Clin. North Am.* 20:789.

Root, A. 1973. The endocrinology of puberty. I. Normal sexual maturation. *J. Pediatr.* 83:1.

Tanner, J. M. 1962. *Growth at adolescence.* Oxford: Blackwell.

ADOLESCENCE

Blos, P. 1962. *On adolescence.* Glencoe, N.Y.: The Free Press of Glencoe.

Conger, J. J. 1977. *Adolescence and youth: psychological development in a changing world,* 2nd ed. New York: Harper & Row.

Erickson, E. H. 1963. *Childhood and society.* New York: Norton.

Erickson, E. H. 1968. *Identity, youth and crisis.* New York: Norton.

Fine, R. N. 1973. What is a normal adolescent? *Clin. Pediatr.* 12:1.

Group for the Advancement of Psychiatry. 1968. Normal adolescence. New York: Charles Scribner & Sons.

Inhelder, B., and Piaget, J. 1958. *The growth of logical thinking from childhood to adolescence.* New York: Basic Books.

—2—
Approaching the Adolescent Patient

Robert L. Johnson, M.D.
Natalia M. Tanner, M.D.

The Office Setting
Time □ Decor □ Office equipment □ Attitude
Parents
Scheduling and Fees
Communication
Confidentiality □ Identity preservation □ Judgmentalism □ Listening
History Taking
Physical Examination
Concluding the Visit

Adolescents may seek health care from a variety of providers, including internists, pediatricians, gynecologists, family practitioners and paraprofessionals, and may present them with a myriad of problems. The goal of the health provider's contact with the adolescent should be to complete a thorough physical and psychosocial evaluation in an atmosphere of trust and confidentiality. The process should be an educational one, through which the adolescent learns to become a better health consumer and a participant in maintaining his or her own wellness.

This chapter and the subsequent one provide guidelines or standards for the primary physician to evaluate not only the acute or chronic problem that brings the adolescent into the health care system but to develop an ongoing plan for integrating the patient into comprehensive care and health maintenance. The approach is flexible, and not all recommendations apply to every adolescent. Many of the suggested procedures will have been accomplished in the continuum of medical care and can be documented by history. Recommendations must be adapted to the patient's maturity, cultural background, and the risk population.

This chapter outlines those considerations important to the successful practice of adolescent health care. These include the office setting, interviewing, conducting the history, and the physical examination. Chapter 3 examines more specific aspects of health maintenance and reviews significant procedures and laboratory tests that should be carried out during the adolescent years.

The Office Setting

A proper setting is vital for an advantageous initial contact. Adolescents respond best if they feel comfortable in the place and time they are to be seen. The physician will be more comfortable if he or she feels properly equipped to meet the adolescents' needs.

TIME

Most adolescents prefer to obtain health care with other individuals of their own age group, or at least not to be the only young person sitting among infants, children, and adults in the waiting room. It usually is impossible to devote an entire practice to adolescent care, but it is possible to set aside a block

8

of appointments exclusively for teenagers. Most appropriately, this will be in late afternoons, evenings, or on Saturdays so as to interfere minimally with school. Following the initial appointment, which parents usually make, it may advance the adolescent's sense of self-control and self-responsibility if he, rather than his parents, makes his own appointments thereafter.

DECOR

Teen-oriented posters and reading materials in the waiting room add to the setting's familiarity and signal that the physician recognizes the uniqueness of this age group and is prepared to respond accordingly. Responding to this need does not require excluding childrens' and adults' interests; a "teen corner" will be sufficient. Decor may also contribute to health education through appropriate posters, displays, and a pamphlet rack.

OFFICE EQUIPMENT

An office set up for adults is equally suitable for adolescents. Pediatricians may need to revise their examining rooms in providing an adult-size examining table with gynecologic stirrups. Special attention should be given to facilities that provide privacy in undressing and dressing. Gowns are necessary for strategic coverage. The only special equipment that may be necessary is several small-sized Peterson speculums for pelvic examinations in virginal and nulliparous girls and materials for culturing *Neisseria gonorrhoeae* and *Candida albicans*, taking Papanicolaou smears, and performing pregnancy tests.

ATTITUDE

Adolescent life-styles and reactions vary substantially from those of adults, including the physician. This difference often creates conflict. Little is to be gained by setting up the patient-physician relationship in such terms; confrontation and power struggles accomplish nothing. The teenager, vigorously trying to find a sense of identity and independence, cannot be expected to modify his or her developmentally derived resistance to paternalism. Thus the physician must be the one to change any rigid positions by becoming aware of defensive stereotypic expectancies concerning adolescent behavior. Most teenagers do well when dealt with through an individualized, collaborative, and negotiated approach. Such physician awareness will prevent many unnecessary conflicts. Further details can be drawn from the section on the therapeutic relationship in Chapter 23.

These matters are not only important for the physician but also for members of the office staff. A hostile receptionist can sabotage the best of physician intents, whereas one who is comfortable with teens and warmly welcoming paves the way for collaboration. Judgmentalism on the part of the office nurse about adolescent sexual behavior, for instance, is equally detrimental. If the physician senses such negativism, several in-service self-awareness sessions may be necessary for all.

Parents

Parents or their surrogates are the most influential individuals in the adolescent's life. The health provider should not interfere with the relationship of parent and child but should facilitate understanding and communication between them. Traditionally, the parent has played the role of health advocate for the child, but this role is often at odds with the health provider's desire to communicate primarily with adolescents as health consumers and to see them alone. Much misunderstanding can be avoided if someone explains this approach and the rationale for it to the parents before the visit.

On the other hand, parents should not be kept in the dark; they are the adolescent's primary support through many life crises, especially those concerning health. Additionally, they may need to communicate to the physician information the teenager overlooked. After seeing the adolescent, we routinely meet with parents in the presence of their child, making sure to tell the teenager what will be said before we talk to them. If parents do not routinely visit with the adolescent, we encourage them to communicate with us by telephone.

Scheduling and Fees

The first full assessment of the teenager will probably require a full hour; it is therefore reasonable to charge a fee comparable to those used for adults.

In a busy practice, a physician may be able to free up more time by training a member of the office staff to complete a historical assessment of the adolescent before the physical examination. This goal can also be accomplished by devising a health inventory form that can be self-administered by the teenager (Figure 2-1).

Return visits for a continuing problem should be scheduled at frequent intervals to improve compliance and understanding. Because these visits are relatively short, the patient should be charged a reduced fee.

Communication
CONFIDENTIALITY
The teenager who is unaccustomed to adolescent practice may feel reluctant to be completely candid

Health Questionnaire

This questionnaire will help us to better know you.

Sometimes it is easier to raise questions you have on your mind this way. Check "YES" or "NO" to the questions on page 1; check the appropriate column for the problems listed on page 2. Hand this paper directly to your physician. You may have it back if you wish.

1. What do you like to be called? _____

2. Why are you coming to the doctor today? _____

_____

	YES	NO
3. Do you have any other things needing medical attention?	☐	☐
4. Do you think you are a healthy person in general?	☐	☐
5. Have you ever been seriously ill, had an operation, or been in the hospital overnight?	☐	☐
6. Do you think you have heart trouble?	☐	☐
7. Do you think you have cancer?	☐	☐
8. Have you ever had low blood or anemia?	☐	☐
9. Are there any foods you can't eat or medicines you can't take because you are allergic to them?	☐	☐
10. Have you ever had a discharge or other problems with your sex organs?	☐	☐
11. Do you have any questions about pregnancy or birth control?	☐	☐
12. Do you have any questions about drinking or drug use?	☐	☐
13. Do you have any questions about smoking cigarettes?	☐	☐
14. Do you have any questions about venereal disease?	☐	☐
15. Do you have any worries about how your body is developing?	☐	☐
16. Are you happy with your weight?	☐	☐
17. Are you happy with your height?	☐	☐
18. Are you absent from school (or job) a lot?	☐	☐
19. Are you having any trouble passing your courses at school?	☐	☐
20. Does anything bother you about school (or job)?	☐	☐
21. Can you talk to your parents about important things or worries?	☐	☐
22. Do you get along with your brothers and sisters?	☐	☐
23. Are there any big problems at home?	☐	☐
24. Do you have any problem making friends?	☐	☐
25. Do you date?	☐	☐
26. Do you go steady?	☐	☐
27. Do you have any worries about your sex feelings?	☐	☐

FIGURE 2-1
A HEALTH QUESTIONNAIRE FOR ADOLESCENTS

This is a list of conditions and problems that sometimes give young people trouble. Check each one as to whether you are troubled by it a lot, once in a while, or never.

	A LOT	ONCE IN A WHILE	NEVER
Skin problems; rashes, pimples	☐	☐	☐
Headaches	☐	☐	☐
Dizzy spells, fainting, blackouts	☐	☐	☐
Eye or vision problems	☐	☐	☐
Do you wear glasses?	☐	☐	☐
Ear or hearing problems	☐	☐	☐
Stuffy, runny, or bleeding nose	☐	☐	☐
Colds or sore throats	☐	☐	☐
Trouble with teeth or gums	☐	☐	☐
Coughing or wheezing	☐	☐	☐
Get out of breath more than friends	☐	☐	☐
Pain or aches in stomach	☐	☐	☐
Vomiting (throwing up)	☐	☐	☐
Diarrhea (loose bowels)	☐	☐	☐
Constipation	☐	☐	☐
Problems with urination (passing water); pain, burning, blood, urinate too often	☐	☐	☐
Pain or aches in back, arms, legs, muscles, or joints	☐	☐	☐
Hay fever, hives, or asthma	☐	☐	☐
Feel upset or nervous	☐	☐	☐
Feel angry	☐	☐	☐
Feel lonely, sad, or depressed	☐	☐	☐
Feel tired all day; no energy	☐	☐	☐
Have problems sleeping	☐	☐	☐
Eat too much or too little	☐	☐	☐
Don't eat right foods	☐	☐	☐
Girls: problems with your period (menstruation)	☐	☐	☐

	YES	NO
Is there anything else your doctor should know about you?	☐	☐
Do you have any other health questions?	☐	☐

Do you wish to make any comments about your health, have concerns about seeing the doctor, being examined, or about this questionnaire? If so, write it here. _____

_____

_____

_____

for fear the information transmitted might be shared with parents or some other authority. The adolescent must be assured of the confidentiality of his or her communication if important information is to be obtained and management is to be effective. When patient and health provider are alone, it is helpful to announce, "I just want to assure you that whatever you tell me is confidential, just between you and me. I won't tell anyone else without your permission." One should, however, add an "out" if the teenager mentions something serious such as suicide; in such cases the physician should add, "But I do reserve the right to tell someone else if I think you might seriously harm yourself." At the end of the patient interview and before bringing parents into the room the health provider should ask, "Is there anything that we have talked about that you would rather I not discuss with your parents?" and be guided accordingly. He or she should also ask permission to reveal information to the nurse or social worker or other professional before doing so. When discussing a sensitive topic such as sexual behavior or drug use, it is best to put away pen and paper and talk to the patient without taking notes.

IDENTITY PRESERVATION

Many health professionals have the false impression that they gain some advantage by identifying with the adolescent in their dress, language, and actions. This is always a mistake. The adolescent expects the physician to be an adult with a considerable degree of knowledge and authority and does not feel more comfortable with an adult who is attempting to be an "aged teeny bopper."

Similarly, the physician must use the language that he or she finds most comfortable. It is not necessary to adopt teenage slang. Doing so will appear artificial and make the visit uncomfortable. At the same time the physician must seek to be understood. Have teenagers repeat explanations in their own terms. If either party fails to understand the other, stop and define terms.

JUDGMENTALISM

A teenager's view of the world and how it operates may differ greatly from the physician's. Imposing your view achieves little beyond creating a contest over control by insisting on your point of view and not listening to the teenager.

LISTENING

A teenager's thoughts and conceptions of an event or symptom may be disorganized and flavored with fantasy. It often takes time to put all the pieces together. Listen carefully, for important clues may be hidden between the lines.

History Taking

A detailed format for history taking is provided in Table 2-1. It includes all the data necessary for a comprehensive evaluation. Physicians differ widely in their practices in this regard but can usually modify their record-keeping system in a compatible manner, whether a structured check-off sheet, computer program, or blank notational page.

Time economy may be achieved through the use of an advanced questionnaire as suggested in Figure 2-1. This format serves two purposes: first, it simplifies the data gathering task and second, it provides adolescents with an opportunity to signal a problem area in a more indirect and impersonal manner, which they might not be able to do in a face-to-face situation. Such a questionnaire should not be overly detailed, and detailed information about intimate matters should not be solicited before the patient has been seen. "Yes"–"No" answers are sufficient to open doors, which then should be explored more fully with the patient.

Although Table 2-1 should be self-evident, a few points need additional clarification:

1. Making the adolescent the prime historian signals that he or she is the health consumer and provides opportunity for communicating confidential matters. Thus the bulk of the history should be taken from the teenager alone, although parental input also will be necessary. Some physicians find it convenient to see the parents first and have the adolescent come at a later time. Others prefer an initial brief visit with parents and adolescents and then to meet with the teenager alone. Whatever the preference, it is desirable *not* to have the patient waiting for extended periods while parents and physician confer together behind a closed door.

2. Adolescents usually are good historians except for early childhood events. Their impressions of symptoms and illnesses, however, often do not come in neat little packages. They need time to express themselves. The physician should also listen carefully, since there may be a hidden agenda. Complaints may seem increasingly specious upon further inquiries. Vagueness or presenting information for an inappropriate or minimal reason may create a feeling that the patient has something more on his or her mind.

3. The adolescent may not be aware of important facts about his or her past history, and such data will need to be obtained from parents. One of the educational responsibilities of the health care

TABLE 2-1
POINTS TO COVER IN THE HEALTH HISTORY OF ADOLESCENTS

1. Current health status
   Chief complaint
   History of present illness
   Other current health problems

2. Past history
   Birth history (place, complications)
   Childhood illnesses
   Hospitalizations (illness, operations, accidents)
   Immunizations (if adolescent unaware, obtain from parents or any other available source and inform adolescent)
   Growth and development (perceived or actual abnormalities, feelings about body, body image concepts as well as specific developmental facts)
   Early childhood development (general parental assessment of physical and emotional progress first year, ages 1–5, and early school years)

3. Family history
   Age, health, and occupation of each family member and other persons in household
   Whereabouts and status of family members not in household
   History of genetically associated or serious communicable diseases

4. Review of systems
   Skin (acne, rashes, warts, fungal infections)
   Lymphatic system (glandular enlargement; unexplained swelling of hands, feet, or legs)
   Head (headaches, alopecia, baldness, nits)
   Eyes (visual acuity, diplopia, blurring, pain, conjunctivitis)
   Ears (auditory acuity, infections, discharge, pain)
   Nose (rhinitis, bleeding, stuffiness, sinusitis)
   Mouth and throat (dental status, last visit to dentist, caries, bleeding gums, herpetic lesions, sore throats)
   Neck (enlarged nodes, thyroid)
   Chest (breast development, gynecomastia, galactorrhea, breast masses, chest pain)
   Lower respiratory tract (hoarseness, cough and characteristics, hemoptysis, dyspnea, pulmonary diseases)
   Cardiovascular system (ever told had murmur, heart disease, or rheumatic fever, palpitations, worries about heart, orthopnea; ever told had high blood pressure, family history of hypertension or early heart attacks if not obtained before)
   Gastrointestinal (abdominal pain, nausea, vomiting, diarrhea, constipation, hematemesis, melena, hepatitis)
   Urinary tract (dysuria, hematuria, renal diseases, enuresis, cystitis)

Reproductive system
   Males: age at onset of genital enlargement, pubic hair; hernia, penile discharge, lesions, venereal disease. Note: sexual behavior can be ascertained here or under dating patterns in psychosocial history, but it must be assessed in every patient and must include use of contraception and paternity)
   Females: age at onset of breast development, pubic hair; age menarche, frequency and duration of menses, *date last menstrual period*, menometrorrhagia, dysmenorrhea, premenstrual tension, vaginal discharge, venereal disease, genital lesions, pelvic inflammatory disease. Note: sexual behavior can be obtained here or under dating patterns in psychosocial history but must be assessed in every patient including use of contraception, past pregnancies, and outcome)
Nervous system (fainting, seizures, paralyses, paresthesias, weakness, incoordination, dizziness)
Musculoskeletal (joint or muscle pain, swollen joints, scoliosis, Osgood-Schlatter's disease (aseptic necrosis of tibial tubercle), chondromalacia, athletic or other injuries, slipped femoral epiphysis)
Hematologic (anemia, coagulopathies, hemoglobinopathies, oncologic disorders)
Allergies (hay fever, hives, asthma, food allergies, medication allergies)
Infectious diseases (tuberculosis, results of past tuberculosis testing, mononucleosis, hepatitis)

5. Habits
   Nutrition (24-hour recall of a normal day)
   Sleep (number of hours, sleep disturbances)
   Substance abuse:
   a. Cigarette smoking (how much, how long, why, attempts to stop)
   b. Alcohol (what substances, how much, how long, is drinking a problem)
   c. Other drugs: marijuana and harder substances (what substances, how much, how long, are drugs a problem)
   Sports and exercise (what activities, how many hours per week, enjoyment)

6. Psychosocial evaluation (note: this is the cornerstone of developmental assessment and detecting mental health and/or behavioral problems. Try to avoid using only open-ended questions. The question, "How are things going at home or school?" is likely to be answered, "O.K." Be specific and follow up with such enquiries as, "Most young people have some problems at home or school. What are yours?")

Continued

TABLE 2-1
POINTS TO COVER IN THE HEALTH HISTORY OF ADOLESCENTS (CONTINUED)

Family: Patient's relationship with mother/father; ask patient to describe what sort of a person the mother/father is; strengths/problems in patient-parent relationship; ability to confide in parents; siblings' relationships to each other and patient. (Note: here and elsewhere it is helpful to define good aspects as well as problematic areas. A therapeutic plan is more often based on what a patient has going for him/her than on attempting to attack vulnerabilities directly.)

Peers: Friends—close/casual; is there one (or more) person(s) the patient can confide anything in; how often does patient see/telephone person; when sees friends—in school only/after school/in own home/friends' homes; peer activities—what do they do when together. (Note: it is essential for adolescents to have effective peer relationships for normal development; isolation should prompt concern; although it may be parentally imposed rather than psychologic predisposition.)

Dating: Ever gone out with boy/girl; ever "gone steady"; ever had sexual intercourse. (Note: young people generally are open about their sexual behavior if you are. Simple inquiries of any patient who has "dated" are effective and need not be defended, e.g., "Have you ever gone out with a boy/girl friend?" If the answer is "no" do not proceed further; if "yes," "Have you and

your boy/girl friend ever gone to bed/had sex together?" If "yes," pursue the following:
a. Comfort of patient with the relationship
b. Has patient ever been pregnant and outcome
c. Possibilities for being pregnant now
d. Contraceptive counseling and prescription
If patient is not dating, establish reason; family won't allow; feels frightened; uncomfortable with opposites; poor interpersonal relationships; homosexual preference. Absent dating in young teens may be no problem; absent dating in older patient worth looking into as a potential problem.

School: Name school attending; grade level; achievement level (passing all courses? marks?). View of school (likes? dislikes?; orderly/disorganized?; gets "hassled/ripped off"?). Gets along with teachers (all/some?); gets along with peers?

Future Plans: Does patient think he/she will graduate from high school? What job plans does he/she have? Further education? Marriage? Where does he/she see self at age 25?

Social, recreational: What does patient do with spare time? What does he/she watch on T.V.? Reading? Hobbies? Special interests? Parties? Sports?

Employment: Ever worked? Full/part time? Paid/volunteer?

provider, however, is making the teenager aware of this information and its importance.

4. Even when alone and assured of confidentiality, some youngsters may find it difficult to talk about highly personal issues. Some specific techniques for drawing out a reluctant youth are found in Chapter 23. Briefly reviewed these are the following:

Announcement: By stating "Many young people today are sexually active/drink alcohol/have problems at home (and so forth) . . . Do you," the physician conveys comfort in discussing controversial behaviors, or at least a nonpunitive and accepting attitude.

Three wishes: "If you could change yourself, your family, your life, and so on, what three things would you wish to change and how?" Such a statement provides direction to a youngster who may have trouble defining his or her concerns.

Indirection: Sometimes it will be easier for the adolescent to talk about friends' behavior than his or her own. Because peer group activity is a strong predictor of the activity of any of its members, it can give indirect evidence of possible patient needs.

Comparative approach: Particularly nonverbal patients may do better with a comparative, "multiple choice" approach. "How would you rate your home, school performance, and so on with that of others?" Better, "Do you feel about the same or more troubled about 'x' than most of your friends?"

Physical Examination

A complete physical examination proceeds along traditional lines and is outlined in Table 2-2. Here, too, the physician is left to construct his or her own best method of recording this data. The following are particular points to be noted in performing the examination:

1. Respect the adolescent's privacy. Use proper draping and avoid unnecessary exposure. Keep the doors to the examining room closed, and do not open them until the teenager is dressed or the curtain of the changing area is pulled. When the physician is of a different sex than the patient, a same-sex chaperone may be advisable in particularly anxious adolescents. A parent should be permitted to remain in the room if the adolescent makes this request.

2. The physical examination is a good teaching

TABLE 2-2
PHYSICAL EXAMINATION OF ADOLESCENTS

Note: It is helpful to accompany the examination with a running commentary as you go along, particularly to point out normal findings: "Your heart is fine. Your blood pressure is perfectly normal. I don't feel anything in your belly that shouldn't be there, etc." If you encounter pathology, you can note this and follow up in postexam discussion. "Your ear looks a little infected. You do have a slight heart murmur. Your liver is a little enlarged. We'll go over this in a minute."

Examination should proceed in a cephalocaudad manner, leaving genitalia until last. Particular points to be emphasized in the adolescent are the following:

☐ *Height, weight, and blood pressure:* B.P. may be somewhat labile; if elevated initially, repeat later when patient is dressed and when anxiety level is lowest

☐ *Physical and mental status:* apparent health, mental functioning, mood, and affect

☐ *Sexual maturation rating* (Tanner stage)

☐ *Skin:* acne—note location, extent, and degree (comedones, pustules, cysts); activity (healing/active)

☐ *Eyes:* visual acuity important; may develop myopia during growth spurt.

☐ *Ears:* auditory acuity (tuning fork, ticking watch)

☐ *Mouth:* dental decay and periodontal disease a major problem

☐ *Thyroid:* enlargement, nodules, bruit

☐ *Breasts:* development, symmetry, masses (usually fibroadenoma)

☐ *Heart:* functional murmurs common

☐ *Abdomen:* Can inspect pubic hair escutcheon for rating maturation at this time. Divert ticklish or tense patients by talking about something pleasant while palpating; "Tell me what you like to do best? Tell me about your best friend. Do you have any pets?" This may help relax the abdominal wall.

☐ *Musculoskeletal:* Scoliosis should be looked for in *all.*

☐ *Genitalia:* Boys always; girls when indicated (e.g., all sexually active girls and those with any symptomatology should have external inspection and internal pelvic exam. Desirably, all adolescent girls should have a pelvic at some time as a matter of routine; between 14 and 16 years is optimal, may encounter problems in those of Hispanic culture and should respect). Daughters whose mothers took diethylatilbestrol (DES) during pregnancy should be referred for culposcopy.

☐ *Rectal:* Sexually active males (may have enlarged prostate from inadequately treated or asymptomatic gonorrhea); symptomatic males; sexually active and symptomatic girls. Introduce for all adolescents at some point in health maintenance plan.

tool, as well as an opportunity to provide useful reassurance. Talking throughout the examination and explaining the procedures increases the teenager's knowledge about his or her body and diminishes the level of anxiety.

3. The touching involved in the physical examination may be sexually stimulating. This is most apparent in teenage males who develop an erection. This type of reaction is usually not a result of feelings about the examiner but rather an uncontrollable natural reflex. It is best not to ignore these reactions but explain them to the teenager in a matter of fact, professional manner. This will lessen embarrassment and misconception.

4. The pelvic examination in girls and the rectal and genital examination in boys are often deleted in an effort to spare the teenager embarrassment. In doing so, the physician misses an important opportunity for reassurance about normal conditions, may overlook significant physical findings, reinforces myths and fantasies about these areas, and conveys the impression that he or she sees the genital region as special and taboo. When the advantages afforded by examination of these parts are explained, the patient usually does not object. Although the pelvic examination should be considered part of the whole and separate consent should not be indicated, it may be appropriate in some families and is a matter for individual assessment.

5. Special attention should be paid to evaluating pubertal development. Figures 2-2, 2-3, and 2-4 provide a guide for this purpose.

Concluding the Visit

Adolescents will imagine the worst if not presented with honest facts; however, such honesty can prompt poor compliance if resulting overconcern produces denial or hypochondriasis. Avoid a conspiracy of silence. Full and careful explanations of procedures in straightforward terms will counter the teenage proclivity for distortion and misinterpretation. Pictures and diagrams are helpful, as is writing things down for later review.

Adolescents need to know what is going on and what the physician thinks about them and their condition in order to feel they are not losing control.

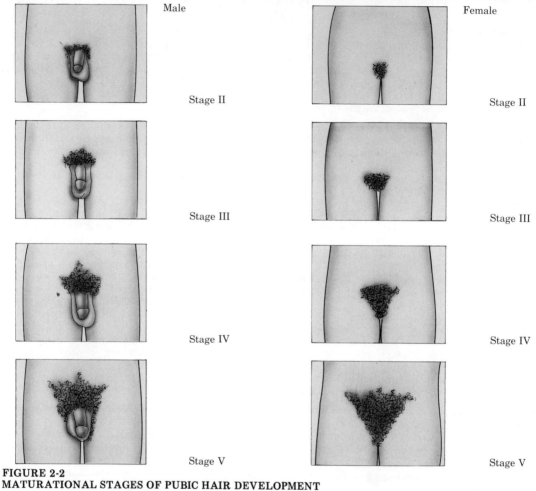

FIGURE 2-2
MATURATIONAL STAGES OF PUBIC HAIR DEVELOPMENT

	MALE	FEMALE
Stage I	Preadolescent; no pubic hair present; a fine vellus hair covers the genital area.	Preadolescent; no pubic hair present; a fine vellus hair covers the genital area.
Stage II	A sparse distribution of long slightly pigmented hair appears at the base of the penis.	A sparse distribution of long slightly pigmented straight hair appears bilaterally along medial border of the labia majora.
Stage III	The pubic hair pigmentation increases; they begin to curl and spread laterally in a scanty distribution.	The pubic hair pigmentation increases; they begin to curl and spread sparsely over the mons pubis.
Stage IV	The pubic hairs continue to curl and become coarse in texture. An adult type of distribution is attained but the number of hairs remains fewer.	The pubic hairs continue to curl and become coarse in texture. The number of hairs continues to increase.
Stage V	Mature; the pubic hair attains an adult distribution with spread to the surface of the medial thigh. Pubic hair will grow along linea alba in 80% of males.	Mature; pubic hair attains an adult feminine triangular pattern, with spread to the surface of the medial thigh.

Adapted from Tanner, J. M. 1962. *Growth at adolescence.* Oxford: Blackwell.

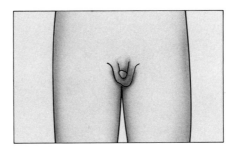

Stage I

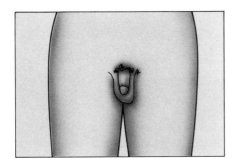

Stage II

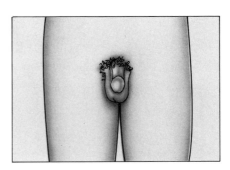

Stage III

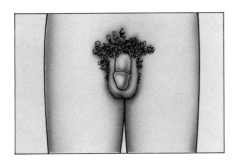

Stage IV

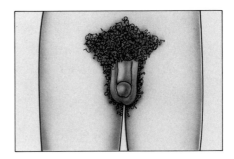

Stage V

FIGURE 2-3
MATURATIONAL STAGES OF MALE GENITAL DEVELOPMENT

Stage I	Preadolescent: testes, scrotum, and penis identical to early childhood.
Stage II	Enlargement of testes as result of canalization of seminepherous tubules. The scrotum enlarges, developing a reddish hue and altering its skin texture. The penis enlarges slightly.
Stage III	The testes and scrotum continue to grow. The length of the penis increases.
Stage IV	The testes and scrotum continue to grow; the scrotal skin darkens. The penis grows in width, and the glans penis develops.
Stage V	Mature: adult size and shape of testes, scrotum, and penis.

Adapted from Tanner, J. M. 1962. *Growth at adolescence.* Oxford: Blackwell.

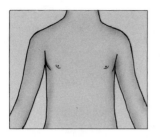 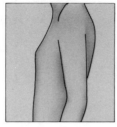 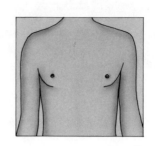 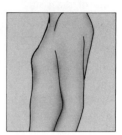

Stage I   Stage II

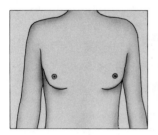 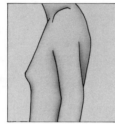 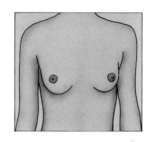 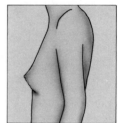

Stage III   Stage IV

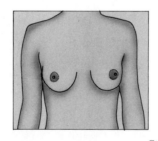 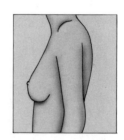

Stage V

FIGURE 2-4
MATURATIONAL STAGES OF FEMALE BREAST DEVELOPMENT

Stage I	Preadolescent; juvenile breast with elevated papilla and small flat areola.
State II	The breast bud forms under the influence of hormonal stimulation. The papilla and areola elevates as a small mound and the areolar diameter increases.
Stage III	Continued enlargement of the breast bud further elevates the papilla. The areolar continues to enlarge, no separation of breast contours is noted.
Stage IV	The areola and papilla separate from the contour of the breast to form a secondary mound.
Stage V	Mature; areolar mound recedes into the general contour of the breast, papilla continues to project.

Adapted from Tanner, J. M. 1962. *Growth at adolescence.* Oxford: Blackwell.

Interpretation of findings and a discussion of plans should be done directly with the adolescent at the end of the visit. Parents can then be brought into the room and nonconfidential matters reviewed. The physician can also effectively reinforce the patient's understanding and sense of control by asking the teenager to repeat comments made to the parents.

In so far as possible, the patient should be in charge of his or her own therapy, for example, taking medication, following regimens, diets, and so forth, although the mother must be involved in special diets, as she usually makes food purchases and prepares meals. Parents should also be advised of therapeutic plans unless they are confidential and be encouraged to allow the patient to exercise self-responsibility. Directions must be given in clear, careful, and unambiguous terms. Patients need to know what to take and why as well as what to do, how to do it, when, and for how long. Write it down. Finally, be sure the patient has enough medication to last.

Future visits should be clearly stated and directions given for interim attention if needed. Try to avoid multiple specialty referrals and/or test procedures within a short span of time. Care needs also should be integrated with school and social activities. Academic achievers should not have matters scheduled during examinations or other critical school times.

Bibliography

Barnes, H. V. 1975. Physical growth and development during puberty. *Med. Clin. North Am.* 59:1305.

Brown, R. T. 1978. Assessing adolescent development. *Pediatr. Ann.* 7:587.

Comerci, G.; Lightner, E. S.; and Hansen, R. C. 1979. *Adolescent medicine case studies.* New York: Medical Examination Publishing Co.

Daniel, W. A., Jr. 1970. *The adolescent patient.* St. Louis: The C. V. Mosby Co.

Gallagher, J. R.; Heald, F. P.; and Garell, D. C. 1975. *Medical care of the adolescent,* 3rd ed. New York: Appleton-Century-Crofts.

Hammar, S. L. 1973. The approach to the adolescent patient. *Pediatr. Clin. North Am.* 20:779.

Kappelman, N. M. 1980. The pediatrician as sex educator and counselor. *J. Current Adoles. Med.* 2:44.

Marks, A. 1980. Aspects of biosocial screening and health maintenance in adolescents. *Pediatr. Clin. North Am.* 27:153.

Marks, A., and Cohen, M. I. 1978. Health screening and assessment of adolescents. *Pediatr. Ann.* 7:37.

Millar, H. E. C. 1975. *Approaches to adolescent health care in the 1970's. (DHEW pub no (HSA) 75-5014)* Washington, D.C.: U.S. Government Printing Office.

Shen, J. T. Y. 1965. Combined private practice of pediatrics and adolescent medicine. *Clin. Pediatr.* 4:286.

Tanner, J. M. 1962. *Growth at adolescence.* Oxford: Blackwell.

—3—
Health Maintenance in Adolescence

Natalia M. Tanner, M.D.

Optimal Health Maintenance Schedule
Components of Health Maintenance

The goals of health maintenance in the adolescent are as follows:

1. To reassure the patient and parents that development is proceeding normally at a time of heightened concern.

2. To institute preventive health and mental health measures by directing attention to biologic and psychosocial high-risk issues and counseling adolescent and parents about them.

3. To educate adolescents about preventive health and mental health, thus inculcating good health behavior patterns and preparing them to be effective health care consumers.

4. The early detection and remediation of biologic problems.

5. The early detection and remediation of psychosocial problems.

Optimal Health Maintenance Schedule

A health maintenance plan for adolescents should begin with the onset of puberty—about age 10 in girls and age 12 in boys. The periodicity of care is mandated by individual need, but annual evaluations are recommended as the minimal standard. The scope of evaluation at any visit also is an individual matter. Some issues, such as pubertal and psychosocial development, need to be reviewed each time; others are required only once during the decade. Table 3-1 presents a health maintenance schedule. Following the approach outlined in Chapter 2 should produce optimal care. If an adolescent enters care at some midway point, any procedure not accomplished or documented by the patient history should be brought up to date, ensuring that the patient is where he or she ought to be on the maintenance plan's continuum.

Components of Health Maintenance

The following comments expand each point in the schedule in the order indicated in Table 3-1.

1. History. The initial history should be completed in the primary encounter. If the patient has been known to the physician since childhood, completing the history is an easy matter. If the adolescent is a new patient, the history will be more time consuming and may require more than a single visit to complete. In either instance, childhood data should not simply be transferred verbatim and applied to the teenager but should be redrafted in a manner appropriate to a new phase in the life-cycle. Keep in mind that the adolescent, not the parent, now becomes the prime historian, and health affairs take on the young person's perspective and are not simply interpretations passed on by adult caretakers.

A concise interval history is adequate for subsequent visits. When the physician is familiar with the patient and has taken the time in the beginning to establish rapport, a short time can be used to maximum advantage to update the history. To this end, it is most productive if the physician spends 80% of annual visits reviewing the patient's concerns and talking to him or her about it, devoting only a small amount of time to the examination itself. The review is much more revealing than the examination, although unfortunately the reciprocal time allocation is the common approach of many physicians.

TABLE 3-1
HEALTH MAINTENANCE SCHEDULE FOR ADOLESCENTS BY AGE

	10	11	12	13	14	15	16	17	18	19	20	21
1. History												
Initial	X or first visit anytime											
Interval	X	X	X	X	X	X	X	X	X	X	X	X
2. Physical examination												
Complete	X		X		X		X		X			X
Assessment	X	X		X	X	X	X	X	X	X	X	X
3. Measurements												
Height	X	X	X	X	X	X	X	X	X	X	X	X
Weight	X	X	X	X	X	X	X	X	X	X	X	X
Blood pressure	X	X	X	X	X	X	X	X	X	X	X	X
4. Developmental appraisal												
Sexual	X	X	X	X	X	X	X	X	X	X	X	X
Skeletal	X	X	X	X	X	X	X	X	X	X	X	X
Dental	X	X	X	X	X	X	X	X	X	X	X	X
5. Mental health												
Discussion/counseling	X	X	X	X	X	X	X	X	X	X	X	X
6. Sensory screening												
Visual acuity	X	X	X	X	X	X	X		X			X
Hearing	X	X	X				X		X			X
7. Immunizations	(Booster—TD 1X) Others as indicated											
8. TB skin test	X		X		X		X		X		X	
9. Hematocrit	X	X	X	X	X		X		X	X		
10. Hgb-electrophoresis	1X as indicated by ethnicity											
11. Urinalysis	X	X	X	X	X	X	X	X	X	X	X	X
12. Urine culture	As indicated											
13. Screen gonorrhea	Annually in sexually active females and males											
14. Serology	X and annually in sexually active females and males											
15. Rubella titer	1X as indicated											
16. Cholesterol and triglicerides	As indicated by family history											
17. Pap smear	As indicated in sexually active females and males X								X	X	X	X
18. G₆PD	1X as indicated by ethnicity											

*Numbers correspond to items in text.

Table 2-2 reviews the data base critical to full evaluation, the physician should refer to it for details. It is strongly suggested that interpretation of this data incorporate a problem-oriented approach.

2. Physical examination. Initially, a full examination should be performed as detailed in Table 2-3. The extent of examination at subsequent visits rests upon the physician's judgment. Certain matters, however, require evaluation each time. These include attention to sexual maturity rating, height and weight, blood pressure, visual acuity, acne, and scoliosis.

3. Measurements

Height and weight: The patient should be completely undressed except for appropriate drapes. Height and weight increments should be noted in sequential, chronologic order on an appropriate graph but interpreted individually in relation to sexual maturity. National Center for Health Statistics growth charts for height and weight (normal value tables in Appendix I) are chronologically derived and do not reflect percentiles in relation to the growth spurt. Thus an artifactual rise in percentile level will be noted if puberty is earlier than the median, whereas youths with later onset will be apparently short.

Body fat: The assessment of fatty tissue in evaluating overweight or obesity is best evaluated by measurement of the triceps skin fold thickness by means of a Lange caliper as in Figure 3-1. (See Table 3 in Appendix I for normal values.)

Blood pressure: Diastolic and systolic levels should be measured in the upper right arm in the sitting position with a cuff covering two-thirds of this area. If the reading is elevated even when the patient is in a reasonably relaxed state, it should be

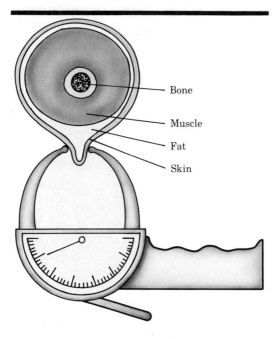

Bone

Muscle

Fat

Skin

FIGURE 3-1
DIAGRAM OF TECHNIQUE FOR
MEASURING THE TRICEPS SKINFOLD
WITH THE LANGE CALIPER

1. The subject stands with his arms hanging loosely at his sides and flexed at 90 degrees.
2. Select the site by determining with a steel tape the midpoint between the tip of the acromion process of the scapula and the olecranon process of the ulna.
3. Grasp a skinfold parallel to the long axis between the thumb and forefinger of the left hand, to depth of about 1 inch, taking care not to include underlying muscle.
4. The calipers are applied at about 1 cm below the operator's fingers at a depth about equal to the skinfold, while the skinfold is still gently held throughout the measurement.
5. Three measurements should be made and the results averaged.

From National Center for Health Statistics. 1974. Skinfold thickness of youths 12–17 years. Series 11, No. 132. (DHEW pub. no. (HRA) 74-1614.). Washington, D.C.: U.S. Government Printing Office.

repeated in all four extremities. The standard adult size (12.5 by 25.5 cm) is suitable for the upper arms; one measuring 17.5 by 35 mm is appropriate for the thighs. The standard adult cuff may give erroneously high results in obese adolescents due to the girth of the arm; with these patients an outsized cuff (14 by 40 cm) should be used.

TABLE 3-2
ADOLESCENT BLOOD PRESSURE LEVELS

Blood pressure (mm Hg)	Normal average	
	Male	Female
Systolic	119 ± 13*	111 ± 12
Diastolic	75 ± 10	72 ± 10
Persistent levels suggesting hypertension = ≥ 2 S.D. above the mean		
Systolic	≥ 145	≥ 135
Diastolic	≥ 95	≥ 92
Persistent levels warranting followup = ≥ 1 S.D. above the mean		
Systolic	≥ 132	≥ 123
Diastolic	≥ 85	≥ 82

From Kilcoyne, M. M.; Richter, R. W.; and Alsup, P. A. 1976. *NY State J. Med.* 76:2002–2006.
*Mean ± 1 S.D.

Blood pressure should be routinely measured at least once a year. Figure 3-2 indicates normal values for males and females on a chronologic basis. The guidelines in Table 3-2 for adolescent blood pressure levels and permissable deviations facilitate detection of an adolescent at possible risk of hypertension. Figure 3-3 offers a protocol for evaluating such an individual, but it should be kept in mind that a single elevated measurement greater than the ninety-fifth percentile does not necessarily reflect disease (also see hypertension entries in index).

4. Developmental appraisal

Sexual: Pubertal maturation should be evaluated according to the scheme proposed by Tanner and defined in detail in Chapter 2 (see Figures 2-1, 2-2, and 2-3).

Musculoskeletal: Skeletal development should be assessed with particular attention to inequities in linear growth of the extremities and the emergence of scoliosis. The spine should be examined by inspection and palpation, first with the patient standing, then bending forward at the waist with palms of the hands together to prevent inadvertent compensation. True scoliosis is revealed by the rotation of the spine on the long axis resulting in an upward thrust of one side of the rib cage over the other and a winging of the scapula on the same side. Compensatory curvature due to unequal leg length does not show such abnormalities but is evident in a pelvic tilt. Sit behind the patient, whose back should be exposed. Place the index fingers along the iliac crest, and sight

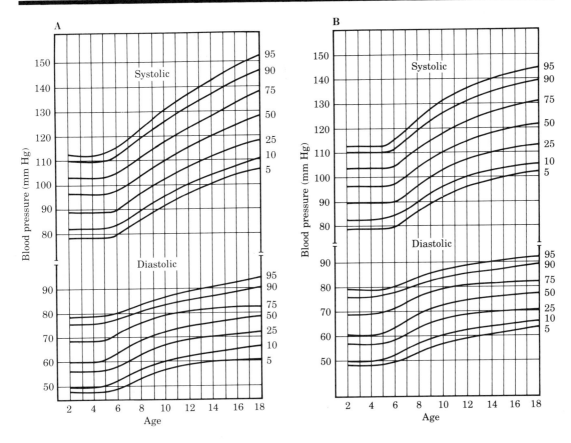

FIGURE 3-2
BLOOD PRESSURE MEASUREMENT
A, Percentiles of blood pressure measurement in males (right arm, seated). B, Percentiles of blood pressure measurement in females (right arm, seated).

From The National Heart, Lung, and Blood Institute's Task Force on Blood Pressure Control in Children. 1977. Report of the task force on blood pressure control in children. *Pediatrics* (suppl.) 59(5):797-820.

down them to determine relative height. Relatively small discrepancies in the elevation of one iliac crest over the other can be detected in this way. Additional clues come from inspecting the relative symmetry of popliteal and gluteal creases.

Assessment of gait should not overlook evidence of pain, limp, genu valgum, or incompletely rehabilitated past injuries with residual, but sometimes subtle, weakness of the affected part. Such abnormalities may be detected in the legs by having the patient stand on one foot at a time and attempt to rise up on tiptoe. A weak extremity is evidenced by relative incompetence in this maneuver. Residual shoulder problems become apparent when one shoulder droops lower than the other without evident spinal curvature.

Dental: The oral cavity should be inspected for hygiene, caries, malocclusion, extractions, developmental aberrations, and traumatic injuries. Examination by a dentist is recommended at least once a year, but semiannual visits are preferable.

5. Mental health. Discussion and counseling by the primary care physician about psychosocial issues is of increasing importance in early pubescence and thereafter. These discussions should include guidance in such matters as sex and drug education, contraceptive counseling, nutrition advice, and parenting. Health education and counseling are most important

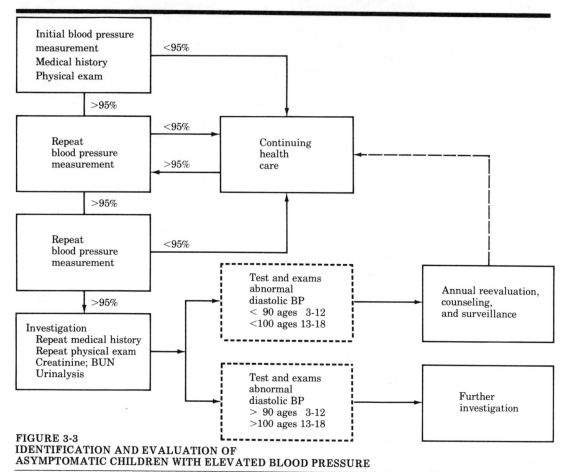

FIGURE 3-3
IDENTIFICATION AND EVALUATION OF
ASYMPTOMATIC CHILDREN WITH ELEVATED BLOOD PRESSURE

From National Heart, Lung and Blood Institute's Task Force on Blood Pressure Control in Children. 1977. Report of the task force on blood pressure control in children. *Pediatrics* (suppl.) 59(5):797–820.

areas of adolescent health care. Preventive as well as therapeutic recommendations in the subject areas mentioned will be found in detail in Chapter 23 and the counseling approach is also outlined extensively.

6. Sensory screening

Vision: Vision should be tested annually, at least until growth is complete. In addition to examining the conjunctivae, sclerae, extraocular muscles (for both phorias and tropias), and fundi, the physician should assess visual acuity using an illuminated Snellen type chart. Such an examination is sufficient to evaluate far vision and detect myopia, the adolescent's most common visual problems, which are caused by rapid orbital growth. Vision testing boxes such as that produced by Titmus should be used to assess near vision, amblyopia, and color perception. Referral to an opthalmologist is indicated for visual

acuity of 20/30 or less in one or both eyes or other possible abnormalities.

Hearing: Audiometric evaluation should be carried out at three-year intervals, using frequencies of 1000, 2000, and 4000 Hertz at 10, 20, and 30 decibels. The normal ear responds to frequencies ranging from 20–20,000 Hertz (although most environmental sounds lie between 400 and 3000 Hertz) at levels between 1 and 20 decibels.

7. Immunizations. The need for assessing immunization status should not be overlooked in adolescence. Too many children are inadequately immunized; even among those who have completed primary schedules, boosters of some vaccines are indicated. Optimally, written documentation of earlier vaccines will be available from parents or from medical or school records. Sometimes such

documentation is not available. When records are missing, patients likely to have received a primary series should receive boosters only. When the probability is low or in question, a full primary series should be given.

Polio (TOPV):

a. Primary. Two doses of trivalent vaccine at 8-week intervals followed by a third dose 6–12 months later.

b. Booster. One dose of TOPV if history is vague or not documented. A booster is recommended by some authorities and not by others if the primary series can be documented.

Tetanus-diphtheria:

a. Primary. Combined tetanus-diphtheria (TD) toxoid, adult type, two doses 6–8 weeks apart followed by one dose in 8–12 months in a patient never or incompletely immunized.

b. Booster. One dose (TD) 10 years after the last booster (or anytime thereafter if missed). (Tetanus only: one dose every 10 years.) (Note: Pertussis vaccine is not indicated in adolescents.)

Measles: A single dose at any age if not given previously or if documentation is uncertain; it may be given in combination with mumps and rubella (MMR), provided precautions for rubella vaccination in adolescent girls are observed. Live attenuated vaccine should be given in any person believed to have received killed measles vaccine or if live attenuated vaccine was given before 12 months of age. Without additional protection such individuals are at risk for atypical measles. Pneumonia may be a complication with acute or residual coin lesions in the pulmonary parenchyma. These lesions suggest metastatic cancer and may inappropriately prompt a thoracotomy. Diagnosis is established by exceptionally high levels of measles antibody in the patient's serum.

Mumps: A previously unimmunized patient of any age should receive a single dose of vaccine, as should patients with uncertain documentation. The vaccine may be given in combination with measles and rubella provided precautions for girls are observed. There is no contraindication to giving mumps vaccine to pubertal boys.

Rubella: Optimally rubella immunization should be administered prepubertally. If the immunization has not been given or if the history is uncertain, it should be given to males of any age. Females should be prescreened with serum hemagglutination inhibition (HI) antibody test to ascertain immunity status and only susceptible individuals (titer 1:8 or less) should be given vaccine and then only if the patient

is not pregnant and if there is no possibility of pregnancy within the ensuing 3 months. Although no infants born to mothers vaccinated with rubella during pregnancy have evidence the rubella syndrome, virus has been recovered from fetal tissues and at least one instance of fetal cataracts has been identified. To avoid the possibility of vaccinating during pregnancy, eligible postmenarcheal females should be vaccinated during the last few days of a regular menstrual period.

Rabies: Some adolescents with wild pets or keen interests in nature are at risk of exposure to rabies. If bitten by skunks, bats, or other wild "reservoir" animals or suspect dogs, the youngster should receive a rabies vaccination. The manufacture of duck embryo rabies vaccine (DEV) was discontinued in the United States on November 30, 1981. Merieux human diploid cell strain rabies vaccine (HDCV) is now licensed for human use in the United States and is the vaccine of choice when given with rabies immune globulin (RIG).

RIG is administered only once at the beginning of treatment. Five 1 ml doses of HDCV are then given intramuscularly (in the deltoid or gluteal region), with the first dose given as soon as possible after exposure and additional doses given on days 3, 7, 14, and 28 thereafter. A serum specimen for rabies antibody should be collected on day 28 at the time of the last dose or 2–3 weeks later. Testing for rabies antibody can be arranged with state departments of health. If an adequate antibody titer is not detected, it should be reported to the state department of health or the Center for Disease Control in Atlanta. A booster dose of HDCV should be given and antibody testing repeated in 2–3 weeks.

8. Tuberculin test. A skin test for tuberculosis is recommended at the first visit and annually thereafter in high-risk populations (those living in high-density areas with significant indigenous rates of tuberculosis, in patients with infected household members, or in members of refugee groups from undeveloped countries). Biennial testing is appropriate for others. Testing gives maximal results if done with 5 TB units of intermediate-strength purified protein derivative (PPD) administered intracutaneously. Although mass testing may necessitate the use of multiprick methods such as the tine or Heaf skin test, the results are less reliable and false-negatives may occur with some frequency. If this method must be used, particular care is needed to ensure that any cleansing agent such as alcohol is thoroughly dry, less the antigenic material become inactivated through denaturation.

All adolescents whose tests convert from nega-

TABLE 3-3
MEAN HEMATOCRIT PERCENTILES
FOR YOUTHS AGED 12-17 YEARS,
BY SEX AND AGE, UNITED STATES, 1966-1970.

Sex	Percentile						
	5	10	25	50	75	90	95
MALE							
12 years	35.2	35.7	33.9	40.5	42.7	44.4	45.7
13 years	36.6	37.9	39.3	41.1	43.0	44.7	45.7
14 years	38.0	38.7	40.2	42.2	43.8	45.8	47.0
15 years	38.4	39.4	41.3	43.2	45.3	48.1	49.1
16 years	39.4	41.0	42.7	44.8	47.1	48.3	49.3
17 years	41.4	42.3	43.4	45.3	47.5	49.1	50.5
18 years	42.8	43.2	44.7	46.3	48.0	48.9	49.7
FEMALE							
12 years	36.4	37.5	38.6	40.2	41.6	42.8	43.5
13 years	37.2	38.0	39.3	40.8	42.4	43.8	45.1
14 years	36.2	37.7	38.9	40.3	42.6	44.6	45.7
15 years	35.9	37.2	38.6	40.3	41.9	44.1	45.6
16 years	36.2	37.2	38.8	40.4	42.6	44.2	45.1
17 years	36.3	37.7	39.2	40.8	42.6	44.1	44.4
18 years	35.7	37.2	39.5	41.1	42.7	44.3	45.6

From National Center for Health Statistics; Hematocrit Values of Youths 12-17 years; United States, Series 11, No. 146, Washington D.C.: U.S. Government Printing Office 1974 (DHEW pub. no. (HRA) 75-1628).

tive to positive or who have a positive test of unknown duration should be evaluated for possible disease; if disease is absent, the patient should be placed on a isoniazid prophylactic regimen for 1 year. The prevalence of positive tuberculin skin tests in the teenage population is low compared to adults —in the range of 7%. Thus any adolescent who is reactive is likely to have a recently positive test and is at highest risk of developing active tuberculosis. Adolescence itself adds additional risk because of rapid growth, particularly if associated with undernutrition and crowded living circumstances.

9. Hematocrit. The hematocrit is the most reliable screening test for anemia. Iron deficiency is not uncommon in adolescence because blood volume expands rapidly, and eating habits are characteristically low in dietary iron. Girls have additional risk factors because of menstrual blood loss. The frequency of checking the hematocrit should parallel the growth spurt; early, mid, and late puberty is optimal. Females should be further tested on an annual basis after menarche until levels are consistently within the normal range and dietary iron is deemed adequate.

Table 3-3 cites hematocrit percentiles by age, but assessment for males, at least, should be based on sexual maturity rating, as Daniels & Brown have demonstrated a much closer relationship with pubertal stages than with age alone. Values rise at each stage until adult levels are achieved coincident with stage V. In girls, hematocrit values gradually increase throughout childhood until puberty begins (stage II) and then stabilizes. Table 3-4 cites fifteenth percentiles in relation to pubertal growth. Levels below these values constitute anemia. This table demonstrates a further significant point. At each stage, black males have lower mean hematocrits than white males. Although black females have lower values than white females in early and midpuberty, by growth's completion both races are equal, although girls remain significantly lower than white or black males.

10. Sickle cell hemoglobinopathy screen. The sickle cell hemoglobinopathy screen is performed one time only when indicated by ethnic origin. Sickle cell anemia is a major health problem of black people in Africa, South America, Central America, the West Indies, and the United States. About one out of every ten black Americans has sickle cell trait, and one out of 400 has sickle cell disease. Less commonly, it is also found in some ethnic groups living around the Mediterranean Sea, such as Greeks, Italians, Sicilians, and Turks.

11. Urinalysis. Urinalysis should be performed annually using a two to five test dipstick.

12. Urine culture. Whether the recommendations for annual urine culture in female children to detect asymptomatic bacteriuria can be extrapolated to adolescent females is not yet clear. Unpublished data (Hofmann) found no instance of this condition in 750 consecutive urine samples from girls 13–18 years of age with negative histories for urinary tract or renal infections or suggestive symptoms. The validity of the results was greatly compromised, however, by a high incidence of grossly contaminated specimens from mixed vaginal and perineal organisms despite the use of the "clean catch" method, in which the patient cleansed the perineum with three iodinated swabs after careful instruction. If the physician elects to perform this test, particular attention to the method of collection to minimize contamination is essential.

13. Cultures for *Neisseria gonorrhoea*. Culture of the endocervix in females and the anterior urethra in males should be performed annually on all sexually active adolescents. Rectal and pharyngeal cultures should be taken on an individual basis, depending on symptomatology and sexual practices. Asympto-

TABLE 3-4
STANDARDS FOR DIAGNOSIS OF ANEMIA IN ADOLESCENCE:
FIFTEENTH PERCENTILES OF HEMATOCRIT VALUES.

Sex maturity rating	Males		Females	
	Black	White	Black	White
1	34.9 (34.3–35.5)*	36.5 (35.1–36.1)	34.0 (33.4–34.6)	35.8 (35.3–36.2)
2	36.0 (35.6–36.4)	36.9 (36.5–37.3)	35.3 (34.9–35.7)	36.6 (36.2–37.0)
3	37.1 (36.7–37.5)	38.2 (37.8–38.6)	36.0 (35.6–36.4)	37.0 (36.5–37.4)
4	38.2 (37.8–38.6)	39.6 (39.2–40.0)	36.2 (35.8–36.6)	36.7 (36.3–37.1)
5	39.3 (38.7–39.9)	40.9 (40.3–41.6)	35.8 (35.2–36.4)	35.9 (35.3–36.6)

From Daniels, W. A., and Brown, R. T. 1979. *J. Current Adol. Med.* 1:5.

*Figures in parentheses are 95% confidence limits.

matic carrier states are more prevalent in females but are not insignificant in males. The incidence has been reported from various series to range from 7%–80% in females and 1.9%–10% in males.

14. Syphilis serology. The syphilis serology should be performed once in early adolescence (if not done before) to detect missed congenital syphilis. Thereafter, it should be performed annually in all sexually active adolescents. The VDRL is the screening test used, but it is not specific and false-positives occur with some regularity. Significant titers should be verified with the antigen-specific fluorescent treponema antibody test (FTA).

15. Rubella titer. Screening for rubella with HI antibody titers is discussed under item No. 4 and immunizations.

16. Cholesterol and triglycerides. Lipid and cholesterol screening are recommended for adolescents with family members having a history of hyperlipidemia, hypercholesterolemia, coronary artery disease evidence before the age of 60 years, diabetes and, possibly, obesity. Genetic penetrance is such that elevation of triglycerides is manifested in early childhood, and a single determination is sufficient for detection. Hypercholesterolemia has delayed penetrance and usually is not detectable until the third decade. Screening for this condition should be carried out periodically in susceptible individuals.

17. Papanicolaou smear. The American Cancer Society's 1980 recommendation for sexually active females younger than 18 years of age is two consecutive annual Pap smears; if both are negative, the test is then required once every 3–5 years. In the non-sexually active female over 18 years of age, with an initial negative screen, the test should be repeated every 3–5 years.

18. Glucose-6-phosphate dehydrogenase. Screening for glucose-6-phosphate dehydrogenase (G_6PD) deficiency should be performed one time in susceptible ethnic groups, such as American blacks, orientals, Greeks, Sardinians, and Italians. This deficiency is associated with hemolytic anemia on administration of certain drugs. It is worldwide in distribution and is estimated to affect 100 million people.

Bibliography

Bailey, E. N.; Keihl, P. S.; Akram, D. S.; et al. 1974. Screening in pediatrics practice. *Pediatr. Clin. North Am.* 21:123.

Brookman, R. R., & Rauh, J. L. 1978. Immunizations of adolescents. *Pediatr. Ann.* 7:614.

Brown, R. 1978. Assessing adolescent development. *Pediatr. Ann.* 7:587.

Committee on Standards of Child Health Care. 1974. Recommendations for preventive health care of children and youth. Amer. Acad. Pediatr. Statement A.A.P. Newsletter (suppl).

Report of the Committee on Infectious Disease, 18th ed. 1977. Am. Acad. of Pediatr.

Report of the Task Force on Blood Pressure Control in Children. 1977. *Pediatrics* (suppl) 59:797.

School Health: A Guide for Health Professionals, 2nd ed. 1977. Appendix C.

Daniels, W. A., & Brown, R. 1979. Adolescent physical maturation. *J. Current Adol. Med.* 1:5.

Discontinuation of Duck Embryo Rabies Vaccine. 1981. *MMWR* 30:407-408.

Fields, C.; Restivo, R. M.; & Brown, M. C. 1976. Experience in mass Papanicolaou screening and cytologic observations of teenage girls. *Am. J. Obstet. Gynecol.* 124:730.

Friedman, I. M., & Goldberg, E. 1980. Reference materials for the practice of adolescent medicine. *Pediatr. Clin. North Am.* 27:153.

Gallagher, R.; Heald, F.; & Garell, D. C. 1975. *Medical Care of the Adolescent,* 3rd ed. New York: Appleton-Century-Crofts.

Greydanus, D. E., & McAnarney, E. R. 1980. The value of Tanner staging. *J. Current Adol. Med.* 2:21.

Heald, F.; Levy, P. S.; Hamill, P. V.; & Rowland, M. 1974. Hematocrit values in youths 12–17 years. DHEW Pub. (HRA) 75-1628, HRA-Nat. Rockville, Md.: Center for Health Statistics.

Hein, K.; Marks, A.; & Cohen, M. I. 1977. Asymptomatic gonorrhea: prevalance in a population of urban adolescents. *J. Pediatr.* 90:634.

Immunization Practices Advisory Committee. 1980. Rabies prevention. *MMWR* 29:265–280.

Kilcoyne, N. M.; Richter, R. W.; & Alsup, P. A. 1974. Adolescent hypertension. I. Detection and prevalence. *Circulation* 50:758.

Klein, J. R. 1980. Update: adolescent gynecology. *Pediatr. Clin. North Am.* 27:141.

Kreuter, A. K., & Hollingsworth, D. R., editors. 1978. *Adolescent obstetrics and gynecology.* Chicago: Year Book Medical Publishers.

Kunin, C. M.; Zacka, E.; & Paquin, A. 1964. Urinary tract infection in school children: an epidemiologic, clinical, and laboratory study. *Medicine* 43:91.

Marketing of Human Diploid Cell Strain Rabies Vaccine. 1982. *MMWR* 31:64.

Marks, A. 1980. Aspects of biosocial screening and health maintenance in adolescents. *Pediatr. Clin. North Am.* 27:153.

Millar, H. E. C. 1975. Approaches to Adolescent Health Care in the 1970s. H.E.W. Washington, D.C.: (HSA) 75-5014.

National Center for Health Statistics. 1976. Growth charts, NCHS percentiles. *Monthly Vital Statistics Report* 25:#3 (Suppl.) (HCA) 76-1120. Rockville, Md.: Health Resources Administration.

PART TWO

GENERAL MEDICAL DISORDERS

Donald E. Greydanus, M.D.
in collaboration with
Adele D. Hofmann, M.D.

-4-
Eyes, Ears, Nose, Mouth, and Throat

The Eyes
Office equipment □ Visual impairment □ Refractive errors □ Strabismus and amblyopia
Nystagmus □ Miscellaneous ocular and pupillary disorders □ Disorders of the eyelids
Disorders of the conjunctivae □ Keratitis □ Uveal tract disorders □ Eye trauma

The Ear
Ceruminosis □ Otitis externa □ Acute suppurative otitis media
Serous otitis media □ Deafness

The Nose
Rhinitis □ Sinusitis

The Mouth, Throat, and Neck
Temporomandibular joint syndrome □ Common disorders of the oral cavity
Pharyngitis □ Differential diagnosis of neck masses

The Eyes

OFFICE EQUIPMENT

The generalist will require additional instruments and supplies to facilitate examination and management of various eye conditions. Many conditions, however, require special treatment skills as well as additional equipment for diagnosis; the following list is not a substitute for appropriate referral to an opthalmologist.

1. Snellen eye chart or vision testing machine (for example, Titmus) for evaluating visual acuity. Referral for refraction is indicated with deviations of more than 20/30 in one or both eyes.

2. Fluorescein paper strips are useful diagnostic tools. When moistened with a drop of water or saline and touched to the inner eyelid margin, dye floods the eye and turns bright fluorescent green wherever the corneal epithelium is damaged.

3. Topical anesthetics can be used in a painful eye to facilitate examination and in any eye during tonometry. Proparacaine (Ophthaine), Alcaine, and tetracaine are three such preparations. Onset of action is 15 seconds, and duration is 15 minutes.

4. Mydriatics dilate the eye, facilitating examination of fundus and relieving ciliary body spasm due to corneal abrasion or foreign body. Preparations include:

a. Tropicamide 0.1% (Mydriacyl); onset of action is 20–30 minutes with duration of 3 hours.

b. Phenylephrine 10%; onset of action is 20–40 minutes with duration of 2 hours.

c. Homatropine, 2%–5%; onset of action in 30 minutes with a duration of 24 hours.

5. Antibiotic ophthalmic ointment or drops can be used, such as neomycin, polymyxin B, or bacitracin, for superficial eye infections. Polysporin or chloramphenicol are alternatives. Neomycin, however, bears a significant risk of a sensitization reaction.

6. The Schiotz tonometer measures intraocular pressure. Values of 20 mm Hg or more exceed the normal range. The *routine* use of tonometry in adolescence, however, is controversial and generally is only indicated when glaucoma is suspected.

VISUAL IMPAIRMENT

A number of conditions can impair vision. Refractive errors are most common in adolescence, particularly myopia. Other causes of vision deficit include amblyopia, trauma, congenital color blindness, albinism, absent iris, cataracts, congenital nystagmus, uncorrected congenital strabismus, keratoconus, absent choroid, macular aplasia, juvenile macular degeneration, and retrolental fibroplasia. Diabetic retinopathy also may be seen in adolescents with long-standing diabetes mellitus. This discussion considers only the more common causes.

REFRACTIVE ERRORS

Glasses. When glasses are prescribed to correct refractive errors in children, compliance usually is not a problem, nor do these individuals object to wearing them during adolescence, since they have already been incorporated into the body image. The situation may differ, however, when refractive assistance is not needed until the teenage years. It is common for a youth, newly discovered to have myopia, to prefer not seeing clearly to suffering a perceived impairment of attractiveness. The primary physician should discuss this matter with the young person before referral for refraction and should review possible methods of handling the problem. It also is important to advise parents that a few extra dollars invested in an attractive pair of glasses, acceptable to the teenager, may be well worth it.

Contact lenses increasingly are a preferred cosmetic alternative for many adolescents. New advances in soft lenses permit quick adaptation, good tolerance, and greater ease in sterilization procedures. Contact lenses are also indicated in certain eye disorders in which satisfactory correction can only be obtained by this method. This includes keratoconus (a conical protrusion of the cornea), irregular or corneal astigmatism, anisometropia (inequality in refractive power between the left and right eye), and an absent lens due to trauma or cataract removal. Persons with marked myopia (3 to 4 diopters or more) experience better vision with contact lenses because the peripheral distortion caused by regular lenses is eliminated. Athletes also may find contact lenses advantageous or even necessary in such sports as football, hockey, and basketball or in others where there is a risk of breakage. Persons who are unable to properly clean and sterilize soft lenses (for example, anyone with limited household facilities such as backpackers or campers) should consider hard lenses, even though adaptation may be more difficult. Contact lenses cannot be used in swimming or skin diving; however, corrective face masks are available.

Myopia. Myopia (nearsightedness) is the most common cause of visual problems in adolescents; it consists of an anatomic disparity between a too-long orbit and the maximal focal length of lens with the focal point (and clearest image) anterior to the retina. Although the condition sometimes begins in childhood, onset is most frequent in puberty due to the marked maturation of facial bones and orbits during these years. Regular vision screening during adolescence is therefore most important in health maintenance.

Signs and symptoms vary from no apparent problem to squinting and specific complaints of not seeing distant lettering clearly (for example, the blackboard in school). Eye fatigue and periorbital pain also may occur. Although the degree of myopia varies greatly from one individual to another, it usually is only mild to moderate and stabilizes once puberty is complete. Rarely, myopia may progress into late adolescence and young adulthood (malignant or progressive myopia). The prognosis in such cases is poor, since not only does the degree of myopia make correction difficult but the risk of retinal detachment is also greater.

Hyperopia. In hyperopia (farsightedness, hypermetropia) the eyeball is shorter than the focal length of the lens, and the focal point is behind the retina. Hyperopia is less apt to be clinically evident than myopia, as accommodation often compensates for the refractive error. Glasses may not be needed. Some individuals, however, experience eye pain, eye fatigue, blurring, or headaches with prolonged eye use at close range. Glasses will correct the situation.

Astigmatism. A disparity and inequality in the refractive ability of the lens in different meridians comprises astigmatism. Vision is blurred to variable degrees. The condition often begins in childhood and usually is associated with hyperopia or myopia. Appropriate refraction improves the situation.

STRABISMUS AND AMBLYOPIA

Strabismus is an imbalance in the eye musculature on one or both sides. It may be evident in overt inward or outward deviation (esotropia, exotropia) or only detected on the cover test in which the patient covers one eye and quickly uncovers it, keeping both eyes open and noting the initial location and any lateral snap to center. The "phorias" (esophoria, exophoria) are not evident when the eye is in use, only at rest. The optical consequences of strabismus (the "tropias" only) is the failure of image fusion and diplopia. This is an unacceptable visual situation perceptually; in response, the image from the affected eye simply is not registered and becomes amblyopic or nonfunctional when both eyes are in use.

Amblyopia also may occur when there is a significant refractive disparity between the eyes (anisometropia), the one with the greater refractive error being perceptually "turned off." Some instances of idiopathic amblyopia may be encountered as well.

Amblyopia must be recognized and corrected before the age of 5 or 6 years if binocular vision is to be restored. Delay past this time results in fixed perceptual monocularity that cannot be corrected. Amblyopia cannot be detected by ordinary vision tests, as the affected eye functions when the other is occluded. Special test methods to detect fusion capacity and binocularity are required.

If amblyopia is missed in childhood, there is little that can be done in adolescence to correct it. Surgical correction of strabismus, however, is indicated for cosmetic reasons.

NYSTAGMUS

Rapid involuntary oscillations of the eye comprise nystagmus. The direction may be horizontal, vertical, or rotary. Movements may be of equal velocity in both directions (pendular nystagmus) or slow in one direction and fast in the other (jerk nystagmus). Vertical nystagmus suggests a midbrain lesion or drug toxicity. Rotary nystagmus is most often associated with labyrinthine disease. Three general categories have been described:

1. Physiologic nystagmus: Mild jerk-type occurring at extremes of lateral gaze.

2. Sensory deprivation nystagmus: Seen with blindness from any cause.

3. Motor imbalance nystagmus: Reflects a defect in the efferent motor neuron system controlling eye movements; further subdivided into the following:

a. Parinaud's syndrome; convergence-refractive nystagmus with midbrain signs.

b. Pathologic vestibular nystagmus: rotary; caused by a lesion in the brain stem or peripheral labyrinthine diseases.

c. Drug-induced: coexisting horizontal and vertical nystagmus may be one sign of barbiturate, antihistamine, or anticonvulsant toxicity.

MISCELLANEOUS OCULAR AND PUPILLARY DISORDERS

Pseudostrabismus: A flat, broad nasal bridge with prominent epicanthal folds giving the appearance of esotropia; ocular motility and vision are normal.

Brown's syndrome: An inability to elevate one or both eyes when in adduction because of restriction of the superior oblique tendon. The cause may be congenital, posttraumatic, or secondary to rheumatoid disease. It is correctable by surgery.

Duane's retraction syndrome: An anomalous innervation and contraction of the medial and lateral recti causing the eye to retract or be pulled back during adduction.

Oculomotor (third cranial nerve) palsy: Unilateral ptosis and mydriasis with exotrophy and poor elevation ability. There is no direct or consensual light reflex. The pupil will constrict with 4% pilocarpine. Causes include trauma, ophthalomoplegic migraine, aneurysm, or tumor.

Trochlear (fourth cranial nerve) palsy: The eye is unable to turn down in the adducted position; the condition can be congenital or due to trauma.

Abducens (sixth cranial nerve) palsy: An inability to abduct the eye. Causes include otitis media, increased intracranial pressure, brain stem neoplasm, viral infection, or Duane's syndrome.

Horner's syndrome: Consists of unilateral ptosis, miosis, and ipsilateral anhidrosis with apparent enophthalmos due to a lesion in any of the three neurons forming sympathetic pathways from the hypothalamus to the eye. The eye will not dilate with 1% hydroxyamphetamine (Paredrine) or 4% cocaine, as will a normal eye.

Adie's tonic pupil: Reflects a lesion in the ciliary ganglion leading to parasympathetic denervation of the pupil. The pupil is large and reacts poorly to light. It is a benign condition that should be differentiated from third nerve (oculomotor) palsy.

Physiologic anisocoria: One pupil is normal in size; the other is larger. Both react normally to light.

DISORDERS OF THE EYELIDS

Blepharitis. Blepharitis, or eyelid inflammation, may be due simply to irritation from an excess of meibomian gland secretion or may reflect a specific local or general disease process. More generalized conditions include seborrheic dermatitis (yellow-gray greasy scales and crusts are present on the eyelids as well as other parts of the body) and pediculosis capitis or pubis (nits on eyelashes, head, or pubic hair). Treatment of blepharitis from either of these conditions is as for the disease in general. Nits can be removed with Florophyl eye ointment.

Bacterial infections of the eyelids are usually due to *Staphylococcus aureus* and evidence greasy, yellow, impetiginous lid margin crusts with thickened lids and absent eyelashes. Small ulcers, styes, chalazia, conjunctivitis, or keratitis may be present as well. Cool water compresses to soften and remove crusts followed by antibiotic ophthalmic ointment or drops are helpful. Bacitracin ophthalmic ointment, Neosporin ophthalmic solution, 10% sulfacetamide ophthalmic ointment, or, 10% or 30% sulfacetamide ophthalmic solution may be used.

Herpes simplex blepharitis is manifested in lid margin vesicles that progress to form confluent crusts. Corneal involvement and keratitis is a possible complication. Adenine arabimosioe (Ara-A) ointment is used by ophthalmologists.

Chalazion. Obstruction to the sebaceous outflow of the meibomian glands results in a granulomatous nodule (chalazion), which may be located at the tarsus midpoint or on the lid margin. Nodules may

TABLE 4-1
CONJUNCTIVAL DISORDERS

Name	Cause	Signs and Symptoms	Treatment
VIRAL CONJUNCTIVITIS General	Echovirus, Coxsackie virus, rubella, variola, and others.	Often seen with upper respiratory tract infection or other, more generalized process; serous conjunctival drainage consisting of monocytes.	Spontaneous clearing without treatment usually seen.
Epidemic keratoconjunctivitis	Adenovirus types 3, 7, 8, 19, and others.	Serous drainage and photophobia; subconjunctival hemorrhage and keratitis possible. Also conjunctival follicles and preauricular lymphadenopathy. Conjunctival scraping shows mononuclear cells and cytoplasmic inclusions. Positive serology.	Cold compresses, topical ophthalmic vasoconstrictors. Refer to ophthalmologist if keratitis is present.
Oculoglandular syndrome (Parinaud's)	*Leptothrix*, *Mycobacterium* tuberculosis, lymphogranuloma venereum, cat scratch virus.	Unilateral conjunctivitis with conjunctival nodules, tender preauricular lymph nodes and fever.	Depends on cause. Note: Many of these agents are not viruses.
CHLAMYDIAL CONJUNCTIVITIS Chlamydial conjunctivitis (trachoma)	Member of trachoma inclusion conjunctivitis (TRIC) group.	Chronic conjunctival erythema, follicles, and papillae slowly develop. Scarring, pannus and blindness may occur. Conjunctival scrapings reveal typical cytoplasmic inclusion bodies. Uncommon in U.S.	Oral sulfonamides or tetracycline for 10 days.
Chlamydial inclusion conjunctivitis (swimming pool conjunctivitis)	TRIC group: *Chlamydia* trachomatis.	Follicular conjunctivitis with enlarged lymph nodes and mucopurulent discharge. Cytoplasmic inclusion bodies seen on smear.	Oral sulfonamides, erythromycin, or tetracycline for 10 days; topical antibiotic treatment used by most.
HERPES SIMPLEX CONJUNCTIVITIS	Herpes simplex virus.	Follicular conjunctivitis often with keratitis. Corneal erosion or ulcer seen on fluorescein stain. Can recur.	Refer to an ophthalmologist.
VERNAL CONJUNCTIVITIS (VERNAL CATARRH)	An allergic reaction.	Seen in spring or summer in individual with personal or family history of allergies. Pruritus, injected conjunctivae, variable stringy white discharge. Cobblestone* conjunctiva, chemosis, and concomitant allergic rhinitis. Scrapings may reveal eosinophilia.	Cold compresses, oral antihistamines, ophthalmic vasoconstrictor (0.1% naphazoline), and steroid.
OTHER Foreign body conjunctivitis	Any foreign body (dust, metal, etc.).	Sudden onset of unilateral eye pain, tearing, and feeling of a large object in the eye.	Evert eyelid and remove with a moistened cotton-tipped applicator; test with fluorescein stain for corneal abrasion.

Continued

TABLE 4-1
CONJUNCTIVAL DISORDERS (CONTINUED)

Name	Cause	Signs and Symptoms	Treatment
Stevens-Johnson syndrome	Unknown; drug sensitivity (antibiotics, anticonvulsants, others), bacteria, and viruses possibly implicated.	Pseudomembranous conjunctivitis with fever, malaise, erythematous papular skin lesions, vesiculobullous lesions of the mucous membranes and anogenital region. Corneal ulcers may be seen.	Systemic steroids, antibiotics, and hydration.
Reiter's syndrome	Unknown; association has been made with sexual contact and acute dysentery.	Urethritis, arthritis, and non-specific conjunctivitis.	Symptomatic; see index.

*Large, flat papillae on the upper tarsal conjunctiva.

be single or multiple, acute or chronic and are only painful if secondarily infected. Conservative treatment involves warm water soaks, gentle massage, and antibiotic ointment (see treatment of blepharitis). If this regimen is effective, slow healing will take place over several weeks. If ineffective, incision and drainage or excision is indicated.

Hordeolum. Hordeolum (sty) is an acute, painful inflammation of the gland of Zeis located at the eyelid margin. The typical course begins with localized erythema and pain followed by a nodular swelling, the formation of a pustule, pointing, and rupture, all taking place over several days. Treatment is as for chalazion. Incision and drainage of a pointing lesion will relieve pain and speed healing. Complications are minimal, although recurrent sties may reflect an underlying eye problem. A careful evaluation for a refractive error or other predisposing cause should be carried out.

DISORDERS OF
THE CONJUNCTIVAE
Conditions involving the conjunctivae may be divided into infectious (bacterial, viral), allergic, traumatic (foreign body), and those reflecting more generalized disorders as in Reiter's syndrome. Bacterial conjunctivitis is discussed in the following section. Other causes are reviewed in Table 4-1.

Staphylococci, streptococci (*Streptococcus viridans, S. pyogenes*), or pneumococci are the most commonly implicated organisms in bacterial conjunctivitis. *Hemophilus influenzae*, Koch-Weeks bacillus (*H. aegyptius*), and the *Neisseria* (*N. gonorrhoeae, N. catarrhalis, N. meningitidis*) may be involved on occasion. Symptoms include pain, irritation, and photophobia; signs include purulent

drainage, swollen eyelids, and injected conjunctivae. If there is a significant hemorrhagic component, the Koch-Weeks bacillus, pneumococcus, or adenovirus may be causal. Membranous conjunctivitis (an adherent membrane over the conjunctiva) is seen, on occasion, with streptococci (or *Corynebacterium diphtheriae* in unimmunized individuals). This condition should not be confused with pseudomembranous conjunctivitis (an easily removed fibrinous exudate), which may be seen with many organisms. Complications of bacterial conjunctivitis include subconjunctival hemorrhage, corneal ulceration, palpebral cellulitis, and cavernous sinus thrombosis. Differential diagnosis includes any other condition that may redden the eye, particularly acute iritis, keratitis, and acute glaucoma (Table 4-2).

Treatment of bacterial conjunctivitis includes the following:

1. Frequent use of a broad-spectrum antibiotic eye drop during the day (q.i.d. or more often) and antibiotic ophthalmic ointment at night (see treatment of blepharitis for useful agents). Continue treatment for 7 days or for at least 2 days after purulent discharge has cleared. Both eyes should be treated, even if only one is symptomatic.

2. Obtain culture from lower eyelid with antibiotic sensitivities; if no improvement occurs with the above regimen in 2 days, change antibiotic accordingly.

3. If due to *N. gonorrhoeae*, condition will need treatment as for systemic disease (see Chapter 17).

4. Supportive measures include avoiding rubbing eyes and the ad lib use of saline or cellulose drops to relieve discomfort.

5. Make sure patient uses separate towel and face cloth to avoid spread to other family members.

TABLE 4-2
CAUSES OF RED EYES

	Acute conjunctivitis	Acute iritis	Keratitis	Acute glaucoma
SIGNS AND SYMPTOMS				
Pain	Minimal	Moderate	Moderate	Variable; mild to severe
Discharge	Variable; moderate with bacterial cause	Tearing but no discharge	Variable	Tearing but no discharge
Vision	Normal	Normal or slightly blurred	Blurred	Moderately blurred
Cornea	Clear	Clear	Cloudy	Cloudy
Pupil size	Normal	Small	Normal or small	Dilated
Pupil light response	Normal	Poor	Poor	Poor
Halo around lights	No	No	No	Yes
Intraocular pressure	Normal	Low	Normal	Elevated
Photophobia	None	Moderate	Moderate	Mild
TREATMENT				
	1. Topical antibiotics	1. Cycloplegics	1. Topical antibiotics	1. Hyperosmotic agents (intravenous mannitol or urea)
	2. Saline irrigation	2. Topical steroids	2. Cycloplegics	2. Diamox
		3. Treat any associated systemic disease		3. Pilocarpine
				4. Surgery

KERATITIS

A red eye with photophobia suggests corneal inflammation, or keratitis, which may be seen as an isolated problem or with conjunctivitis and iritis (inflammation of the iris and ciliary body). Causes of keratitis include trauma (producing corneal ulceration with secondary bacterial or fungal infection), hypersensitivity reaction to bacterial conjunctivitis (particularly with staphylococci and manifested in superficial marginal ulcers), and viral agents (herpes simplex, herpes zoster, variola, rubella, adenovirus). Pain and photophobia are variable. Differential diagnosis is given in Table 4-2. Fluorescein staining may reveal injury to the corneal epithelium.

Smears and cultures are indicated to identify the causal agent if it is believed to be bacterial; treatment is then instituted with an appropriate antibiotic ophthalmic preparation. Viral cultures are indicated if this class of microorganism is suspected. Cycloplegic medication and surgery may be required. If the condition fails to respond promptly to antibiotic treatment, referral to an ophthalmologist is indicated. Corneal scarring and compromised vision are possible.

UVEAL TRACT DISORDERS

The uveal tract is comprised of the iris, ciliary body, and choroid. Anterior uveitis involves structures anterior to the lens; posterior uveitis involves structures behind the lens, such as the vitreous and choroid.

Iritis (with the iris the only site of inflammation) and iridocyclitis (involvement of the iris and ciliary body) are component entities of the broader, all inclusive, disorder of anterior uveitis. Iridocyclitis (iritis, anterior uveitis) may be a complication of conjunctivitis or keratitis of any etiology; it is a common accompaniment of corneal trauma (foreign body ulceration). It may be seen as an isolated ocular phenomenon in tertiary syphilis, tuberculosis, and brucellosis. Iridocyclitis also may be a manifestation of various systemic disorders, such as ankylosing spondylitis, juvenile rheumatoid arthritis, Reiter's syndrome, ulcerative colitis, sarcoidosis, and Behçet's syndrome. The eye signs may antecede (and thus be of diagnostic importance) or follow systemic manifestations. Differential considerations are reviewed in Table 4-2. Cases due to easily treatable underlying causes (bacterial conjunctivitis, minor trauma) should quickly respond to appropriate treatment; others should be referred. If at all in doubt about the cause of eye pain or its treatment, it is far better to err on the side of caution and send the patient to an opthalmologist at once.

Posterior uveitis also is known as choroiditis, or chorioretinitis and retinochoroiditis, as the retina also is frequently involved. In adolescence, this condition, although rare overall, is most commonly due to *Toxoplasma gondii.* The organism usually is acquired congenitally and remains asymptomatic until the second or third decade of life, when visual impairment suddenly develops due to a focal, exudative inflammation of the retina and choroid. This acute phase subsides over several weeks and vision improves, but residual choroidal scarring may preclude the return of fully normal sight. Recurrences occur with variable frequency unless the organisms can be eliminated. Treatment consists of a complex and lengthy treatment regimen involving pyrimethamine (Daraprim), sulfonamides, and prednisone and should be carried out with ophthalmologic consultation. Other less common causes of chorioretinitis that may be encountered in the adolescent include *Toxocara canis* or *T. cati, Treponema pallidum, Mycobacterium tuberculosis,* fungi (*Aspergillus, Coccidioides, Histoplasma*), *Brucella, Entamoeba histolytica, Onchocerca volvulus,* and sarcoidosis.

EYE TRAUMA

Injuries to the eye are frequent in adolescents and vary from simple injuries caused by foreign bodies, with or without corneal abrasions and ulcers, to penetrating wounds, lacerations, and avulsion. Fortunately, the former are infinitely more common. Anything more than the most superficial injury should be referred to an ophthalmologist. Blunt eye trauma may cause hyphema requiring ophthalmologic consultation.

Corneal trauma. Simple corneal injuries most often result from particulate foreign bodies or scratches from tree branches, fingernails, animal claws, and so forth. Management should include the following:

1. Examine the eye for any foreign body in the conjunctival sac or embedded in underside of upper eyelid and remove if found (Table 4-1).

2. Examine the cornea under magnification for embedded foreign body. Ensure (through use of varying diopters of ophthalmoscope) that object has not penetrated below corneal surface. Remove the object with saline-moistened cotton applicator if nonpenetrating; refer to ophthalmologist if it is penetrating. A slit-lamp examination is important.

3. Apply moistened fluorescein strip to eyelid margin and examine cornea for bright green areas, which indicate epithelial injury (whether foreign body present or not).

4. Apply antibiotic ophthalmic ointment and occlusive eye patch (gauze pad) for 24 hours if any injury is present.

5. Prescribe cellulose ophthalmic drops q.i.d. and ad lib for discomfort for several days.

6. Reexamine eye in 2–3 days; repeat step 2 to evaluate healing. Recovery should be prompt with notable symptomatic improvement overnight.

7. Failure of prompt improvement suggests a missed foreign body, more serious injury than originally thought, secondary infection, or development of iridocyclitis. Referral to an ophthalmologist is indicated.

Subconjunctival hemorrhage. Rupture of a small blood vessel may be due to any of a number of conditions: surface trauma, blunt blows, and conjunctivitis are most common. The hemorrhage is clearly visible in the scleral region and may almost obliterate all white areas. Because it is startling, it usually causes the patient more worry than pain. Examination reveals a normal cornea and internal eye structures. Other causes of a red eye should be ruled out (Table 4-2). No treatment for the hemorrhage itself is needed; it will resolve spontaneously within a few days. Attention should be directed at any underlying cause and to ensuring that no serious injury occurred.

Vision-compromising injuries. Although the management of severe eye injuries is a matter for the ophthalmologist, the primary care physician may well have a significant supporting role, particularly in counseling the adolescent. Avoiding discussion of what may be a devastating loss is a common pitfall of the health provider and only makes the adolescent's course more difficult. The patient must be apprised of the situation in honest albeit gentle terms. If the best recommendation is to remove the eye, the patient should be actively involved in this decision and be the one to finally agree. Virtually all adolescents will make the appropriate choice when they understand return of vision is not possible and are aware of the excellent cosmetic results that can be achieved by a prosthesis (reference to Sammy Davis, Jr., and his accomplishments despite only one eye can be reassuring). The advantage of this approach is that the teenager, perceiving himself or herself to have made the best decision and to have remained in control, is far less likely to invoke denial, projection, or acting out—all maladaptive coping mechanisms. Rather, he or she can quickly get on to the business of mourning and working through the loss in a constructive, adaptive manner.

The Ear

CERUMINOSIS

Ceruminosis (excessive cerumen formation) usually is idiopathic and is an insignificant physiologic variant unless it impacts and occludes the ear canal. A foreign body, dermatosis, infection, or canal stenosis are causes in some cases and should either be ruled out or, if present, considered in the management plan. Signs and symptoms of ceruminosis vary from none at all to fluctuating hearing levels or consistent hearing loss and/or popping sounds on swimming or washing the ear.

Treatment consists of softening and lysing the impaction by one of several methods. The least expensive is the twice daily instillation of acetic acid (white household vinegar) or mineral oil, using a wick of cotton or gauze to keep the impaction moist; it will gradually soften after 5–7 days and can be flushed out with gentle tepid water irrigation using a bulb syringe. More rapid results can be obtained by flooding the ear with 10–15 drops of a lytic agent (Cerumenex or Debrox drops), allowing them to stand for 15–30 minutes and then irrigating as above. This procedure can be repeated once or twice a day for 3–4 days if needed. A few individuals may develop contact dermatitis with the use of these agents (Cerumenex in particular), and proper caution should be given. Resistant cases may need to be treated by direct removal with a curette under magnification.

OTITIS EXTERNA

Important factors in the normal defense mechanisms of the external ear canal include epithelial integrity and an acid pH. Anything that alters these factors may result in infection and inflammation. The most common cause in adolescents is "swimmer's ear," in which water retained after swimming causes epithelial maceration and damage and converts the acid environment into an alkaline one. Acute otitis externa also may result from a foreign body, laceration, or abrasion (for example, using a hard object to clean ears), exposure to purulent drainage from otitis media with perforation, or compromised host defense. Causal organisms may be bacterial, fungal, or viral. Localized infections of hair follicles of the external ear, or furunculosis, also can be seen. Less commonly, eczema, seborrhea, or neurodermatitis may involve the ear canal as a primary process, and variable degrees of secondary infection may occur. A necrotizing (malignant) otitis externa with tissue destruction and granulation may be seen in diabetes mellitus. This is a serious condition that may extend to involve the parotid gland and seventh nerve, thus warranting immediate hospitalization. Herpesvirus otitis manifests in a cluster of vesicles progressing to painful ulcers and may progress further to involve the auditory nerve and geniculate ganglion with deafness, vertigo, facial paralysis, and ear pain resulting (Ramsay-Hunt syndrome).

Signs and symptoms of acute diffuse otitis externa include a swollen, painful, erythematous canal with increased pain on movement of the pinna and, occasionally, on opening the jaw. The frequent presence of purulent or cheesy material can make it difficult to discriminate between this condition and acute otitis media with perforation. Regional lymphadenopathy is possible, particularly if the infection is due to a gram-positive organism. Yellow or white spots on the cerumen indicates fungal overgrowth and sometimes is seen in chronic forms of swimmer's ear.

Treatment of acute otitis externa is as follows:

1. Clean canal with alcohol or Burow's solution (aluminum acetate); a moistened wick of cotton or gauze may be necessary for 24 hours if swelling is severe.

2. Apply Cortisporin otic solution (4 drops t.i.d.) or VōSol HC otic solution (5 drops q.i.d.) until the condition is cleared, usually 2–5 days. A moistened wick may be useful; it should be remoistened every 4–6 hours and changed once a day.

3. Treat other coexistent problems:

a. Incision and drainage of fluctuant furuncles (aseptic technique).

b. Systemic antibiotics if acute regional lymphadenopathy is pronounced (penicillin V, 250 mg or 400,000 U q.i.d. × 7 days p.o.) or dicloxacillin sodium, 250 mg q.i.d. × 7 days p.o.).

c. Relieve pain with Auralgan otic solution, mild analgesics, and local heat.

4. If recurrent or resistant to the above measures, reevaluate the condition for some underlying precipitating cause such as overexposure to water, foreign body, improper cleansing techniques, ceruminosis, dermatoses, or diabetes mellitus.

Prophylaxis for swimmer's ear should be instituted even after a single episode if the adolescent plans to spend a good bit of time in the water. The procedure is simple and inexpensive: a few drops of a 1:1 mixture of 70% rubbing alcohol and white household vinegar are instilled in each ear shortly after swimming. The alcohol mixes with any retained water, reduces surface tension, and facilitates drainage and drying. It also acts as a mild antiseptic. The vinegar restores an acid pH.

ACUTE SUPPURATIVE OTITIS MEDIA

Bacterial infection of the middle ear is common in infants and young children. It is less common in adolescents because first, the eustachian tube increases in length and angulation with pubertal growth, minimizing opportunities for ascending infection; and, second, lymphoid tissue shrinks, decreasing the potential for adenoidal obstruction to middle ear drainage. Therefore, when acute otitis media is seen in the teenage years, some other underlying factor is apt to be operative. Such factors include eustachian tube dysfunction, trauma, and compromised host defenses, although idiopathic cases do occur.

More commonly, adolescents present with one or more of the long-term complications of inadequately treated childhood disease. Chronic perforation with chronic infection (usually with an antibiotic resistant gram-negative organism) and/or cholesteatoma, chronic mastoiditis, "glue ear," and deafness all may be seen.

When acute suppurative otitis media does occur in the adolescent, pneumococcus is the most common cause, but *H. influenzae* or group A beta-hemolytic streptococcus also may be encountered. If bullous lesions on the tympanic membrane are a dominant feature, the offending organism often is *Mycoplasma pneumoniae*, although other infecting agents may well be implicated, including *Staphylococcus aureus*, *S. epidermis*, *Neisseria Branhamella catarrhalis*, or viruses (parainfluenza, adenovirus, coxsackie virus, or rhinovirus).

Symptoms include ear pain with or without hearing loss, fever, malaise, respiratory tract infection, or cervical lymphadenopathy. Examination reveals injection, thickening, and bulging of the tympanic membrane with a decreased light reflex, and blunting or loss of bony landmarks. Conductive hearing loss and decreased motility of the tympanic membrane may be noted as well. If perforation has occurred, it may be evident or may be obscured by purulent material in the canal. Fluid-filled blebs on the tympanic membrane may indicate middle ear fluid and bullous myringitis.

Differential diagnosis is primarily between acute suppurative otitis media and serous otitis media. Diagnosis can be difficult and may require aspiration and culture of middle ear fluid, which is sterile in the second condition. Confusion, however, is introduced by the fact that sterile fluid also may be present in the postsuppurative middle ear for a number of weeks following successful treatment.

A 10-day course of antibiotics is the mainstay of treatment. Penicillin V (250 mg q.i.d.) is the drug of choice for pneumococcal and streptococcal infections, while ampicillin (250–500 mg q.i.d.), amoxicillin (250 mg t.i.d.), penicillin plus a sulfonamide (sulfisoxazole, 1 g q.i.d.), or erythromycin (500–1000 q.i.d.) plus a sulfonamide (as Pediazole) are useful in *H. influenzae* infection. Bullous myringitis (*M. pneumoniae*) may respond to erythromycin. Cefaclor and trimethoprim-sulfamethoxazole are also useful antibiotics in treating otitis media.

Tympanocentesis for fluid culture and antibiotic sensitivities is indicated in resistant cases. Inadequate treatment may lead to any of the aforementioned chronic conditions as well as labyrinthitis, meningitis, brain abscess, lateral sinus thrombosis, and sixth and seventh nerve palsies. Prophylactic use of a suitable antibiotic may be indicated in recurrent cases. If unresponsive to antibiotic treatment, the possibility of serous otitis media should be considered.

SEROUS OTITIS MEDIA

Serous otitis media is also known as middle ear effusion, secretory otitis media, glue ear, middle ear catarrh, or tubotympanitis. Although most common in children under the age of 5 years, it is seen on occasion in adolescence; 3% of all cases occur in those over age 12. It is characterized by the presence of sterile fluid in the middle ear, which may be one of three types:

1. Serous effusion: A yellow or clear transudate of low viscosity, which is seen in classic acute serous otitis media, often following an upper respiratory tract infection.

2. Mucoid effusion (glue ear): Cloudy, thick fluid, sometimes appearing as tenacious rubbery material adherent to (and limiting motion of) ossicles. It is due to active secretion by middle ear glandular epithelium.

3. Bloody effusion: Bleeding due to trauma (such as a blow to the ear), barotrauma (scuba diving), or coagulopathy. The tympanic membrane has a bluish appearance due to blood in middle ear behind it.

Conditions that may predispose to serous otitis media include inadequately treated acute suppurative otitis media, repeated episodes of barotrauma, trauma of other origin, allergy, eustachian tube obstruction from adenoidal hypertrophy or nasopharyngeal polyps, and compromised host defenses. The fundamental problem appears to be eustachian tube dysfunction resulting in inadequate ventilation of the middle ear space, persistent negative pressure, and resultant fluid formation.

Serous otitis usually presents as hearing loss with or without ear pain. The tympanic membrane may appear yellow or grayish, retracted or bulging, and may have a diminished or absent light reflex. Diminished tympanic membrane mobility (as demmonstrated on pneumatic otoscopy) and a conductive hearing loss of 10–40 decibels are common. These signs, however, are not always distinctive and tympanocentesis or impedance audiometry may be required to demonstrate the presence of middle ear fluid.

A major complication of serous otitis is glue ear with significant hearing loss. Cholesteatoma formation also is possible and usually requires surgical excision. Both of these complications may present in adolescence as a carryover from earlier childhood-onset disease.

Various treatment regimens have been tried with inconclusive results. No one regimen is clearly superior, and none are predictably effective. Considerable controversy surrounds the management approach. Various combinations of pseudoephedrine and antihistaminics are commonly used, but controlled clinical trials have found these agents to be ineffective; they do not alter the course or outcome in any significant way. Patients with an allergic overlay may benefit from a hyposensitization program. Exercises aimed at improving eustachian tube function also have been tried with variable results; these include balloon blowing, gum chewing, Valsalva maneuver, and autoinflation therapy.

Myringotomy with insertion of ventilating tubes will improve hearing immediately, but long-term benefits are unclear and a variety of procedure-related complications can occur, including general anesthesia risks, purulent otitis media, persistent perforation following tube removal, membrane formation at insertion sites, cholesteatoma formation, tympanosclerosis, foreign body reaction, and further hearing loss. Tonsillectomy and adenoidectomy have not been shown to improve this disorder and probably are not indicated.

DEAFNESS

Hearing loss is a common entity in the population at large, occurring in 13 million individuals in the United States. Although deafness largely affects older people, adolescents may have hearing loss for a number of reasons. The loss may be *conductive* (impaired sound transmission through the external ear canal or middle ear) for any of the reasons described in the previous section or *sensorineural* (disorder of the organ of Corti, the auditory nerve or both). Auditory nerve disorders may be isolated congenital or hereditary defects or may be but one element of a disease complex. Table 4-3 lists conditions associated with sensorineural hearing loss.

TABLE 4-3
CAUSES OF SENSORINEURAL HEARING LOSS

1. Congenital
   a. Isolated idiopathic defect
   b. Rubella syndrome
   c. Syphilis

2. Postnatal, nongenetic
   a. Infectious. Chronic or recurrent otitis media including a variable complication of viral infections such as measles, mumps, influenza
   b. Metabolic. As a variable manifestation of hypothyroidism, hyperparathyroidism, hyperlipoproteinemia, chronic renal disease
   c. Trauma. Acoustic nerve injury from continuous loud noise, fractures
   d. Neoplasm. Neoplasm, acoustic neuroma, other ear tumors, leukemia, lymphoma
   e. Ototoxic drugs. Aminoglycosides, furosemide, aspirin, lead, mercury, others
   f. Neurologic disorders. Multiple sclerosis, Friedreich's ataxia
   g. Ménière's disease

3. Postnatal, genetic
   a. Familial progressive sensorineural deafness
   b. Otosclerosis (usually not manifested until third decade or later)
   c. As a variable component of many syndromes: Waardenburg, Pendred, progressive retinitis pigmentosa (Usher), glomerulonephritis with nerve deafness (Alport), albinism, Alström, Hurler, Refsum, von Recklinghausen, trisomy 13–15, and trisomy 18

Diagnosis. The type of deafness may be indicated by the use of a tuning fork (the Weber and Rinne tests). A conductive hearing loss is indicated in the Weber test (vibrating tuning fork pressed to the midforehead) when the sound is directed to the poorer ear rather than being centrally perceived; a sensorineural loss is indicated if the sound is directed to the better ear. In the Rinne test (evaluating air versus bone conduction by comparing the sound of a tuning fork held just outside the ear with that when pressed to the mastoid), a conductive loss is indicated if bone conduction is louder and longer than air conduction; the opposite is true in a normal ear and with sensorineural loss if combined with diminished overall hearing.

Further discrimination as to the type and magnitude of deafness requires audiometric study. The magnitude of the loss in decibels (db) can be classified as follows:

10–26 db loss	Hearing still essentially normal; may have slight difficulty in classroom or situations where there is a high level of background noise.
27–40 db loss	Mild hearing loss; has difficulty with faint or distant speech; may benefit from a hearing aid if loss approximates 40 db.
41–55 db loss	Has difficulty with conversations beyond 3–5 feet.
56–70 db loss	Moderately severe hearing loss; only understands loud conversation.
71–90 db loss	Severe hearing loss; hears only shouted or amplified speech.
Over 90 db loss	Extreme hearing loss.

Conductive loss generally has a more favorable outlook than sensorineural loss in that it is usually responsive to medical and surgical intervention or hearing aid support. Further, as conductive forms are acquired later rather than earlier in life, there is little problem with speech acquisition. Prognosis in sensorineural types is more variable. Congenital defects (usually either isolated or secondary to the rubella syndrome), if of 56 db or more, pose serious problems to communication and speech acquisition. In addition to amplification, special educational, recreational, social, and psychologic support systems are essential. When little assistance is forthcoming from a hearing aid, a major decision needs to be made as to whether the affected individual is going to try to learn to speak, even if haltingly and atonally, or whether communication will be by signing. The deaf adolescent has additional needs in ensuring that he or she has appropriate opportunity to pursue developmental tasks, gain a healthy sense of identity and self-esteem, and become autonomous. These concerns are particularly likely to be overlooked in deaf adolescents in institutional settings (schools for the deaf) and are most notably ignored in the area of sexuality education and exploring heterosexual intimacy at an appropriate level.

Acoustic trauma. Exposure to loud, amplified music (or other sounds) for a period of several hours predictably results in a measurable decrease in sensorineural hearing from injury to the organ of Corti. Complete recovery will ensue if sufficient time (5–7 days) is allowed for healing before reexposure. Frequent repetitive episodes without a rest interval, however, can result in permanent hearing loss. Young people who are members of music groups and practice frequently should either keep the volume of amplifiers down or wear ear protectors. Ear protectors also should be worn by any working youth ex-

posed to high levels of industrial noise. Attendance at a rock concert, if not a nightly event, could result in transient but not permanent loss. On the other hand, constant playing of a high wattage output stereo system at maximum volume may cause permanent damage. Young people should be appropriately advised and their music habits assessed as a component of preventive health care. Those who have a significant degree of exposure would be well advised to have audiometric evaluation once or twice a year.

The Nose

RHINITIS

The differential diagnosis of rhinitis includes the common cold, allergic rhinitis, vasomotor rhinitis, sinusitis, excessive use of sympathomimetic nasal drops or sprays, side effects of certain drugs (for example, reserpine), withdrawal from narcotic addiction, nasal foreign body or obstruction (septal deviation, polyp), and leakage of cerebrospinal fluid secondary to a fracture through the cribriform plate. The common cold, allergic rhinitis, vasomotor rhinitis, and sinusitis are most frequently seen in adolescents. Little need be said in this volume about the first entity.

Allergic rhinitis. Allergic rhinitis (hay fever) frequently begins during the adolescent years and tends to occur more frequently in females than males. An earlier childhood onset is possible, but in this instance there is no sex predilection. A watery or mucoid rhinorrhea with variable degrees of sneezing, itchy nose and/or eyes, lacrimation, and conjunctival injection or edema occurs in individuals who are sensitive to such allergens as house dust, mold spores, animal dander, and pollens (grasses, trees, flowers). A history of association between symptoms and exposure to one of these precipitants often can be obtained, as for example, a seasonal occurrence with pollen allergy, exacerbation of dust or mold sensitivity when housecleaning, or increased irritation in the presence of cats or dogs when animal dander is the culprit. A personal or family history of other atopic conditions, including eczema and bronchial asthma, is common.

Diagnosis is based on history and the finding of pale boggy swollen turbinates. Other associated stigmata may be noted on occasion: allergic "shiners" (dark areas under the eyes), the allergic "salute" (frequent wiping of a dripping nose with the back of the hand), a transverse nasal crease (from frequent salutes pushing up the tip of the nose), an adenoidal facies, or a high arched palate. Wright-stained smears of nasal mucus often demonstrate increased eosinophiles, a helpful finding in ambiguous cases. More specific information about the precise nature of precipitants in a particular case may be forthcoming from skin testing, radioallergosorbent testing (RAST), and provocative nasal challenge tests.

Treatment includes the following:

1. Environmental control aimed at minimizing exposure to dust, molds, danders, pollens, low humidity, noxious fumes, and pollutants.

   a. Furnishing the bedroom simplex with fully washable bedding and hypoallergenic pillows and mattress (foam rubber, synthetic fibers); eliminating dust-catchers such as drapes, upholstered furniture, high-pile rugs, and collections of stuffed animals; vacuuming frequently; dusting only with damp cloths moistened by polish or water, never dry.

   b. Air conditioning, air filters, and humidifiers (30%–40% humidity optimal); changing furnace filters frequently if the heating system is forced hot air.

   c. Dehumidifying damp, mold-producing areas such as the basement and washing walls with antimold chemical.

   d. Avoiding bringing pets, flowers, and so forth into the home if known to be precipitants; painting or fumigating the household only when the patient is away.

2. Symptomatic medication with antihistamines, decongestants, expectorants, and analgesics, singly or in combination. Many products are available such as Actifed, Sudafed, Dimetapp, and Ornade. Avoid the overuse of nasal decongestant sprays.

3. Steroids (prednisone, dexamethasone nasal spray) may be used temporarily in recalcitrant cases. Keep in mind that steroids administered in nasal sprays are well absorbed systemically even if not intended to be.

4. Antibiotics are indicated for secondary infection (see discussion of acute sinusitis).

5. Desensitization frequently is helpful.

Complications include purulent rhinitis, sinusitis, nasal polyposis, and serous otitis media. The prognosis varies but spontaneous resolution is unlikely if signs and symptoms have been present for more than 4 or 5 years.

Vasomotor rhinitis. Rhinorrhea as an exaggerated response to such stimuli as air pollutants, chilling, fatigue, medication, emotional stress, menses, or dry air is termed vasomotor rhinitis. Allergic rhinitis is excluded by the history and absence of demonstrable atopy. Therapy often is not necessary, but any oral decongestant may be used for symptomatic relief;

known precipitants should be avoided if possible. Nasal sprays or drops should be avoided and the patient cautioned against their excessive use, which will exacerbate the condition by causing a reactive rhinitis.

Epistaxis. The most common cause of nosebleeds is local trauma or irritation of the anterior nasal septum. Nose picking, excessive drying due to low humidity, and rhinitis from any cause are the usual precipitants. Rhinitis may be due to upper respiratory tract infections, allergies, excessive use of vasoconstrictive nose drops with rebound hyperemia, or sniffing cocaine or glue. Trauma is another frequent, but usually obvious cause. Rarely, staphylococcal infections of the nasal vestibule, juvenile polyps (often associated with allergic disorders), adolescent angiofibromas, malignant melanoma, hypertension, or bleeding disorders may be implicated.

Diagnosis usually can be established by the history and physical examination alone. Local causes commonly produce hyperemia of the septal mucosa, with or without a demonstrable bleeding point or scab. If suggested by severe, protracted, recurrent nose bleeds, evaluation for nasal tumors may require special techniques to visualize the posterior nasal cavity. Bleeding disorders and hypertension should be suggested by additional relevant findings.

Acute epistaxis usually can be arrested simply by applying pressure through pinching the nares together for several minutes. Resistant cases may be treated by packing with petroleum jelly gauze or cotton soaked in a 2% solution of 1–2% cocaine plus 1:1000 epinephrine. Other methods include using a cotton ball soaked with 0.25% phenylephrine or 1% Lidocaine, as well as packing with Gelfoam or topical thrombin. Posterior nasal packing (gauze pad or balloon tampon) may be required for more proximal bleeding. Preventive measures for local causes include cutting finger nails, discouraging picking, application of petroleum jelly to the anterior nares at night, and increased humidification. Attention also should be given to any coexistent rhinitis.

SINUSITIS

Infection of the sinuses is a common disorder in adolescents. Likely pathogens include *Streptococcus pyogenes*, *S. pneumococcus*, *S. aureus*, *H. influenzae*, and various anaerobic bacteria. The maxillary and frontal sinuses are most apt to be involved. Acute sinusitis is manifested in a dull midfacial pain or ache due to swelling and blockage of the sinus ostia. The sinus mucosae are acutely inflamed, and the sinus cavities may be filled with purulent exudate. Severe throbbing pain exacerbated by percussion over the involved sinus is characteristic. Maxillary sinusitis also may manifest in pain in the upper canines and lateral incisors. Photophobia, fever, leukocytosis, and malaise frequently are seen. Resolution occurs within 10–14 days after the initiation of antibiotic and decongestant therapy. Subacute sinusitis is suggested by the persistence of a purulent nasal discharge following an episode of acute sinusitis. Pain is not common. Sometimes other nasal conditions such as septal deviation or polyps are contributing factors. Chronic sinusitis is characterized by persistent nasal discharge that does not resolve with medical treatment. Sometimes this may present as a postnasal drip with a chronic tickling cough due to irritation of the posterior pharyngeal wall; it may be worse on arising in the morning and "productive" while asleep due to pooling of secretions. Recurrent headache also can occur. Allergic factors may be contributory, and allergic rhinitis may coexist. Pain, tenderness, and throbbing generally are not seen.

Ethmoid and sphenoid sinusitis are less common than maxillary or frontal involvement and more difficult to detect. Sphenoid disease tends to manifest in vague or generalized symptoms with diffuse or occipital headaches or alternatively, a constant, deep, boring pain located in the orbital, temporal, or neck regions. Effects on the second, third, fourth, or sixth cranial nerve are manifested by appropriate neurologic dysfunction. Purulent material usually is noted above the middle meatus in the posterior choanae. Although often missed as a separate entity, sphenoid sinusitis frequently presents in combination with more obvious maxillary-frontal disease or both, a fortuitous situation that should lead to consideration of this diagnosis. Ethmoid sinusitis usually presents with deep, constant pain in or behind the eyes that is accentuated by ocular motion. There may be tenderness to pressure over the medial canthal region and glabella. Upper eyelid edema, photophobia, and lacrimation are other occasional signs. As in sphenoid sinusitis, purulent material may be noted high in the posterior nasal cavity.

The most common complications of acute sinusitis (of any location) is progression to the subacute or chronic form. Less common complications include orbital or periorbital cellulitis, osteomyelitis, cavernous sinus thrombosis, brain abscess, meningitis, epidural or subdural abscess, and mucocele.

Treatment depends on the particular stage. Acute sinusitis is managed as follows:

1. Analgesics (aspirin, acetaminophen, codeine, or meperidine)

2. Decongestants

a. Nasal sprays; ¼%–½% phenylephrine hydrochloride (Neo-Synephrine), or 0.05% naphazo-

line hydrochloride, 0.05% oxymetazoline, and others

b. Systemic medications (Actifed, Sudafed, Ornade, or others)

3. Antibiotics

a. Oral penicillin V, 250–500 mg q.i.d. × 10–14 days

b. Erythromycin, 500 mg q.i.d. × 10–14 days

c. Ampicillin, 500 mg q.i.d. × 10–14 days (or amoxicillin)

d. Others as indicated by culture and sensitivities

4. Supportive measures (local heat, rest, air humidification, hydration)

Subacute forms may be caused by organisms resistant to the antibiotic used. A 2–3 week course of a different antibiotic selected on the basis of cultures and sensitivities may be helpful. Failure of treatment in either subacute or chronic disease should prompt a search for any complicating factors (allergy, obstruction) and their correction. In the absence of such factors, serious degrees of chronic sinusitis will require surgical resection of chronically inflamed mucosae, improvement of drainage, and so forth. Irrigation may be helpful in some cases but should not be done during the acute phase.

The Mouth, Throat, and Neck
TEMPOROMANDIBULAR JOINT SYNDROME

The temporomandibular joint (TMJ) syndrome is characterized by pain on motion of the jaw and, frequently, a "locking" of the temporomandibular joint on opening. Various organic factors may be involved, from arthritis to malocclusion or subluxation of the TMJ meniscus (this is the only joint other than the knee to have a meniscus). Adolescents, however, infrequently evidence underlying pathology other than malocclusion or subluxation. Rather, most cases seem to be due to spasm and fatigue of the muscles of mastication. Emotional tension reflected in unconscious clenching of the jaw, or bruxism, is thought to be a significant contributing factor. Adolescents who undergo orthodontia may be at increased risk of the TMJ syndrome later in life.

Symptoms are usually unilateral and include pain and tenderness in and around the joint on the affected side and difficulty in chewing. Limited jaw motion, clicking sounds, and crepitation also may occur. Physical examination corroborates these complaints. A click alone, however, is not diagnostic, as it may be a normal physiologic finding. X-ray films usually either are normal or demonstrate restriction of forward condylar motion; rarely, actual bone dis-

TABLE 4-4
DIFFERENTIAL DIAGNOSIS OF EXUDATIVE, DIFFUSE, OR MEMBRANOUS PHARYNGITIS

Cause	Description	Treatment
Group A beta-hemolytic streptococcus	Exudative, diffuse, or membranous type. Other features: strawberry tongue, tender anterior cervical lymphadenopathy, fever, and leukocytosis. Minimal coryza and cough. Positive throat culture. Scarlet fever rash can occur.	1.2 million U benzathine penicillin IM or oral penicillin, 250 mg q.i.d. $\times$ 10 days; erythromycin, 250 mg q.i.d. $\times$ 10 days.
Infectious mononucleosis (Epstein-Barr virus)	Exudative, diffuse, or membranous erythema. Periodic fever, lymphadenopathy (especially anterior cervical), splenomegaly, absolute lymphocytosis, positive heterophil agglutination test (or other serologic evidence of infectious mononucleosis).	Supportive
Gonococcal pharyngitis (*N. gonorrhoeae*)	Exudative pharyngitis or diffuse erythema of the oropharynx associated with anterior cervical lymphadenopathy and history of oral sex with an infected sexual partner. May also be asymptomatic.	Difficult to treat. Variable regimens tried. High failure rates with ampicillin or spectinomycin hydrochloride. See Chapter 17 for treatment of gonococcal infections.
Adenovirus pharyngitis	Common cause of nonstreptococcal exudative pharyngitis; diffuse erythema also noted, with fever, coryza, and cough.	Supportive
Acute lymphonodular pharyngitis (Coxsackievirus A_{10})	Raised, white or yellow lesions with surrounding erythema on the posterior pharynx.	Supportive
Herpangina (Coxsackievirus A)	Papulovesicular lesions on the pharynx.	Supportive
Hand, foot, and mouth disease (Coxsackievirus A_{16})	Vesicular and ulcerative lesions in the mouth and pharynx with vesicular eruptions over hands and feet.	Supportive

ease may be detected. The TMJ syndrome often is misdiagnosed as migraine or tension headache, otitis media, sinusitis, impacted wisdom tooth, or dental abscess.

Treatment consists of putting the jaw at rest. Soft foods, local heat, aspirin (analgesic and anti-inflammatory agent), muscle relaxants (diazepam), gentle massage, biofeedback relaxation techniques (to minimize jaw clenching and bruxism), and avoiding opening the jaw widely can be helpful. Treatment may be required for a number of weeks, and the condition may recur. In resistant cases more vigorous investigation for meniscus dislocation, malocclusion, or emotional tension is indicated; if present, these conditions must be dealt with appropriately. Unless specific pathology is identified requiring operative intervention, surgery should be avoided, since it is rarely helpful and bears a significant risk of inadvertent facial nerve injury.

COMMON DISORDERS OF THE ORAL CAVITY

Chelitis: Scaling and cracking of the lips in windy or cold weather; may involve the corners of the mouth. Treat with an emollient lip balm (ChapStick).

Cheilosis: Fissuring, pain, and erythema of corners of lips and mouth due to bacterial or fungal infection or, rarely, vitamin deficiency. Treat with topical antibiotics, fungicidal cream (MicaTin, Lotrimin), or vitamins as indicated.

Herpes labialis (fever blister): Recurrent outcroppings of clusters of painful vesicles at lip border due to herpesvirus, type I. The vesicles, which often appear with systemic stress (colds, influenza, febrile illnesses, emotional stress), progress to shallow ulcers and then form a crust. No specific treatment is available; the outbreak usually runs a self-limited course of 6–10 days. Topical anesthetics (Benzocaine gel) may give temporary relief. Immunocomprised individual with herpes labialis may benefit from application of 5% acyclovir ointment.

Aphthous ulcer (canker sore): One or several painful, small white ulcers with an erythematous border appear on the buccal mucosa and gingivae. The sores tend to recur in susceptible individuals and may be triggered by acute illness, local trauma (including orthodontia), and physical or emotional stress. The cause is unknown but may be a variant of recurrent herpetic infections. Treatment is generally ineffective. Topical anesthetics (Benzocaine in Orabase, Xylocaine 2% viscous solution, etc.) provide temporary relief. Limiting the diet to soft foods and drinking citrus juices through a straw will help reduce pain. Healing occurs spontaneously in 7–10 days.

Aphthous stomatitis: An acute viral enanthem with multiple small ulcers similar to those described for aphthous ulcer but more numerous and disseminated throughout the mouth. The course is self-limited with healing in 7–10 days. Symptomatic topical treatment may be helpful in relieving pain. Attention should be given to fluid maintenance, as the patient may well limit intake due to discomfort. Recurrences are not common.

Mucocele: A mucus-containing cyst involving one of the minor salivary glands in the region of the tongue and on the inner lips due to the traumatic rupture of the gland's secretory duct. It is of little consequence except for associated discomfort. The only effective treatment is by surgical excision.

Fordyce granules: Multiple, yellow-white granular lesions on the buccal mucosa and inner lips. These granules actually are sebaceous glands and are more prominent in adolescence or adulthood due to gland hypertrophy beginning in puberty.

Dental conditions: The highest rate of cavity formation occurs in adolescence. In addition, inadequate childhood care and poor oral hygiene leave many teenagers with major dental and periodontal problems, including severely carious, broken, and missing teeth and chronic gingivitis. Malocclusion also becomes more pronounced at this time due to maturation of facial features. Impacted wisdom teeth are another frequent concern. Attention to these issues and institution of good oral hygienic practices and regular evaluation by a dentist are important elements of health maintenance to be reinforced by the primary care physician.

PHARYNGITIS

Complaints of sore throat are ubiquitous and may accompany colds, excessive smoking, inadequate humidity while sleeping, shouting and yelling, as well as specific infectious conditions. Table 4-4 re-

---

TABLE 4-5
DIFFERENTIAL DIAGNOSIS
OF CERVICAL MASSES

LYMPHATIC, INFECTIOUS MASSES
Viral upper respiratory tract infections
Infectious mononucleosis
Reactive to infections of ears, pharynx, teeth, scalp
Suppurative adenitis (usually secondary to conditions cited in above).
Tuberculosis; atypical mycobacteria
Fungi (histoplasmosis, coccidioidomycosis)
Cat scratch fever

LYMPHATIC, NONINFECTIOUS MASSES
Hodgkin's disease
Lymphoma
Leukemia
Sarcoidosis

EXTRALYMPHATIC MASSES
Bronchial cleft cyst
Hygroma
Enlarged thyroid gland; thyroiditis, colloid goiter, hyperthyroidism, tumor.
Ectopic thyroid nodule
Enlarged parotid gland; parotitis (mumps, bacterial), parotid duct stone, tumor
Lipoma, fibroma, dermoid cyst

---

views the various types of exudative or diffusely erythematous pharyngitis that may be encountered frequently in adolescence. More rarely, pharyngitis due to *M. pneumoniae, Fusobacterium necrophorum* (Vincent's angina), or *Toxoplasma gondii* may be seen. Kawasaki disease (mucocutaneous lymph node syndrome) is more frequently encountered in children but may appear in the teenager on occasion. Diphtheria should never be overlooked as a possibility in patients with an uncertain history of immunizations and a particularly severe infection.

In diagnosing a possible streptococcal pharyngitis, it is impossible to discriminate between bacterial and some viral infections on clinical grounds alone; the presence or absence of exudate is not a reliable sign. Controversy exists as to whether antibiotics should be started at once in all patients with suspected streptococcal throats and discontinued if the culture is negative or whether the reciprocal course is more appropriate (waiting 24 hours until a provisional culture report is obtained before determining whether an antibiotic is needed). We advocate the latter course provided the physician has ready access to culturing facilities and good communication with the patient. It imposes no greater risk of complications, avoids unnecessary administration of antibiotics, and is much more cost effective.

DIFFERENTIAL
DIAGNOSIS OF NECK MASSES

Many diseases are manifested by enlarged cervical lymph nodes, either localized or part of a generalized lymphadenopathy. Other extralymphatic conditions also may present as a cervical mass. Table 4-5 cites the differential diagnosis relevant to the adolescent. Refer to the index for discussions of specific issues.

Bibliography

THE EYES

Angle, J., and Wissman, D. A. 1980. The epidemiology of myopia. *Am. J. Epidemiol.* 111(2):220-227.

Baum, J. L. 1978. Ocular infection. *N. Engl. J. Med.* 299(1):28-31.

Catalano, J. D., editor. 1977. Pediatric ophthalmology. I and II. *Pediatr. Ann.* 6(1):5-136 and 6(2):10-144.

Cohen, K. L., and Hyndiuk, R. A. 1978. Ocular emergencies. *Am. Family Phys.* 18(4):178-184.

Gellady, A. M.; Shulman, S. T.; and Ayoub, E. M. 1978. Periorbital and orbital cellulitis in children. *Pediatrics* 61(2):272-277.

Greydanus, D. E.; Noble, K. G.; and Hofmann, A. D. 1977. Chorioretinitis in the adolescent: two case presentations with discussion. *Pediatrics* 60(6):884-892.

Mathalone, M. B. R. 1981. Ophthalmic emergencies. *Practitioner* 225:1151-1155.

Middleton, D. B., and Ferrante, J. A. 1980. Periorbital and facial cellulitis. *Am. Family Phys.* 21(2):98-103.

Moore, R. A., and Schmitt, B. D. 1979. Conjunctivitis in children. *Clin. Pediatr.* 18(1):26-32.

Rush, J. A. 1980. Pseudotumor cerebri. Clinical profile and visual outcome in 63 patients. *Mayo Clin. Proc.* 55:541-546.

Thatcher, R. W. 1978. Treatment of acute gonococcal conjunctivitis. *Ann. Ophthalmol.* 10:445-449.

Waring, G. O., and Bodai, B. I. 1978. The red eye. *J. Family Pract.* 7(4):825-883.

THE EAR

Chui, R. 1982. Otitis media. *Primary Care* 9(2):401-412.

Farmer, H. S. 1981. A guide for treatment of external otitis. *Am. Family Phys.* 21(6):96-101.

Greydanus, D. E.; O'Connell, E. J.; and McDonald, T. J. 1977. Middle ear effusions: current concepts. *Mayo Clin. Proc.* 52:497-503.

Harrison, R. J. 1979. Current concepts in the management of hearing loss. *Am. Family Phys.* 19(1):135-142.

Johnson, J. T., and Rood, S. R. 1981. Epistaxis management. *Postgrad. Med.* 70(5):231-235.

Meyers, A. D. 1977. Practical ENT. Managing cerumen impaction. *Postgrad. Med.* 62(1):207-209.

Obiako, M. N. 1981. Malignant external otitis. *Practitioner* 225:1617-1618.

Paparella, M. M. 1977. Hearing loss. The physician's responsibility. *Postgrad. Med.* 62(4):94-98.

Paradise, J. L. 1980. Otitis media in infants and children. *Pediatrics* 65(5):917-943.

Rowe, D. S. 1975. Acute suppurative otitis media. *Pediatrics* 56(2):285-294.

Stool, S. E. 1981. Symposium on pediatric otolaryngology. *Pediatr. Clin. North Am.* 28(4):727-1016.

Vernon, M.; Griffin, D. H.; and Yoken C. 1981 Hearing loss. *J. Family Pract.* 12(6):1053-1058.

Wright, D. 1981. Sinusitis: acute and chronic. *Practitioner* 225:1555-1564.

Zack, B. G. 1982. Otitis media: diagnosis and treatment. *Drug Therapy* 12(2):83-91.

THE NOSE

Healy, G. B. 1981. Acute sinusitis in childhood. *N. Engl. J. Med.* 304(13):779-780.

Mullarkey, M. F. 1981. A clinical approach to rhinitis. *Med. Clin. North Am.* 65(5):977-986.

Strome, M. 1976. Rhinosinusitis and mid-facial pain in adolescents. *Practitioner* 217:914-918.

THE MOUTH, THROAT, AND NECK

Guralnick, W.; Kaban, L. B.; and Merrill, R. G. 1978. Temporomandibular joint afflictions. *N. Engl. J. Med. Med.* 299(3):123-129.

Josell, S. D., and Abrams, R. G. (editors). 1982. Symposium on oral health. *Pediatr. Clin. North Am.* 29(3):427-770.

Nizel, A. B. 1977. Preventing dental caries. *Pediatr. Clin. North Am.* 24(1):141-156.

Tice, A. W., and Rodriguez, V. L. 1981. Pharyngeal gonorrhea. *J.A.M.A.* 246(23):2717-2719.

–5–
The Thorax

Disorders of the Breast
Evaluation and examination □ Congenital anomalies
Precocious or delayed breast development □ Asymmetric breast development
Underdeveloped breasts □ Virginal hypertrophy □ Breast masses
Mastodynia □ Galactorrhea □ Gynecomastia
Chest Pain
Differential diagnosis □ Mitral valve prolapse syndrome
Spontaneous pneumothorax □ Tietze's disease
Anterior chest wall syndrome □ Miscellaneous

Disorders of the Breast

Examination of the breast is an important yet often neglected aspect of the physical examination in adolescence. The first appearance of the breast bud heralds the onset of puberty. Once the process begins, the female must begin to formulate a new identity as a young adult and contend with emerging sexuality. These issues, together with the erotic mystique ascribed to the female breast, heighten the embarrassment of the teenaged girl during examination, and possibly that of the physician as well. There is great concern and fear over breast cancer among adolescents as well as adults. Any abnormality may be believed malignant, even if the worry remains unspoken. Thus the breast is an emotionally charged aspect of the physical examination from many aspects, making it all the more important to carry it out with tact and sensitivity.

Adolescence also is an effective time to introduce the concept of routine breast self-examination. Establishing the pattern of checking each month at a regular time gives the female an awareness of what her normal breast is like and increases her sensitivity to abnormalities in later life when early cancer detection is a critical matter. This can be explained at some point in midadolescence or slightly later, when abstract thought has developed, enabling the patient to perceive long-range benefits more clearly. Reinforcement can be achieved by giving the patient a pamphlet describing and illustrating the breast self-examination. One such publication is available free from the American Cancer Society; another from the National Cancer Institute (see Appendix II).

EVALUATION AND EXAMINATION

Historical points relate not only to the parameters of any symptoms such as pain, lesions, discharge, and so forth, but also to age of pubertal onset, rate of breast growth, and menstrual history, including the last menstrual period. (Note that complaints of breast pain may be a symptom of pregnancy.) The method of conducting the examination is outlined in Table 5-1.

The adolescent's concerns may relate to inappropriate breast size relative to the perceived ideal, asymmetric development, delayed or precocious development (see Chapter 12), painful breasts, and various breast lesions. These concerns may not always be verbalized because of embarrassment. The patient often presents with a screen complaint (some other, less anxiety-producing reason for the visit), not revealing her true concern until a later time. On occasion she may simply wait and see if the physician discovers the "problem" independently. If exceptionally large, small, or asymmetric breasts are noted on examination, it is well to raise the issue in the postexamination discussion even if the patient has not done so herself. All that is often needed is a simple review of the situation, coupled with the reassuring statement that these are common problems that worry many girls. The patient usually is relieved; if she continues to be concerned, she is then able to discuss her feelings more easily.

CONGENITAL ANOMALIES

Absence of nipples (athelia) or breast tissue (amastia) or the presence of accessory nipples (polythelia) or

TABLE 5-1
OUTLINE OF THE BREAST EXAMINATION

1. Inspect the patient when she is sitting
   With her arms at her side.
   With her arms pressed against her hips.
   With her arms raised.
   While she bends forward.

2. Observe for
   Pubertal status of each breast.
   Asymmetry.
   Palpable lesions (check each quadrant).
   Nipple discharge.
   Supraclavicular and axillary masses.

3. Inspect patient when she is supine
   Place a small pillow under the side of the breast being evaluated.
   Examine the inner aspect of the breast with her arms raised.
   Examine the outer aspect with her arms at her sides.
   Examine the nipple and areola with the arms raised.

breast tissue (polymastia) are uncommon anomalies but may be noted on occasion. Polythelia and/or polymastia are more common than absence of tissue. The accessory tissue usually is rudimentary but invariably is located along the embryonic milk line running from axilla to groin. These are benign lesions, although surgical excision may be indicated for cosmetic purposes.

PRECOCIOUS OR DELAYED BREAST DEVELOPMENT
See Chapter 12.

ASYMMETRIC BREAST DEVELOPMENT
Asymmetric breast development is a relatively common complaint and may occur as early as the time of breast bud appearance. Breast development on one side several months before development on the other is a common physiologic variation. There may be additional concern because the breast bud does not have characteristic consistency of the more mature breast, but rather is a tender, firm discrete discoid mass measuring 2—3 cm in diameter. Some patients may believe this to be a tumor. Biopsy for histologic diagnosis is contraindicated, as it will impair or destroy future development of a normal breast.

Asymmetrical development in the phase of rapid breast growth (Tanner stages II–IV) also is a normal physiologic variant. The more slowly growing breast usually catches up with the more rapidly growing one in time. Reassurance and a padded brassiere to establish outward symmetry is the treatment of choice. Some girls may be tempted to try breast pumps, massage, and other bogus advertisements in various lay magazines that claim the ability to augment breast size. The girl should be cautioned against developing false hopes.

Permanent breast asymmetry is far less common than the transient form; however, inequality in an adolescent who has achieved Tanner stage V development for two or more years is unlikely to resolve. Although further increase of breast size caused by fat deposition during the balance of the teenage years may minimize the degree of disproportion, only rarely will it disappear altogether. Treatment, if desired, is by breast augmentation of the smaller side. Where asymmetry is marked, most young women want this procedure but may be too embarrassed to suggest it. Intervention should be deferred until the late teen years, however, to permit maximal development and optimal correction.

UNDERDEVELOPED BREASTS
The normally developed adolescent girl who complains of too small breasts also is a common event. Much importance is placed on physical appearance in adolescence, and the teenager who perceives herself to be inadequately endowed may feel diminished in attractiveness and femininity. Treatment consists of careful explanation of pubertal events, thorough examination, and reassurance that breast size has little to do with the patient's potential as a woman, whether in relation to sexual intimacy, pregnancy, or lactation. Surgical augmentation can be performed, but as no deformity is involved (as in asymmetry), this procedure should only be embarked upon in adulthood; too many fantasies and shifts in concerns are at work during adolescence for a truly rational decision to be made.

Breast atrophy is a different matter and may be seen in any condition associated with marked weight loss, such as crash dieting, anorexia nervosa, or chronic organic illness. Treatment focuses on the underlying problem.

VIRGINAL HYPERTROPHY
Breast tissue in some adolescents is hypersensitive to estrogens, which produce massive diffuse enlargement. The usual history is of a normal thelarche followed by explosive bilateral or, occasionally, unilateral mammary enlargement. Complications include significant neck and back strain, impairment

of physical and athletic function, intertrigo, local pain, skin ulceration, and significant general discomfort, which is exacerbated by a tight brassiere. Considerable psychological embarrassment and self-consciousness almost always are present as well, the adolescent having long been the butt of numerous crude comments and sexual innuendos. Mild regression of breast tissues may occur in late adolescence, but this is unlikely to return the breasts to normal proportions. If the condition is handicapping, surgical reduction is indicated at any time, regardless of age or Tanner stage, in order to restore physical mobility and minimize psychologic trauma. Several points should be recognized by the girl in giving her informed consent: first, if done early in adolescence, enlargement may recur for a few years more, possibly necessitating additional surgery; second, the situation may be aggravated by oral contraceptives, and if birth control is needed some other method may be best; third, reduction usually requires the reimplantation of nipples at a higher location; in this event, however, lactation and nursing a child will not be possible.

BREAST MASSES

Cancer is exceptionally rare in adolescents, but it has been reported in the literature and does enter into the differential diagnosis. However, most masses in the adolescent breast are benign. Far and away the most common (between 80% and 90%) are fibroadenomas. The balance are predominantly cysts. Occasionally, cystosarcoma phylloides, intraductal papillomas, hemangiomas, lymphangiomas, and lipomas may be seen. Cystosarcoma phylloides is a rapidly growing, multitumored, painless lesion sometimes presenting with a bloody nipple discharge. It is comprised of epithelial and stromal elements and 85%–90% are benign.

Fibroadenoma. Fibroadenoma is the most common lesion seen in adolescents and is entirely benign. It can appear any time after the onset of puberty but is more frequently seen during the later teen years. It presents as a slowly enlarging, rubbery, well-demarcated, and encapsulated nontender mass. Usually it is single and located in the upper outer quadrant, but multiple and bilateral fibroadenomata are not uncommon and any quadrant may be involved. A single tumor usually measures 2–3 cm at discovery and, although it may remain unchanged in size for some period of time, it also may grow to 10–15 cm or more. Differential considerations include any of the masses mentioned in the preceding paragraph. Rapidly enlarging lesions are of the most concern

and should be distinguished from virginal hypertrophy, giant (juvenile) fibroadenoma (a rare variant of the ordinary type), and the rare case of adenocarcinoma or cystosarcoma phylloides.

Fibroadenomas would not need to be removed unless painful or of such size as to be disfiguring if the diagnosis were easy to verify. Short of biopsy, however, it is difficult to rule out the possibility of malignancy; even if uncommon, it still can occur. Some delay is acceptable to observe the lesion for several months if it is discrete, well demarcated, freely movable, and without any of the signs associated with breast cancer. A number of fibroadenomas (and cysts as well) will spontaneously involute during this time. If size does not decrease over 4–6 months or if progressive enlargement occurs over 2–4 months, simple excision is the most reassuring course.

Cystic breast disease. Single or multiple cysts also can be encountered in the adolescent but far less commonly than adenomas. Cysts usually contain variable amounts of a sterile, watery fluid, which may be clear, brownish, or blood-tinged. Cysts can be classified as fibrocystic disease with multiple small cysts, solitary large or "blue-domed" cysts containing bloody fluid, simple single cysts, or galactoceles.

Fibrocystic disease, although more frequent in women over 35, may present in the adolescent girl as firm, mobile, cordlike nodularities distributed diffusely throughout the breast. Premenstrual tenderness and change in breast size during the menstrual cycle are characteristic. Differential diagnosis is primarily between this condition and physiologic premenstrual mastodynia; a biopsy may be required. Simple cysts frequently resolve spontaneously. It is worthwhile to observe any single, discrete mass for two or three menstrual cycles before removal (for the same reasons an adenoma is removed). Diffuse fibrocystic disease, of course, cannot be treated effectively by surgery unless extensive, and the procedure is difficult at best. Heat, a firm and supporting brassiere, and mild analgesics may be helpful. The use of cyclic hormone therapy (oral contraceptives) to inhibit progesterone secretion may give relief, as cysts are more painful in the late (secretory, progestational) phase of the menstrual cycle.

Breast abscess. Presenting much as does an abscess in any part of the body, a breast abscess is a tender, cystic, or fluctuant mass with erythema and increased heat of the overlying skin. Lesions may be single or multiple, with varying degrees of cellulitis and regional adenopathy. Although an abscess may be idiopathic, recognized causes include cutaneous infections, lactation and breast-feeding, foreign body, trauma, epidermal cysts, and chronic illness with reduced host defenses. It should be noted that trauma must be something more than that sustained in ordinary rough and tumble activity; there is no evidence of an increased incidence of breast abscesses (or any other breast lesion) in girls involved in competitive athletics.

Staphylococcus aureus is the most common causative organism, but gram-negative bacteria (*Escherichia coli, Pseudomonas*) may be involved in 25% of the cases and should be suspected, particularly when surrounding cellulitis is marked.

Treatment consists of incision and drainage, antibiotics, heat, and analgesics. Broad-spectrum agents should be chosen to cover both gram-positive and -negative organisms. These are best administered intravenously unless the abscess is small and well localized and cellulitis is minimal or absent. Oral antibiotics should be continued for several weeks or even longer until all signs have completely cleared. Relapses have been reported to occur in up to 50% of cases. Residual scarring may result and appear as a small nubbin of tissue; this should not be mistaken at a later date for a fibroadenoma. Scarring is most apt to occur when trauma (with associated fat necrosis) was the precipitating cause or when an inadequately treated abscess became chronic or recurrent.

MASTODYNIA

Breast pain is a common complaint. It may be seen with any breast lesion and frequently occurs as a component of the normal menstrual cycle. Most breast pain in adolescents is of organic origin and is seldom hysterical, imaginary, or psychosomatic. It should be taken seriously and responded to appropriately. Careful examination is indicated to rule out a mass or fibrocystic disease. Various causes of chest pain, as outlined in the next section, also should be excluded. A history of regularly occurring tenderness and congestion during the several days just before a menstrual period (as a single finding or in combination with other symptoms of premenstrual tension) comprises premenstrual cyclic mastodynia. Examination reveals tender, rubbery nodules premenstrually, which disappear postmenstrually. This condition may be difficult to differentiate from fibrocystic disease on any other than a statistical basis; premenstrual cyclic mastodynia is much more common. Treatment consists of heat, firm support, analgesics and, in persistent and particularly discomforting situations, a trial of cyclic hormonal therapy (this may be indicated in any event if the girl is sexually active).

GALACTORRHEA

Galactorrhea is characterized by the abnormal secretion of breast milk, that is, at any time other than during postpartum lactation and nursing. It is most often due to pregnancy-related elevation of prolactin levels and may be seen as a persistent condition following miscarriage, therapeutic abortion, or delivery without nursing. Increased prolactin levels also are seen with pituitary adenomas and the administration of certain drugs. Heavy marijuana smoking has been implicated, although not proven, and is a controversial cause of galactorrhea in females and gynecomastia with or without galactorrhea in males. Oral contraceptives, phenothiazines, reserpine, spironolactone, estrogens, and methyltestosterone, among a wide variety of other drugs, taken singly or in combination, may induce galactorrhea as well. In addition, increased prolactin levels may be encountered with hypothalamic injury (infection, tumor, surgery), hypothyroidism, anxiety, and depression. Galactorrhea also may occur as a result of end-organ hypersensitivity to normal prolactin levels; this may be idiopathic or due to intercostal nerve stimulation as in herpes zoster or thoracic surgery. Thus elevated prolactin levels suggest a more serious underlying cause and recommend further investigation for pituitary or hypothalamic lesions, thyroid disfunction or an historical search for implicated drugs. Normal prolactin levels reassuringly indicate a benign end-organ cause.

Treatment depends on the final diagnosis. Ergotoxine, L-dopa, and bromocriptine have been used in some adult patients to inhibit excessive prolactin secretion with variable success, although bromocriptine has not yet received FDA approval for use in children. Surgery to remove a prolactin-secreting tumor or lactating tissue is necessary on occasion. Little can be done for low prolactin types.

GYNECOMASTIA

Transient breast development is noted in two-thirds or more of adolescent males. It characteristically occurs during early puberty at Tanner stage II–III, lasts for a number of months, and gradually disappears within a year after onset. It most commonly begins unilaterally, then progresses to bilateral involvement. The most common type consists of a small, tender, firm, discoid subareolar mass measuring 2–3 cm in diameter, which is referred to as type I gynecomastia. Rarely, a more generalized glandular enlargement is noted approximating the Tanner stage III or even stage IV breast development seen in adolescent girls; this is referred to as type II gynecomastia or macromastia. Lesser degrees of type II may or may not clear with time whereas more advanced degrees frequently persist.

Although gynecomastia usually is a normal physiologic variant (probably due to increased sensitivity of rudimentary breast tissue to pubertal hormonal changes and alterations in the testosterone-estrogen ratio) other conditions must be ruled out. Klinefelter's syndrome may present with gynecomastia and small testes. Other pituitary-gonadal endocrinopathies also may be implicated. The administration of a wide variety of drugs also has been implicated; these include estrogens (which may be taken as "street" drugs by some "gay" youths), testosterone, chorionic gonadotropins, corticosteroids, tricyclic antidepressants, insulin, methadone, marijuana (controversial), amphetamines, cimetidine, and digitalis. Pseudogynecomastia may occur in obese adolescent males with the deposition of fat in the breast region or in muscular youths. Consideration of nonphysiologic reasons is particularly indicated when gynecomastia appears at some time other than between Tanner II and IV developmental stages.

Treatment of physiologic gynecomastia consists, first, of reassuring the boy that his hormones have not gone awry and that some mysterious internal confusion has not mixed up his sex. The horrifying fantasy of turning into a girl is real; despite the ubiquitous nature of this problem it is not a matter of common teenage knowledge. Mild forms, or stage I gynecomastia, require nothing more. Boys who are singularly upset or bordering on homosexual panic (a not uncommon normal developmental stage in the young adolescent that is apt to be exacerbated by gynecomastia) may need additional counseling, emotional support, and a gym excuse (based on some other less compromising cause) to avoid the overwhelming anxiety that may be encountered in the locker room. Type II gynecomastia deserves surgical correction as soon as it is apparent that resolution will not occur, that is, after observation for 6–12 months.

Chest Pain
DIFFERENTIAL DIAGNOSIS

The various causes of chest pain are cited in Table 5-2. The most problematic differential is between the relatively rare instance of cardiovascular disease without murmurs (yet capable of producing pain) and the ubiquitous, benign idiopathic anterior chest wall syndrome so common among adolescent girls and, occasionally, adolescent boys. Most other causes have additional historical or physical signposts pointing the way to the correct diagnosis. It is useful to note that thoracic wall pain tends to be fairly well localized to specific intercostal spaces, whereas visceral pain from the heart, lungs, or esophagus

TABLE 5-2
DIFFERENTIAL DIAGNOSIS
OF CHEST PAIN IN ADOLESCENCE

THORACIC WALL DISORDERS
Idiopathic chest pain syndrome of adolescence (anterior chest wall syndrome)
Trauma (fractures of ribs, clavicles, or sternum; intercostal muscle strain; muscle hematoma or abscess)
Tietze's syndrome (costochondritis)
Slipped rib syndrome
Xiphoidalgia
Cervical rib
Pyogenic chondritis
Intercostal nerve neurofibroma or ganglioneuroma
Rib tumor (benign, malignant)

BREAST DISORDERS
Physiologic, cyclical
Mammary hyperplasia
Fibrocystic disease
Fibroadenoma

PULMONARY DISEASE
Pleurodynia (epidemic myalgia)
Bronchitis
Pleurisy, pneumonia
Asthma
Pneumothorax
Pulmonary embolism

CARDIAC DISEASE
Pericarditis
Myocarditis
Mitral valve prolapse syndrome
Idiopathic hypertrophic subacute stenosis
Aortic valve stenosis

MISCELLANEOUS
Thoracic outlet syndrome (brachial plexus compression due to a cervical rib or tight scalenus anterior muscle)
Leukemia
Sickle cell disease
Herpes zoster
Cervical osteoarthritis
Cervicodorsal nerve root irritation syndrome (nerve root inflammation with spasm of associated intercostal muscles)
Scalenus anterior compression
Osteomyelitis
Presternal edema of mumps
Disk space infection
Reflex esophagitis (heartburn)
Hiatal hernia
Peptic ulcer
Cholecystitis
Hyperventilation syndrome
Pancreatitis
Fitz-Hugh–Curtis syndrome (perihepatitis in association with pelvic inflammatory disease)
Precordial catch syndrome
Idiopathic

tends to be deep and poorly localized but with the potential for referred pain to almost any of the skin dermatomes supplied by the same spinal nerves. Those conditions that are most likely to be confused with each other are reviewed in the following sections. Other related conditions germane to the adolescent will be found in the index.

The major significance of chest pain in the teenage years is the frequency of this complaint and the conviction of each adolescent who experiences it that he or she has heart disease or, in girls, breast cancer. Thorough and careful examination with running commentary as to normal findings is indicated, first to ensure no pathologic condition is missed and, second, to relieve the patient of unnecessary worry by reassurance.

MITRAL VALVE PROLAPSE SYNDROME
Perhaps as many as 15% of otherwise healthy teenagers and young adules have the mitral valve prolapse syndrome (MVPS), in which mitral valve leaflets (especially posterior) project or prolapse into the left atrium toward the end of systole. This condition may be congenital or acquired, idiopathic or related to rheumatic or viral myocarditis and is more common in females. Variable chest pain may be the only sign. It is often described as a stabbing left precordial pain lasting hours to days. Sometimes severe chest discomfort develops, as well as palpitations and specific cardiac arrhythmias. Auscultation may reveal a midsystolic click with a late systolic murmur, but sometimes only the click is heard. The click may appear earlier and the murmur last longer with the patient in a standing rather than recumbent position. The chest roentgenogram is normal, and the ECG often shows T-wave inversion with variable arrhythmias possible. Diagnosis is established by echocardiogram demonstrating prolapse. The course is generally benign, but bacterial endocarditis, serious cardiac arrhythmias, and sudden death have been reported. Antibiotic prophylaxis before surgical or dental procedures is recommended. Propranolol is effective in relieving the chest pain and many of the associated arrhythmias.

SPONTANEOUS PNEUMOTHORAX
Severe, sharp, unilateral chest pain with variable degrees of dyspnea and cyanosis in a young, apparently "healthy" individual is the usual presentation for spontaneous pneumothorax. Often this is in a tall, asthenic, and athletic male. Adolescence is a common time of appearance. Examination reveals variable degrees of respiratory distress with increased resonance on percussion and reduced breath sounds and fremitus on auscultation. The chest roentgenogram is confirmatory, with evidence of air on one side and displacement of mediastinal structures. Treatment consists of placing a chest tube that is connected to a positive-pressure apparatus to reexpand the lung. A very small pneumothorax may only need observation. Recurrences may occur, but there is no evidence that activity should be curtailed on this count. Most cases are idiopathic and thought due to the rupture of small congenital blebs. Trauma also may predispose to this problem. In addition, spontaneous pneumothorax may be a complication of cavitary pulmonary tuberculosis, staphylococcal pneumonia, or other serious lung disease. Appropriate diagnostic steps should be taken, including a tuberculosis skin test, if any of these conditions are serious possibilities.

TIETZE'S DISEASE
Tietze's disease is also called the costosternal syndrome, costochondritis, and a host of other terms. It refers to a painful, nonsuppurative, fusiform swelling of the upper costal cartilages, usually at the costochondral junction.

Usually only one rib is involved, the second costal cartilage being the most frequent site, but the third, fourth, and/or others may be affected in some cases. It is most commonly, but not exclusively, seen on the left side and sometimes may be bilateral. An upper respiratory tract infection may be an associated factor, with exacerbation on coughing, sneezing, inspiration, recumbency, bending, exercise, barometric changes, and even anxiety. Both sexes are affected, and the incidence is highest in the third to fourth decade of life. However, the common complaint of chest pain in teenagers is often ascribed to this condition, although usually without clear evidence of costochondral junction swelling and tenderness. In such instances, the anterior chest wall syndrome is a more likely diagnosis. The cause of Tietze's disease is unknown, and it is unclear if a specific joint space or the surrounding ligaments are inflamed. The pain can be mild or severe and may even radiate to the shoulder or arm. Pressure over the area causes pain. Roentgenograms of the area or bone biopsy are normal.

Although this is a benign disorder, it may recur or run a chronic and persistent course, lasting months to years. The differential diagnosis includes any entity in Table 5-2. Treatment includes reassurance, local heat, salicylates, local anesthetics or hydrocortisone injections and, in extreme cases, local surgical excision.

ANTERIOR CHEST WALL SYNDROME
The term anterior chest wall syndrome refers to idiopathic chest pain of thoracic origin. The pain is most often localized to the precordium or left para-

sternal region in the second, third, or fourth inter-costal space. Sometimes left shoulder or left arm pain also occurs. The pain, which is unpredictable and may occur at rest or be exertionally induced, may be described as sharp and stabbing or as a duller ache lasting a few minutes, hours, or a day. Chest wall tenderness may be detected when firm, steady pressure is applied to the specific area; however, examination may be entirely negative. There is no evidence of specific costochondral disease. The cause is unknown and there probably are multiple contributing factors, including intercostal muscle strain and psychogenic factors. It most commonly occurs in adolescent girls at the end of puberty, and one cannot help but contemplate the possible con-tribution of breast development. It also could be a variant of Tietze's syndrome, without demonstrable costochondral junction swelling. The condition is benign, and unless other complaints or findings suggest further investigation, chest roentgenogram, electrocardiogram, or both are not indicated. Treat-ment consists simply of reassurance with particular emphasis on the absence of cardiac disease; many adolescents with this condition genuinely fear they have angina, even if they do not admit it to the physician. Some attention should be given to psy-chogenic factors, but many of these patients are well adjusted and without any singular stress or evidence of an emotional basis. Symptoms usually clear spontaneously within 6–12 months. No limita-tion of activity or medication is warranted.

MISCELLANEOUS

A cervical rib is a congenital, unilateral or bilateral, fibrous or bony extension from the seventh cervical vertebra. It may cause local pain but more often produces pain and parasthesias in the ipsilateral arm due to brachial plexus pressure; vasomotor or vascu-lar symptoms also are seen due to blood vessel com-pression.

The precordial catch syndrome refers to recur-rent episodes of brief, sharp, left-sided precordial pain in young adults, sometimes with adolescent onset. The pain is mild to severe, lasts for 30–60 seconds, and is described as stabbing or needlelike. It may occur with rest or mild activity and may worsen with inspiration or poor posture. The pain is localized to the left sternal border or cardiac apex area and does not radiate. Affected individuals are healthy, with normal physical examination results. No treatment other than reassurance is needed. The difference between this condition, the anterior chest wall syndrome, and a variant of Tietze's syndrome without costochondral swelling is obscure. Treat-ment here also is by reassurance. The slipping rib syndrome (Davies-Colley syndrome; rib-tip syn-drome; clicking rib syndrome) is another obscure cause of chest pain. Symptoms result from an ab-normal degree of mobility of the anterior intercostal articulations of the lower ribs (8–10), with one or more ribs (usually only the eighth) slipping over another. The condition usually is unilateral and may be associated with trauma. The pain is described as burning, sharp, and stabbing and may be epigastric as well as lower thoracic in location. Radiation to the back sometimes is seen. Rest, bending, or twist-ing may exacerbate the discomfort. Nausea, emesis, and intercostal muscle spasms can occur. Hooking fingers over the inferior rib margin of the involved side and pulling anteriorly will produce the char-acteristic pain. Repeating this process on the other side elicits no pain. Roentgenograms are normal. Treatment involves local anesthetic infiltration and/or surgical resection of the involved ribs.

Bibliography

BREAST AND CHEST DISORDERS

Ashikari, W.; Jun, M. Y.; Farrow, J. H.; et al. 1977. Breast carcinoma in children and adolescents. *Clin. Bull.* 7(2):55-62.

Brown, R. T. 1981. Costochondritis in adolescents. *J. Adol. Health Care* 1:198-201.

Carlson, H. E. 1980. Gynecomastia. *N. Engl. J. Med.* 303(14):795-799.

Daniel, W. A., and Mathews, M. D. 1968. Tumors of the breast in adolescent females. *Pediatrics* 41(4):743-749.

Dewhurst, J. 1981. Breast disorders in children and adolescents. *Pediatr. Clin. North Am.* 28(2):287-308.

Driscoll, D. J.; Glicklich, L. B.; and Gallen, W. J. 1976. Chest pain in children: a prospective study. *Pediatrics* 57(5):648-651.

Epstein, S. E.; Gerber, L. H.; and Borer, J. S. 1979. Chest wall syndrome. A common cause of unex-plained cardiac pain. *J.A.M.A.* 241(26):2793-2797.

Falk, R. H., and Hood, W. B. 1981. Mitral valve pro-lapse: striking a therapeutic balance. *Drug Therapy* 11(9):125-134.

Gelfand, M. L.; Kronzon, I.; DeCarolis, P.; et al. 1980. Mitral valve systolic click syndrome. *Am. Family Phys.* 21(5):135-141.

Greydanus, D. E., and McAnarney, E. R. 1982. Menstruation and its disorders in adolescence. *Curr. Probl. Pediatr.* 12(10):1-61.

Heinz, G. J., and Zavala, D. C. 1977. Slipping rib syndrome. Diagnosis using the "hooking maneuver." *J.A.M.A.* 237(8):794-795.

Knorr, D., and Bidlingmaier, F. 1975. Gynaecomastia in male adolescents. *Clin. Endocrinol. Metabol.* 4(1):157-171.

Levey, G. S., and Calabro, J. J. 1962. Tietze's syndrome: report of two cases and review of the literature. *Arthrit. Rheum.* 5(3):261-269.

Mitchell, G. W. 1977. The gynecologist and breast disease. *Clin. Obstet. Gynecol.* 20(4):865-880.

Naggar, C. Z. 1979. The mitral valve prolapse syndrome: spectrum and therapy. *Med. Clin. North Am.* 63(2):337-353.

Scheinman, M. M. 1976. Finding the cause of chest pain. *Consultant* 16(11):49-57.

Schydlower, M. 1982. Breast masses in adolescents. *Am. Family Phys.* 25(2):141-148.

Seashore, J. H. 1975. Breast enlargements in infants and children. *Pediatr. Ann.* 4(10):8-47.

Sparrow, M. J., and Bird, E. L. 1978. "Precordial catch": a benign syndrome of chest pain in young persons. *N.Z. Med. J.* 88:325-326.

Teasdale, C., and Baum, M. 1976. Breast cancer in a schoolgirl. *Lancet* 2(2):627.

Turbey, W. J.; Buntain, W. L.; and Dudgeon, D. L. 1975. The surgical management of pediatric breast masses. *Pediatrics* 56(5):736-739.

Wilcox, P. M., and Ettinger, D. S. 1977. Benign breast disease: diagnosis and treatment. *Primary Care* 4(4):739-754.

CHEST PAIN

Brown, R. T. 1981. Costochondritis in adolescents. *J. Adol. Health Care* 1:198-201.

Corso, P. J. 1978. Chest trauma. *Primary Care* 5(3):543-555.

Driscoll, D. J.; Glicklich, L. B.; and Gallen, W. J. 1976. Chest pain in children: a prospective study. *Pediatrics* 57(5):648-651.

Elmore, M. F., and Lehman, G. A. 1978. Chest pain. *Pediatrics* 61(1):143-144.

Epstein, S. E.; Gerber, L. H.; and Borer, J. S. 1979. Chest wall syndrome: a common cause of unexplained cardiac pain. *J.A.M.A.* 241(26):2793-2797.

Falk, R. H., and Hood, W. B. 1981. Mitral valve prolapse: striking a therapeutic balance. *Drug Therapy* 11(9):125-134.

Gill, G. V. 1977. Epidemic of Tietze's syndrome. *Br. Med. J.* 2:499.

Haller, J. A., and Shermeta, D. W. 1975. Major thoracic trauma in children. *Pediatr. Clin. North Am.* 22(2):341-347.

Heinz, G. J., and Zavala, D. C. 1977. The slipping rib syndrome: diagnosis using the "hooking maneuver." *J.A.M.A.* 237(8):794-795.

Kayser, H. L. 1956. Tietze's syndrome. A review of the literature. *Am. J. Med.* 21:982-989.

Levey, G. S., and Calabro, J. J. 1962. Tietze's syndrome: report of two cases and review of the literature. *Arthrit. Rheum.* 5(3):261-268.

Miller, A. J., and Texidor, T. A. 1955. Precordial catch: a neglected syndrome of precordial pain. *J.A.M.A.* 159:1364-1365.

Naggar, C. Z. 1979. The mitral valve prolapse syndrome: spectrum and therapy. *Med. Clin. North Am.* 63(2):337-354.

Palmer, E. 1978. Two causes of nonvisceral abdominal wall pain. *Am. Family Phys.* 17(4):115-116.

Rib pain (editorial). 1976. *Br. Med. J.* 1:358-359.

Rosenow, E. C.; Osmundson, P. J.; and Brown, M. L. 1981. Pulmonary embolism. *Mayo Clin. Proc.* 56:161-178.

Scheinman, M. M. 1976. Finding the cause of chest pain. *Consultant* 16(11):49-57.

Sparrow, M. J., and Bird, E. L. 1978. "Precordial catch": a benign syndrome of chest pain in young persons. *N.Z. Med. J.* 88:325-326.

Wolf, E., and Stern, S. 1976. Costosternal syndrome: its frequency and importance in differential diagnosis of coronary heart disease. *Arch. Intern. Med.* 136:189-191.

–6–
The Lower Respiratory Tract

Bronchitis
Bronchiectasis
Pneumonia
Pulmonary Tuberculosis
Asthma
Exercise-induced asthma □ Complications and prognosis □ Treatment
Pleurodynia
Pulmonary Embolism
Cystic Fibrosis
Unusual Disorders Associated with Chronic Pulmonary Disease
Kartagener's syndrome □ Middle lobe syndrome □ Goodpasture's syndrome
Idiopathic pulmonary hemosiderosis □ Wegener's granulomatosis
Alpha-1-antitrypsin protein deficiency □ Hypertrophic osteoarthropathy
Hemoptysis

Bronchitis

Acute bronchitis, either bacterial or viral, is a common disease in adolescents. It usually involves other portions of the respiratory tree as well, particularly the trachea (tracheobronchitis). Precipitating factors in otherwise healthy adolescents include upper respiratory tract infections, air pollution, noxious fumes (sulfur dioxide, ammonia, chlorine, sulfuric acid), and cigarette smoke. Allergic conditions and chronic sinusitis also are implicated. Any of the preceding factors may damage the bronchi by increasing mucus-secreting goblet cells or decreasing ciliated cells, which consequently impairs respiratory tract defense mechanisms.

The onset of bronchitis is marked by a dry, hacking nonproductive cough, frequently in association with coryza. The cough gradually produces variable types of mucus. In bacterial bronchitis the mucus tends to be purulent, even blood-streaked, whereas viral forms are more likely to be accompanied by whitish sputum. Sternal chest pain or shortness of breath may be present on occasion, although the pain is more likely to be from intercostal muscular strain from coughing than of pulmonary

parenchymal origin. Coarse rhonchi are frequently heard on auscultation. Fever is variable, as is the white blood cell count and erythrocyte sedimentation rate, which tend to follow the differential patterns seen in viral and bacterial infections. The chest roentgenogram usually is negative. Resolution ordinarily occurs over several weeks, but sometimes the cough persists for much longer, even for months. In this instance additional differential considerations most commonly include a low-humidity environment, asthma, chronic sinusitis, substance misuse (cigarette or marijuana smoking, glue or cocaine sniffing), air pollution, cough tic or habit cough, or progression of the original bronchitis into a more chronic form. Among the less common considerations are bronchiectasis, cystic fibrosis, tuberculosis, alpha-1-antitrypsin deficiency, and congestive heart failure. A prolonged episode of severe, paroxysmal coughing with wheezing for several weeks comprises the pertussislike syndrome and is thought to be caused by adenovirus or echovirus. Pertussis itself is rare today among immunized populations. Adenovirus 21 also has been implicated in bronchiolitis obliterans, a rare condition in which an episode of acute bronchitis rapidly progresses over several weeks to chronic pulmonary disease with bronchiectasis. However, chronic bronchitis from any cause can result in a similar picture if it persists over months and years. This event, however, is an uncommon complication in adolescents who do not have any underlying pulmonary or immunologic disorder.

Treatment of nonbacterial bronchitis (nonpurulent sputum, minimal or absent fever, minimal signs of toxicity, normal to low white blood cell count, and normal erythrocyte sedimentation rate, and so forth) is purely symptomatic. Antibiotics are added (after culturing the sputum) when a bacterial agent is suggested by fever, toxicity, purulent sputum, and an elevated white blood cell count and erythrocyte sedimentation rate (Table 6-1). Prolonged treatment or prophylactic antibiotics may be necessary in some cases. Desensitization for coexistent allergic conditions also can be helpful in those chronic or recurrent conditions in which allergy appears to be a contributing factor.

Bronchiectasis

Bronchiectasis is characterized by an irregular patulous widening of bronchi and bronchioles and increased secretion and pooling of mucus leading to chronic airway infection. Involvement may be limited to a single segment or a single lobe or be more widespread. Although bronchiectasis is uncommon in adolescents, it may be encountered as a complication of pulmonary infections (tuberculosis, measles, bronchopneumonia, aspergillosis), cystic fibrosis, foreign body aspiration, trauma, postsurgical atelectasis, middle lobe syndrome, Kartagener's syndrome, and severe chronic bronchitis.

The most predominant symptom is a chronic cough with production of large amounts of sputum, often purulent. The cough tends to be most marked in the morning following the pooling of secretions overnight. Other signs and symptoms may include fever, recurrent episodes of bronchitis or pneumonia (bacterial or viral), chronic sinusitis, and hemoptysis. Physical findings vary. The examination may be entirely negative or only reveal a few scattered rhonchi. At the other end of the spectrum, generalized wheezing, rhonchi, a flat thorax, deviated mediastinum, clubbing, and cyanosis indicate severe disease. Cor pulmonale also is a possible complication of advanced bronchiectasis.

H. influenzae, pneumococci, and staphylococci are the most common organisms cultured from the sputum. The chest roentgenogram may reveal increased coarse lung markings; any coexistent parenchymal disease also will be evident. Bronchoscopy

---

TABLE 6-1
TREATMENT OF ACUTE BRONCHITIS

1. Antitussives and expectorants separately or in combination. Do not oversuppress cough reflex, and avoid antitussive use entirely when thick bronchial secretions are part of an underlying process such as asthma or cystic fibrosis.
   a. Oral antitussives
      □ Codeine, 15-20 mg every 6-8 hr as needed
      □ Hydrocodone bitatrate 5 mg every 4-6 hr as needed
      □ Dextromethorphan, 15-20 mg every 6 hr as needed (in proprietary cough mixtures)
   b. Oral expectorants (may make the patient with a harsh cough more comfortable, but of no proven therapeutic value in the course of the disease; no longer has FDA endorsement)
      □ Glyceryl guaiacolate (Guaifenesin), 100 mg every 3-6 hours
      □ Proprietary cough mixtures

2. Antibiotics for mucopurulent bronchitis
   a. Tetracycline, 250-500 mg q.i.d. × 7-10 days (avoid if patient is pregnant due to effects on fetus)
   b. Ampicillin, 250-500 mg q.i.d. × 7-10 days
   c. Erythromycin, 250-500 mg q.i.d. × 7-10 days

3. General measures
   a. Humidification of sleeping environment
   b. Avoiding secondary irritants such as cigarette smoke
   c. Avoiding antihistamines, as they dry secretions

---

and bronchography provide definitive diagnosis of the abnormal bronchi.

Treatment is directed at minimizing the pooling of secretions and recurrent infection through postural drainage and oral, parenteral, or aerosol antibiotics. Attention also is given to underlying disease states such as cystic fibrosis and exacerbating factors such as those cited for bronchitis. Complications of bronchiectasis include recurrent pneumonia, hemoptysis, lung or brain abscess, empyema, pneumothorax, and secondary amyloidosis.

Pneumonia

Pneumonia (infection of the lung parenchyma) is not uncommon in even healthy adolescents. Viral forms are most frequently seen. When bacterial pneumonia does occur, pneumococci and mycoplasma are the predominant causal organisms, although a wide variety of other agents are implicated on occasion (Table 6-2). Symptoms vary from a moderately severe cough with minimal systemic signs to a hacking cough,

TABLE 6-2
ETIOLOGY OF PNEUMONIA

BACTERIAL
Pneumococcal (*Streptococcus pneumoniae*)
Mycoplasma pneumoniae
Hemophilus influenzae
Staphylococcus
Streptococcus
Gram-negative penumonia (*Klebsiella, Pseudomonas, Escherichia coli*)
Legionnaire's disease

VIRAL
Influenza virus
Parainfluenza
Adenovirus
Coxsackievirus
ECHOvirus
Respiratory syncytial virus
Myxovirus
Picornavirus
Measles
Varicella

PULMONARY TUBERCULOSIS

FUNGAL
Histoplasma capsulatum
Coccidioides immitis
Nocardia

OTHER
Psittocosis
Toxoplasma gondii
Pneumocystis carinii

dyspnea, fever, and chills; viral infections tend to be less severe than bacterial (Table 6-3). Treatment of viral pneumonia is supportive and symptomatic. Management of bacterial pneumonias is outlined in Table 6-4.

Pulmonary Tuberculosis

Although considerably less common today than 50 years ago, pulmonary tuberculosis still occurs with sufficient frequency to warrant its consideration in the differential diagnosis of pulmonary disease. Adolescents comprise a group at relative risk due to the physical stresses of pubertal growth. Those of the inner city living under crowded circumstances are most vulnerable. It also constitutes a major health problem among refugees from underdeveloped countries.

Pulmonary tuberculosis is divided into primary and postprimary (secondary) forms. In primary tuberculosis, airborne organisms from an infected individual enter the lung and establish a granulomatous lesion; usually this is in a lower lobe and is accompanied by regional hilar lymph node enlargement. The patient usually is asymptomatic but may have a mild cough and/or modest fever and malaise. Initially, the tuberculin skin test is negative, not becoming positive until after 3–8 weeks. The chest roentgenogram demonstrates a lower lobe infiltrate with hilar adenopathy (the primary complex); with time, calcification may be noted as well.

Postprimary pulmonary tuberculosis occurs

TABLE 6-3
COMPARISON OF VIRAL AND BACTERIAL PNEUMONIA

	Viral pneumonia	Bacterial pneumonia
INCIDENCE	Frequent.	Comparatively infrequent; mycoplasma and pneumococcal pneumonias predominate.
SYMPTOMS AND SIGNS	Often begins with an upper respiratory tract infection that gradually worsens. Cough may be protracted, but symptoms relatively mild; pneumonia due to measles or varicella, however, can be severe, as can any of the viral infections in immunologically deficient individuals.	Abrupt onset with more severe symptoms. Cough may produce blood-streaked, purulent sputum. Mycoplasma pneumonia tends to be milder than other bacterial forms and more like viral types.
CHEST ROENTGENOGRAM	May be negative or demonstrate patchy, diffuse, or interstitial infiltrates.	Often more signs of consolidation. Lobar involvement common in pneumococcal pneumonia.
TREATMENT	Symptomatic.	Antibiotics. Drainage of pleural effusion if present.
COMPLICATIONS	Rarely myocarditis, pericarditis, and encephalitis.	Empyema, lung abscess relatively common; less commonly septicemia, endocarditis, or meningitis.

TABLE 6-4
BACTERIAL PNEUMONIAS

Type of pneumonia	Description and comments	Treatment
Mycoplasma pneumoniae	Most common cause of pneumonia in patients 5-15 years of age and a frequent cause in older teenagers and young adults. Severe headache develops, followed by persistent cough, chest pain, myalgia, and malaise. Symptoms classically outweigh signs. Interstitial or bronchopneumonic pattern of consolidation noted on roentgenogram, with rare pleural effusion. Diagnosis is by culture or complement fixation titers. Cold agglutinins often positive but nonspecific. Major symptoms last 2-10 days, but the cough may persist for weeks. Rare complications include hemolytic anemia, thrombocytopenia, erythema nodosum, Stevens-Johnson syndrome, cerebral ataxia, peripheral neuropathy, transverse myelitis, and Guillain-Barré syndrome.	Early treatment with erythromycin (40 mg/kg/day or 250-500 mg q.i.d. p.o. $\times$ 5 days) may shorten the course. Tetracycline also has been used. Both agents effective in vitro, but evidence for in vivo benefit less clear.
Pneumococcus (*Streptococcus pneumoniae*)	One of the most common types. Purulent sputum with numerous gram-positive diplococci, polymorphonuclear leukocytes, and small amount of blood. A lobar or bronchopneumonia pattern of consolidation often seen on roentgenogram. May be confused with pulmonary embolism and infarction. Pneumococcal vaccine (Pneumovax) should be given to individuals at high risk (e.g., with asplenia, sickle cell anemia, the nephrotic syndrome, congestive heart failure, chronic pulmonary disease, diabetes mellitus, and compromised host). Avoid vaccine in pregnancy.	A 10-day course of: 1. Penicillin (drug of choice) a. 400,000 units q.i.d. p.o. (Pen V) *or* b. 600,000 units b.i.d. IM or IV (Pen G) *or* 2. Erythromycin 250-500 mg q.i.d. p.o. *or* 3. Cephalexin (Keflex), 50 mg/kg/day or 250-500 mg q.i.d. p.o. (up to 4 grams per d). *or* 4. Sodium cephalothin (Keflin), 100 mg/kg/day or 500-1000 mg q.i.d. IV
Hemophilus influenzae	Less common, but incidence in adolescents may be increasing. Primarily a complication of chronic bronchitis or other chronic lung disease. Diagnosis is by culture (sputum, blood). Ampicillin-resistant strains encountered with rising frequency.	A 14-day course of: 1. Ampicillin, 100-200 mg/kg/day or 2-4 g/day p.o. IV *and/or* 2. Chloramphenicol, 100 mg/kg/day (observe for aplastic anemia) *and/or* 3. Tetracycline 1-2 g/day (as supplement, not alone)
Staphylococcus aureus	Infrequent cause; most often seen in debilitated individuals or those with chronic pulmonary disease. Heavy purulent sputum with masses of gram-positive cocci in clumps. Produces a necrotizing picture with pseudocysts (pneumatoceles), cavities, abscesses, effusions, and empyema. Staphylococcal septicemia with spread to liver, kidneys, spleen, meninges, etc., may occur.	A 2-3 week course of: 1. Penicillinase-resistant, semisynthetic penicillins a. Methicillin (Staphcillin); 1 g q 4 hr IM or q 6 hr IV *or* b. Oxacillin (Prostaphlin), 150 mg/kg/day, or 1 g q 4 hr Im or IV *and/or* 2. Keflin (cephalexin) 500-1000 mg q 4 hr IV *and/or* 3. Penicillin G, 12-20 million units per day IV; also thoracentesis for pleural effusion and open drainage for emphyema.
Streptococcus	Infrequent cause of pneumonia. Lobar or bronchopneumonic pattern seen.	IV penicillin as per pneumoccal pneumonia.

when a primary complex is reactivated and progresses to one or more of the following: lobar pneumonia, bronchopneumonia, cavitary disease, and endobronchitis. Hematogenous dissemination from a primary or secondary pulmonary lesion may involve virtually any organ system, including cervical lymph nodes (lymphadenitis), meninges, kidney, and joints. Miliary spread also can occur but is uncommon in adolescents who are immunologically intact. Tuberculosis from some other portal of entry than the lungs, for example, the gastrointestinal tract, is rare today. Postprimary disease is not an invariable event and occurs in an unpredictable manner. It is most likely to appear during.the year following initial exposure, but individuals subject to particular physical stress (puberty, pregnancy, debilitating disease) also are prone regardless of the interval since exposure. Dominant symptoms of pulmonary extension are a productive cough, fever, night sweats, and weight loss. Erythema nodosum also may occur. Hemoptysis is a frequent manifestation of cavitary and endobronchial disease. Pneumothorax is another possible complication. Manifestations of miliary disseminated tuberculosis depend on the organ systems involved; tuberculous meningitis is similar to other meningeal infections, albeit somewhat more insidious in onset. However, these forms of disease are infrequently seen in adolescents.

Chest roentgenograms will demonstrate the type of secondary involvement present in the given case plus old evidence of the primary complex. Pneumonitis, with or without cavitation, tends to involve the upper lobes, while miliary disease is seen as diffuse infiltrates throughout the lung field. The differential diagnosis includes pneumonitis from any of the agents listed in Table 6-2, lung abscess, foreign body reaction and fungal infections (histoplasmosis, blastomycosis, actinomycosis).

Patients with pulmonary tuberculosis are only contagious during the postprimary stage. Infectivity depends upon the total number of organisms dispersed into the air, duration of exposure, and closeness of contacts. Thus family members and intimate friends are at significant risk, whereas those more distant (such as school mates) are considerably less so. Treatment with an appropriate agent renders the patient noninfectious within a relatively short period of time—a matter of several weeks—but many school districts require a negative culture before a student is allowed to return to the classroom.

Many adolescents have neither primary nor postprimary disease but give evidence of exposure by virtue of a positive skin test. The Tine tuberculosis skin test is used for mass screening. (Note: the fore-arm should be thoroughly dried before testing if first cleansed with alcohol, as alcohol can denature the antigenic material and result in a false-negative.) Greater reliability is achieved with the intradermal use of 0.1 ml of 5 IU potency fresh purified protein derivative (PPD). All individuals with a positive or questionable Tine test should be tested with PPD, which is the procedure of choice in those with suspected disease or definitive exposure. A position reaction is defined by induration (not erythema alone) of 10 mm or more appearing after 48-72 hours. Induration of 5-9 mm is a borderline or doubtful reaction, and the test should be repeated. Persons vaccinated with bacillus of Calmette-Guérin (BCG), as is common in some European and many Asian, African, and Latin American countries, also will give a positive reaction to the Tine test or PPD, but in most instances the induration does not exceed 8 mm. A reaction of 10 mm or more, even with a history of BCG vaccination, probably represents exposure, and prophylaxis is indicated if BCG has never been given (see below). Atypical mycobacteria also may cause positive tests, although these infections are more likely to produce cervical adenitis, bronchitis, osteomyelitis, arthritis, or meningitis than pulmonary parenchymal disease. The PPD test will be negative even in the presence of active disease if it is of recent onset or if the patient is receiving steroids or is anergic from some other cause. Measles frequently temporarily inhibits PPD reactivity, as does immunization with live measles vaccine. Other acute febrile illnesses and severely debilitating states can interfere transiently as well. Whether the patient actually has a negative skin test (and thus no tuberculosis) or is anergic is best determined by testing for other commonly encountered delayed hypersensitivity reactions, for example, with the Schick test in individuals immunized for diphtheria or with Candida skin tests.

In patients with a suggestive history and suspicious roentgenogram, regardless of skin test results, further investigation requires the microscopic examination of three sputum specimens (or early morning gastric washings in patients unable to produce sputum) prepared with Ziehl-Neelsen stain. At least 20 minutes should be spent looking for acid-fast bacilli and the total number seen recorded. Sputum, gastric washings, and other suspect body fluids (for example, urine, joint aspirate, pleural effusion, cerebrospinal fluid) should be cultured for tubercle bacilli (Mycobacterium tuberculosis) as well. Although it usually takes 6 weeks for a culture to become positive, this is an essential step to a confirmed diagnosis.

Treatment of tuberculosis employs one or more

TABLE 6-5
ANTITUBERCULOSIS DRUGS

Drug	Dosage	Duration	Side effects
Isoniazid (INH)	5–10 mg/kg p.o. up to 300 mg maximum given in a single dose daily.	6–12 months for treatment of positive tuberculin reaction; longer if there is postprimary disease. Supplement with 50–100 mg pyridoxine/day to prevent peripheral neuritis.	Hepatitis or transient liver enzyme elevations, peripheral neuritis, optic neuritis, hypersensitivity reaction (fever, dermatitis), agranulocytosis. Because of the rare possibility of fatal hepatitis, it is important to monitor liver function tests.
Rifampin	10–20 mg/kg p.o. up to 600 mg maximum given in a single dose daily.	Used in postprimary disease for several months or longer, depending upon extent of involvement. Often used with INH; sometimes with ethambutol.	GI disturbances, hepatitis, thrombocytopenia, immunosuppression, hypersensitivity reaction, and menstrual disturbances, among others.
Ethambutol	15 mg/kg p.o. given in a single dose daily. Not FDA-approved for use in individuals under 13 years of age.	As for rifampin.	Optic neuritis (check vision regularly), dermatitis, GI disturbances, and mental confusion, among others.
Streptomycin	20–40 mg/kg IM up to a maximum of 1 g/day given in 3 or 4 divided doses.	Generally limited to a short course of treatment in patients with advanced postprimary disease and/or organisms resistant to other drugs. Commonly used in combination with one or more of the above.	Ototoxicity (nausea, emesis, vertigo, hearing loss), nephrotoxicity, dermatitis, and thrombocytopenia, among others.

of the drugs listed in Table 6-5. Prophylactic treatment with isoniazid and pyridoxine supplement should be given for 6–12 months in any adolescent with a positive PPD skin test, even in the face of a negative chest roentgenogram, as well as in those with a primary complex. This will prevent further progression of the disease. Compliance often is a problem in adolescents who feel well; they are likely to be "forgetful" in denying their difference from peers. Time should be spent with patient explaining the situation and in working out a schedule he or she feels is manageable. It is ill advised to invest responsibility in parents, unless this is viewed as helpful by the adolescent. Monitoring urine for isoniazid content may or may not be useful and also should be reviewed with the patient as to acceptability; it should not be employed in a mood of coercive surveillance, as most young people are quite adept at circumvention. If compliance becomes a serious problem, an alternative for converters without primary disease is to check chest roentgenograms at 3-month intervals for a year or until pubertal growth is complete, whichever is

longer. Prophylaxis, however, always is preferred in individuals less than 25 years of age.

Treatment of postprimary disease usually employs two or more antituberculosis drugs. Isoniazid plus rifampin and/or ethambutol is a common combination. Prednisone, 1 mg/kg/day, is often added with pleural or endobronchial involvement.

Prophylaxis also should be considered for household members, close friends, and dating partners of patients with recently diagnosed secondary pulmonary tuberculosis. Mass BCG vaccination is widely practiced in many countries as previously noted. It appears to provide a fair degree of protection against the development of primary and secondary disease but the degree of protection is controversial. BCG is not widely employed in the United States because of the uncertain protection and the considerable confusion it introduces into mass skin test screening programs. There may be validity, however, for BCG vaccination of certain high-risk individuals such as those subject to constant exposure or those in whom isoniazid prophylaxis cannot be used because of adverse reactions or poor compliance.

Asthma

Asthma, the most common chronic lung disorder of adolescents and a major cause of school absenteeism, is a diffuse, reversible obstructive airway disease in which hyperactivity of bronchial beta-adrenergic receptors results in excessive mucus production, bronchial edema, and bronchospasm. The condition is due, in part, to an IgE antigen-antibody reaction involving bronchial mast cells, causing release of histamine, bradykinin, and other inflammation-inducing substances. Both extrinsic and intrinsic factors contribute to this reaction. Extrinsic factors include allergy to pollens, molds, animal danders, and/or house dust; upper respiratory tract infections (usually viral); cold air or cold drinks; exercise; air pollutants (particularly sulfur dioxide); atmospheric weather changes; cigarette smoke; ingestion of certain drugs such as aspirin, indomethacin, and propranolol; and, possibly, food allergies. Intrinsic factors are less well specified but include genetic, familial, and psychosomatic issues. The assignation of an intrinsic cause often is one of exclusion and is made in those individuals for whom no extrinsic cause can be found.

Asthma may begin in childhood, adolescence, or adulthood. When present from early life, adolescence can be a pivotal time during which asthma often improves or worsens. Manifestations of an acute attack vary from a brief period of mild wheezing to a medical emergency with severe hypoxia. Symptoms include the sudden onset of shortness of breath, wheezing, a choking feeling, chest tightness, chest pain, and cough. When the reaction is severe, the patient also experiences acute apprehension and feelings of suffocation. A single episode may last from only a few hours to a number of days. The frequency varies from only once or twice a year to nearly every day. A good index of overall dysfunction is the number of school days missed because of asthma and how often medication is required for relief, either self-administered or during emergency room visits. Detailed inquiry about associated intrinsic and extrinsic factors often is revealing as well and is essential for effective management.

Physical findings of note generally are present only during an attack and relate to its severity; the examination at other times tends to be entirely normal. Some degree of wheezing is invariably present during an acute episode and is an important diagnostic sign. It characteristically occurs in the expiratory phase, which is prolonged. Intercostal and sternal retractions and the use of accessory muscles of respiration increase with the degree of obstruction. Cyanosis, chest distention, and absence of wheezing are other signs of an advancing state and may presage respiratory failure. Death is a possible but uncommon outcome. If an upper or lower respiratory tract infection or hay fever has been contributory, signs of these conditions will be present as well.

Arterial blood gases may reveal an initial decrease in PCO_2 due to hyperventilation, but this shortly will become abnormally high in association with a decreased PO_2 as air exchange becomes further impaired. Characteristic findings on testing pulmonary function are a low forced volume during the first second of the expiratory phase, a decreased peak expiratory flow rate, decreased vital capacity, elevated residual volume, and elevated functional residual capacity. A chest roentgenogram often demonstrates peribronchial thickening with hyperinflation of the lungs.

EXERCISE-INDUCED ASTHMA

Exercise-induced asthma is a variant of some significance in adolescents due to the importance of athletics in this age group. It occurs in most individuals with classic asthma and in 40% of those with hay fever or allergic rhinitis. Viral respiratory tract infections, cold air, or airborne allergens may exacerbate this reaction. Characteristically, bronchospasm and wheezing develop 5–10 minutes after initiating physical activity with the heart rate exceeding 170 beats per minute. These developments are associated with a drop in lung function of 15% or more. Symptoms resolve spontaneously within 15–30 minutes after stopping exercise. Diagnosis is by history and by replicating the situation in the office setting. The patient exercises to an extent sufficient to raise the heart rate to 170 beats per minute. Lung function before and after exercise is evaluated with a recording spirometer or Wright peak flowmeter.

COMPLICATIONS AND PROGNOSIS

Complications of severe asthma include pneumonia, atelectasis, pneumothorax or, rarely, pneumomediastinum. In long-standing disease with frequent, protracted attacks, irreversible emphysematous lung changes may occur. In this instance, the chest roentgenogram demonstrates a persistent increase in the anteroposterior diameter and hyperaeration of the lungs even when the patient is not experiencing an attack. Bronchiectasis is another long-range possibility.

Although a variety of other conditions may produce a picture resembling asthma, expiratory wheezing in the absence of other pulmonary pathology and the rapid response to bronchodilators effectively differentiate this condition from such diseases as cystic fibrosis, bronchiectasis, endobronchial tuberculosis, foreign body reaction, pneumonia, bronchitis, and others.

The long-term prognosis for an individual with asthma is as variable and unpredictable as are the manifestations of an acute attack. The majority of individuals seem to improve over time or are effectively controlled by medication. Severe, frequent episodes, however, may lead to permanent lung damage. As previously noted, matters often change during adolescence for better or worse, and it is particularly difficult to anticipate the ultimate course during these years. But a dire prognosis should not be made for the occasional adolescent with relatively mild childhood asthma who suddenly experiences an increase in the number and severity of attacks. The reasons for this are not clear, but the normative heightening of intrinsic stress during adolescence may have a bearing. Most patients in this group sooner or later return to a more benign and easily managed course.

TREATMENT

Acute asthma is treated with varying combinations of adrenergic agents, hydration, xanthines, oxygen and, in resistant cases, corticosteroids (Table 6-6). One initial treatment protocol for an acute episode is as follows:

1. Epinephrine, 0.3-0.4 ml of 1:1000 dilution subcutaneously, every 20-30 minutes for one to three doses until a response is achieved. Alternatively, terbutaline sulfate, 0.25 mg subcutaneously, is given every 15-30 minutes.

2. Adrenergic aerosol, 0.2-0.5 ml in 2.5 ml saline, may be given in conjunction with the above and repeated once in 30 minutes (see Table 6-6). This can be done in the emergency room, as it is desirable to avoid admission if at all possible.

3. If responsive, maintain patient at home with:
a. A stat dose of epinephrine HCl, 0.1-0.3 ml of a 1:200 dilution subcutaneously. (Sus-Phrine)
b. Theophylline, 3-6 mg/kg, every 6 hours p.o. Adjust subsequently for maintenance if indicated (see Table 6-6).
c. Oral metaproterenol, 20 mg t.i.d.-q.i.d. or terbutaline, 2.5-5.0 mg t.i.d.-q.i.d., may be given at the same time or added if wheezing recurs.
d. Instructions to maintain hydration with the fluid intake of 3 liters or more per day.
e. Instructions for alleviating precipitating factors and using a humidifier.
f. Institution of antibiotics if bacterial infection coexists.

If the patient does not respond to these measures within 30-60 minutes (as in status asthmaticus) or has (a) severe asthma without wheezing (indicating advanced airway obstruction; (b) a PO_2 less than 60-65 mm Hg; (c) a PCO_2 over 45-50 mm Hg; or (d) pneumothorax, admission to the hospital is indicated. Management is as follows:

1. IV aminophylline, 5-7 mg/kg, diluted in saline and run in over 15-30 minutes. Continue with intravenous administration of 5 mg/kg q 6 hours or 0.6-0.9 mg/kg/hr (or an amount resulting in therapeutic serum levels of 10-20 mg/ml).

2. Nebulized bronchodilator inhalation (1:200 isoproterenol aerosol or 0.5% metaproterenol solution) for 5 minutes every 30 minutes × 4, then every 2 hours as necessary. Stop at any time the pulse rate exceeds 190/min.

3. IV steroids: dexamethasone phosphate, betamethasone phosphate, or hydrocortisone hemisuccinate (see Table 6-6).

4. Hydration:
a. 2500 ml/m^2/24 hours given as 5% glucose for severe dehydration.
b. Add potassium (2 mEq/100 ml) and sodium (3 mEq/100 ml) to the hydration solution.
c. Watch for possible inappropriate antidiuretic hormone secretion (decreased serum sodium and plasma osmolality, increased urine osmolality).
d. Reduce fluid intake to maintenance as hydration improves.

5. Sodium bicarbonate is helpful in severe metabolic acidosis (0.3 × kg × base excess). Give half intravenously at once and the other half after further arterial blood gases.

6. Oxygen.

7. Ventilatory support may be necessary. Intubate if PCO_2 over 50-55 mm Hg.

8. Chest tube and positive suction for pneumothorax.

Patients with frequent severe attacks should be on maintenance theophylline or aminophylline with the addition of beta-adrenergic medications (metaproterenol, terbutaline) as needed (see Table 6-6). Beclomethasone dipropionate or cromolyn sodium inhalation may be helpful for some patients in preventing attacks or reducing their frequency and severity. But the chronic use of *systemic* corticosteroids should be avoided if at all possible.

Patients with only infrequent or mild episodes of asthma may be effectively managed on an as needed basis with one of the many available pharmaceutical products containing theophylline or aminophylline alone or in combination with sympathomimetic

TABLE 6-6
ASTHMA MEDICATIONS

Drug	Initial dose	Maintenance dose	Mechanism of action	Comment
Epinephrine: Adrenalin, 1:1000 aqueous solution	0.3-0.4 ml SQ	None. May be repeated q 15-30 minutes 3-4 times.	Sympathomimetic amine, which acts as a beta- and alpha-adrenergic agonist.	Most common first step in treatment of an acute asthma attack. Tachycardia and arrhythmia occur with excessive dose or individual patient hypersensitivity.
Sus-Phrine, 1:200 solution	0.1-0.3 ml SQ	None. May be repeated every 6 hours for several doses.	A longer acting epinephrine than the aqueous form.	Commonly used to sustain effects of aqueous form in breaking up acute attack.
Isoproterenol (Isuprel) 1:200 dilution aerosol	0.2-0.3 ml aerosolized in 2.5 u saline taken in 5-15 deep inhalations.	Used with nebulizer q 4-6 hours p.r.n.	Sympathomimetic amine acting on beta-adrenergic receptors to relax bronchial muscle.	Severe paroxysmal airway resistance may occur if excessive doses given. Prescription may be abused by patient and resultant death possible.
Theophylline or aminophylline (85% theophylline)	5-7 mg/kg p.o. or IV.	5 mg/kg/q.i.d. up to 200 mg t.i.d.-q.i.d. p.o. for long-term maintenance. Adjust dose to obtain therapeutic serum levels of 10-20 μg/ml % with 3 day intervals between increments. Slow-release capsules given 1-2 times a day may improve effects and/or compliance.	Xanthine derivative inhibiting production of phosphodiesterase with increased cylic AMP output and suppression of inflammatory mediator release (histamine, bradykinin, etc.).	Drug of choice in maintenance treatment of moderate-to-severe asthma. Side effects often noted at higher levels, including nausea, gastrointestinal irritation, and tachycardia. Arrhythmias, convulsions, and respiratory arrest are possible toxic complications. Addition of ephedrine or phenobarbital of no proven further benefit.
Metaproterenol sulfate (Alupent)*	20 mg p.o. or 2-3 inhalations of metered dose inhaler.	20 mg t.i.d. or q.i.d. or 2-3 inhalations of metered dose inhaler q 4 h p.r.n., not to exceed 12 inhalations/day,	Sympathomimetic amine and potent beta-adrenergic stimulant.	Often used as an adjuvant to theophylline. Caution should be taken against patient abuse of inhalant form.
Terbutaline sulfate (Bricanyl)	0.25 mg SQ with repeat dose in 15-30 minutes if needed, or 2.5-5.0 mg p.o.	Ages 13-15: 2.5 mg t.i.d. p.o.; ages 16 and over: 2.5-5.0 mg. t.i.d.	Sympathomimetic amine that is a beta-adrenergic agonist with preferential effects on beta-receptors.	Not recommended for patients under age 13. Tachycardia, anxiety, tremor, arrhythmias, and headache can occur, as with other sympathomimetic amines.
Cromolyn sodium (Intal with Spin haler)	One inhalation of a 20 mg capsule (delivers ¼ of the total capsule contents).	1 capsule 3-4 times/day by Spin haler.	Exact mechanism unclear. Seems to suppress the allergic reaction and inhibits release of inflammatory mediators. Not effective in an acute episode.	The capsule is crushed in the Spin haler, and the contents are inhaled with a single deep breath. Must be used for several weeks before full effect achieved. Used as a prophylactic agent to prevent or reduce number of asthma attacks. Bronchospasm, nasal congestion, pharyngeal irritation may be complications.

*Other aerosol medications include isoetharine, albuterol and fenoterol.

Continued

TABLE 6-6
ASTHMA MEDICATIONS (CONTINUED)

Drug	Initial dose	Maintenance dose	Mechanism of action	Comment
Beclomethasone dipropionate (Vanceril inhaler)	84 μg (2 inhalations) t.i.d. by aerosol.	Two inhalations (84 μg) t.i.d. or q.i.d. with a daily range of 2–16 inhalations adjusted according to need.	Antiinflammatory steroid given by way of inhaler. Precise antiasthmatic mechanism unclear. Systemic absorption seems to be minimal.	Not for acute asthma. Often of benefit in steroid-dependent patients. Withdrawal of systemic steroids and addition of Vanceril must be done carefully to avoid adrenal insufficiency. Complications include candidiasis and aspergillosis of the mouth, pharynx, and larynx (respond to antifungal medications and/or withdrawal of Vanceril).
Cortico-steroids	Given by IV drip $\times$ 2 days. a. Prednisone, 40 mg/day b. Dexamethasone phosphate, 0.3 mg/kg, then 0.1 mg/kg q.i.d. c. Hydrocortisone succinate, 7 mg/kg at first dose then 5 mg/kg q.i.d.	Undesirable to maintain with steroids. Taper initial dose slowly over 1 week. If necessary for long-term control, use lowest effective oral dose and an alternate-day regimen when possible. Oral Prednisone dose: 1–2 mg/kg/day.	Unclear; may stimulate production of cyclic AMP, which suppresses release of inflammatory mediators.	Used primarily in treatment of status asthmaticus. Generally takes 6–12 hours for an effect. Long-term use employs p.o. rather than IV forms. Side effects of long-term use are numerous and should be carefully considered before using. Alternate-day therapy recommended. Maintenance makes for additional problems in rendering the patient steroid-dependent and minimizing effects in treating status asthmaticus.

drugs. Newer and more selective adrenergic agents include albuterol (oral or aerosol) and fentoterol (aerosol). The conjoint use of sedatives is no longer commonly recommended. In any event, it is unlikely that adolescents will comply with daily maintenance therapy when not singularly discomforted by their diseases. If an association exists between upper respiratory tract infections and asthmatic episodes, antiasthmatic medication should be instituted at the first signs of such an infection and not delayed until wheezing starts. Antihistamines are helpful when hay fever coexists but should be used with caution due to their drying effect on bronchial mucus.

Certain drug and cross-drug reactions should be kept in mind. Aspirin, indomethacin (and, possibly, other antiinflammatory agents), propranolol, and morphine may induce an asthmatic attack in some individuals. Monoamine oxidase inhibitors and tricyclic antidepressants may act synergistically with sympathomimetic drugs, increasing the risk of hypertension or cardiac arrhythmias.

Individuals with exercise-induced asthma may benefit from one of the following schedules (see Table 6-6 for dosage):

1. Beta-adrenergic agonists (oral metaproterenol or terbutaline) taken 30–60 minutes before exercise; alternatively, isoetharine or isoproterenol aerosol inhaled just before exercise.

2. Theophylline or aminophylline, 30–60 minutes before exercise.

3. Cromolyn sodium, within 30 minutes of exercise.

Alternatively, the sport may be changed to one less likely to precipitate an asthmatic episode, for example, swimming in contrast to bicycling or running. This is not always possible in the committed athlete and from a psychologic perspective, it is best to encourage athletic accomplishment in adolescents rather than impose strictures.

Attention to extrinsic precipitants (as identified by history and skin testing) by avoiding exposure or hyposensitization is as important for control as medication. General environmental measures can be helpful as well and include hypoallergenic (synthetic) pillows, mattresses, and blankets or enclosing ordinary bedding in plastic covers; eliminating dust catchers such as draperies, upholstered furniture, shag rugs, quantities of stuffed animals in the patient's bedroom; scrupulous attention to maintaining the bedroom dust-free by vacuuming frequently and dusting only with dampened cloths; installing air conditioning and electronic air filters; treating damp areas in the household to eliminate mold; and avoiding household pets or flowers.

Psychotherapy often is indicated in patients with significant psychologic problems that contribute to the asthma itself or that create secondary effects such as the debilitation, isolation, and depression that accompany severe disease. In every case, counseling the patient and parents is essential. The young person must continue to pursue normal developmental tasks to the degree his or her condition permits, and parents must be helped to avoid overprotectiveness and overpermissiveness. Chapters 1 and 21 offer specific information to these ends.

Pleurodynia

Pleurodynia (epidemic myalgia), a group B Coxsackie virus infection, frequently occurs in epidemics during the summer and fall. It most commonly affects adolescents and young adults and is characterized by the acute onset of fever, headache, and severe pleuritic chest pain. The pain often is described as knifelike and more severe on inspiration; the interscapular area or nape of the neck also may be involved. The patient usually evidences difficulty in breathing and has splinting and chest wall tenderness over the affected area. A friction rub in the lower half of the chest is common. The chest roentgenogram is negative and laboratory data do not contribute to the diagnosis. This disease usually is self-limited, with full recovery in 3-7 days; treatment is purely symptomatic. Orchitis, aseptic meningitis, and pericarditis, however, are rare complications. The major implications of this usually benign disease rests in differentiating it from more serious causes of pleuritic pain.

Pulmonary Embolism

Pulmonary embolism is a rare condition in adolescents but is included here as a possible complication of deep leg vein thrombophlebitis, which may be seen in teenage females taking oral contraceptives, in young people subject to prolonged immobilization, and in patients with sickle cell disease or lower extremity circulatory disorders. Signs and symptoms of pulmonary embolism are sudden chest pain, dyspnea, hemoptysis and, sometimes, syncope. Fever, wheezing, tachycardia, and an increased second heart sound in the pulmonic area also may be noted. Cardiorespiratory failure is possible.

Laboratory data indicating significant embolism are a decrease in arterial PaO_2 to less than 80 mm Hg, increased fibrin split products, and nonspecific electrocardiogram changes with general T wave inversion, a large S wave in lead I, ST depression in lead II, and a large Q wave in lead III. The chest roentgenogram often demonstrates a lower lobe infiltrate that is adjacent to the pleura. A lung scan or pulmonary arteriography offers more precise information on the infarct's location and extent. Treatment consists of anticoagulation therapy, starting with heparin and gradually shifting to coumadin on the fifth day, with the latter continued as long as is clinically indicated by the pulmonary pathology, associated thrombophlebitis, and underlying cause. Pulmonary endarterectomy and inferior vena cava ligation may be necessary in selected instances. Females on oral contraceptives should discontinue this drug and be switched to an alternative method of birth control. Nonsexually active females should be similarly advised for the future.

Cystic Fibrosis

Cystic fibrosis, a hereditary, multisystem disease of the exocrine glands, predominates in Caucasians, is transmitted as an autosomal recessive gene, and occurs in one out of 2000 live Caucasian births. The classic triad consists of chronic pulmonary disease and elevated sweat chloride in all patients and pancreatic insufficiency in 85%. Penetrance is variable, with some individuals having only mild pulmonary disease, whereas others are in difficulty from infancy. Other features of this disease, which may be seen on occasion, include intestinal and rectal prolapse, cirrhosis, pancreatitis, nasal polyposis, pansinusitis, short stature, and delayed puberty. Approximately 85% of males with cystic fibrosis are sterile due to an abnormality or absence of the spermatic collecting system, but testosterone production remains intact. Females may have endocervical polyps and dry, viscous cervical mucus that impairs sperm migration, but the majority are fertile and capable of bearing children when these impediments are overcome. Although most cases of cystic fibrosis are diagnosed in childhood, discovery may not occur until adolescence, either because the degree of involvement is relatively mild or because this etiology was overlooked until pubertal delay prompted reevaluation.

Cystic fibrosis should be considered a possibility

in any adolescent with undiagnosed chronic pulmonary disease or evidence of malabsorption. Lung problems are due to the production of abnormally viscous mucus leading to mucoid impaction, secondary infection, and ultimate tissue destruction with bronchiectasis. Symptomatology varies but may include a chronic, productive cough, dyspnea, hemoptysis, and/or recurrent bouts of bronchitis, pneumonia, or atelectasis. Pneumothorax, hyperinflation, and hilar adenopathy also may be seen. Clinical and x-ray findings are compatible with the specific type of pulmonary complication present. Cultures commonly reveal *Staphylococcus aureus* or *Pseudomonas aeroginosa*, but virtually any bacterial pathogen may be involved. Malabsorption is evident in steatorrhea with characteristic foamy, bulky, foul-smelling stools and increased stool fat, together with poor weight gain (see Chapter 8).

Diagnosis is confirmed by a positive sweat test using quantitative pilocarpin iontophoresis. The collection of 100 mg of sweat is preferable, although 50 mg usually will suffice. A sweat chloride of over 60 mEq/L in children or 70–75 mEq/L in adults is significant. Values between 50–70 mEq in an adolescent are equivocal, and the test should be repeated; most individuals who have cystic fibrosis exhibit sweat chloride levels between 80–120 mEq/L. A false-positive test may be encountered in untreated adrenal insufficiency, ectodermal dysplasia, nephrogenic diabetes insipidus, glucose-6-phosphate dehydrogenase deficiency, the mucopolysaccharidoses, malnutrition and, sometimes, hypothyroidism.

An experienced specialist should probably handle the therapy for the pulmonary aspects of this disease. Management regimes are complex, employing varied combinations of postural drainage, expectorants, oral and aerosol antibiotics on a daily basis, and early treatment of secondary infections. It should be noted, however, that agents that suppress the cough reflex and/or dry up mucus are to be avoided. Pancreatic insufficiency is treated with oral extracts of animal pancreas (Viokase tablets, Cotazym capsules), increased vitamins, and a high-protein, low-fat diet with medium-chain triglyceride supplementation. Two to 4 g/day of supplemental salt should be given to patients at times of increased sweat production (fever, heavy exercise, prolonged exposure to heat) to avoid heat prostration (see Chapter 18).

Psychosocial issues are those relevant to any chronic disease as outlined in Chapter 21. Additional counseling will be needed for infertile males.

Unusual Disorders Associated with Chronic Pulmonary Disease

Although this group of diseases is rare in adolescents, they may be seen on occasion and enter into a differential consideration of undiagnosed chronic lung problems.

KARTAGENER'S SYNDROME

Kartagener's syndrome consists of dextrocardia, chronic sinusitis, or (less commonly) agenesis of the frontal sinuses and bronchiectasis. Whether bronchiectasis is primary or secondary to chronic sinus infection is not entirely clear. Nasal polyposis, chronic otitis media, lymphosarcoma of the small intestine, impaired spermatogenesis, and cystic fibrosis are relatively rare complications. Treatment is directed at the bronchiectasis and sinusitis.

MIDDLE LOBE SYNDROME

Persistent extrinsic obstruction of the middle lobe bronchus results in chronic middle lobe pneumonitis and atelectasis. Hilar lymphadenopathy from tuberculosis or neoplasm is the most frequent cause. Treatment is directed at the underlying pathology producing obstruction, although persistent atelectasis or pneumonitis may require surgical removal of the affected part.

GOODPASTURE'S SYNDROME

Glomerulonephritis in combination with diffuse pulmonary alveolar inflammation and hemorrhage comprises Goodpasture's syndrome, an autoimmune disease, although involvement of the two organ systems need not coincide. A cough, hemoptysis, and dyspnea may be the only presenting symptoms, and evidence of renal disease may not appear for weeks or months. Treatment with steroids and immunosuppressive agents has been tried with variable results. Renal failure can be severe and may require dialysis or transplantation.

IDIOPATHIC PULMONARY HEMOSIDEROSIS

In idiopathic pulmonary hemosiderosis, thought to be an immunologic disorder, lung lesions similar to those in Goodpasture's syndrome occur but without renal involvement. Diffuse infiltrates are noted on the chest roentgenogram, and a lung biopsy reveals hemosiderin-laden macrophages. This condition may be confused with polyarterritis nodosa or anaphylactoid purpura. The prognosis generally is poor, the patient experiencing a slowly progressive downhill course. Steroids and immunosuppressive agents have been tried but with limited success.

TABLE 6-7
EVALUATION AND DIFFERENTIAL DIAGNOSIS OF HEMOPTYSIS

---

1. Establish that the substance in question is blood via a guaiac test.
2. Discriminate between hematemesis, epistaxis, and hemoptysis.
   a. Hematemesis is characterized by dark red or brownish blood mixed in mucus having an acidic pH. Food particles frequently are present as well. A Gram stain reveals no organisms.
   b. In epistaxis, relatively pure, bright red blood is evident in the pharynx and nasal cavity during an acute episode. The actual bleeding site usually is evident as an active bleeding point or, if bleeding has stopped, a scabbed-over area on the anterior nasal septum.
   c. Hemoptysis usually presents with a frothy, bright red mucus having an alkaline pH. The blood persists in coughed up material for a somewhat longer time than with either of the above. A Gram stain reveals many organisms.
3. Laboratory evaluation:
   a. White blood count, hematocrit, erythrocyte sedimentation rate.
   b. Examine sputum with Gram and Ziehl-Neelsen stains; culture for bacteria (including tuberculosis) and, if indicated, fungi.
   c. Chest roentgenogram, including anteroposterior and lateral views. Tomograms, sonography, lung scans, and computerized axial tomography offer noninvasive methods for further imaging.
   d. In instances of *recurrent* hemoptysis undefined by the preceding, fiberoptic bronchoscopy and bronchography are indicated. A single episode, however, does not warrant invasive procedures and may be idiopathic.
   e. Sputum cytology is indicated if neoplasm is suspect.
   f. A lung biopsy may be performed if the diagnosis still is obscure but only if prior tests suggest this will be productive, no bleeding disorder is present, and hemoptysis has occurred more than once.
4. Differential diagnosis:
   a. Primary infections. Bronchitis, pneumococcal pneumonia, necrotizing pneumonia (*Klebsiella, Staphylococcus, Pseudomonas*), tuberculosis.
   b. Underlying mechanical pathology with secondary infection; bronchiectasis, cystic fibrosis.
   c. Immunologic disorders. Wegener's granulomatosis, Goodpasture's syndrome, idiopathic pulmonary hemosiderosis, polyarteritis nodosa.
   d. Cardiovascular disorders. Severe mitral stenosis with pulmonary hypertension, pulmonary arteriovenous fistula.
   e. Pulmonary embolism with infarction. Usually secondary to deep leg vein thrombophlebitis.
   f. Neoplasm. Primary, metastatic.
   g. Trauma.
   h. Bleeding diathesis. Clotting factor deficiency, thrombocytopenia, excessive anticoagulation for some other problem.
   i. Idiopathic. Some (usually single, nonrepetitive) episodes of hemoptysis defy diagnosis.

WEGENER'S GRANULOMATOSIS

Wegener's granulomatosis, also known as lethal midline granuloma, is also an immunologically related condition. It is marked by the appearance of destructive granulomatous lesions involving the nose, pharynx, sinuses, and lungs with progressive generalized vasculitis. Renal damage ultimately develops. Diagnosis is by biopsy. Steroids and immunosuppressive agents have been used in treatment but with questionable benefit (also see Chapter 16).

ALPHA-1-ANTITRYPSIN PROTEIN DEFICIENCY

Alpha-1-antitrypsin protein deficiency, a hereditary enzymatic disorder, is first manifested in the neonatal period with hepatitis. Pulmonary emphysema, cirrhosis, or both appear in adolescents or adults as later complications. Diagnosis is indicated by abnormally low serum levels of the alpha-1-antitrypsin protein using immunologic methods. No treatment is currently available.

HYPERTROPHIC OSTEOARTHROPATHY

Clubbing of the fingers, painful periostitis of the long bones, and polyarthritis comprise the basic clinical picture in hypertrophic osteoarthropathy. Bronchiectasis, lung neoplasms, lung abscess, tuberculosis, or pneumonia are also often associated with the condition, as is gynecomastia and ulcerative colitis. The etiology is obscure. Treatment is directed at the infections, or at inflammatory or neoplastic pathology.

Hemoptysis

Hemoptysis can be a particularly distressing symptom of lower respiratory tract disease because of its implications for serious underlying pathology. Some patients present with hemoptysis as the only sign, which makes diagnosis more problematic. Table 6-7 offers a protocol for evaluation.

Bibliography

Adult and teenage cigarette smoking patterns. 1977. *MMWR* 26:160.

Bywater, E. M. 1981. Adolescents with cystic fibrosis: psychosocial adjustment. *Arch. Dis. Child.* 56(7):538–543.

Cassell, G. H., and Cole, B. C. 1981. Mycoplasmas as agents of human disease. *N. Engl. J. Med.* 304:80–89.

DiSant'Agnese, P. A., and Davis, P. B. 1979. Cystic fibrosis in adults. 75 cases and a review of 232 cases in the literature. *Am. J. Med.* 66:121–132.

Eigen, H. The clinical evaluation of chronic cough. 1982. *Pediatr. Clin. North Am.* 29(1):67–78.

An index predicting relapse and need for hospitalization in patients with acute bronchial asthma. *N. Engl. J. Med.* 305(14):783–788.

Glassroth, J.; Robins, A. G.; and Snider, D. E. 1980. Tuberculosis in the 1980's. *N. Engl. J. Med.* 302(26):1441–1450.

Honicky, R. E. 1977. Cystic fibrosis. *Primary Care* 4(4):693–703.

International symposium on Legionnaire's diseases. 1979. *Ann. Intern. Med.* 90:491–707.

Leffert, F. 1980. The management of acute severe asthma. *J. Pediatr.* 96(1):1–12.

Leffert, F. 1980. The management of chronic asthma. *J. Pediatr.* 97(6):875–885.

Lerner, A. M. 1980. The gram-negative bacillary pneumonias. *D.M.* 27(2):1–56.

Marks, M. I. 1981. The pathogenesis and treatment of pulmonary infections in patients with cystic fibrosis. *J. Pediatr.* 98(2):173–179.

McAlister, A. L.; Perry, C.; and Maccoby, N. 1979. Adolescent smoking. *Pediatrics* 63(4):650–658.

Muldoon, R. L.; Jaecker, D. L.; and Kiefer, H. K. 1981. Legionnaire's disease in children. *Pediatrics* 67:329–332.

Pagono, J. S., and Sarubbi, F. A. 1972. Pneumonia. *Am. Family Phys.* 6(6):84–92.

Parsons, G. H., and Lillington. 1978. Hemoptysis. *J. Family Pract.* 7(2):353–359.

Putnam, J. S., and Tellis, C. J. 1978. Hemoptysis. *Primary Care* 5(1):67–80.

Putnam, J. S., and Tuazon, C., editors. 1980. Symposium on infectious lung diseases. *Med. Clin. North Am.* 64(3):317–574.

Raffin, T., and Roberts, P. 1982. The prevention and treatment of status asthmaticus. *Hosp. Pract.* 17(2):80A–80Z.

Rosenow, E. C. 1981. Pulmonary embolism. *Mayo Clin. Proc.* 56:161–178.

Shramp, H. 1975. Coughing in childhood. *J. Family Pract.* 2(1):55–58.

Smoking and cancer. 1982. *MMWR* 31:77–80.

Taussig, L. M. 1981. Chronic bronchitis in childhood: what is it? *Pediatrics* 67(1):1–5.

Weinberger, M.; Hendeles, L.; and Ahrens, R. 1981. Clinical pharmacology of drugs used for asthma. *Pediatr. Clin. North Am.* 28(1):47–76.

Weinberger, M.; Hendeles, L.; and Ahrens, R. 1981. Pharmacologic management of reversible obstructive airways disease. *Medical Clin. North Am.* 65(3):579–613.

–7–
The
Cardiovascular System

Heart Murmurs
Innocent murmurs □ Mitral valve prolapse
Murmurs of congenital heart disease □ Murmurs of acquired heart disease
Arrhythmias
Rheumatic Fever
Major manifestations □ Diagnosis □ Treatment
Subacute Bacterial Endocarditis
Hyperlipidemia
Hypertension
Essential hypertension □ Management
Peripheral Vascular Disease
Thrombophlebitis □ Primary lymphedema □ Raynaud's disease

Heart Murmurs

NORMAL MURMURS

Fifty percent to 85% of healthy individuals have innocent (benign, functional, normal, physiologic) murmurs at some time during their childhood and adolescence. With few exceptions, these murmurs are soft (grade 3/6 or less*), well localized, short, poorly transmitted, and vary with respiration. They are further classifiable into ejection murmurs, venous hums, carotid bruits, and cardiorespiratory murmurs (Table 7-1).

Systolic murmurs that are holosystolic, harsh, transmitted beyond the precordium, or louder than 3/6; any diastolic murmur; and murmurs of any type associated with other signs of heart disease signify an organic origin. Uncertainty as to whether a murmur is benign or organic warrants evaluation by a chest roentgenogram, electrocardiogram (ECG), and other specialized tests as indicated (sonogram, echocardiogram, phonocardiogram).

*Grading scale of murmurs according to intensity: grade 1/6 = difficult to hear, not heard by every examiner; grade 2/6 = soft murmur, heard by most examiners; grade 3/6 = easily heard by all examiners; grade 4/6 = loud murmur with a thrill; grade 5/6 = loud murmur heard with edge of stethoscope just touching chest; grade 6/6 = loud murmur heard with stethoscope off the chest wall.

It is extremely important, however, that the evaluation of a probable functional murmur not create undue anxiety or alarm. Adolescents and their parents commonly overreact in an excessively protective manner if there are *any* intimations of possible heart disease, no matter how remote. The heart is, of course, perceived as the most vital body organ, with compromised function a threat to life. Moreover, adolescents generally do not discriminate between coronary vascular disease and its potential for sudden, unexpected death in adults and the less catastrophic forms of cardiac disease common to their own age group. Silence on the part of the physician is likely to be misinterpreted by the patient as indicating something is very wrong. Thus even somewhat more extended examinations of the heart than is customary require explanation. Following the examination, the nature of the murmur, its probable genesis, and the absence of concern about coronary disease should be carefully reviewed in some detail. It is also important to advise both youth and parents that no curtailment of activity is indicated and normal pursuits should be fully pursued. This message usually needs to be reinforced over several visits, as overriding anxiety may distort matters greatly the first time around.

Two other conditions should be considered in evaluating a possible functional murmur:

TABLE 7-1
CLASSIFICATION OF INNOCENT (FUNCTIONAL) MURMURS

Name	Description	Cause	Differential diagnosis
Vibratory systolic ejection murmur (Still's)	Early to mid 1/6-3/6 systolic, low-pitched murmur often in the third to fifth left intercostal space in a line from the sternal border to the apex. Described as a musical, groaning or twanging "fiddle string." Often heard best with the stethoscope bell. Disappears with a Valsalva maneuver or when patient is upright.	Vibration of the pulmonic valve or of the chordae tendineae in the ventricular cavity.	1. Idiopathic hypertrophic subaortic stenosis. 2. Aortic stenosis. 3. Pulmonary valve stenosis. 4. Mitral insufficiency.
Pulmonary ejection murmur	Early to mid 1/6-3/6 systolic, crescendo-decrescendo murmur in the second or, occasionally, third left intercostal space. Heard only in the supine position. Also, a normal widening of the pulmonic valve sound with inspiration and narrowing with expiration is present.	Turbulent flow through a normal pulmonary valve. Seen with any condition increasing pulmonary flow: anemia, anxiety, exercise, or fever. Straight-back syndrome brings this murmur out.	1. Pulmonary valve stenosis. 2. Secundum atrial septal defect. 3. High, small ventricular septal defect. 4. Idiopathic pulmonary artery dilatation. 5. Coarctation of the aorta.
Jugular venous hum (bruit de diable)	Continuous (systolic and diastolic), 1/6-3/6, medium-pitched, humming murmur best heard at the heart base and over jugular veins. Disappears with digital pressure over the jugular vein, when the patient turns his/her head to the same side or when lying down. This is the only innocent *diastolic* murmur. A continuous venous thrill above the right clavicle can be felt 1/3 of the time in the sitting position.	Rapid return of cerebral venous blood through the jugular vein and vena cava into the right atrium.	1. Patent ductus arteriosus. 2. Arteriovenous fistula.
Carotid bruit	Early to mid 1/6-2/6 systolic ejection murmur loudest over the carotid arteries in the neck and heard only faintly (or not at all) over the aortic area.	Due to turbulence of blood flow through normally tortuous carotid arteries.	1. Aortic stenosis.
Cardiorespiratory murmur	Mid to late 1/6-3/6 systolic murmur heard over any part of the precordium or at the heart margins. Can be a short, high-pitched screeching murmur, which is loudest in inspiration, occurs in synchrony with the heart beat, and sometimes is called a "systolic whoop." Murmur disappears with cessation of respiration. Often varies in its timing.	Originates at the interface between the heart and the lungs. Sometimes indicates the presence of pulmonary consolidation, atelectasis, or pleural or pericardial adhesions.	1. Late systolic murmur syndrome of mitral regurgitation. 2. Pleuropericardial rub.

1. The straight-back syndrome: In this condition, there is a loss of normal thoracic curvature and a marked decrease in the anteroposterior diameter of the chest. This causes normal heart sounds to seem unusually loud.

2. The systolic click-late systolic murmur syndrome: This situation is evidenced by a late apical murmur preceded by a systolic click. The P waves are inverted in the left precordial leads of an ECG. Usually this is a benign finding, but it may signify

pathology, in some cases associated with rheumatic heart disease or Marfan's syndrome and a prolapsed mitral valve. It also has been noted to be a sex-linked inherited trait in females.

MITRAL VALVE PROLAPSE

Mitral valve prolapse is now recognized as one of the more common cardiac abnormalities. It has particular relevance for adolescents and young adults, as symptoms, if they are going to occur, tend to first appear during these years. It affects females more often than males and seems to have a genetic association. Some 6% of individuals with Marfan's syndrome develop mitral valve prolapse.

The basic pathology consists of myxomatous degenerative changes in the mitral valve and lengthening of the chordae tendineae, which leads to ballooning, prolapse, and various paroxysmal arrhythmias. In asymptomatic individuals the only indication of this lesion may be the signs described for the systolic click-late systolic murmur syndrome. Variations in the timing of the click or intensity of the murmur in response to maneuvers that alter left ventricular volume or pressure are characteristic of prolapse and are unlikely to occur with idiopathic forms. Symptoms, when present, include episodes of anginalike pain and palpitations due to tachyarrhythmias. Bradycardia also may occur. These may or may not be exacerbated with exercise.

Diagnosis is by echocardiography demonstrating abnormal valve leaflet movement. A random ECG may demonstrate an abnormal rhythm, but a Holter monitor for 24 hours or longer may be necessary for detection. An exercise stress test can be useful in planning treatment, which is indicated only if arrhythmias are present, and the patient is symptomatic. Propranolol is the drug of choice in the minimum effective dose; this may vary from 30–400 mg per day in three to four divided doses. Phenytoin and quinidine also may be helpful. Antibiotic prophylaxis against bacterial endocarditis is indicated for invasive procedures, including dental extraction. Valve replacement may be necessary in the rare instance of severe insufficiency. Exercise and sports need not be restricted unless resulting in arrhythmia, nor is pregnancy contraindicated.

MURMURS OF CONGENITAL HEART DISEASE

Murmurs of congenital heart disease are reviewed in Table 7-2. Although most are diagnosed in childhood, coarctation of the aorta and, less commonly, aortic stenosis may be missed and only discovered during adolescence or young adulthood.

Management generally is best supervised by a cardiologist. The degree of limitation experienced depends on the extent of the lesion, the presence or absence of pulmonary hypertension, and the degree of cardiac decompensation, if any. How much activity needs to be limited is highly individual and is based on tolerance, except in aortic stenosis. Individuals with this lesion usually are asymptomatic, although the degree of stenosis usually increases with age and strenuous athletics such as football, wrestling, or basketball may produce myocardial ischemia and anginal pain. These activities are usually best proscribed. The degree of ischemic potential may be illuminated by an ECG taken during an exercise stress test and the demonstration of ischemic ST and T wave changes. In general it is important not to restrict an adolescent's activity any more than is absolutely required. One can create far more problems of a psychologic nature by limiting a teenager's involvement in sports because of heart disease than by working matters out on an individual tolerance basis.

MURMURS OF ACQUIRED HEART DISEASE

Mitral valve damage is the most frequent cause of an acquired organic murmur and most often is due to rheumatic fever; sometimes it may be encountered in Marfan's syndrome as well (see discussion of mitral valve prolapse). Regurgitation is the more common manifestation in adolescence, although stenosis ultimately occurs in half of all affected individuals and may appear late in the second decade. Classic mitral regurgitation is characterized by a soft S_1, a loud blowing holosystolic murmur at the apex with transmission to the left axilla, a wide, split S_2, an S_3 gallop, and a short diastolic rumble. Stenosis presents with a loud, delayed, snapping S_1, a mitral opening snap that follows S_2, and a low-pitched diastolic rumble localized in the mitral area; the murmur is loudest in early diastole and best heard in the lateral decubitus position.

Aortic or tricuspid damage is a possible consequence of rheumatic fever and may be encountered in adolescence, but the rarity of this occurrence warrants omission of further discussion here.

Arrhythmias

With the exception of ventricular ectopic beats, cardiac arrhythmias are relatively uncommon in adolescence. On occasion, however, they may be implicated as the cause of dizziness, "blackout" spells, or faints, all of which are common complaints in the adolescent. Although such symptoms usually

TABLE 7-2
COMMON CONGENITAL HEART DISEASES

Name	Clinical features	Complications
Ventricular septal defect	Loud, harsh pansystolic murmur best heard in the lower left sternal border with wide transmission. A systolic thrill may be felt. A loud murmur with a small defect is called the bruit de Roger. Large defect may be associated with a loud single S_2 over the pulmonary area (indicating pulmonary hypertension) and also a short, low-pitched diastolic murmur over the mitral area. Bilateral atrial and ventricular enlargement can be noted in the chest roentgenogram and ECG.	1. Congestive heart failure (CHF) 2. Subacute bacterial endocarditis (SBE) 3. Pulmonary hypertension
Atrial septal defect	Soft pulmonary ejection murmur with a systolic pulmonary thrill and a widely split S_2. Often associated with a low-pitched, early diastolic murmur (rumble) over the xyphoid or midleft sternal border (due to increased tricuspid valve flow). Increased pulmonary vascular markings and right ventricular hypertrophy noted on chest roentgenogram and/or ECG.	Uncommon (CHF, SBE, pulmonary hypertension possible)
Aortic stenosis (valvular)	Loud, harsh, crescendo-decrescendo murmur over the aortic area, with wide transmission to the neck vessels and precordium. Can also note an early systolic ejection click and a thrill in the aortic area. The blowing diastolic murmur and diastolic thrill of aortic insufficiency may be noted in severe cases. Left ventricular hypertrophy seen on chest roentgenogram and ECG.	Sudden death, SBE, CHF (left ventricular), arrhythmias
Patent ductus arteriosus	Loud, continuous (systolic-diastolic), crescendo-decrescendo murmur best heard over the pulmonary area, and often with a systolic thrill at the site of maximum intensity. This "machinery" murmur reaches its peak intensity in late systole, wanes in mid to late diastole, and does not vary with position change. Wide pulse pressure and a loud S_2 are noted. Chest roentgenogram may show calcium deposits in the dilated ductus. ECG is variable.	SBE, pulmonary hypertension, CHF
Coarctation of the aorta	Loud systolic murmur over the interscapular area and left supraclavicular area in association with delayed leg pulses and hypertension in the arm(s). Widespread, soft systolic bruits are present, reflecting collateral circulation. Chest roentgenogram reveals posterior rib notching and dilated aorta.	SBE (on associated bicuspid aortic valves), hypertension, and dissecting aneurysm or rupture (including involvement of associated circle of Willis aneurysm).
Pulmonary stenosis (valvular)	Loud, harsh, ejection murmur with diminished S_2 over the pulmonic area, systolic ejection click, and thrill. Chest roentgenogram and ECG demonstrate right ventricular hypertrophy.	SBE, CHF

are functional, it is appropriate at least to think of an arrhythmia in the differential diagnosis. Increasing attention is being given to paroxysmal types, recognizing that they occur more frequently (albeit still relatively rarely) than formerly thought, particularly in relation to mitral valve prolapse (see previous discussion). Table 7-3 reviews the diagnostic features of all but ectopic foci, which are discussed in the following section. Evaluation of a suspected arrhythmia warrants more than a single ECG if the first is unrevealing. Continuous recording over a period of time with a Holter monitor can be helpful. In general Propranolol (Inderal) is very effective for paroxysmal atrial tachycardia, whereas phenytoin (Dilantin)

TABLE 7-3
CLASSIFICATION OF CARDIAC ARRHYTHMIAS

Name	Definition	Description	Treatment
Sinus bradycardia	Regular heart rate under 60 per minute	A normal finding in athletes, consequent to training and improved cardiac output. Pathologically, can be due to certain drugs (digitalis, propranolol, morphine, reserpine or prostigmine) or is idiopathic. An AV nodal block may be thought to be sinus bradycardia initially. Heart rate increases with exercise or in response to atropine. Failure of response may indicate the sick sinus syndrome. Symptoms in non-athletes (due to slow heart rate) include dizziness, syncope, angina pectoris, and congestive heart failure. Treatment is necessary if these develop.	1. Often not necessary 2. Atropine 3. Pacemaker 4. Isuprel (isoproterenol) is used for nodal bradycardia with hypotension.
Sinus tachycardia	Regular heart rate over 100 per minute	Usually transient, secondary to exercise, fright, emotional upset, or fever. Precipitating causes also include hypotension, congestive heart failure, and thyrotoxicosis.	1. Usually transient 2. Treat underlying cause 3. Carotid sinus massage 4. Digitalis
Sinus arrhythmia	Irregular sinus rate, which varies with respiration (increases at the end of inspiration and decreases at the end of expiration)	This is a normal phenomenon related to vagal tone changes.	Not necessary
Paroxysmal supraventricular tachycardia	Rapid heart rate (150–250/min) due to SA node stimulation or AU node stimulation, PAT (paroxysmal nodal tachycardia)	Usually transient, secondary to the same stimulants as for sinus tachycardia. Some patients are prone to repeated attacks, which must be treated to convert to a normal rhythm (under 100 beats per minute). Dyspnea, palpitations, diaphoresis, light-headedness, and syncope can be noted. More serious arrhythmias, cerebral ischemia, or heart failure are also possible. May be due to digitalis toxicity or associated with the Wolff-Parkinson-White syndrome.	1. Measures to increase vagal tone: carotid sinus massage, Valsalva maneuver, or eyeball pressure for 15 sec 2. Quinidine sulfate 3. Digitalis 4. Propranolol 5. Procainamide hydrochloride 6. Verapamil 7. Endophonium
Atrial flutter	Rapid irregular heart rate (250–350/min) due to ectopic atrial pacemaker	Often see a saw-tooth pattern on ECG. A serious arrhythmia requiring immediate treatment. Often progresses into serious ventricular arrhythmias.	1. Digitalis 2. Quinidine sulfate 3. Electrical cardioversion
Atrial fibrillation	Rapid irregular heart rate (over 400/min) due to multiple ectopic atrial pacemakers	Chaotic atrial pattern on ECG. Immediate treatment needed.	1. Digitalis 2. Electrical cardioversion 3. Propranolol

Continued

TABLE 7-3
CLASSIFICATION OF CARDIAC ARRHYTHMIAS (CONTINUED)

Name	Definition	Description	Treatment
Ventricular flutter	Rapid irregular heart rate (200–300/min) due to ectopic ventricular pacemaker	Characteristic "sine-wave" pattern on ECG. Requires immediate treatment.	1. Lidocaine 2. Procainamide hydrochloride 3. Propranolol 4. Quinidine sulfate 5. Electrical cardioversion
Ventricular fibrillation	Rapid irregular heart rate due to multiple ectopic ventricular pacemakers	"Bag of worms" appearance on ECG. Cardiac arrest imminent.	1. Electrical cardioversion 2. Treat cardiac arrest: Advanced cardiac life support *and* a. 500 mg calcium chloride IV b. 0.5–1.0 mg 1:10,000 epinephrine solution IV c. 0.5–1 mEq/kg sodium bicarbonate (8.4% solution) IV q 10–15 min. d. Vasopressors e. Lidocaine hydrochloride f. Procainamide (Pronestyl) g. Bretylium
Atrioventricular blocks		Heart rate is regularly slowed in 2nd degree and irregularly slow in 3rd degree. Digitalis or propranolol aggravate and exercise-induced tachycardia improve 1st degree block. The *Wenckebach phenomenon* is when the PR interval in a 2nd-degree block progressively lengthens with each beat until a ventricular response is dropped. The *Stokes-Adams syndrome* occurs in 3rd-degree blocks, when flow to the brain is so diminished (40–45 beats/min or less) as to produce episodes of dizziness and syncope.	1. Isoproterenol 2. Pacemaker
First degree	Prolonged PR interval on ECG of over 0.2 seconds		
Second degree	Two or more atrial impulses required to produce one ventricular response		
Third degree	Total block; ventricles act independent of atria		
Wolff-Parkinson-White syndrome	Due to an accessory conduction bundle (Kent's) found in up to 3–4% of "normal" ECG tracings. Results in a short PR interval less than 0.12 sec and a prolonged QRS segment.	Generally asymptomatic but may lead to recurrent episodes of supraventricular tachycardia.	1. Prophylactic treatment with quinidine and digitalis or propranolol 2. Surgical interruption of accessory bundle of Kent

Continued

TABLE 7-3
CLASSIFICATION OF CARDIAC ARRHYTHMIAS (CONTINUED)

Name	Definition	Description	Treatment
Prolonged QT syndrome	Found on routine ECG	Usually an incidental finding. Warrants evaluation as may be associated with sudden death syndromes, mitral valve disease, hypokalemia, administration of quinidine or phenothiazines, the Ward-Romano syndrome, and the Jervell and Lange-Nielsen syndrome.	1. Evaluate for associated cardiac disease
Sick sinus syndrome	Inappropriate bradycardia due to decreased sinus node automation or impaired sinus node conduction	May manifest in sinus arrest or sinoatrial exit block. Does not revert to normal rate with exercise or atropine.	1. None necessary in mild cases 2. Pacemaker in symptomatic patients

should be considered for digitalis-induced arrhythmias. The clinician should be aware of newer antiarrhythmic drugs that are now being introduced, such as Verapamil (for P.A.T.) and Bretylium (for ventricular fibrillation).

The premature firing of an ectopic focus prompts a contraction that appears earlier than usual in the cardiac cycle (premature ectopic beat). The following beat often is delayed and tends to be more forceful than normal. This sequence is experienced by the patient as a "skipped beat" or "palpitation." Foci may be atrial, in the AV node or ventricular, with the latter the most common site.

Premature ventricular contractions (PVCs) occur in 2% of healthy individuals and are not indicative of disease per se. Precipitating factors include stress, tobacco, caffeine, alcohol, anoxia, sympathomimetic drugs, and digitalis toxicity. Occasional PVCs are benign and require no intervention. Concern is warranted in the following circumstances:

1. More than 6 PVCs occur per minute.
2. Multifocal PVCs are noted on the ECG.
3. There are runs of four or more PVCs in succession, comprising ventricular tachycardia.
4. The PVCs do not disappear on exercise to a point sufficient to raise the heart rate to 140 per minute or more.
5. If the PVC falls on a T wave.

Treatment under any of the preceding circumstances consists of avoiding associated precipitants and using such medications as lidocaine (Xylocaine), quinidine, or procainamide (Pronestyl).

Rheumatic Fever

Rheumatic fever develops one to several weeks after an untreated (or incompletely treated) episode of group A beta-hemolytic streptococcal pharyngitis and represents an antigen-antibody hypersensitivity response rather than a direct infectious process. The most significant symptoms and signs are listed in Table 7-4. Less specific symptoms that also may be seen include nausea, vomiting, abdominal pain, epistaxis, pneumonia, and weight loss.

Children and adolescents ages 6–19 years of age are at greatest risk, with a peak incidence between 6 and 9 years. Any patient who has had a previous attack is at even greater risk of recurrence if challenged again by a streptococcal pharyngitis. The frequency of rheumatic fever is considerably less today than it was 30–40 years ago due to the advent of antibiotics and the effective treatment of streptococcal disease. In many communities it is a rarity. Nevertheless, inadequate treatment of streptococcal pharyngitis continues to occur through failure of patient, parent, or physician to take appropriate steps. Subsequently, rheumatic fever remains the leading cause of acquired heart disease in adolescents. Active disease is most prevalent in certain pockets in the southeast and among inner city and other poverty groups, among whom health care tends to be episodic and crisis oriented.

MAJOR MANIFESTATIONS
Carditis. Fifty percent of patients with acute rheumatic fever develop some degree of carditis, although the predilection for carditis is greater in younger patients, and it is less commonly seen in adolescents with a first attack. Two or more attacks, however, bear an increasing likelihood of cardiac involvement. The severity is highly variable and may be manifested by ECG changes only (prolonged ST segment, P wave

changes) or by pericarditis, myocarditis, endocarditis, and failure. Clinical signs vary from none to changing heart murmurs, poor heart sounds, gallop rhythms, AV blocks, cardiomegaly, pericardial friction rubs, and/or pericardial effusion. The nature and extent of permanent damage depends on the severity of the initial attack and the number of subsequent attacks. The mitral valve is most likely to be damaged with an initial insufficiency later followed by stenosis. Aortic regurgitation is next in order of frequency. Bacterial endocarditis is a major complication of valvular injury.

Arthritis. Seventy-five percent of patients with acute rheumatic fever develop arthritis. Usually one or several large joints (knees, ankles, wrists, elbows) become swollen, tender, and hot in a migratory manner, although almost any joint can be involved. Symptoms may last several days to several weeks and clear without sequelae. Aspirin administration rapidly improves the symptoms. In the adolescent population, it is important to discriminate rheumatic fever arthritis from septic arthritis due to *Neisseria gonorrhoeae*. These two conditions may mimic each other, and the consequences of missing gonococcal arthritis can be a destroyed joint. In the absence of definitive clinical findings distinguishing one from the other, an arthrocentesis with a cell count, Gram stain, and culture can be revealing. Additional differential considerations include other causes of septic arthritis, osteomyelitis, rheumatoid arthritis, serum sickness, sickle cell crisis, Henoch-Schönlein purpura, rubella arthritis, and others.

Chorea. Chorea (Sydenham's chorea, St. Vitus dance) is a relatively uncommon manifestation, occurring weeks or months after streptococcal pharyngitis. It is characterized by continuous purposeless choreiform movements, poor neuromuscular coordination, and emotional lability. It may coexist with mild carditis but more often is the only manifestation. The differential diagnosis includes simple restlessness, habit tics, athetosis, benign familial chorea, Wilson's disease, Huntington's chorea, and Gilles de la Tourette syndrome. Symptoms may last several weeks or months and can be exceptionally handicapping. Sedation and padding to protect from injury may be required. Chorea ultimately clears spontaneously and is without sequelae.

Subcutaneous nodules. Subcutaneous nodules are firm and nontender, 0.1–1 cm in diameter, and situated on the extensor surfaces of joints (elbows,

---

TABLE 7-4
MANIFESTATIONS OF RHEUMATIC FEVER

MAJOR MANIFESTATIONS
1. Carditis
2. Arthritis
3. Chorea
4. Subcutaneous nodules
5. Erythema marginatum

MINOR MANIFESTATIONS
1. Clinical
   a. Previous rheumatic fever or rheumatic heart disease
   b. Arthralgias
   c. Fever
2. Laboratory tests
   a. Leukocytosis
   b. Elevated erythrocyte sedimentation rate
   c. Elevated C-reactive protein
   d. Prolonged PR interval on ECG

SUPPORTING EVIDENCE OF STREPTOCOCCAL INFECTION
1. Positive throat culture for group A beta-hemolytic streptococcus
2. History of recent scarlet fever (streptococcal pharyngitis with a strawberry-red tongue, circumoral pallor, and diffuse, erythematous punctiform rash over the trunk and inner arms followed by desquamation in 1–2 weeks)
3. Increased titer to streptococcal antibodies
   a. Antistreptolysin 0 (over 250–500 Todd units)
   b. Antistreptokinase
   c. Antihyaluronidase
   d. Anti-DNAase B (antidesoxyribonuclease B)
   e. Anti-DPNase (anti-diphosphopyridine nucleotidase)

---

wrists, knees), scalp (occiput), scapulae and/or spinous processes of the thoracic and lumbar vertebrae. They are freely movable, and the overlying skin is unaffected. Although most commonly seen in rheumatic fever, nodules also can occur in systemic lupus erythematosus, scleroderma, polyarteritis nodosa, and Henoch-Schönlein purpura. Differential considerations include granuloma annulare, sarcoidosis, subcutaneous fat necrosis, infectious nodules of mycobacterium or fungi, erythema nodosum, and neoplastic nodules. The primary significance of rheumatic nodules is in aiding the diagnosis. They themselves are inconsequential and resolve spontaneously over time.

Erythema marginatum. Seen only in 10% of patients with rheumatic fever, erythema marginatum is a rash consisting of migrating, fleeting, faint, reddish mac-

TABLE 7-5
TREATMENT SCHEDULES FOR RHEUMATIC FEVER AND ITS MANIFESTATIONS

Manifestation	Therapy	Comments
Acute phase: any symptoms or signs	1.2 million units benzathine penicillin IM once; or 250 mg (400,000 U) oral penicillin q.i.d. × 10 days; or 250 mg erythromycin q.i.d. × 10 days	Goal is to eradicate all streptococcal organisms whether pharyngitis present or not. Sulfonamides or tetracycline not recommended as not always effective.
Prophylaxis: following any manifestation(s)	1.2 million units benzathine penicillin IM once a month; or 125 mg (200,000 U) oral penicillin daily; or 1 g sulfadiazine p.o. daily	Initiate after 10-day acute treatment phase. Continue indefinitely if heart disease present or at least 10 years if no heart disease. Goal is to prevent streptococcal infection and possibility of a recurrent attack.
Carditis, mild	Bed rest Salicylates (60 mg/lb/day in divided doses up to 10 g/day maximum); to avoid gastric symptoms, give with meals or with sodium bicarbonate or use buffered form	Optimum salicylate level is 25–30 mg/100 ml; follow blood levels taken 2–3 hours after a meal, increasing aspirin intake every 3–5 days until desired level obtained. Nausea, emesis, tinnitus, hyperpnea, or decreased auditory acuity suggest aspirin toxicity. Prednisone use in mild carditis is controversial and usually not recommended.
Carditis, severe (pericardial effusion or congestive heart failure)	Bed rest Salicylates as above Prednisone, either high or low dose: a. Low dose: 2 mg/kg/day × 4-6 weeks b. High dose: 2.5–4 mg/kg/day × 7 days	There is no evidence that prednisone improves residual damage.
Residual rheumatic heart disease	Activity limitations according to the American Heart Association classification and recommendations Prophylaxis	An adolescent should not be limited in activity any more than absolutely necessary. Guard against overprotectiveness. Keep possibility of complicating subacute bacterial endocarditis in mind.
Arthritis	Salicylates as for mild carditis Bed rest of possible but not proven value	Primary benefit of salicylates in acute rheumatic fever probably is in relation to arthritis and fever.
Chorea	Phenobarbital, diazepam and haloperidol have been used.	No proof that any medication is effective. Bed rest is of value to prevent patients from harming themselves.
Subcutaneous nodules	None	Do not confuse with nodules due to other causes; see text.
Erythema marginatum	None	Rarely seen in other disorders.

ules with pale centers and annular or serpiginous borders located on the trunk and/or the proximal portions of the extremities. The rash is nonpruritic, nonindurated, may blanch on pressure, and is brought out by heat. Differential considerations include urticaria, erythema multiforme, and erythema nodosum.

DIAGNOSIS

The diagnosis of rheumatic fever is based on the Jones criteria. The patient must at least demonstrate two major manifestations or one major and two minor manifestations as listed in Table 7-4. These criteria should be strictly applied and overdiagnosis avoided. Committing a patient to needless antibiotic

TABLE 7-6
ANTIBIOTIC SCHEDULES FOR THE TREATMENT OF SUBACUTE BACTERIAL ENDOCARDITIS

Organism	Antibiotic	Duration of treatment
Streptococcus viridans	Penicillin G; 200,000–300,000 U/kg/day IV in 4–6 divided doses up to a maximum of 16–20 million U/day. Streptomycin 30 mg/kg/day IM in 2 doses may be added optionally.	Penicillin: 4–6 weeks Streptomycin: 2 weeks
Staphylococcus aureus	Penicillin G as above if organism sensitive; otherwise use nafcillin or oxacillin 150–200 mg/kg/day IV in 4 divided doses. If methicillin-resistant use vancomycin 50 mg/kg/day IV in 4 divided doses. Cephalosporins may be used, as: cephalothin, cefazolin, cephalexin, cephradine or others.	6–8 weeks; all drugs
Hemophilus influenzae	Ampicillin 150 mg/kg/day IV in 4 divided doses; or chloramphenicol 100 mg/kg/day IV in 4 divided doses. (Note: recent ampicillin-resistant strains have been identified; sensitivities are particularly important)	6–8 weeks (note: observe closely for early signs of chloramphenicol toxicity and bone marrow suppression)
Pseudomonas aeruginosa	Carbenicillin 400–600 mg/kg/day IV in 4 divided doses with or without Gentamicin 4–6 mg/kg/day IV in 2–3 divided doses	6 weeks or more
Unknown organism	Penicillin G + oxacillin + Gentamicin IV in doses as given above	6–8 weeks

prophylaxis and inflicting the psychologic consequences of believing onself to have a condition that potentially leads to heart disease are a high price to pay for casual diagnosis.

Eighty percent of patients with rheumatic fever have evidence of recent streptococcal infection in a positive antistreptolysin 0 titer; an additional 15% have a positive anti-DNAase B test, particularly in chorea. There are other streptococcal antibodies as well.

Differential considerations relating to specific manifestations have already been listed. Other considerations include systemic lupus erythematosus, subacute bacterial endocarditis, and sickle cell disease.

TREATMENT
Therapy for the various phases and manifestations of rheumatic fever is outlined in Table 7-5. Prophylaxis is particularly significant during the first 1–2 years after the first attack, when recurrences are most frequent. It is recommended that monthly intramuscular benzathine penicillin G (Bicillin) be given during this time rather than oral penicillin (with the possibility of inconsistent compliance), as it affords a better guarantee of effective blood antibiotic levels at all times. Thereafter oral medication can be used, but it is wise to work out a convenient schedule with the adolescent to minimize forgetfulness.

Subacute Bacterial Endocarditis
Subacute bacterial endocarditis (SBE) is characterized by bacterial vegetations located in the chambers of the heart, usually on a damaged valve, or on a prosthetic valve or rim of a septal defect. Indeed, it is uncommon for this condition to occur in the absence of a cardiac defect and associated aberrant blood flow. An exception to this rule is in intravenous injection of contaminated heroin or other abused substances. In this instance, vegetations tend to be right sided and on the tricuspid valve in contrast to the left-sided mitral involvement most commonly seen with cardiac defects.

The onset of SBE often is subtle. Signs and symptoms include fever, petechiae, splinter hemorrhages in nail beds, heart murmurs (either those of the original abnormality or changing murmurs), splenomegaly, and Osler's nodes (tender subcutaneous embolic lesions in fingers and toes). Advanced cases may demonstrate clubbing, joint swelling, or heart failure. Septic emboli may cause pulmonary, cerebral or renal abscesses, mycotic aneurysms, microinfarcts, and other evidence of embolic phenomena and disseminated infection.

Endocarditis should be suspected in adolescents having any of the above in association with a congenital lesion, rheumatic heart disease and inconsistent antibiotic prophylaxis, or intravenous drug abuse. Diagnosis is based on a positive blood culture. Multiple specimens should be taken to ensure recovery of the offending organism, particularly at times of fever spikes. *Streptococcus viridans* is implicated in 50%–80% of the cases, but *Staphylococcus piedermis (albus)*, Group D streptococci (enterococci), and many other bacteria (including *Neisseria gonorrhoeae* and *Chlamydia trachomatis*) may be involved on occasion. Other significant laboratory data include leukocytosis, an elevated erythrocyte sedimentation rate, and microscopic hematuria.

Differential considerations are legion and include acute rheumatic fever, systemic lupus erythematosus, sickle cell disease, drug reactions, periarteritis nodosa, and many others.

Treatment is outlined in Table 7-6. Even with treatment, the mortality rate can be as high as 25%. Prevention, therefore, is an important aspect of management. Any patient at risk of SBE and undergoing a dental procedure (extraction, gingival resection), surgery of the respiratory tract (v. tonsillectomy), or a more major operation, should receive antibiotic prophylaxis (Table 7-7). Patients at risk include those with valvular heart disease, congenital heart disease, prosthetic heart valves, a previous history of endocarditis, idiopathic hypertrophic aortic stenosis, or mitral valve prolapse syndrome with mitral insufficiency, and those who have undergone repair of a patent ductus arteriosus or atrial septal defect within the previous 6 months.

Hyperlipidemia

Genetically determined, primary hyperlipidemia comprises a major risk factor for the early development of coronary artery disease. Detection and intervention in adolescence can be an important preventive step. Although controversy surrounds the definition of abnormally high lipids, it is generally agreed that fasting serum cholesterol levels over 200–230 mg and serum triglycerides over 110–140 mg/ml are above the normal adolescent range.

Secondary hyperlipidemia may be seen with

TABLE 7-7
ANTIBIOTIC PROPHYLAXIS
FOR PATIENTS AT RISK OF SBE
AND UNDERGOING DENTAL PROCEDURES
OR UPPER RESPIRATORY TRACT SURGERY*

Agent and dose given 30–60 min before procedure	Agent and dose given q.i.d. × 2 days following procedure
Aqueous penicillin G, 1 million U + procaine penicillin G, 600,000 U IM	Penicillin V, 500 mg p.o.
OR	
Penicillin V, 2 g p.o.	Penicillin V, 500 mg p.o.
OR	
Aqueous penicillin G, 1 million U + procaine penicillin G, 600,000 U + streptomycin, 1 g IM	Penicillin V, 500 mg p.o.
OR (if allergic to penicillin)	
Erythromycin, 1 g p.o.	Erythromycin, 500 mg p.o.
OR (if allergic to penicillin)	
Vancomycin, 1 g IV	Erythromycin, 500 mg p.o.

*Note: For antibiotic prophylaxis schedules in more major procedures see Kaplan, E. L., et al. 1977. *Circulation* 56:139A–143A.

such diseases as diabetes mellitus, hypothyroidism, the nephrotic syndrome, chronic renal disease, and obstructive liver disease or with the administration of such drugs as oral contraceptives, glucocorticoids, and alcohol. Management is directed at the underlying cause with only minimal, if any, attention required by the elevated lipids.

The five classic types of primary hyperlipidemia are outlined in Table 7-8. Types IIA, IIB, and IV account for 95% of all adult cases. Types IV and V are characterized by delayed penetrance and are not usually manifested until the third decade; occasionally they may be detected in late adolescence. Types IIA and IIB are evident in childhood and therefore are present in the adolescent as well. Type IV is chemically detectable by midpuberty (Tanner stage III), and clinical features develop in adulthood.

The diagnosis should be considered in any adolescent or young adult who has a close (first-degree) relative under age 50–55 with coronary artery disease (heart attack, angina, died of cardiovascular disease) or when hyperlipidemia is a known family trait. If fasting serum cholesterol, triglyceride levels, or both are elevated, underlying diseases as noted should be ruled out. Further analysis for lipoproteins should be carried out to ascertain the precise type.

Symptoms and signs of the hyperlipidemias vary and depend on type and duration. Most adolescents have no clinical evidence and appear normal in all respects. Those with relatively long-standing lipid elevations may evidence xanthomas (eruptive in type I, tendinous in type IIA and IIB, palmar in type III). Types IV and V are not usually seen during the teenage years, and xanthomas are not evident until adulthood. Corneal arcus is another common sign. There also is a significant association with diabetes mellitus, myxedema, pancreatitis, porphyria, and jaundice. Aortic stenosis is sometimes seen in young people with type IIA or IIB disease. Lipidemia retinalis is a reported finding in types I and V.

Specific treatment measures are outlined in Table 7-8. General measures include controlling blood pressure, maintaining ideal body weight, discouraging cigarette smoking, and encouraging regular physical exercise. Even with these measures, it may not be possible to achieve "normal" lipid levels. Indefinite monitoring of diet and drug regimens should be carried out at 3–12 month intervals, with the shorter time preferred until the young person is able to comply reasonably well. Management should be with the patient directly, although the parents' help will be needed to see that appropriate foods are available. Significant problems will be encountered if the adolescent feels he or she is selectively different than peers or other family members, particularly when he or she feels well and is not yet cognitively mature enough to contend with possibilities of disease in the far future. The physician also needs to empathize with the plight of the hyperlipidemic adolescent at a time in life when it can be difficult to follow a special diet. Tolerance of regimen lapses is necessary. It may be a number of years—probably not until young adulthood—before sustained compliance can be achieved.

Hypertension

Although some debate exists over just when blood pressure is elevated, systolic pressures over 140 mm Hg and diastolic pressures over 90 mm Hg are at or above the ninetieth percentile for adolescents and generally considered to be in the hypertensive range (see Chapter 3 and Appendix I). Estimates of the prevalence of hypertension in adolescents range from 1%–11.5%; 90% or more of these cases are "essential" or "idiopathic." Many instances of borderline

or mildly elevated pressures are of the labile variety and probably do not have clinical significance. Adolescents with labile hypertension experience a rise in pressure under stressful circumstances, such as a physical examination. Several repeated measurements during and at the end of the examination or, if necessary, three to four measurements at weekly intervals generally accustom the patient to the procedure sufficiently to alleviate anxiety and reveal normal values.

ESSENTIAL HYPERTENSION

Essential hypertension usually is asymptomatic during the adolescent years and is only detectable by routine blood pressure screening. Those with hypertension consequent to specific disease states (Table 7-9) more commonly are symptomatic, presenting with headaches, dizziness, or blurred vision as the pressure increases. With levels above 100 mm Hg diastolic, the patient may develop seizures, focal neurologic signs, retinal changes (narrow arterioles, hemorrhages, exudates), reduced renal function, left ventricular hypertrophy, pulmonary edema, cardiac failure, and/or cerebral vascular accidents. Evaluation of persistently (nonlabile) elevated blood pressure is outlined in Table 7-10.

MANAGEMENT

Management of hypertension depends, first, on the underlying cause and, second, on the degree of elevation. General measures include the following:

1. Identifying and treating any associated disease state (Table 7-10).

2. Promoting weight reduction, if indicated, and maintaining ideal body weight.

3. Avoiding compounds that exacerbate hypertension (for example sympathomimetics, oral contraceptives, steroids, amphetamines).

4. Encouraging relaxation or biofeedback techniques (see Benson, H. 1977. *N. Engl. J. Med.* 296: 1152).

5. Limiting free salt (no salt shaker) for levels under 140/100; reducing salt intake to 2–5 g per day for higher levels.

6. Instituting antihypertensive medication (Table 7-11) beginning with one of the diuretics (for example, hydrochlorothiazide) for levels over 140/ 100 and increasing to maximum dose before adding other drugs. A variety of alternative regimens have been recommended. One option is as follows:

a. Thiazide diuretic to maximum dose (use furosemide if creatinine clearance is reduced).

b. If ineffective, gradually add methyldopa to maximum dose.

TABLE 7-8
PRIMARY HYPERLIPIDEMIA: DIAGNOSIS AND MANAGEMENT

Type	Lipid elevations	Lipoprotein elevations	Dietary management
I	Triglyceride ↑↑ Cholesterol ↑ or →	Chylomicra (extremely low density) ↑↑↑	Decrease dietary fat to 30 g/day. Abstain from alcohol.
IIA	Cholesterol ↑	Beta lipoprotein (low density) ↑↑	Limit cholesterol to 300 mg/day. Decrease saturated fats to under 40% of total fat intake. Maintain on a 2:1 polyunsaturated to saturated fat ratio.
IIB	Triglyceride ↑ Cholesterol ↑	Beta lipoprotein ↑ Pre-beta lipoprotein (very low density) ↑	As for IIA, plus reduction of sugar and alcohol intake.
III	Triglyceride ↑ Cholesterol ↑	Beta lipoprotein variant; ("broad B")	As for type IIB.
IV	Triglyceride ↑	Pre-beta lipoprotein ↑↑	Reduce carbohydrates to 40% total caloric intake. Reduce sugar and alcohol. Control diabetes mellitus when present.
V	Triglyceride ↑↑ Cholesterol ↑ or →	Pre-beta lipoprotein ↑ Chylomicra ↑	Reduce fat to 25% of total caloric intake; carbohydrates 50% of total caloric intake. Limit alcohol.

↑ = increased   → = normal

c. If ineffective, gradually add or substitute propranolol hydrochloride to maximum dose (particularly useful in high renin output hypertension).

d. If ineffective, gradually add or substitute guanethidine. Reserpine, spironolactone, hydralazine, and others also have been used with success.

7. Secure consultation if patient resists normalizing blood pressure by these measures. Review the possibility of having overlooked some cause other than essential hypertension.

Patients with blood pressures of 200/114 or higher are in imminent danger of serious complications and should be hospitalized at once. One or more of the antihypertensive agents listed in Table 7-12 should be instituted promptly, and evaluation for an underlying cause carried out. There are newer antihypertension agents that may be used for youths in the near future. These include prazosin, captopril, and metoprolol.

Ongoing management of essential hypertension must be life-long, which can be difficult. Adoles-cents, just as adults, find it hard to limit salt intake, lose weight if obese, or take medication on a daily basis, particularly when they feel well. Considerable patience and empathy are needed to establish such a plan. This should be worked out with the adolescent directly, not through his or her parents; it is important not to place management in the midst of intergenerational contests over control and the emancipation process. The physician also should expect considerable variance in the degree of compliance and should try to avoid coercion, scare tactics, or scolding when lapses occur. A better way is to offer positive encouragement of the adolescent's efforts to do better and to communicate a sense of tolerance and understanding that it can take time for the young person to modify his or her life patterns according to this new need.

Peripheral Vascular Disease
THROMBOPHLEBITIS

Phlebitis (inflammation only), thrombophlebitis (inflammation with occlusion), and phlebothrombosis (occlusion only) are variations on a theme. Involve-

TABLE 7-8
PRIMARY HYPERLIPIDEMIA: DIAGNOSIS AND MANAGEMENT

Drug Therapy	Comments
None	Rare Low risk for coronary artery disease Medication not helpful
1. Cholestyramine (Questran), 16–36 g/day with or without beta-siterol, 9–39 g/day 2. D-thyroxine, 4–6 mg/day	Common; autosomal dominant High risk for coronary artery disease Cholestyramine tastes terrible; mix with cookies. Side effects include constipation, nausea, bloating, mild steatorrhea D-thyroxine should not be used if hypertension or heart disease coexistent
Clofibrate, 1–2 g/day and Cholestyramine 16–36 g/day	Common; autosomal dominant High risk for coronary artery disease Clofibrate lowers triglyceride levels; side effects include cholelithiasis, myositis, rashes, nausea, diarrhea, weight gain, gynecomastia, arrhythmias. Reduce dose with renal failure.
Clofibrate, 1–2 g/day	Rare; high risk for coronary artery disease
Clofibrate, 1–2 g/day with or without nicotinic acid, 3–6 g/day	Common; autosomal dominant; usually not manifested until late adolescence or adulthood High risk for coronary artery disease If nicotinic acid used start with 300 mg/day, as may be poorly tolerated with flushing, abnormal liver function, elevated blood sugar, gastrointestinal distress, elevated uric acid.
As for type IV; add norethindrone acetate for females	Rare; usually not manifested until late adolescence or adulthood. Low risk for coronary artery disease. Drug therapy used to prevent recurrent attacks of pancreatitis.

ment may be superficial (usually branches of the greater or lesser saphenous system or upper extremity veins) or deep (usually the popliteal and calf veins, sometimes iliac or femoral veins).

Superficial thrombophlebitis is most commonly seen following trauma and often is caused by an indwelling intravenous catheter. Tenderness and erythema of the involved vein and surrounding cellulitis are diagnostic. Improvement usually follows removal of any offending agents (such as a catheter), elevation, and heat. Failure to respond to these measures may indicate a septic process requiring antibiotic coverage.

Factors contributing to the development of deep thrombophlebitis include prolonged immobilization (as with leg casting), pregnancy, the use of oral contraceptives, and postsurgical situations. Calf pain, tenderness and, sometimes, edema of the involved leg with distended superficial veins are characteristic signs. Increased pain with dorsiflexion of the foot (Homan's sign) is an important diagnostic finding when present. Phlebography or ultrasound have been used to confirm the diagnosis in questionable cases. Immediate treatment is indicated to avoid pulmonary emboli and relieve pain. The patient should receive anticoagulation therapy, first with heparin and then coumadin, with the latter maintained for several weeks to months. Additional acute measures include bed rest and elevation of the extremity. Fibrinolytic agents (urokinase, streptokinase) have been used with variable success.

PRIMARY LYMPHEDEMA
Impaired return of lymph fluid due to abnormalities of the lymphatic capillaries and the accumulation of fluid in dependent parts may first appear in childhood (Milroy's disease), in late childhood or adolescence (lymphedema praecox), or in adulthood (lymphedema tarda). A history of infantile lymphedema of the hands and feet is one of the classic features of ovarian dysgenesis (Turner's syndrome) and is of historical significance in any adolescent female with delayed puberty for whom this diagnosis is being entertained.

Lymphedema praecox is characterized by lymphatic vessel aplasia, hypoplasia, and/or varicosity

---

TABLE 7-9
DIFFERENTIAL DIAGNOSIS OF SECONDARY HYPERTENSION

RENAL DISORDERS
Pyelonephritis
Glomerulonephritis, acute and chronic
End-stage renal disease
Polycystic kidneys
Hydronephrosis
Obstructive uropathy
Lupus nephritis
Hemolytic uremic syndrome
Anaphylactoid purpura
Neoplasm
Trauma
Radiation nephritis
Renal transplant

VASCULAR DISORDERS
Renal artery stenosis (Goldblatt kidney)
Fibromuscular dysplasia of the renal artery
Renal vein or artery thrombosis
Coarctation of the aorta
Takayasu's disease (inflammatory disease of aorta
and major branches)
Fistula
Aneurysm

CENTRAL NERVOUS SYSTEM DISORDERS
Encephalitis
Poliomyelitis
Guillain-Barré syndrome
Trauma
Tumor or other space-occupying lesion
Lead encephalitis

ENDOCRINE DISORDERS
Cushing's syndrome
Hyperthyroidism (systolic only)
Adrenogenital syndrome (some forms)
Pheochromocytoma
Hyperaldosteronism

DRUGS AND OTHER INGESTANTS
Oral contraceptives
Vitamin D toxicity
Reserpine overdose
Methyldopa overdose
Amphetamine overdose
Ergotamine overdose
Corticosteroid excess (and DOCA)
Sodium bicarbonate toxicity
Sympathomimetic drugs (e.g., ephedrine sulfate)
Lead, mercury poisoning

MISCELLANEOUS (transient or sustained)
Too small blood pressure cuff; pseudohypertension
Postgenitourinary surgery
Postorthopedic surgery
Idiopathic hypercalcemia
Hypernatremia
Neurofibromatosis
Anxiety
Amyloidosis
Polyarteritis nodosa
Tuberous sclerosis
Marfan's syndrome
Stevens–Johnson syndrome
Turner's syndrome
Congenital rubella syndrome
Familial dysautonomia
Pseudoxanthoma elasticum
Burns
Acute bacterial endocarditis
Porphyria
Homocystinuria
Carcinoid syndrome
Sipple syndrome
Toxemia of pregnancy
Leg traction (stretching of the femoral nerve)

---

beginning in adolescence. It occurs three times more often in females than males. Regional trauma or infection may be precipitants. Examination reveals firm, rubbery, gravity-dependent, nonpitting edema of one or both lower extremities. In addition to fluid accumulation, cellulitis and lymphangitis are major complications.

In considering the diagnosis of a primary lymphedema, the following conditions should be ruled out: congestive heart failure or renal failure, myxedema, deep cavernous hemangioma, deep venous thrombosis or thrombophlebitis, and lymphatic blockage due to neoplasms, surgery, radiotherapy, recurrent regional infection or inflammation, motor paralysis, and filariasis. Fluid aspiration and analysis affirming the lymphatic origin, lymphangiography and possibly, venography are indicated when the etiology is unclear.

Treatment of primary lymphedema includes elevating the affected extremity(s) as much of the time as possible, massage, tight elastic stockings, diuretics, a low-salt diet, and antibiotic treatment of intercurrent infections. Unfortunately, this regimen is not always helpful. Moreover, the condition tends to be progressive. An alternative is surgical excision of abnormal tissue, but this too is a difficult procedure and often has poor cosmetic results.

TABLE 7-10
EVALUATION OF HYPERTENSION (NONLABILE)

HISTORY (noteworthy points):
Symptoms of headache, dizziness, syncope, blurred vision
Drugs being taken, including oral contraceptives
Family history of hypertension, renal disease, pheochromocytoma or adrenogenital syndrome

PHYSICAL EXAMINATION (noteworthy points):
Vital signs, including several blood pressure determinations during and at end of examination. Take pressures (with proper cuffs) in both upper and lower extremities.
Fundi for hemorrhages, exudates, arteriolar narrowing or nicking
Cardiovascular system including all major pulses.
Abdomen: bruits, masses, enlarged kidney(s)
Neurologic system
Striae or abnormal fat distribution

LABORATORY TESTS (initial):
Routine (hemoglobin or hematocrit, white blood count, and urinalysis with microscopic examination)
Erythrocyte sedimentation rate
Urine culture (with antibiotic sensitivities for any significant organisms)
Blood urea nitrogen and creatinine

LABORATORY TESTS (as indicated by other positive findings and/or hypertension of 140/95 or more):
1. Renal system
   a. Electrolytes, pH, bicarbonate
   b. Intravenous pyelogram (rapid sequence)
   c. Serum protein and electrophoresis

d. Cholesterol and triglycerides
e. Alkaline phosphatase (note: will be high during growth, see Appendix I)
f. Plasma renin; split renin determination from renal veins
g. Intravenous saralasin infusion (detects high angiotensin II levels)
h. Renal ultrasound
i. Isotope renograms
j. Renal biopsy
2. Cardiovascular or renal–vascular systems
   a. Chest roentgenogram
   b. Electrocardiogram
   c. Renal arteriogram
3. Endocrine system
   a. Plasma cortisol
   b. Urine 17-hydroxycorticosteroids, 17-ketosteroids
   c. Urine catecholamines and metanephrines
   d. Urine VMA (vanillymandelic acid)
   e. Serum calcium and phosphorus
   f. Serum parathyroid hormone
   g. Urine homovanillic acid
   h. Urine aldosterone
4. Miscellaneous
   a. 5-hydroxy indole acetic acid (carcinoid syndrome)
   b. Skull roentgenograms, CAT scan
   c. Antinuclear antibody, lupus erythematosus preparations
   d. As indicated by suspected underlying disease state

RAYNAUD'S DISEASE

Raynaud's disease is a relatively rare chronic disorder of the digital vasculature with a female-male ratio of 5:1. The onset usually is in adolescence or young adulthood. A typical attack begins with blanching and numbness of the fingers and, in half the patients, the toes (the vasoconstrictive phase). This is followed by cyanosis due to stagnation of blood and then, within minutes, by a vasodilatory phase with hyperemia, throbbing pain, tingling, swelling, and increased local heat lasting 5-10 minutes more. Sometimes the hands, wrists, ankles, and face may be involved as well. Attacks are unpredictable and of variable frequency, although they are often induced by cold or emotion and relieved by heat or rest. The etiology is unknown but a hyperresponsiveness of the involved vasculature to normal reflex sympathetic nerve activity has been postulated. Complications of chronic disease (frequent attacks for 1-4 years or more) include thin, tapered fingers with smooth shiny skin and curved

nails and recurrent episodes of localized infection, blisters, or gangrene.

Diagnosis is based on the clinical picture; laboratory tests are unrevealing. Raynaud's *disease*, however, should not be confused with Raynaud's *phenomenon*, which is sometimes seen with collagen disorders, repetitive trauma (typing, piano playing), occlusive arterial disease, myxedema, pulmonary hypertension, thoracic outlet compression syndrome, polycythemia vera, paroxysmal hemoglobinuria, chronic leukemia, carpal tunnel syndrome, and ergot or methysergide intoxication. These should be ruled out.

Treatment includes avoiding cold, trauma, vasoconstrictor substances (nicotine, tobacco), and any associated emotional precipitants. In addition to heat and rest, catecholamine depletors or vasodilators can be used (reserpine, tolazoline hydrochloride, phenoxybenzamine hydrochloride, cyclandelate, methyldopa). Regional sympathectomy is another alternative in extreme and unresponsive cases.

TABLE 7-11
ANTIHYPERTENSIVE DRUGS

Drug	Mechanism of action	Starting dose	Maximum dose	Side effects	Comments
Chlorothiazide (Diuril)	Thiazide diuretic; decreases vascular resistance, decreases plasma volume	6–10 mg/kg/day	20–30 mg/kg/day (1000 mg/day); 2 daily doses	Hypokalemia, hyperglycemia, hyperuricemia, thrombocytopenia, alkalosis	Useful for mild essential hypertension or as an adjunct to other regimens
Hydrochlorothiazide (Hydrodiuril)	As above	1 mg/kg/day	2 mg/kg/day (100 mg/day); 2 daily doses	As above	As above
Spironolactone (Aldactone)	Potassium sparing diuretic; decreases plasma volume	2 mg/kg/day	3 mg/kg/day (200 mg/day); 3–4 daily doses	Avoid in renal failure; may cause hyperkalemia	Potassium supplement not necessary
Triamterene (Dyrenium)	As above	2 mg/kg/day	4 mg/kg/day (300 mg/day); 1–2 daily doses	As above	As above
Furosemide (Lasix)	Loop diuretic; decreases plasma volume	0.5 to 1 mg/kg/day	2 mg/kg/day (80 mg/day); 2 daily doses	Hypokalemia, hyperuricemia, alkalosis, volume depletion, ototoxicity	Potent diuretic; useful if creatinine clearance is reduced
Hydralazine (Apresoline)	Vasodilator agent; relaxes arteriolar smooth muscles; decreases peripheral resistance	1 mg/kg/day	3 mg/kg/day (300 mg/day); 4 daily doses	Tachycardia, flushing, nasal dryness, lupus syndrome	Useful adjunct with diuretics
Reserpine (Serpasil)	Depletes nerve endings of catecholamines; decreases peripheral vascular resistance	0.01 mg/kg/day	0.02 mg/kg/day (0.25–0.5 mg/day);	Nasal stuffiness, depression, tachycardia, diarrhea	Reduces renin levels; useful in hypertensive crisis (0.07 mg/kg IM or IV q 4–6 hrs)
Methyldopa (Aldomet)	Peripheral norepinephrine depletion; decreases peripheral vascular resistance	10 mg/kg/day	50 mg/kg/day (3000 mg/day); 2–3 daily doses	Orthostatic hypotension, bradycardia, sedation, diarrhea, abnormal liver function tests, positive Coombs test	Reduces renin levels Emergency dose: 250–500 mg IV over 30 minutes
Propranolol hydrochloride (Inderal)	Beta-adrenergic blocker; reduces peripheral vascular resistance	1–2 mg/kg/day	7–10 mg/kg/day (400–500 mg/day); 3–4 daily doses	Hypotension, bradycardia, bronchospasm, syncope, hypertrichosis	Lowers renin levels; avoid with asthma, heart block, or heart failure
Guanethidine (Ismelin)	Blocks chemical neurotransmission at the sympathetic nerve endings; depletes norepinephrine; reduces peripheral vascular resistance	0.2–0.5 mg/kg	2 mg/kg/day (50–75 mg/day); 1 daily dose	Orthostatic hypotension, bradycardia, postexertional syncope	Avoid with pheochromocytoma and MAO inhibitors
Clonidine (Catapres)	Alpha adrenergic blocker	0.1 mg b.i.d.	0.4 mg/kg/day 2 daily doses	Sedation, emesis, dry mouth	Rebound hypertension with withdrawal of medication

TABLE 7-12
DRUGS FOR EMERGENCY TREATMENT OF HYPERTENSION (HYPERTENSIVE CRISIS)

Drug	Dosage	Onset of action	Side effects
Diazoxide (Hyperstat)	2–5 mg/kg, IV push (75–300 mg)	Immediate, lasts 4–5 hr	Tachycardia, elevated blood sugar, weight gain (sodium and water retention), profound hypotension, burning at injection site
Hydralazine (Apresoline)	0.25 mg/kg IV or IM (10–20 mg); repeat q 4–6 hr	10–20 minutes, lasts 4–6 hr	Tachycardia, headache, emesis, psychotic reactions
Prazosin (Minipress)	1–5 mg p.o.	30 minutes to 2 hr, lasts 6–24 hr	Tachycardia, sedation, emesis, fluid retention, profound hypotension
Sodium nitroprusside (Nipride)	0.5–10 μg/kg/min as a continuous IV infusion	Immediate onset, lasts 2–4 min	Tachycardia, nausea, hypothyroidism, thiocyanate poisoning

Bibliography

Bailie, M. D., and Mattioli, L. F. 1980. Hypertension: relationships between pathophysiology and therapy. *J. Pediatr.* 96(5):789.

Benson, H. 1977. Systemic hypertension and the relaxation response. *N. Engl. J. Med.* 296:1152.

Engle, M. A. 1981. Heart sounds and murmurs. *Pediatr. Ann.* 10(3):18.

Engle, M. A. 1981. The adult with congenital heart disease. *D.M.* 29(1):3–59.

Faigel, H. C. 1977. Hyperlipidaemia. *Practitioner* 218:238.

Falk, R. H., and Hood, W. B. 1981. Mitral valve prolapse: striking a therapeutic balance. *Drug. Ther.* 11(9):125.

Gettes, L. S. 1981. Physiology and pharmacology of antiarrhythmic drugs. *Hosp. Pract.* 16(10):89.

Havel, R. J. 1982. Symposium on lipid disorders. *Med. Clin. North Am.* 66(2):317–550.

Hazzard, W. R. 1976. A pathophysiologic approach to managing hyperlipemia. *Am. Family Phys.* 14:78.

Hoffman, G. S. 1980. Raynaud's disease and phenomenon. *Am. Family Phys.* 21:91.

Johnson, C. M., and Rhodes, K. H. 1982. Pediatric endocarditis. *Mayo Clin. Proc.* 57(2):86.

Johnson, W. D. 1978. Antibiotic prophylaxis of bacterial endocarditis. *Primary Care* 5:597.

Jones Criteria (revised) for guidance in the diagnosis of rheumatic fever. 1965. *Circulation* 32:664.

Kaplan, E. L.; Anthony, B. F.; Bisno, A.; et al. 1977. Prevention of bacterial endocarditis. *Circulation* 56:139A.

Kaplan, E. L. 1978. Acute rheumatic fever. *Pediatr. Clin. North Am.* 25:817.

Loggie, J. M. H., editor. 1978. Symposium on hypertension in childhood and adolescence. *Pediatr. Clin. North Am.* 25:1–186.

Margolis, S. 1975. The hyperlipoproteinemias in adolescence. *Med. Clin. North Am.* 59:1359.

McCracken, D., and Everett, J. E. 1976. An investigation of the incidence of cardiac murmurs in young healthy women. *Practitioner* 216:308.

McCrory, W. (editor). 1982. Childhood hypertension. *Pediatr. Annals* 11(7):581–628.

Murphy, G. K. 1978. Sudden death in adolescence. *Pediatrics* 61(2):206.

Nademanee, K., and Singh, B. N. 1982. Advances in antiarrhythmic therapy. The role of newer antiarrhythmic drugs. *J.A.M.A.* 247:217.

Nora, J. J. 1980. Identifying the child at risk for coronary disease as an adult: a strategy for prevention. *J. Pediatr.* 97:706.

Pruitt, A. W. 1981. Pharmacologic approach to the management of childhood hypertension. *Pediatr. Clin. North Am.* 28(1):135.

Riemenschneider, T. A. 1978. Heart murmurs in infants and children. *J. Family Pract.* 6:151.

Rowland, T. W. 1981. Physical fitness in children: implications for the prevention of coronary artery disease. *Curr. Probl. Pediatr.* 11(9):3–54.

Silver, D., and Harrington, M. P. 1977. Thrombophlebitis: prevention, recognition and management. *Primary Care* 4:585.

Whelton, P. K. 1981. Mild hypertension: is it important? *South Med. J.* 74:979.

—8—
The Gastrointestinal Tract

The Alimentary Tract
Peptic ulcer disease □ Inflammatory bowel disease □ Other diarrheal disorders
Gastrointestinal polyps □ Anorectal disease □ Constipation
Acute abdominal conditions □ Abdominal masses □ Chronic abdominal pain
Hepatic and Pancreatic Disorders
Overview □ Hepatitis A □ Hepatitis B □ Chronic hepatitis
Fitz-Hugh–Curtis syndrome □ Cholecystitis □ Pancreatitis

The Alimentary Tract

PEPTIC ULCER DISEASE

Ulcers of the stomach or duodenum are related to many factors, including increased gastric secretions (hydrochloric acid, pepsin, gastrin), decreased mucosal defense mechanisms, genetic predisposition, and ingestion of various drugs (cigarette smoking, aspirin, coffee, alcohol, steroids). The role of psychologic stress is controversial; emotional factors clearly may exacerbate an existing ulcer, but it is less clear that they may cause one in the absence of other contributing factors. Multiple peptic ulcers are seen with severe physical stress (burns, septicemia, surgery) and in the rare Zollinger-Ellison syndrome (gastrin-secreting pancreatic tumors and extreme gastric hyperacidity).

Ulcers are relatively common in adolescents and are almost always duodenal. Symptoms approximate those seen in adults and are less apt to be as ambiguous or silent as in childhood. The pain is sharp and burning or dull, epigastric in location, and it often radiates to the back. It most frequently occurs at night and both before meals and 2–3 hours after. Ingesting coffee, alcohol, aspirin, or spicy foods usually increases pain, whereas bland foods and antacids relieve it. (In contrast, even bland foods tend to produce immediate pain with a gastric ulcer.) Physical findings generally are limited to epigastric tenderness. Laboratory evaluation may indicate chronic and/or acute blood loss with guaiac positive stools (which may be tarry), a microcytic, hypochromic anemia, and reticulocytosis. Table 8-1 presents the differential diagnosis of peptic ulcer disease and includes any condition manifested by epigastric pain or gastrointestinal bleeding.

Although most adolescents with an ulcer present with a history of gradually progressive symptoms over several weeks or months, they also may present as an acute abdominal emergency manifested by hemorrhage or perforation and shock. In these situations, there may or may not have been a prior history suggestive of chronic ulcer disease. Signs of peritonitis predominate in perforation, and free air may be present on an abdominal x-ray. Hematemesis usually accompanies hemorrhage. Gastric aspiration confirms the source, with bright red blood present if bleeding is current and coffee ground material if blood has been in the stomach a longer time. Intestinal obstruction also is a possible, but rare, complication.

Perforation requires immediate surgery for repair once the patient has been stabilized. It may be desirable to perform a highly selective vagotomy at the same time; scarring and adhesions tend to preclude its later performance even if warranted by recurrent disease. A more extensive vagotomy will then be all that is possible. Hemorrhage usually responds to conservative management with iced saline lavages, frequent doses of an antacid (Table 8-2), 30 ml every 1–2 hours, and cimetidine, 300 mg q.i.d. Additional measures include blood transfusions and intravenous fluid and electrolytes. Rarely, hemorrhage will require surgery.

Chronic peptic ulcer disease is diagnosed by an

TABLE 8-1
DIFFERENTIAL DIAGNOSIS
OF PEPTIC ULCER DISEASE

A. Major causes of abdominal pain
1. Functional dyspepsia, chronic gastritis
2. Peptic ulcer disease
3. Cholecystitis with or without cholelithiasis
4. Pyelonephritis
5. Pancreatitis
6. Appendicitis
7. Hiatal hernia
8. Benign tumor of the small intestine
9. Anaphylactic purpura
10. Abdominal epilepsy

B. Major causes of upper gastrointestinal bleeding
1. Esophageal varices
2. Peptic ulcer disease
3. Gastritis or stress gastric ulcer
4. Esophagitis
5. Trauma
6. Mallory-Weiss syndrome
7. Clotting abnormalities

upper gastrointestinal x-ray series and endoscopy if x-rays are inconclusive; the finding of a deformed bulb on roentgenogram indicates past or present disease, and only a definitive crater confirms an active ulcer. Stool guaiac tests will identify occult bleeding. Angiography may be helpful when a history of possible bleeding suggests impending erosion of a significant blood vessel.

Management of a chronic duodenal ulcer combines the use of antacids, cimetidine, and dietary modification. Constipation tends to occur with the use of antacids high in aluminum content, whereas increased magnesium may prompt diarrhea. Alternating or combining both types may eliminate these problems. Hydroxide preparations should not be used with tetracycline since they impair the absorption of tetracycline. Calcium carbonate antacids can cause hypercalcemia if taken in large amounts over time. This problem may be exacerbated if calcium carbonate intake is accompanied by drinking substantial quantities of milk and may give rise to the *milk-alkali syndrome* (hypercalcemia, azotemia, mild alkalosis). Kidney damage is possible if this situation is missed and left uncorrected.

Cimetidine is a histamine-2 receptor antagonist and a potent inhibitor of gastric acid secretion. Usual dosage is 300 mg q.i.d. (with meals and at bedtime) for 4–8 weeks. Although side effects are uncommon if use is restricted to the recommended dose and period of administration, gynecomastia, mental disturbances (agitation, delirium, hallucinations, coma),

neutropenia, dermatitis, muscular pain, mild elevation of creatinine, elevated liver enzymes, interference with B_{12} absorption, and sterility in males have all been reported.

Aspirin, alcohol, cigarettes, and spicy foods should be avoided. A moderately bland, low roughage diet with frequent meals and snacks (milk, crackers, bread and butter) is tolerated well. Alternative medications and those being considered for the future include anticholinergics, such as propantheline bromide (ProBanthine), colloidal bismuth, carbenoxolone, prostaglandin analogs, and sulpiride. Surgery (vagotomy, pyloroplasty, gastrojejunostomy, partial gastrectomy) is reserved for those with intractable disease or severe complications. Generally the prognosis is good; many adolescents with peptic ulcer disease improve rapidly with treatment and may return to an average diet without medication after a few months. Recurrences are possible but by no means the rule.

INFLAMMATORY BOWEL DISEASE

Regional enteritis. Regional enteritis (Crohn's disease, granulomatous ileocolitis), a chronic exacerbating and remitting disease, is characterized by patchy, granulomatous inflammation involving the intestinal mucosa, submucosa, and deeper wall structures (in contrast to the mucosa only in ulcerative colitis). Adolescence is a common time of onset. Often there is a positive family history. Although the distal ileum is most frequently involved, virtually any portion of the large and small bowel may be affected, including the rectum and perianal region. Complications include fissures, abscesses, ulceration, obstruction, and fistulas of any involved segment. Symptomatology is diverse, and variably includes fever, anorexia, weight loss, anemia, abdominal pain, diarrhea, bloody stools, and constipation. The patient may have a tender abdomen with cramps, bloating, and/or tenesmus. Extragastrointestinal tract manifestations such as hepatitis, arthritis, spondylitis, tenosynovitis, uveitis, dermatitis (erythema nodosum, pyoderma gangrenosum), and clubbing are common. In some instances, these conditions antecede the manifestations of bowel disease. In contrast to ulcerative colitis, the onset of regional enteritis is more insidious, but it also tends to have a more debilitating course, resulting in a greater degree of growth retardation, delayed sexual maturation, abdominal pain, and anorexia. There also is a greater frequency of extraintestinal features.

Physical findings are related to the progress of the disease and vary from only mild abdominal tenderness early in the course to abdominal masses

TABLE 8-2
SELECTED ANTACID MEDICATIONS: THEIR COMPOSITION AND DOSAGE

Medication	Composition	Dosage
Amphojel	Aluminum hydroxide gel	*Suspension:* 2 tsp 5–6 times/day, including h.s. *Tablets:* 2 tablets 5–6 times/day, including h.s.
Gaviscon	Aluminum hydroxide gel, with magnesium trisilicate and alginic acid, among other components	*Liquid:* 1–2 T q.i.d. (after meals and h.s.) *Tablets:* 2–4 tablets q.i.d. (after meals and h.s.)
Gelusil (Gelusil-M or Gelusil-II contains higher concentrations of ingredients)	Aluminum hydroxide, magnesium hydroxide, simethicone*	*Liquid:* 2 tsp q.i.d. (p.c. and h.s.) *Tablets:* 2 tablets q.i.d.(p.c. and h.s.)
Maalox	Magnesium and aluminum hydroxide	*Suspension:* 2–4 tsp q.i.d. (20–60 min p.c. and h.s.) *Tablets* (No. 1): 2–4 tablets q.i.d. (20–60 min p.c. and h.s.) *Tablets* (No. 2): 1–2 tablets q.i.d. (20–60 min p.c. and h.s.)
Maalox Plus	Magnesium and aluminum hydroxide with simethicone*	*Suspension:* 2–4 tsp q.i.d. (20–60 min p.c. and h.s.) *Tablets:* 2–4 tablets q.i.d. (20–60 min p.c. and h.s.)
Mylanta (Mylanta-II contains higher concentrations of ingredients)	Aluminum hydroxide and magnesium hydroxide with simethicone*	*Liquid:* 1–2 tsp q 2–4 hours between meals and h.s. *Tablets:* 1–2 tablets q 2–4 hours between meals and h.s.
Riopan (Riopan Plus: magaldrate with simethicone*)	Magaldrate	*Suspension:* 1–2 tsp between meals and h.s. *Chew tablets:* 1–2 tablets between meals and h.s. *Swallow tablets:* 1–2 tablets between meals and h.s.

*Simethicone is an antiflatulant; it may help relieve gas pains, flatulence, and distention.

(representing inflamed loops of bowel or abscesses), perianal disease, and signs of extraintestinal complications. Laboratory data include anemia, and elevated erythrocyte sedimentation rate, and evidence of malabsorption (low blood levels of folate, B_{12}, carotene, and albumin). A barium enema (with influx into the distal ileum) or an upper gastrointestinal series (with small bowel follow-through) demonstrates irregular, patchy areas anywhere in the intestinal tract (predominantly the ileum) with narrowing of the lumen, a "cobblestone" appearance to the mucosa and ulcerations. Fissures, fistulas, and/or pseudodiverticulitis also are seen in advanced disease. The mesentery thickens, and mesenteric lymph nodes enlarge. Sigmoidoscopy and sometimes colonoscopy confirm the presence of granulomatous inflammation. A biopsy from an appropriate site is often diagnostic.

The differential diagnosis includes any condition resulting in chronic diarrhea (see following sec-

tions) or producing similar extraintestinal signs. The irritable bowel syndrome, lactase deficiency, and ulcerative colitis are particularly apt to be confused with regional enteritis early in the course until definitive studies are carried out. Acute terminal ileitis caused by *Yersinia enterocolitica* may produce an acute disease with a red, swollen terminal ileum and cecum and mesenteric lymphadenitis. Signs and symptoms of anorexia nervosa also may be misleading on occasion.

Treatment consists of rest, sulfasalazine (Sulfasalazine, Azulfidine) 3–5 g/day for acute disease tapered to 1–2 g/day total for a more extended time (see ulcerative colitis) and a diet high in protein, carbohydrates, and calories (but low in residue) with iron and vitamin supplementation. Prednisone is also used. However, treatment often is unsatisfactory. Lomotil (diphenoxylate hydrochloride with atropine) to control diarrhea may be used but only with caution, as megacolon and obstruction can result from excessive or prolonged administration. Cholestyramine also has been tried but has significant limitations in its propensity for producing steatorrhea. Total parenteral alimentation and liquid elemental diets (for several weeks or months) have been used with some success. Surgical removal of diseased areas may be necessary and is indicated in instances of medical failure when growth is seriously impaired or symptoms are severely debilitating. Unfortunately, 30% of operative cases develop disease in another segment at a later time. If remission can be achieved by medical or surgical means, a variable amount of catchup growth can be expected. Such growth will be maximal and close to normal expectancies if the patient is in early puberty at disease onset. Possibilities for normal physical development diminish with increasing age.

Prognosis is highly variable. Some patients have chronic, active disease for years and are severely disabled; others have only periodic exacerbations and are able to lead full and productive lives. Even if the disease is well controlled or in sustained remission, it warrants life-long monitoring, as the risk of later bowel cancer is increased. However, this risk is not as great as with ulcerative colitis, and prophylactic surgery generally is not carried out.

Ulcerative colitis. Ulcerative colitis is a chronic, diffuse inflammation of the gastrointestinal mucosa (in contrast to regional ileitis that involves all wall layers). The disease may be limited to the rectum, but variable amounts of the colon usually are involved as well. Onset in adolescence and young adulthood is common. Frequently, there is a familial history of the condition. Initial symptoms and signs may be insidious (50%), acute (30%), or fulminant (20%). Diarrhea and rectal bleeding are frequent presenting complaints and are usually more pronounced than in regional ileitis. Other manifestations include nausea, vomiting, fever, anorexia, weight loss, abdominal pain, growth failure, megacolon, and bowel perforation. But perianal disease, fissures, fistulas, or abscesses (as in regional ileitis) are not encountered. Extraintestinal features, however, are similar; migrating arthritis, arthralgias, hepatic disease, erythema multiforme, erythema nodosum, pyoderma gangrenosum, skin abscesses, and eczema may be seen and also may precede onset of bowel disease on occasion.

Significant laboratory findings include anemia, elevated erythrocyte sedimentation rate, and evidence of malabsorption (low blood levels of folate, B_{12}, carotene, and albumin). Barium enema, proctosigmoidoscopy, or colonoscopy demonstrates a friable, erythematous, and inflamed mucosa with loss of normal haustral markings. The disease begins at the anorectal margin and extends in a continuous and symmetric, rather than patchy, manner. Biopsy reveals a chronic inflammatory process of the mucosal layer. Major differential considerations include regional ileitis, the infectious diarrheas, the irritable colon syndrome, intestinal polyps, gonococcal proctitis, Meckel's diverticulum, and other causes of diarrhea or rectal bleeding.

Treatment is similar to that for regional enteritis. Sulfasalazine, a nonabsorbable compound, acts as an intestinal antiinflammatory agent and is useful in some cases at a dosage of 3-5 g/day in four divided doses for acute disease, with 1-2 g/day adequate for long-term maintenance. This drug's effectiveness generally is greater in ulcerative colitis than in regional enteritis. Significant side effects include nausea, emesis, frontal sinus headache, dermatitis, hemolytic anemia, and aplastic anemia. Prednisone, 1-2 mg/kg/day, may be given for 4-6 weeks, then tapered to a lower total dose of 10-15 mg/day for a more prolonged period. Prednisolone enemas can be beneficial in severe proctitis. Tranquilizers, sedatives, opiate antidiarrheal drugs, and antispasmodics are useful adjuncts in some cases, although caution is indicated in the use of opiates such as Lomotil (see discussion of regional enteritis). Various nutritional supplements (iron, vitamins) albumin, and/or blood may be needed when debility and malnutrition is marked. Elemental diets may be helpful in some resistant cases. Total parenteral alimentation has been used to advantage in patients with particularly severe disease. The role of antibiotics (tetracycline, ampicillin, sulfonamides) and azathioprine is unclear at present; all have been tried but with variable results. Recent studies implicate a possible beneficial effect with metronidazole or cromolyn sodium. Surgery (colectomy with ileostomy) may be necessary for uncontrolled disease with severe debility, severe growth failure, toxic megacolon, and unacceptable steroid side effects in disease only manageable by this drug. In any event, colectomy usually is indicated as a prophylactic measure at some point in adolescence or young adulthood (preferably the latter for psychologic reasons) due to the significant risk of malignant degeneration after 10-15 years of active disease. Annual colonoscopy and biopsy of suspicious areas can be helpful in maintaining bowel integrity as long as possible.

Prognosis is variable, with some patients experiencing easy control and only periodic exacerbations, if any. Others continue with unremitting disease until surgery is carried out. Surgical intervention should not be delayed long enough to irreversibly retard growth or permanently impair psychosocial

TABLE 8-3
DIFFERENTIAL DIAGNOSIS (PARTIAL) OF DIARRHEAL DISORDERS

1. Infectious gastroenteritis (viral, bacterial, parasitic, food poisoning)
2. Irritable bowel syndrome
3. Inflammatory bowel disease
4. Lactase deficiency
5. Celiac disease
6. Cystic fibrosis
7. Other malabsorption syndromes
8. Pseudomembranous enterocolitis
9. Various endocrinopathies
10. Drugs (antibiotics, laxatives, magnesium antacids, alcohol, diuretics, adrenergic blockers, heavy metal poisoning, and others)
11. Some systemic illnesses and major organ system diseases (collagen disorders, congestive heart failure, renal failure, Whipple's disease, medullary carcinoma of the thyroid, carcinoid syndrome, Zollinger-Ellison syndrome, and others)
12. Postgastrointestinal surgical complications (dumping syndrome, postcolectomy)
13. Laxative abuse in anorexia nervosa
14. Withdrawal from narcotic addiction

TABLE 8-4
USEFUL PROCEDURES IN THE DIAGNOSIS OF CHRONIC DIARRHEA

1. Complete blood count and erythrocyte sedimentation rate
2. Urinalysis
3. Serum calcium, protein, electrolytes, carotene
4. Prothrombin time
5. Stool examination
   a. Contents: fat, pus, bacteria, pH
   b. Occult blood
   c. Ova and parasites
   d. Culture
   e. 72-hour collection for stool fat
6. Roentgenographic evaluation (upper gastrointestinal series with small bowel follow-through, barium enema)
7. Colonoscopy with biopsy
8. Duodenal aspirate and biopsy
9. Lactose tolerance test
10. Endocrine profile
11. Specific tests as indicated by signs of extra-bowel disease
12. Laparoscopy, exploratory laparotomy

development. The results of colectomy can be so dramatic in a return to feeling well, resumption of growth, and improved quality of life that the problems encountered with a colostomy or ileoproctostomy are an acceptable price to pay. In contrast to regional enteritis, excision usually is curative if all involved bowel is removed.

OTHER DIARRHEAL DISORDERS

Overview and differential diagnosis. Diarrhea defines the frequent (three or more times daily) passage of unformed or liquid stool, often with increased volume and increased loss of water, electrolytes, and nutrients. The diarrhea can be either enteric (identifiable by the presence of undigested food) or colonic and due to increased water secretion, impaired fluid absorption, or both. The course may be acute and just a few days in duration or chronic, with exacerbations and remissions over years. Acute infectious gastroenteritis, acute food poisoning, and the irritable bowel syndrome are by far the most common causes of diarrhea in adolescence, as they are for the population at large. More serious diseases seen with some frequency in this age group primarily include ulcerative colitis and regional enteritis. Differential considerations are cited in Table 8-3; various laboratory tests that may be useful in diagnosis are given in Table 8-4.

Treatment depends on the etiology, although many cases of acute infectious or toxic diarrhea are manageable by the use of antidiarrheal medications (Table 8-5) and attention to fluid and electrolyte balance alone. Some controversy exists over the use of antidiarrheal medications in acute food poisoning out of the concept that this is a self-limited condition in any event and slowing the rate of bacterial endotoxin elimination simply protracts the course. Used as adjuncts, these agents may also benefit chronic diarrhea.

Irritable colon syndrome. Irritable colon (bowel) syndrome is an idiopathic and, probably, functional condition characterized by episodic diarrhea with or without abdominal pain and with or without alternating episodes of constipation. Blood in the stools, fever, weight loss, or other systemic signs are usually absent. It occurs relatively frequently in adolescents and young adults. An antecedent history of additional gastrointestinal disturbances or migraine headaches in the patient or other family members is common. Examination may reveal hyperactive, loud bowel sounds (borborygmi) due to aerophagia and intestinal hyperperistalsis. Laboratory studies are within normal limits. Small bowel barium studies may or may not demonstrate an abnormally rapid intestinal transit time.

There is no proven treatment. Diet manipula-

TABLE 8-5
ANTIDIARRHEAL MEDICATIONS

Medication	Dosage
Konsyl (brand of psyllium hydrophilic mucilloid)	1 tsp in 1/3 glass water 1–3 times/day
Paregoric (camphorated tincture of opium)	4 ml t.i.d. or q.i.d.
Codeine sulfate or phosphate	32–64 mg t.i.d. or q.i.d.
Lomotil (diphenoxylate hydrochloride with atropine sulfate)	10–20 mg/day in 3–4 divided doses until control develops; then 5 mg b.i.d. for maintenance
Imodium (loperamide hydrochloride)	4 mg in the morning, up to 16 mg/day
Miscellaneous (Kaopectate, Pepto-Bismol, many others)	

tion may be beneficial by eliminating those foods that seem to exacerbate the situation. Coffee, cold or carbonated beverages, and flatus-forming foods are often implicated. Antidiarrheal agents offer symptomatic relief, as do laxatives if constipation also is a significant feature. Mild tranquilizers, sedatives, and antispasmotic agents (Donnatal) also may have a place, with the first two groups of drugs indicated when stress appears to play a significant role. When stress is a factor, counseling or definitive psychotherapy may be warranted if significant environmental factors or psychologic difficulty is present. It is equally important to reassure the patient and his or her parents, conveying the benign nature of this condition.

Lactase deficiency. Some individuals (primarily those of black, Asian, or Jewish ethnicity) are genetically predisposed toward developing lactase deficiency during later childhood or adolescence. Less commonly, this deficiency may be congenital or secondary to severe acute gastroenteritis, celiac disease, tropical sprue, or gastrointestinal surgery. Symptoms include diarrhea, cramping, bloating, and flatulence after lactose (milk sugar) ingestion; in the absence of lactase, this sugar is converted to lactic acid which, in turn, increases the osmotic load of intestinal contents with a resultant increased secretion of fluid into the lumen.

Diagnosis is suggested by the clinical association between symptoms and lactose (milk) intake and absence of symptoms on a lactose-free diet. The stool pH usually is acid (under 6.0) and may demonstrate the presence of reducing substances with Clinitest tablets. Additional procedures useful in cases of obscure origin include an oral lactose tolerance test (positive if the blood sugar fails to rise by 25%), a breath-hydrogen test analyzing the amount of H_2[51] in the breath after a lactose load, and analysis of intestinal biopsy for lactase and disaccharidase content. Satisfactory treatment usually is achieved by eliminating or reducing the intake of milk and other lactose-containing foods or by oral administration of lactase.

Malabsorption diseases. Pancreatic disease (cystic fibrosis), intestinal disease (sprue, regional enteritis, lactase deficiency, giardiasis, lymphoma), and liver disease (biliary cirrhosis) may impair nutrient absorption with resultant weight loss, debility, and frequent frothy, bulky, foul-smelling and light-colored stools (steatorrhea). Clinical findings relate to the underlying cause and possible associated malnutrition. Laboratory evaluation reflects malabsorption with (a) iron-deficiency anemia, (b) low levels of serum iron, folate, vitamin B_{12}, total protein, albumin, and carotene, and (c) an increased content of stool fat and starch. Treatment is directed at the underlying cause and at improving nutritional status by appropriate nutrient and enzyme replacement therapy; supplementation with fat-soluble vitamins (A, D, E, K) should not be overlooked. Cholestyramine may improve the steatorrhea.

Antibiotic-associated colitis. Many antibiotics can produce a diarrheal state of variable severity by suppressing normal intestinal flora and the subsequent overgrowth of toxin-producing *Clostridium difficile*. Symptoms of antibiotic-associated colitis (pseudomembranous enterocolitis) include fever, diarrhea, abdominal pain, generalized toxicity, and leukocytosis. Yellow-white raised, exudative plaques (pseudomembranes) on the mucosa usually are noted on sigmoidoscopy. Treatment consists of discontinuing the implicated antibiotic. Severe cases may benefit from alternate antibiotic treatment aimed at eradicating *C. difficile*; vancomycin (Vancocin), 500 mg q.i.d. × 7–10 days, is effective. Metronidazole (Flagyl) may also be used.

Acute gastroenteritis. Gastroenteritis usually is transmitted by the ingestion of water or food contaminated by any one of many implicated organisms, but transmission through sexual relationships is increasingly recognized as a possible mode. Symptoms generally occur a few hours or a day after exposure and are manifested in the rapid onset of nausea, vomiting, and profuse diarrhea. Most cases, however, rapidly improve in several days without specific treatment.

The disease may be caused directly by the growth of toxin-producing organisms in the intestinal tract (infectious gastroenteritis) or by consuming a toxin-containing food in which the organism has been incubating for some time (toxic gastroenteritis, food poisoning). Inadequately refrigerated foods that require considerable handling in their preparation are notorious sources; custards, pastry cream filling, ham and potato salads, and poultry stuffings often are implicated.

Treatment usually is supportive with attention to maintenance of fluid and electrolyte balance through oral administration of suitable liquids (Pedialyte, Lytren, carbonated soft drinks, Gatorade) or intravenous therapy if dehydration is marked. Antidiarrheal medications may be helpful and include Pepto-Bismol (bismuth subsalicylate), Kaopectate with aluminum hydroxide, paregoric, Lomotil, and loperamide among others (Table 8-5). Opiate derivatives (paregoric, Lomotil, loperamide) should be avoided in patients suspected of having shigellosis or salmonellosis, as these preparations may exacerbate either disease. Some of the more important bacterial causes of acute gastroenteritis that may be seen in adolescents are discussed in the following paragraphs (for discussions of giardiasis and amebiasis, see Chapter 15). Viral agents, including rotavirus, parvovirus, ECHO virus, adenovirus, and coxsackievirus, also are frequently involved.

Escherichia coli is an important cause of "traveler's diarrhea" due to its wide distribution in water and food. The incubation period is 6–8 hours. Symptoms include nausea, vomiting, watery diarrhea, abdominal cramps, and low-grade fever. Stool culture is positive for *E. coli*. Treatment is supportive, with resolution occurring in 3–7 days, although some cases may be more prolonged. Prophylactic treatment with doxycycline, 100–200 mg once a day, protects for the duration of treatment and 2 weeks thereafter; this may be useful for individuals traveling to endemic areas, primarily underdeveloped countries.

Ingestion of contaminated water or food contaminated with *Salmonella* results in fever, emesis, and a watery, mucoid diarrhea after an incubation period of 1–2 days. Bloody stools are not as common as with shigellosis, but large numbers of leukocytes are seen on microscopic examination. Diagnosis is by stool culture demonstrating one of the many species that may be involved. The course is usually self-limiting, lasting 2–5 days, unless *S.*

typhimurium is involved, in which case typhoid fever results. With typhoid fever or with septicemia accompanying gastroenteritis due to any species of this organism, treatment with ampicillin is indicated (1 g intravenously every 4 hours for 7 days; then 500 mg by mouth every 6 hours for 7 days more). Other occasional complications include osteomyelitis (particularly in individuals with sickle cell disease) and meningitis; here either ampicillin or chloramphenicol is the drug of choice with treatment schedules appropriate to the site of infection.

Bacillary dysentery is manifested by high fever, emesis, and voluminous watery stools following ingestion of *Shigella*-contaminated food or water and an incubation period of 8–40 hours. Symptoms progress to tenesmus and mucoid, bloody diarrhea; leukocytes are prominent on microscopic examination. Diagnosis is by stool culture demonstrating *S. dysenteriae, S. flexneri, S. boydii,* or *S. sonnei.* Specific treatment is with 2.5 g of tetracycline given in a single dose or ampicillin, 500 mg q.i.d. × 5 days. Strains resistant to these antibiotics usually respond to daily treatment with two double-strength tablets (160 mg/800 mg) of trimethoprim-sulfamethoxazole. Symptoms generally abate in 4–10 days.

Clostridium perfringens, a strict anaerobe, is an important cause of food poisoning. Some 8–14 hours after ingesting toxin-containing food, the patient experiences the sudden onset of nausea, vomiting, abdominal pain, and watery diarrhea; leukocytes and blood usually are absent from the stools. Recovery generally is rapid with marked improvement after just 1 day. Treatment, if needed at all, is symptomatic. *C. perfringens* also is implicated in gas gangrene and necrotizing enteritis, but these are uncommon disease entities and not complications of simple food poisoning. Nor should this condition be confused with that caused by *C. botulinum,* or botulism, which is a far more serious condition with muscle paralysis in addition to gastrointestinal symptoms, frequently resulting in death.

Staphylococcus aureus also is a common cause of food poisoning and is frequently implicated in epidemics following parties or picnics. Severe vomiting, abdominal pain, and variable degrees of diarrhea are experienced 1–6 hours after ingesting toxin-containing food. Stools are loose or watery but only rarely contain pus or blood. Recovery usually occurs within 4–24 hours. Treatment is supportive, if needed at all.

Yersinia enterocolitica, a gram-negative coccobacillus, is increasingly recognized as a human pathogen. Illnesses now attributed to *Yersinia* include gastroenteritis, a pseudoappendicitis syndrome, hepatitis, nonsuppurative or suppurative polyarthritis, polyarthralgia, erythema nodosum, urethritis, and possibly Reiter's syndrome.

Gastrointestinal disease generally appears after an incubation period of 4–10 days. Symptoms variably include emesis, abdominal pain, and profuse watery diarrhea. Stools contain leukocytes but usually not blood. The course commonly lasts 1–3 weeks; less commonly, symptoms may be more prolonged and/or particularly severe with gastrointestinal ulceration, perforation, and peritonitis. Sometimes none of these manifestations are present except for abdominal pain due to mesenteric lymphadenitis or terminal ileitis, mimicking an acute abdominal condition requiring surgery. Diagnosis is by a positive stool culture. Antibiotics are not necessary for mild disease. Chloramphenicol, gentamicin, or colistin may be tried in severe or prolonged infection, although none are of proven efficacy.

Campylobacter (subspecies jejuni or fetus) recently has been recognized as an important cause of acute diarrheal illness. Watery diarrhea followed by blood-streaked stools and severe mid-abdominal pain follow an incubation period of 2–10 days. Additional symptoms include fever, malaise, headache, and chills. Diagnosis is by a positive stool culture. Most patients recover without sequellae in several days, but progression to a chronic diarrhea is seen on occasion. Treatment of mild cases is symptomatic, if needed at all. Ampicillin, erythromycin, chloramphenicol, tetracycline, or aminoglycosides may be used in chronic or severe disease. Campylobacter also may be the causal organism in some cases of septicemia, endocarditis, meningitis, thrombophlebitis, salpingitis, peritonitis, and septic arthritis.

GASTROINTESTINAL POLYPS

Diagnosis of rectal bleeding. Although not common, polyps of the gastrointestinal tract can occur in adolescents. Their significance rests in being a major cause of rectal bleeding and, even in the absence of symptomatology, in the risk of malignancy associated with some juvenile and hereditary forms.

The differential diagnosis of rectal bleeding, or melena, is given in Table 8-6. Blood loss may be acute or chronic, visible or occult, external to or mixed with stool. Gastrointestinal bleeding from the stomach, small intestine, or right colon tends to be tarry, whereas that from the left colon, sigmoid, rectum, and perianal region tends to be red. Acute blood loss may lead to an initial elevation of hematocrit, platelets, and blood urea nitrogen, but these values drop as plasma volume reexpands. Other signs

TABLE 8-6
DIFFERENTIAL DIAGNOSIS OF
LOWER GASTROINTESTINAL BLEEDING

1. Hemorrhoids
2. Anal fissures
3. Gastrointestinal polyps
4. Inflammatory bowel disease
5. Infectious proctitis (gonococcal, amebic, others)
6. Systemic disease (Henoch-Schönlein syndrome, hemolytic-uremic syndrome, bleeding diathesis, polyarteritis nodosa, uremia, drugs, others)
7. Infectious diarrhea
8. Endometriosis
9. Diverticulitis
10. Intussusception
11. Hepatic dysfunction
12. Ingestion of rough foods
13. Upper gastrointestinal bleeding
14. Meckel's diverticulum
15. Colonic tumors
16. Pseudobleeding from ingestion of beets

of acute blood loss are tachycardia, hypotension, and elevated white blood count. Chronic blood loss may be accompanied by hypochromic anemia, an elevated reticulocyte count, and low serum iron.

Diagnosis and detection of the bleeding site are directed by clinical signs. Bleeding secondary to a peptic ulcer generally is ruled out by the absence of blood in gastric aspirates with confirmation through a negative endoscopy and/or upper gastrointestinal x-ray series. Rectal examination, colonoscopy, and barium x-ray examinations (including air contrast studies) are useful in lower intestinal or colonic disease. Celiac and mesenteric arteriography may be revealing when other, lower-risk procedures have failed. A technetium study may help detect Meckel's diverticulum. The following laboratory tests also should be considered: complete blood count, erythrocyte sedimentation rate, liver function tests, blood urea nitrogen, creatinine, clotting studies (bleeding time, clotting time, prothrombin time, and partial thromboplastin time), and others as indicated by preliminary differential indications. When all else fails, laparoscopy or laparotomy may be necessary for a final diagnosis. If the bleeding is acute, typing and cross-match for possible blood transfusions also should be carried out.

Juvenile or inflammatory polyps. Single, sometimes multiple, polyps develop during the first decade of life. Seventy-five percent are located within 25 cm of the anus and are readily detectable by rectal and sigmoidoscopic examination. Symptoms generally are limited to bright red, postdefecatory blood streaking and need to be differentiated from anal fissures and hemorrhoids (see page 95). The lesions are benign and can be removed easily by fiberoptic colonoscopy. As more than one polyp may be present, the rest of the colon should also be examined at the same time. Occasionally, a more extensive, generalized inflammatory polyposis may be seen. This is a benign condition and not associated with malignant change.

Familial adenomatous polyposis of the colon. Familial adenomatous polyposis of the colon is an autosomal dominant disorder manifested by multiple sessile or pedunculated adenomas disseminated throughout the colon and rectum. They occur by late childhood or early adolescence, although symptoms of rectal bleeding and diarrhea may not be evident until a later time. Carcinoma of the bowel develops in 80% of these individuals by young adulthood; 40% have evidence of malignant changes at the time of first diagnosis. A total colectomy or subtotal colectomy with ileoproctostomy is indicated in late childhood or early adolescence. All family members should be screened for this disorder with colonoscopy or barium enema.

Peutz-Jegher's syndrome. Peutz-Jegher's syndrome, an autosomal dominant disorder, is characterized by multiple hamartomatous polyps located primarily, but not exclusively, in the jejunum. Mucocutaneous pigmentation of the buccal, perioral, periorbital, or perianal regions and of the digits and/or of the colonic mucosa itself are classic additional findings and, when noted on a routine physical examination, mandate intestinal evaluation. But this pigmentation, although present in childhood, may fade by adolescence; the history thereby assuming particular importance. Symptoms may be absent or include gastrointestinal bleeding, tarry stools, anemia, or recurrent intussusception.

These polyps are capable of malignant degeneration, but the risk of colon cancer is low, and prophylactic bowel resection usually is not done, although a life-time monitoring plan is indicated. It is important that counseling be rendered in a manner that promotes compliance with such a plan but not to the point of producing cancer phobia. Adolescents tend to have exaggerated fears about malignancy even when entirely healthy and are likely to amplify these fears way out of proportion when there is, in fact, legitimate cause for concern. Inadequate counseling can easily result in debilitating, but wholly unnecessary, emotional distress. Some of the counseling principles set forth in Chapters 21 and 23 will be useful here.

Gardner's syndrome. Gardner's syndrome also is an autosomal dominant disorder that may first be noted in adolescence. Multiple small and large bowel polyps develop in association with dental anomalies, osteomas of facial and other bones, and such soft tissue lesions as sebaceous cysts, lipomas, fibromas, leiomyomas, and dermoids. There is a high risk of colon carcinoma in the postadolescent period, and prophylactic subtotal colectomy with ileoproctostomy is indicated in young adulthood.

Lymphoid nodular hyperplasia. Small sessile polypoid lesions of the colon and rectum may present with painless bleeding. They are comprised of hypertrophied lymphatic germinal follicles or thick mucosal folds infiltrated with lymphocytes. Their clinical significance rests in the degree of associated blood loss; steroid enemas may be helpful if such loss is severe.

Hemangiomas. Although not strictly classifiable as a polypoid lesion, single and multiple hemangiomas of the bowel may manifest in abdominal pain, intussusception, and lower gastrointestinal bleeding. Large cavernous hemangiomas also can occur, particularly in the rectum. Diagnosis is by barium x-ray studies and visceral angiography. Hereditary hemorrhagic telangiectasia (Rendu-Osler-Weber syndrome) is characterized by multiple small angiomas of the skin, mucous membranes, tongue, nasal mucosa, lips, fingertips, and gastrointestinal tract.

Malignant carcinoid syndrome. Malignant carcinoid syndrome is a symptom complex characterized by a serotonin-secreting carcinoid tumor in the ileum with metastases to the mesenteric lymph nodes and liver. Carcinoid tumors of other locations and tricuspid or pulmonic valvular lesions also may occur. Symptoms reflect elevated serotonin levels in tachycardia and flushing, as well as gastrointestinal disease in diarrhea, abdominal pain, bloating, melena, tenesmus, and so forth. There are many variants of this syndrome; although the prognosis is generally poor, occasional patients do well.

ANORECTAL DISEASE

Proctitis. Inflammation of the rectum in otherwise healthy adolescents usually is due to *Neisseria gonorrhoeae*. Proctitis also may be a manifestation of inflammatory bowel disease, amebiasis, shigellosis, herpes progenitalis, syphilis, lymphogranuloma venereum, and beta-hemolytic streptococcal infection. *Chlamydia trachomatis* has been cultured in some cases of proctitis and recently proven as a cause. Signs and symptoms include painful defecation, tenesmus, variable amounts of rectal mucus and pus, and occasionally blood streaking of the stool or on wiping. Diagnosis is by history (including sexual contact), microscopic examination of the stool for *Entamoeba histolytica*, and both aerobic and anaerobic stool cultures, including media appropriate for *N. gonorrhoeae* (Thayer-Martin, others). Dark-field examination for *Treponema* spirochetes should be done if genital or perianal ulcers are present; syphilis serology should be obtained in any case. Other sexually transmitted diseases should be looked for as well. Treatment is directed at the causal organism; antibiotic schedules for *N. gonorrhoeae* are reviewed in Chapter 17.

Gonococcal proctitis in males frequently is consequent to homosexual activity. In females, the disease may occur from anogenital sexual contact or simply from rectal contamination by infected vaginal secretions. This disease in either sex is cause for further investigation into sexual behavior and possible associated problems. Proctitis in a young adolescent male, for instance, may not simply indicate a voluntary homosexual relationship but also sexual abuse, exploitation, or prostitution. Anogenital sexual relations may have the same abusive implications for female adolescents.

Anal fissures and hemorrhoids. Superficial tears or erosions (fissures) at the mucocutaneous junction of the anus, manifesting in pain and blood streaks on defecation, are most commonly associated with constipation or are idiopathic. But the possibility of their occurring as a result of anal intercourse, either heterosexual or homosexual, should not be overlooked. Less commonly, fissures may occur with any of the various rectal and colonic diseases previously discussed.

External hemorrhoids (varicosities of the anorectal veins) and anal tags may produce similar symptoms and have similar etiologies. In addition, hemorrhoids are common in late pregnancy. Only rarely do they indicate collateral circulation secondary to portal obstruction, although this can be a complication in older adolescents and young adults with long-standing alcoholism and consequent cirrhosis.

Examination may reveal a fissure, protruding hemorrhoid, or anal tag (representing healed, past hemorrhoidal disease). Fissures, however, are not

TABLE 8-7
DIFFERENTIAL DIAGNOSIS OF PRURITUS ANI

1. Chronic scratching
2. Poor hygiene
3. Constipation
4. Diarrhea
5. Diet
6. Hemorrhoids/anal fissures
7. Fungal infections (*Candida albicans*, *Trichophyton rubrum*)
8. Enterobiasis (pinworm)
9. Contact dermatitis (soaps, perfumes, perineal deodorant sprays, bubble bath)
10. Hyperhidrosis
11. Tight clothes
12. Pediculosis
13. Scabies
14. Secondary to vaginitis (*Candida*, *Trichomonas*)
15. Condylomata acuminata
16. Proctitis
17. Hypertrophied anal papillae
18. Fistulas and other rectal disease, including prolapsed rectum
19. Erythrasma due to *Corynebacterium minutissimum*
20. Amebiasis
21. Syphilis

always visible, although blood streaking on the examining finger is suggestive. Guaiac tests for blood are negative if the sample is taken from the interior of a stool specimen.

Treatment of fissures or hemorrhoids consists of warm sitz baths, topical anesthetics (Americaine hemorrhoidal, Anusol, Nupercaine, Xylocaine ointment or suppositories), stool softeners such as docusate sodium (Colace; 100–200 mg at bedtime), glycerine suppositories to ease defecation, and correction of any underlying constipation (see following discussion of constipation). Surgical excision of chronic fissures or hemorrhoids resistant to medical treatment may be necessary.

Pruritus ani. Anal itching can be an acute or chronic problem and occurs with many conditions (Table 8-7). Treatment consists of proper hygiene, topical anesthetics (see preceding section), and attention to the precipitating cause. Temporary use of a steroid cream also is helpful.

CONSTIPATION
Constipation is marked by the difficult passage of inspissated stools at infrequent intervals. Abdominal cramps relieved by defecation, anal fissures, and

hemorrhoids are common symptoms and signs. Almost every case of constipation in adolescents is functional. Symptoms usually have been present intermittently for years, and other family members often have similar difficulty. Additional historic features include low daily fluid intake, a diet low in roughage, irregular stooling time, and frequent ignoring of the defecatory urge.

The differential diagnosis includes narcotic abuse, Hirschsprung's disease, hypothyroidism, hypercalcemia, anal or rectal stenosis, skeletal muscle defects of the abdominal wall, and scleroderma. It also may be a variable feature of regional enteritis or the irritable colon syndrome. A functional etiology usually is evident from the history and physical examination alone. Specific tests for organic etiology should be performed when suggested by clinical findings.

Treatment of functional constipation is aimed at correcting dietary inadequacies and poor bowel habits. The following is a helpful protocol in many instances:

1. Two tablespoons milk of magnesia plus 200 mg (two capsules) of Colace (docusate sodium and a stool softener) at bed time for the first 2–3 weeks. Dulcolax (two 5 mg tablets or one 10 mg suppository), mineral oil (1 tablespoon in orange juice), or Metamucil powder (one packet dissolved in water taken t.i.d.) may be substituted for milk of magnesia if the latter is ineffective or poorly tolerated. Many other laxative preparations are available; most may be used safely for short periods, but bulk and stool-softener types are preferred for chronic administration.

2. Establish a regular time for a daily bowel movement 30–45 minutes after eating to capitalize on the gastrocolic reflex. A glycerine suppository inserted 10 minutes before going to stool may be helpful, particularly if defecation is difficult or painful. The patient should remain at stool for 20 minutes each time with periodic defecatory attempts even if there are no results. Morning is preferable, but after dinner can be a satisfactory alternative if more convenient for the adolescent's schedule (and, thus more likely to improve compliance.

3. Increase dietary intake of fruits and foods with high residue such as leafy vegetables, salads, and bran.

4. Increase fluid intake to 64 ounces (eight glasses) per day; any liquid except milk is satisfactory. Increase further at times of high fluid loss, as during strenuous exercise or on hot days.

5. Gradually taper milk of magnesia (or other laxative) after 2–3 weeks and discontinue after approximately 1 month. Maintain Colace at bed time for 1–2 months more (it has no pharmacologic action, and only acts as a wetting agent aiding in the maintenance of soft stools) but at a dosage of 100 mg; gradually taper and discontinue.

ACUTE ABDOMINAL CONDITIONS

The causes of acute abdominal conditions are legion (Table 8-8) and include many medical as well as surgical disorders. Some conditions manifest in recurrent bouts of abdominal pain, others in just a single episode. Recurrent pain for which no organic cause is readily apparent often is ascribed to psychogenic factors. Although these may well be operative, a diagnosis of emotional etiology can only be reached after careful exclusion of alternatives.

A wide variety of procedures and tests may be employed in establishing the diagnosis, although a judicious rather than "shotgun" selection should be based on historic and physical clues. A partial list includes a complete blood count, erythrocyte sedimentation rate, urinalysis, urine culture, stools culture, stool guaiac, stool ova and parasites, tuberculosis skin test, intravenous pyelogram, upper gastrointestinal x-ray series with small bowel follow-through, barium enema, proctoscopy, sigmoidoscopy, colonoscopy, and endoscopy. In addition, new advances in ultrasonography and computerized axial tomography are making these procedures increasingly useful in diagnosing abdominal pathology. In some cases laparoscopy or even laparotomy may be necessary.

It also is important not to overlook the pelvic examination in both virginal and sexually active adolescent females. A number of pelvic conditions enter into the differential diagnosis (Table 8-8). (Note: Pelvic inflammatory disease may occur in nonsexually active girls as well as in those who are sexually active.)

Inflammation of the appendix is the classic cause of an acute abdominal condition requiring surgery. The incidence peaks in early adolescence and continues to be an important consideration throughout the second decade. Appendicitis occurs more frequently in males than females. The earliest symptom is periumbilical, epigastric, or generalized abdominal pain, often insidious in onset. Typically the pain becomes increasingly severe and localizes in the right lower quadrant; the patient is reluctant to move and prefers to lie with knees bent. Fever, anorexia, nausea, and vomiting are frequently noted as well.

Physical examination reveals generalized tenderness on palpation with the greatest intensity in the right lower quadrant. Peritoneal irritation is mani-

TABLE 8-8
DIFFERENTIAL DIAGNOSIS OF ACUTE ABDOMINAL CONDITIONS

Organ system	Disorder	Organ system	Disorder
Gastrointestinal tract	Appendicitis Mesenteric lymphadenitis *Yersinia* ileitis Inflammatory bowel disease Peptic ulcer disease, with or without perforation Acute gastroenteritis and food poisoning *Campylobacter* enteritis Postsurgical adhesions Meckel's diverticulum Diverticulitis Peritonitis Intussusception Incarcerated hernia (femoral, inguinal); diaphragmatic hernia	Cardiopulmonary system	Acute pericarditis Pneumonia Pulmonary infarction Pneumothorax Mediastinitis
		Musculoskeletal system trauma	Intraabdominal trauma Abdominal muscle strain; rectus sheath hematoma Vertebral disk space infection
Liver/Pancreas	Hepatitis Fitz-Hugh–Curtis syndrome Cholecystitis Pancreatitis	Systemic syndromes	Diabetic ketoacidosis Hemolytic-uremic syndrome Henoch–Schönlein syndrome Acute intermittent porphyria Systemic lupus erythematosus Polyarteritis nodosa Familial Mediterranean fever Familial hyperlipidemia Hereditary angioneurotic edema Acute rheumatic fever Sickle cell anemia Infectious mononucleosis Acute lymphoblastic leukemia
Female reproductive tract	Pelvic inflammatory disease Ectopic pregnancy Mittelschmerz Endometriosis Torsion or rupture of ovarian cyst		
		Miscellaneous	Narcotic withdrawal Heavy metal poisoning Abdominal migraine Abdominal epilepsy
Renal/Genitourinary tract	Urolithiasis, nephrolithiasis Pyelonephritis Prostatitis		

fested in guarding, rebound tenderness, muscular rigidity, and decreased bowel sounds. Often there is a positive psoas sign (extension of the right hip stretching the psoas muscle, which is inflamed by the overlying appendix, and thus produces pain). Findings may be less clear when there is a retrocecal appendix; in this instance right-sided tenderness on rectal examination becomes a particularly important finding provided pelvic inflammatory disease is ruled out in females.

The white blood count usually is elevated (up to 20,000/mm^3) with a shift to the left, whereas urinalysis results are normal. A flat plate and upright film of the abdomen may reveal cecal distention and, sometimes, intestinal air-fluid levels. Occasionally an appendiceal fecalith may be noted.

If the diagnosis initially is unclear, the patient may be hospitalized, maintained on intravenous fluids, and observed. A significant number will improve within 24 hours, some other condition having masqueraded as appendicitis. The differential diagnosis of such conditions is presented in Table 8-8, but the primary contenders in adolescence are mesenteric lymphadenitis, pelvic inflammatory disease, mittelschmertz, ectopic pregnancy and, possibly, *Yersinia* enteritis, perforated peptic ulcer, or inflammatory bowel disease. Complications of appendicitis include perforation, peritonitis, pelvic abscess, and adhesions. Death is rarely encountered today. Treatment is by surgical removal with antibiotic therapy and drainage if peritonitis is present. Prognosis is excellent with full recovery expected.

ABDOMINAL MASSES

By far the most common abdominal mass encountered in adolescence is physiologic and limited to the female sex: pregnancy. The gravid uterus can be palpated at the pelvic brim around the fourth month. The other most frequent cause of an abdominal "mass" in this age group is inspissated stool in the

TABLE 8-9
FEATURES DIFFERENTIATING ORGANIC AND FUNCTIONAL ABDOMINAL PAIN

Pain factors	Organic	Functional
Nature	Consistent	Often variable, inconsistent
Location	Tends to stay in same place	Tends to vary; sometimes cannot describe well
Time of day	May be replicable, occurring under similar circumstances	Often highly variable or clearly related to stress
Effect on sleep	May wake up	Rarely wakes
Precipitants	May be specific, e.g., food	Tends not to be specific unless related to stress
Relief	May have specific measures, e.g., antacids, aspirin	Rarely relieved by other than rest, time
Time between onset and seeking of medical help	Usually only a few weeks	Presence for months or years common
Impact on activity	Often seriously interferes	May interfere; often does not
Level of patient concern	High	Variable; may be indifferent
Weight	May evidence loss	Rarely any documented loss
Associated symptoms	Tend to relate to single organ system; consistent with underlying pathology	Multiple organ system complaints common; inconsistent with pathophysiologic principles

colon. Hepatomegaly, splenomegaly, or both may be encountered in a number of diseases, including hemolytic disorders and metastatic disease, although viral hepatitis or infectious mononucleosis are much more likely to be the cause.

Otherwise, most intraabdominal lesions seen in this age group are not palpable and remain hidden because of their location and small size. Occasionally, fibrotic areas of bowel manifested as firm, ropy segments may be encountered in regional ileitis. Some ovarian cysts may become quite large (10 cm or more in diameter) and be felt as firm, cystic, smooth-walled masses in the lower abdomen, located in the midline or slightly to one side. As these cysts easily rupture spontaneously (without serious consequence), they may be present on one examination only to disappear subsequently.

All in all, the search for masses by abdominal palpation alone is singularly unrevealing. The yield may be enhanced by a pelvic examination in a female and a rectal examination in the male.

CHRONIC ABDOMINAL PAIN
Recurrent or chronic abdominal pain is one of the more ubiquitous symptoms in adolescents, particularly females. It often defies diagnosis and commonly leads to frustrating multiple diagnostic procedures

without achieving resolution. The major challenge is to discriminate between organic pathology and functional or psychogenic pain. The history is particularly helpful (significant differential points are reviewed in Table 8-9). Regrettably, these are not invariably distinguishing, and crossovers do occur. Functional pain, for example, sometimes may masquerade as an acute abdominal condition; a seemingly psychogenic condition may in fact be due to regional ileitis. Such conflicting possibilities of course, constitute the fundamental dilemma.

In approaching chronic abdominal pain, it is helpful if the evaluation follows a logical, pragmatic plan (Figure 8-1), avoiding more major procedures without reasonable indication yet taking significant differential considerations into account (Table 8-10). Even if the patient has an organic condition, he or she usually is not harmed by being observed until vague or ambiguous symptoms and signs become more specific. Weight loss (documented—not by patient report alone), debility, and/or an elevated erythrocyte sedimentation rate are significant differential clues. Although a urinalysis (and, possibly, a urine culture) is indicated routinely, hidden renal disease rarely is the cause of idiopathic abdominal pain in adolescence and remains low on the differential list if there is no prior history of a renal tract

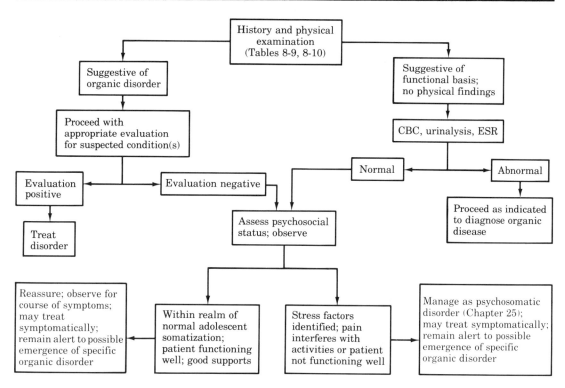

FIGURE 8-1
FLOW CHART FOR THE EVALUATION AND MANAGEMENT OF CHRONIC ABDOMINAL PAIN

disorder. Congenital problems should make their appearance well before this age. Some controversy exists over asymptomatic bacteriuria in adolescent females and, if it exists, over its significance. In any event, this is not a common cause of chronic abdominal pain. A sexual history, however, should not be overlooked; chronic, low-grade pelvic inflammatory disease is one of the more difficult conditions to distinguish from a functional basis for lower abdominal pain.

Even if the patient's pain is functional (psychogenic), the patient still perceives it as real, nor does he or she make any association between the symptoms and emotional stress. It is essential that the pain be accepted on the patient's terms without debunking or implying that it is all in the patient's mind. Indeed, such pain may well be mediated through a biologic pathway, as with the spastic bowel syndrome. Hasty psychiatric referrals made before motivational groundwork has been laid often are rejected, the patient and parents feeling the

physician to be insensitive and disbelieving. This then leads to the common situation of the family's continued "shopping" in a fruitless search for an organic answer.

It will be useful to take adequate time in the beginning to respond to the pain itself, ensuring that the patient feels his or her complaints are taken seriously. At the same time, psychosocial evaluation and counseling about identified problems can be instituted (Chapter 23). After dealing with each aspect for several visits, patient insight as to the association between symptoms and life events usually can be achieved. In cases in which this is not possible, it is perfectly feasible to manage the pain on a symptomatic basis while dealing with stress factors in a separate manner. When the latter are resolved, the former generally will be unconsciously surrendered. If counseling is unavailing after several months, a mental health referral is indicated and usually will be accepted.

In some cases, no apparent psychologic stress

TABLE 8-10
COMMON CAUSES OF CHRONIC ABDOMINAL PAIN IN ADOLESCENCE

Disorder	Key symptoms and signs	Diagnostic measures
Chronic gastritis	Usually burning epigastric pain; may be peri-umbilical as in children. Occurs several hours after meals; relieved by ingestion of bland food. Sometimes exacerbated by stress. Major differential, peptic ulcer; symptoms tend to be less severe, less well defined.	Clinical trial with bland diet and ant-acids. Stool guaiac negative.
Peptic ulcer	As above; usually more severe. May have melena, history of hematemesis, anemia.	Upper GI series or endoscopy; stool guaiac.
Cholecystitis	Sharp or dull, colicky or persistent RUQ pain in a female. Classically exacerbated on inges-tion of fatty foods. A positive family history or hemolytic disorder commonly present. Physical exam variably reveals RUQ tenderness.	Sonography, cholecystogram.
Hepatitis	Epigastric pain, anorexia, sometimes vomiting. May have history of jaundice, light stools, dark urine, injection of drugs. Physical exam may reveal RUQ tenderness, enlarged liver.	SGOT, SGPT, other liver function tests. Hepatitis B antigen/antibody studies and mononucleosis tests may help specify type. Liver biopsy may be necessary if evidence of chronic hepatitis.
Fitz-Hugh–Curtis syndrome	Epigastric pain, RUQ tenderness in sexually active female. Commonly associated with pelvic inflammatory disease. More likely to be acute rather than chronic situation.	Liver enzymes; ESR and WBC may be elevated. Technetium or gallium scan may be consistent with perihepatic inflammation. Laproscopy reveals adhesions.
Regional ileitis	Generalized crampy pain. Variable diarrhea, anorexia, and/or weight loss. Pain dysfunc-tional; patient usually appears chronically ill.	Barium enema with ileocecal reflux. GI series with small bowel follow-through. Stool guaiac, ESR, and WBC may be abnormal. Colonoscopy with biopsy.
Ulcerative colitis	Generalized crampy pain with bloody diarrhea.	Barium enema, colonoscopy with biopsy, stool guaiac.
Constipation	Episodic sharp crampy pains, often in RLQ. History of infrequent and painful defecation. Sometimes blood streaking on toilet tissue, hemorrhoids. Stool palpable in colon, rectum.	Clinical trial with constipation treat-ment plan.
Chronic pelvic inflammatory disease	Variable pelvic pain, sometimes dyspareunia in sexually active female. History of incomplete-ly treated acute P.I.D. common. Pelvic exam may reveal adnexal masses, tenderness.	Sonography; culdoscopy/laparoscopy with culture in confusing or persistent cases. ESR may be elevated.
Dysmenorrhea	Crampy pelvic pain occurring at menses.	History.
Endometriosis	Severe dysmenorrhea.	History, sonography (sometimes reveals cysts), laparoscopy.
Mittelschmertz (rupture of ovarian follicle)	Episode of sharp lower abdominal pain (1-2 days) in midcycle of menstruating female.	History.
Pregnancy	Missed menstrual period(s).	Pelvic examination, pregnancy test.
Spastic bowel syndrome	Highly variable and inconsistent pain patterns. Often exaggerated by stress.	Absence of history or physical findings suggestive of above, plus history of stress association. Proceed with more invasive test, ruling out other conditions only if clinically justified.
Psychogenic abdominal pain	As for spastic bowel syndrome; may be same condition.	As above.

can be identified, and the patient seems to be doing well in all life parameters, to have good family and environmental supports, and to be only minimally inconvenienced by the symptoms. This situation usually reflects normal adolescent somatization. Young people in the midst of pubertal and psychosocial development tend to be hypersensitive and hyperresponsive to the minor gastrointestinal discomforts we all are heir to. Normal psychologic tensions also are easily expressed in somatic form consequent to the heightened focus on the body and body image issues. Here, all that is needed is reassurance, modest continuing support, and periodic review. Symptoms usually clear within a few months in parallel with the resolution of current developmental conflicts.

Hepatic and Pancreatic Disorders

OVERVIEW

Hepatitis (A, B, or non-A, non-B) is the second most common form of liver inflammation seen in adolescents, exceeded only by infectious mononucleosis (Chapter 15). Other viral agents that may produce liver disease on occasion include rubella, herpes simplex, varicella, cytomegalovirus, coxsackievirus, adenovirus, influenza, and mumps. Additional causes of hepatic injury are syphilis, tuberculosis, toxoplasmosis, schistosomiasis, ascariasis, amebiasis, various fungal diseases, certain medications (sulfonamides, aspirin, acetaminophen, isoniazid, propylthiouracil, nitrofurantoin, tetracycline, phenothiazines, phenytoin, haloperidol, oral contraceptives, among others), and the abusive sniffing of chlorinated hydrocarbons as may be found in cleaning fluids. Differential considerations also include gonorrheal perihepatitis (Fitz-Hugh–Curtis syndrome), Wilson's disease (hypercupremia), and Gilbert's disease (glucuronyl transferase deficiency).

Signs and symptoms of liver disease are variably manifest in right upper quadrant tenderness, hepatomegaly, anorexia, vomiting, clay-colored stools, dark urine, and jaundice. Abdominal pain, when present, may be exacerbated by eating and relieved by the knee-chest position. Splenomegaly also may be seen. Laboratory evidence of hepatic dysfunction includes elevated liver enzymes (SGOT, SGPT, LDH), alkaline phosphatase, urinary urobilinogen, and serum bilirubin. (Note: alkaline phosphatase normally exceeds standard adult values during growth; see Appendix I). Clotting studies may show an increased prothrombin time and partial thromboplastin time. The sedimentation rate and white blood cell count vary and depend more on the causal agent than the nature and degree of liver damage.

HEPATITIS A

Hepatitis A (infectious hepatitis, short incubation hepatitis, MS-1 infection) virus has an incubation period of 15–50 days and usually is transmitted by the fecal-oral route, although other mechanisms are possible, including parenteral administration (contaminated needles, infected blood or blood components), the consumption of virus-bearing shellfish from sewage-polluted waters, and through intimate contact of mucous membranes as in sexual intercourse.

In addition to the general clinical features of liver disease as already described, the patient may experience fever, malaise, lethargy, and posterior cervical lymphadenopathy. Significant laboratory findings frequently include an elevated erythrocyte sedimentation rate and abnormal liver function studies. Clotting dysfunction is less common, but a prolonged prothrombin time is particularly significant as the marker separating benign from clinically concerning disease. Major differential considerations in adolescents are other forms of viral hepatitis, infectious mononucleosis, and the Fitz-Hugh–Curtis syndrome. (Other conditions that may be encountered are cited in the overview.) The diagnosis of hepatitis A is confirmed by culturing the virus from feces or blood during late incubation or in the acute phase.

Asymptomatic and anicteric forms of the disease are common, whereas the presence of extrahepatic symptoms (arthritis, urticaria, erythema nodosum) or the progression to fulminant or chronic hepatitis is rare. Even if symptomatic, the course is relatively mild, but the patient may fatigue easily for several months.

Treatment is supportive with a high protein diet and rest. Intravenous fluids and electrolytes may be necessary if vomiting and dehydration are pronounced. Alcohol and oral contraceptives should be avoided for approximately 6 months. Stool and urine precautions are indicated for several weeks to prevent spread to other household members. (Note: There is little risk to those not in a close living relationship, such as class-mates in school.) Immediate contacts (family, dating partner, intimate friends, co-group home residents) should receive immune serum globulin prophylaxis intramuscularly at a dosage of 0.01–0.02 ml/kg or, alternatively 0.5 ml/kg for persons weighing under 50 pounds, 1 ml/kg if between 50–100 pounds and 2 ml if over 100 pounds. Higher doses (0.04–0.06 ml/kg or 1 ml, 2.5 ml, and 5 ml per kilogram for the above weight groups, respectively) are given to individuals who plan to be in tropical areas or developing countries for 3 or more months.

TABLE 8-11
INTERPRETATION OF HEPATITIS B ANTIGEN AND ANTIBODY TESTS*

HBsAg	Anti-HBc	Anti-HBs	Clinical interpretation
Negative	Negative	Negative	No hepatitis B infection past or present
Positive	Negative	Negative	Very early acute hepatitis B
Positive	Positive	Negative	Acute hepatitis B infection or carrier
Negative	Positive	Negative	Early convalescent or immune hepatitis B; not infectious
Negative	Positive	Positive	Past hepatitis B infection; immune
Negative	Negative	Positive	Past hepatitis B infection; immune

*HBsAg, hepatitis B surface antigen; anti-HBc, antibody to hepatitis B core antigen; anti-HBs, antibody to hepatitis B surface antigen.

Note: HBsAg is detectable early in the disease followed by a rise in anti-HBc, the anti-HBs, which neutralizes the virus. HBsAg usually disappears as anti-HBc rises but may persist indefinitely in some individuals and indicates the carrier state. Both antibodies also may persist for years.

HEPATITIS B

Hepatitis B (serum hepatitis, long incubation hepatitis, MS-2 infection) infection is most commonly transmitted by exposure to viral-bearing serum through the use of contaminated needles and by transfusions of whole blood or blood fractions (for example, cryoprecipitate, albumin, packed red cells). Fecal-oral spread and sexual transmission, however, also are possible routes. Symptomatology is similar to that of hepatitis A but with a longer incubation period (40–180 days). The onset tends to be more insidious, but the overall course often is more severe with a higher incidence of fulminant and chronic forms. Extrahepatic manifestations (arthritis, urticaria, erythema nodosum) are more common, occasionally anteceding signs of liver disease itself. Pruritus also is a more frequent feature.

Individuals at high risk of developing hepatitis B include those who are using illicit drugs by a parenteral route ("skin popping," "mainlining"), persons receiving frequent transfusions of whole blood or any if its component parts (patients with hemophilia, hemolytic anemia, aplastic anemia), and those with impaired immunity. Health professionals also are vulnerable if inadvertently innoculated with infected blood. Laboratory data are similar to those found in hepatitis A, although the erythrocyte sedimentation rate is more likely to be normal.

Various viral antigens may be identified in the patient's blood (Table 8-11). Surface antigen (HBsAg) is the more sensitive indicator of whole virus and, if present in the serum for 6 months or more, confirms that the patient has become a carrier, an event occurring 10% of the time. Carriers not only pose problems in transmitting disease to others but they themselves are at risk of ultimately developing chronic liver disease.

Most cases of hepatitis B resolve after 3–6 months without sequellae. Treatment is supportive as for hepatitis A. Prolonged posthepatic asthenia (excessive fatigue despite normal liver function tests) is common. A few individuals develop chronic persistent hepatitis, a benign and ultimately resolving situation in which liver enzymes remain elevated for 6–8 months while the patient is otherwise well (activity need not be restricted during this time). A rare patient will develop chronic active hepatitis (see following section) or acute fulminant hepatitis. In the second instance the patient often (but not invariably) has compromised immunity due to some other cause. Fulminant disease rapidly progresses to liver failure and the myriad of complications that may accompany this condition; these range from intravascular coagulation or the hemolytic uremic syndrome to all of the metabolic consequences of severely impaired hepatic function. Death is common.

Persons exposed to a contaminated needle or having sexual intercourse with an infected individual and those requiring frequent transfusions of whole blood or blood components should receive prophylaxis. This may be problematic, as high levels of hepatitis B antibody usually are not present in standard gamma globulin preparations (as is true for hepatitis A), and hepatitis B immune globulin is not always readily available. The prophylactic dose of hepatitis B immune globulin is 0.05–0.07 ml/kg given intramuscularly with a repeat dose in 25–30 days. Maximum benefit is achieved if given within 7 days of exposure. In light of the high price of this preparation, it would be most cost-effective to first check that the contact case does indeed have circulating antigen present (HBsAg). In its absence, the contact case either has hepatitis B in a noninfectious stage or another form for which B immune globulin is not indicated. Standard gamma globulin may be given at the same dose and schedule if the immune type is not available, but the degree of protection is unpredictable. Recently the FDA has licensed a Hepatitis B vaccine and has recommended its use for certain individuals at high risk for hepatitis (hospital workers, male homosexuals, drug users, sex partners of carriers who are HBsAg positive, neonates of carrier mothers and others.) See the reference by Krugman. Additional protection for patients requiring transfusions is achieved by prescreening all blood donors for HBsAg.

CHRONIC HEPATITIS

Individuals with elevated liver function test results for 4-6 months or longer have chronic hepatitis by definition. This is an all-inclusive general term for a number of forms of liver disease with similar clinical manifestations but differing histopathology. The term includes chronic active hepatitis, chronic persistent hepatitis, subacute hepatitis with bridging necrosis, subacute hepatitis with multilobular necrosis, postnecrotic cirrhosis, and massive hepatic necrosis.

Excluding the benign and ultimately self-limiting chronic persistent form, chronic active hepatitis is the next most common of these variations. Not only is this a possible complication of viral hepatitis but it also is sometimes seen in association with acne, obesity, chronic lymphocytic thyroiditis, rheumatoid arthritis, secondary amenorrhea, pleurisy, chronic diarrhea, Sjögren's syndrome, and other conditions. Recurrent episodes of anorexia, jaundice, right upper quadrant tenderness, hepatomegaly, and pruritus are characteristic. Estrogen appears to be a predisposing factor, accounting for the greater incidence of this condition in females and the likelihood of exacerbation with exogenous estrogen administration (oral contraceptives).

A wide variety of laboratory abnormalities may be detected, regardless of the type of chronic disease that exists singly or severally. These include abnormal liver function and clotting studies, an elevated erythrocyte sedimentation rate, elevated immunoglobulins, a positive LE preparation, and positive tests for smooth muscle antibodies, antimitochondral antibodies, and antinuclear antibodies. A liver biopsy usually is required to establish the precise diagnosis. Other causes of chronic liver impairment such as Wilson's disease, Gilbert's disease, cystic fibrosis, and alpha-1-antitrypsin deficiency, should be ruled out. The prognosis is variable but usually guarded; progression to cirrhosis and liver failure or hepatocellular carcinoma with time is common. Steroids and other immunosuppressive drugs may improve poor function, but whether they alter the ultimate course or not is uncertain.

FITZ-HUGH-CURTIS SYNDROME

N. gonorrhoeae and C. trachomatis may escape from the female pelvic organs via the fallopian tube, travel up the right colonic gutter, and seed on the surface of the liver capsule, producing inflammation and, occasionally, subphrenic abscess. The condition (the Fitz-Hugh-Curtis syndrome, or gonorrheal perihepatitis) is manifested by acute, sharp, severe right upper quadrant pain, sometimes radiating to the right shoulder. Other symptoms and signs variably include fever, nausea, vomiting, abdominal rebound, and/or rigidity, a right costal margin friction rub, pleurisy, and pleuritic chest pain. There may or may not be a symptomatic genital infection at the same time.

The erythrocyte sedimentation rate usually is elevated and tends to be higher than that seen with viral hepatitis (40 mm/hour or more). Commonly, liver function tests are entirely normal or only evidence a transient rise of liver enzymes. Serum amylase may be elevated in some cases. Ultrasonography and a technetium scan may or may not demonstrate perihepatic exudate or an abscess. Laparoscopy, however, is definitive and reveals perihepatic inflammation and adhesions. Cervical cultures for gonorrhea usually are positive, at least in the acute stage.

The differential diagnosis includes other causes of right upper quadrant abdominal pain such as hepatitis, cholecystitis, pancreatitis, peptic ulcer disease, pyelonephritis, pleurisy, pneumonia, pleurodynia, and pulmonary embolism.

CHOLECYSTITIS

Although a relatively rare disease in otherwise healthy adolescents, inflammation of the gallbladder (cholecystitis) is seen with sufficient frequency to warrant consideration when symptoms and a positive family history suggest this diagnosis. However, this is a common condition in teenagers with chronic hemolytic disorders (particularly sickle cell disease) in whom the formation of gallstones (cholelithiasis) is a frequent complication. Other factors implicated in the development of stones and inflammation are familial predisposition, recent dieting, pregnancy, oral contraceptives, parasitic infections, scarlet fever, salmonellosis, choledochal duct cyst, biliary tract malformations, cystic fibrosis, oxalosis, cystinosis, acute lymphoblastic leukemia, and abdominal trauma.

Cholecystitis usually occurs in the presence of cholelithiasis. Manifestations of chronic disease include episodic right upper quadrant or epigastric pain, nausea, occasional vomiting, flatulence, and exacerbation of the symptoms on ingestion of fatty foods (fatty food intolerance). The differential diagnosis primarily includes peptic ulcer disease and hepatitis, but adhesions due to Fitz-Hugh–Curtis syndrome, chronic pancreatitis and, sometimes, regional ileitis or giardiasis may give a similar picture. Acute cholecystitis is an acute abdominal condition with fever, severe persistent pain, nausea, vomiting, right upper quadrant tenderness, and abdominal guarding and tenderness. Icterus may be noted when the choledochal duct is obstructed by inflammation or stones.

An oral cholecystogram (in a nonicteric patient) or intravenous cholangiogram (in an icteric patient) usually demonstrates cholelithiasis, a nonfunctional gall bladder, or both. The white blood cell count, erythrocyte sedimentation rate, bilirubin and alkaline phosphatase levels may be elevated, particularly in an acute attack. (Note: Alkaline phosphatase normally exceeds standard adult values during the growth spurt and should be measured against adolescent values; see Appendix I.) Treatment is by cholecystectomy in the acute or postacute period together with the administration of broad-spectrum antibiotics in acute disease. Medical dissolution of gallbladder stones with chenodeoxycholic acid is under investigation.

PANCREATITIS

Inflammation of the pancreas may occur in association with many conditions, but most cases in adolescents are related to viral infections (mumps, infectious mononucleosis, coxsackievirus, hepatitis B, rubella, mycoplasma) or to drugs (alcohol, corticosteroids, oral contraceptives, chlorothiazide, immunosuppressive agents). Rarer precipitating factors include abdominal trauma, hyperlipidemia (particularly types IV and V), pregnancy, diabetes mellitus, peptic ulcer disease, systemic lupus erythematosus, porphyria, cystic fibrosis, biliary tract disease, hyperparathyroidism, and septic shock. In a certain number of cases no cause can be found.

The course may be acute or chronic, mild or severe, recurrent or only a single episode. Symptoms include nausea, vomiting (often exacerbated by eating), fever, and constant right upper quadrant or epigastric pain with tenderness, which may radiate to the back. Some relief may be obtained by the knee-chest position. Significant laboratory data include leukocytosis, elevated serum amylase and lipase levels, elevated amylase clearance, and an amylase/creatinine clearance ratio greater than 5.5%. The serum amylase often is elevated only during the first few days, but the amylase clearance tends to remain abnormal for a somewhat longer time. Evaluation of pancreatic exocrine function and structure may be indicated in chronic or recurrent disease and includes the pancreozymin test, a 72-hour stool specimen for fat analysis, abdominal x-rays, pancreatic scan, ultrasonography, computerized axial tomography, and/or pancreatic biopsy.

Treatment is supportive. Pancreatic secretion should be minimized by giving nothing by mouth, instituting nasogastric drainage, and administering anticholinergic drugs. Intravenous fluid and electrolyte replacement should take gastric as well as other body losses into account. The pain often is sufficiently severe to require analgesia and sedation. Surgery may be necessary in resistant cases.

Bibliography

Ackley, A., and Gocke, D. D. 1980. Viral hepatitis. *Am. Family Phys.* 21:156.

Angelides, A., and Fitzgerald, J. F. 1981. Pharmacologic advances in the treatment of gastrointestinal diseases. *Pediatr. Clin. North Am.* 28(1):95–112.

Arko, F. R. 1980. Anorectal disorders. *Am. Family Phys.* 22:121.

Bain, H. W. 1974. Chronic vague abdominal pain in children. *Pediatr. Clin. North Am.* 21:991.

Ballantine, T. V. N. 1981. Appendicitis. *Surg. Clin. North Am.* 61:1117.

Bartlett, J. G. 1981. Antibiotic-associated pseudomenbranous colitis. *Hosp. Pract.* 16(12):85.

Brown, R. B. 1980. Vesicular and ulcerative infections of the mouth and oropharynx. *Postgrad. Med.* 67:107.

Cartwright, G. E. 1978. Diagnosis of treatable Wilson's disease. *N. Engl. J. Med.* 298:1347.

Czaja, A. J., and Davis, G. L. 1982. Hepatitis Non A, Non B: Manifestations and implications of acute and chronic disease. *Mayo Clin. Proc.* 57:639–652.

Dhar, G. J., and Soergel, K. H. 1979. Principles of diarrhea therapy. *Am. Family Phys.* 19:164.

Farmer, R. G.; Ferguson, R.; and Sivak, M. O., editors. 1981. Update on digestive disorders. *Primary Care* 8:179.

Feinberg, L. E. 1980. Treating duodenal ulcer: antacids or cimetidine? *Am. Family Phys.* 21:83.

Fitzgerald, J.; Angelides, A.; and Wyllie, R. 1981. The hepatitis spectrum. *Curr. Probl. Pediatr.* 11(11):3–51.

Fitzgerald, J. F., and Clark, J. H. 1982. Chronic diarrhea. *Pediatr. Clin. North Am.* 29(1):221–232.

Graham, J. 1978. Rectal bleeding. *J. Family Pract.* 7:169.

Grand, R. J., and Homer, D. R. 1975. Approaches to inflammatory bowel disease in childhood and adolescence. *Pediatr. Clin. North Am.* 22:835.

Greydanus, D. E., and McAnarney, E. R. 1982. Menstruation and its disorders in adolescence. *Curr. Probl. Pediatr.* 12(10):1-61.

Gunn, A. A. 1981. Acute cholecystitis. *Practitioner* 225:491.

Isenberg, J. I. 1981. Peptic ulcer. *D.M.* 3-58.

Janowitz, H. D. 1982. Inflammatory bowel disease. *Adv. Intern. Med.* 27:205.

Jordan, S. C., and Ament, M. E. 1977. Pancreatitis in children and adolescents. *J. Pediatr.* 91:211.

Klein, H. 1982. Constipation and fecal impaction. *Med. Clin. North Am.* 66(5):1135-1141.

Kohl. S. 1979. Yersinia enterocolitica infections in children. *Pediatr. Clin. North Am.* 26:433.

Krugman, S. 1982. The newly licensed hepatitis B vaccine: characteristics and indications for use. *J.A.M.A.* 247:2012-2015.

Kurfees, J. F. 1981. Acute pancreatitis. *Am. Family Phys.* 23:154.

Leevey, C. M., editor. 1979. Symposium on treatment of liver disease. *Med. Clin. North Am.* 63:477.

Painter, N. S. 1978. Constipation. *Practitioner.* 224:387.

Schoenfield, L. J. 1982. Gallstones and other biliary diseases. *Clinical Symposia (Ciba).* 34(4):2-32.

Silen, W. 1980. The prevention and management of stress ulcers. *Hosp. Pract.* 15:93.

Silverberg, M., editor. 1977. Liver diseases in infancy and childhood. *Pediatr. Ann.* 6(5):8-113.

Snydman, D. R. 1982. Campylobacter gastroenteritis. *Am. Family Phys.* 25:133.

Steinheber, F. U. 1973. Medical conditions mimicking the acute surgical abdomen. *Med. Clin. North Am.* 57:1559.

Thomas, J. G. 1981. The ABC's of viral hepatitis—recent advances in laboratory differential diagnosis. *Primary Care* 8:643.

Thomford, N. R. 1979. Appendicitis. *Contin. Educ. Family Phys.* 11(12):49.

Winship, D. H., editor. 1980. Symposium on inflammatory bowel disease. *Med. Clin. North Am.* 64:1021-1232.

–9–
The Genitourinary Tract

Urinary Tract Infections
Cystitis □ Diagnosis □ Treatment
Asymptomatic bacteriuria □ Pyelonephritis
Renal Disease
Proteinuria □ Hematuria □ Glomerulonephritis
Nephrotic syndrome □ Nephrolithiasis
Enuresis
Male-Specific Sexually Transmitted Diseases
Nonspecific urethritis □ *Chlamydia trachomatis* urethritis
Reiter's syndrome □ Behçet's syndrome
Scrotal Disorders
Hydrocele □ Varicocele □ Spermatocele
Testicular torsion □ Acute epididimytis □ Testicular neoplasms
Prostatitis
Miscellaneous Disorders
Balanoposthitis □ Hypospadius □ Cryptorchidism □ Priapism

Urinary Tract Infections

CYSTITIS

Dysuria, frequency, hesitancy, urgency and occasionally, lower abdominal pain, low-grade temperature elevation, and gross hematuria are characteristic symptoms of acute bacterial cystitis. This condition should not be confused, however, with the urethral syndrome in which similar symptoms are due to irritation (bacterial, chemical, or mechanical) of the urethra alone.

Some 10%–20% of all females experience at least one episode of acute cystitis during their reproductive years. It is three to five times more common in females than in males. The relatively shorter female urethra and the proximity of the meatus to vaginal and rectal microorganisms predispose to ascending infection in a manner not experienced by males. Poor perineal hygiene, tight panty hose, fecal contamination, and vulvovaginitis are some of the common precipitating factors. The frequent association with coitus signals the additional need to inquire about sexual behavior and to determine the need for sex counseling and contraception. In contrast, cysti-

tis in the male is much more likely to be due to an abnormality of the genitourinary tract than a confluence of external factors (Table 9-1).

DIAGNOSIS

Laboratory support for the diagnosis of a urinary tract infection (UTI) includes pyuria of over 10 white blood cells per high-power field of spun urine sediment, a positive Gram stain with one or more bacterium per high-powered field of uncentrifuged urine and, most importantly, a positive urine culture with antibiotic sensitivities identifying the causal organism.

Ordinarily, a culture with over 10^5 bacterial colonies per cubic centimeter is required to establish the presence of infection. A 10^4–10^5 colony count, however, may be significant, particularly if the specimen was obtained by catheterization or needle aspiration or if the recovered organism is gram-positive, such as a coagulase-negative *Staphylococcus*. On the other hand, a *single* culture of 10^5 colonies per cubic centimeter of any of the Enterobacteriaceae—*Escherichia coli* in particular—may not be significant. A

TABLE 9-1
PRECIPITATING FACTORS
IN ACUTE OR CHRONIC CYSTITIS

FEMALES
1. Anatomic short urethra
2. Poor perineal hygiene
3. Coital irritation, change of coital patterns, new sexual partner ("honeymoon cystitis")
4. Vulvovaginitis
5. Vaginal or rectal colonization with pathogenic bacterial serogroups (viz. *E. coli*)
6. Pregnancy (abnormal ureteral peristalsis)
7. Bladder contamination secondary to douching
8. Vaginal foreign body

MALES OR FEMALES
1. Urologic abnormality with stasis and/or obstruction (urethral stenosis, abnormal valves, neurogenic bladder, ectopic ureter, nephrolithiasis, etc.)
2. Vesicoureteral reflux (primary or secondary to infection)
3. Instrumentation of the urethra (medical, masturbatory)
4. Urethral foreign body
5. Urethral trauma
6. Other foci of infection (direct extension from kidney, prostate, or hematogenous spread from distant site)
7. Lowered host resistance to infection
8. Presence of secretory IgA in bladder or urethra
9. Multiple antibiotic usage and development of resistant organisms
10. Infrequent or incomplete voiding on voluntary basis.

single positive culture correlates with true infection in four out of five cases with false-positives in 20%. Two positive cultures recovering the same organism increases the probability of infection to 95%. Mixed cultures, even if of substantial counts, usually indicate contamination. Obviously, some caution is indicated in interpreting culture results.

E. coli is the most common cause of isolated episodes of acute cystitis, being implicated 90% of the time. Chronic or recurrent infection, however, may be due to any of a wide variety of organisms in addition to *E. coli*, including *Klebsiella, Enterobacter, Enterococcus, Pseudomonas, Serratia*, and others. Recurrent infection may be with the same (relapse) or different (reinfection) agent; occasionally, two or more pathogenic strains are present at the same time, particularly after multiple antibiotic administration.

A single isolated episode of cystitis in females does not necessarily require investigation for an ana-tomic cause, particularly if external precipitants are identified. Two to three episodes of cystitis in a female within a span of 12–24 months, however, is clear indication for a full evaluation, including intravenous pyelography, cystoscopy, and a voiding cystourethrogram. In males, only one episode warrants a full evaluation due to the greater likelihood of a urogenital abnormality.

TREATMENT

In addition to attending to any identified precipitants, the infection itself should be treated by administering an appropriate antibiotic for 7–10 days (Table 9-2). A single-dose treatment procedure for cystitis (as 3 grams of amoxicillin) has been used by some clinicians and may become more common in the future. A cure may be claimed if the urine becomes sterile within 2 weeks, although a marked reduction in the urinary bacterial count will occur in 48 hours with an effective agent. Clinicians should be aware of new cephalosporins which are becoming available; these include cefoxitim, cefotaxime, cefoperazone, moxalactam, and others. They may have a therapeutic role in infections resistent to the antibiotics listed in Table 9-2.

Females who have recurrent episodes of cystitis despite the absence of any genitourinary abnormality may benefit from antibiotic prophylaxis (Table 9-2). When coitus appears to be a major contributing cause, 50 mg of nitrofurantoin or one-half tablet of trimethoprim-sulfamethoxazole taken immediately after coitus may be preventive.

ASYMPTOMATIC BACTERIURIA

The presence of 10^5 colonies per cubic centimeter of the same bacterial strain in three consecutive midstream urine specimens comprises asymptomatic bacteriuria in those without symptoms. This occurs in 1.2% of prepubertal school girls, but the incidence in adolescent females is difficult to ascertain due to the problem of vaginal contamination even in clean-catch specimens. Asymptomatic bacteriuria is uncommon in males.

Predisposing factors in some cases include pregnancy, urologic abnormalities, diabetes mellitus, and indwelling urethral catheters. But many cases, particularly in females, are idiopathic. Persistent bacteriuria should be evaluated according to the guidelines recommended for recurrent cystitis.

The significance of asymptomatic bacteriuria in the individual with a normal genitourinary tract is unclear. Affected sexually active females appear to have a higher incidence of postcoital cystitis, and those who are pregnant are more likely to develop pyelonephritis. In the latter instance, there may be

TABLE 9-2
ANTIBIOTICS AND OTHER AGENTS OF USE IN TREATING URINARY TRACT INFECTIONS

Drug	Therapeutic dose (p.o.)	Prophylactic dose (p.o.)
Sulfisoxazole*	One dose of 75 mg/kg; then 150 mg/kg/day up to 1 g q.i.d.	—
Sulfamethoxazole*	One dose of 60 mg/kg; then 60 mg/kg/day up to 1 g t.i.d.	1 tablet daily (h.s.)
Ampicillin*†	100 mg/kg/day up to 500–1000 mg q.i.d.	—
Amoxicillin	250–500 mg t.i.d.	—
Tetracycline*§	10–20 mg/kg/day up to 250–500 mg q.i.d.	—
Carbenicillin† (indanyl sodium)	1–2 tablets q.i.d.	—
Cephalexin†	25–50 mg/kg/day up to 250–500 mg q.i.d.	250 mg q.i.d.
Cephradine†	25–50 mg/kg/day up to 250–500 mg q.i.d.	—
Nitrofurantoin	5–7 mg/kg/day up to 100 mg q.i.d.	50 mg daily (h.s.)
Nalidixic acid	55 mg/kg/day up to 1 g q.i.d.	500 mg q.i.d.
Methenamine mandelate	500–1000 mg q.i.d.	500–1000 mg q.i.d. (acidify the urine)
Methenamine hippurate	—	1 g b.i.d. (acidity the urine)
Trimethoprim-sulfamethoxazole*‡		
Regular strength: 80 mg trimethoprim, 400 mg sulfamethoxazole	2 tablets b.i.d.	½ tablet daily (h.s.)
Double strength: 160 mg trimethoprim 800 mg sulfamethoxazole	1 tablet b.i.d.	—

*Appropriate agents for most episodes of acute cystitis (e.g., *E. coli*).

†Agents that are safe to use if renal insufficiency is present.

‡Best agent for males with cystitis secondary to prostatitis; most effective in penetrating and sterilizing prostatic secretions.

§Do not use in pregnancy, as tetracycline is deposited in fetal teeth and bones.

an increased risk of infection to the fetus as well. Treatment of asymptomatic bacteriuria in otherwise healthy individuals is controversial. A course of antibiotics can be tried and prophylaxis considered if bacteriuria recurs.

PYELONEPHRITIS

Symptoms of acute cystitis together with fever, chills, costovertebral tenderness, elevated white blood cell count, elevated erythrocyte sedimentation rate, and positive urine cultures (see discussion of cystitis) are characteristic findings in acute pyelone-phritis (infection of the renal pelvis and medulla). Sometimes the presentation is less clear, with only a low-grade fever, simple backache, and/or abdominal pain.

Contributing causal factors are similar to those for cystitis, although there is a much higher association with urogenital abnormalities in females as well as males. Here, too, *E. coli* predominates in isolated episodes, but other agents also are likely to be involved in chronic disease. Vesicoureteral reflux may occur due to bacterial endotoxin inhibition of ureteral peristalsis, even in individuals with normal

TABLE 9-3
DIAGNOSTIC PROCEDURES
FOR PERSISTENT PROTEINURIA*

1. Repeat urinalysis to ensure abnormal findings are not transient.
2. Evaluate for orthostatic proteinuria by comparing daytime (upright) and nighttime (recumbent) urine specimens.
3. 24-hour urine collection (no preservative needed) for total protein and, possibly, protein electrophoresis.
4. Urine culture for bacteria plus antibiotic sensitivities; also culture for tuberculosis or fungi if clinically suspect.
5. Complete blood count and erythrocyte sedimentation rate.
6. Serum blood urea nitrogen and creatinine.
7. Total serum protein, serum albumin.
8. Creatinine clearance.
9. Serum protein electrophoresis.
10. Serum complement (C_3, C_4 particularly) and cryoimmunoglobulin.
11. Other blood tests: electrolytes, calcium, phosphorus, alkaline phosphatase, cholesterol, hepatitis antigen, liver function tests, LE preparation, antinuclear antibody, rheumatoid factor, ASO titer, streptozyme and other antistreptococcal antibody tests, VDRL.
12. Clearance ratio for IgG and albumin or urine FDP (fibrin-fibrinogen degradation products); the higher the level, the greater the nonselectivity of the proteinuria.
13. Intravenous pyelogram (with radionuclear studies if visualization is poor); ultrasound and/or computerized axial tomography (CAT).
14. Inferior vena cavagram or selective renal venogram if renal vein thrombosis a consideration.
15. Renal biopsy.

*Steps 1–7 comprise a reasonable initial test battery to be performed in any evaluation; the remaining tests are selected according to diagnostic suspicions and clinical judgment.

ureters. Differentiation between upper and lower urinary tract infection is not always possible on clinical grounds alone. Evaluation of lactic dehydrogenase isoenzymes, immunofluorescent antibodies coating bacteria in the urine, and direct ureteral cultures may aid in this distinction.

Mild cases can be treated with oral antibiotics (Table 9-2) for 7–10 days on an ambulatory basis. Recent studies in adults also indicate that single-dose antibiotic therapy may be effective. If compliance is poor, this may be worth trying, provided followup cultures can be obtained. Those who are acutely ill and toxic warrant hospitalization. Following blood

and urine cultures, intravenous treatment with an agent such as ampicillin (2 g IV q 6 hr) should be instituted until the patient is afebrile for 24 hours or more; this is then followed by oral antibiotics (Table 9-2) for a combined total treatment period of 10–14 days. Gentamicin and/or tobrymycin may be needed to treat some infections due to gram negative organisms. A complete urologic evaluation is usually indicated at some point in patients of either sex after even an isolated acute episode. Chronic pyelonephritis is a complex, poorly understood entity. It often appears due to the combination of antibiotic resistant gram-negative organisms and urologic obstruction.

Renal Disease

Kidney disease is frequently silent until impaired function is sufficient to produce such specific clues as edema, uremia, oliguria, hypertension, or colic from urolithiasis. Many renal disorders have presented in childhood and, for the adolescent, pose the serious problems of chronic or even end-stage renal disease, dialysis, and transplantation. Other disorders do not initiate until the teenage years, with diagnostic and early treatment issues predominating as clinical concerns. This section primarily discusses the latter situation, but reference should be made to Chapter 21 on chronic illness for issues relevant to adolescents with long-standing disease.

PROTEINURIA

Transient proteinuria is a relatively common event in many healthy individuals. Fever, strenuous exercise, extreme cold, and, possibly, emotional stress are thought to be contributing factors. The upper limits of normal for urinary protein loss have not been uniformly set, but most agree that the daily loss of over either 100 mg/m^2 or 200 mg total exceeds the normal range and requires further evaluation.

Vigorous exercise may be associated with proteinuria of up to 300 mg/day along with a few hyaline or granular casts and hematuria, but it clears within 24 hours. False-positive tests may occur in patients taking tolbutamide, large doses of one of the penicillins, or in those using sulfosalicylic acid. The administration of organic iodine compounds for diagnostic x-ray procedures may result in transient pseudoproteinuria with a positive heat-coagulation test but a negative dip-stick test.

Orthostatic (postural) proteinuria is characterized by a two to ten times greater excretion of urinary protein when upright than when recumbent. It may be persistent, intermittent, or transient and rarely exceeds levels of 1 g/day. Occurring in 20%

of normal individuals, this condition is thought to have no clinical significance. Diagnosis is by excluding pathologic reasons for the proteinuria and by the absence of protein in urine produced while lying down (for example, a first morning urine specimen collected before rising).

Persistent, chronic proteinuria may be due to various drugs, cardiac disease, pregnancy, or urologic abnormalities as well as primary renal disease. Benign persistent proteinuria has been described but is a diagnosis of exclusion after full evaluation and careful followup has failed to reveal any other cause. The loss of more than 1 g/day, however, is most likely due to renal parenchymal disease to be pursued according to guidelines offered in Table 9-3.

HEMATURIA

The presence of gross or microscopic blood in the urine may be due to any of a number of factors (Table 9-4). It should be kept in mind, however, that factitious hematuria occurs in females from 1–2 days before menstruation until 1–2 days thereafter and may be accompanied by factitious proteinuria as well. Products that give the urine a reddish, smokey, or dark appearance also should be ruled out, for example, urate crystals, beets, porphyrin compounds, bile, free heme, and myoglobin.

Transient hematuria is a frequent occurrence and usually of little clinical significance except as an indicator of other possible problems. It is commonly seen with urinary tract infections, generalized infections, or infections of other organ systems such as the respiratory tract, either bacterial or viral (adenovirus in particular). Hematuria also may occur with the ingestion of certain drugs (sulfonamides, cyclophosphamide, penicillin) and following trauma (both recognized and unrecognized as may occur in contact sports). Vigorous exercise or a period of strenuous training can cause hematuria and may be accompanied by proteinuria and casts as well, but the condition invariably clears within 24 hours.

Several forms of persistent or recurrent hematuria have minimal clinical significance. This includes benign familial hematuria and essential (benign, idiopathic) hematuria. The latter is without genetic predisposition: it may be an isolated finding or, in males, may be seen in association with upper respiratory tract infections.

Persistent or recurrent hematuria warrants a thorough investigation for an underlying cause. Evaluation includes those procedures outlined for proteinuria (Table 9-3) together with clotting studies, platelet count, tuberculin test, and urologic studies of the lower urinary tract (cystogram, voiding cystourethrogram).

TABLE 9-4
DIFFERENTIAL DIAGNOSIS
OF HEMATURIA (PARTIAL LIST)

1. Urinary tract infection (cystitis, urethritis, prostatitis, pyelonephritis)
2. Essential hematuria (idiopathic, recurrent)
3. Benign familial hematuria
4. Glomerular or tubular diseases
5. Hemorrhagic disorders (coagulopathies, platelet deficiency or dysfunction)
6. Hemoglobinopathies (viz. sickle cell disease)
7. Hemolytic-uremic syndrome
8. Henoch-Schönlein syndrome
9. Trauma
10. Systemic diseases (viz. systemic lupus erythematosus)
11. Nephrolithiasis
12. Urethral or bladder foreign body
13. Renal neoplasm
14. Renal tuberculosis
15. Subacute bacterial endocarditis
16. Various infectious diseases (mumps, rubeola, upper respiratory infections)
17. Leukemia
18. Allergic reactions (drugs, insect bites, etc.)
19. Alport's syndrome (chronic hereditary nephritis with nerve deafness)
20. Polycystic kidney disease

Treatment depends on the underlying cause. Hematuria per se is rarely sufficient to cause serious blood loss with shock or anemia.

GLOMERULONEPHRITIS

Poststreptococcal glomerulonephritis is the most commonly encountered form of this condition (Table 9-5) in children and younger adolescents. It is rooted, like the other forms, in immunologic mechanisms and demonstrates a diffuse glomerular and interstitial proliferative cellular response. The onset is 5–21 days following a streptococcal pharyngitis or pyoderma and often is heralded by the abrupt appearance of hematuria (red, brown, or smokey urine). Variable degrees of proteinuria, reduced serum complement, azotemia, edema, and hypertension are other clinical signs. Streptococcal antibodies (streptolysin 0, streptokinase, hyaluronidase, DNAase, NADase) are usually elevated. Acute renal failure, uremic encephalopathy, and the nephrotic syndrome are possible complications. Treatment is symptomatic plus antibiotics to eliminate any residual streptococcal infection. There appears to be no benefit from enforced bed rest or steroids. Most patients recover without sequelae and appear clinically well within 2–3 weeks, although

TABLE 9-5
OUTLINE OF GLOMERULONEPHRITIS

Type	General description	Treatment	Prognosis
Minimal change glomerulonephritis (nil lesion)	A common type of glomerulonephritis causing 70% of cases of nephrotic syndrome in children and 20% in adults. Formerly known as lipoid nephrosis. Renal function often remains good. A preceding history of upper respiratory infection, allergic exposure, or immunizations is common.	Steroids: 40–60 mg/m^2/day. High protein diet, restricted salt intake, diuretics.	Usually good response to steroids and good prognosis.
Focal sclerosing glomerulonephritis	Often presents with the nephrotic syndrome; occasionally with hypertension, elevated creatinine, or hematuria. Can be seen with heroin addiction, familial nephrotic syndrome, or chronic pyelonephritis.	As above.	Less responsive to steroids. Slow progression to renal failure common.
Membranous glomerulonephritis	Often presents with the nephrotic syndrome and hematuria with cylindruria. May be primary, or secondary to SLE, hepatitis B, drugs, sickle cell disease, Sjögren's syndrome, and others.	As above.	1/3, spontaneous remission. 1/3, features of the nephrotic syndrome remain but renal function normalizes. 1/3, steady progression to renal failure.
Membranoproliferative (mesangiocapillary) glomerulonephritis	Variable presentation with hematuria, nephrotic syndrome, or renal failure. Type I is associated with normal complement levels; type II with low levels of C_3 and partial lipodystrophy of face and upper torso; type II peaks in adolescence.	Cyclophosphamide Coumadin Dipyridamole	Variable. Poor prognosis if multiple crescents are present on renal biopsy. Recurrent bacterial infections with type II.
Diffuse proliferative glomerulonephritis	Presents with microscopic hematuria and proteinuria, occasionally as rapidly progressive glomerulonephritis. Poststreptococcal glomerulonephritis is the main example. Glomerulonephritis associated with subacute bacterial endocarditis or infected atrioventricular shunts has a similar histologic picture.	Usually supportive. Hypertension or edema may develop and requires treatment.	95% have an apparent recovery; 30% of older patients *may* develop a slowly progressive glomerulonephritis with renal failure in 20–25 years.
Focal proliferative glomerulonephritis (IgA/IgG nephritis or Berger's disease)	Frequently presents as recurrent, gross hematuria, often after an upper respiratory infection, gastroenteritis, extreme exertion, or cold exposure. Microscopic hematuria often persists. Nephrotic syndrome occasionally seen.	Supportive	Most have a benign course. 5%–10% have renal deterioration over many years.
Rapidly progressive (crescentic) glomerulonephritis	This is not a histologic diagnosis but a clinical term in which epithelial crescents are noted on biopsy. Can be primary or secondary. Often presents as acute nephrotic syndrome which worsens. Can be seen with Goodpasture's syndrome, Henoch-Schönlein nephritis, polyarteritis nodosa.	Variable	Rapid progression to renal failure in weeks to months (especially if over 50% of the glomeruli have crescents).

hematuria and proteinuria may persist for months. There is no increased risk of recurrence when rechallenged by a streptococcal infection, as in rheumatic fever, and prophylaxis is not indicated. Recent studies, however, suggest that individuals who have a history of streptococcal glomerulonephritis in earlier years are more likely to develop hypertension as an adult. Few patients with acute glomerulonephritis progress to a subacute or chronic form with progressive renal impairment.

Table 9-5 reviews other types of glomerulonephritis that may be encountered. Membranoproliferative (mesangocapillary) glomerulonephritis, type II, classically peaks in incidence during adolescence and is therefore particularly noteworthy. Diagnosis usually requires a renal biopsy. In addition to primary disease, secondary causes of glomerulonephritis also should be considered in the diagnosis. These include lupus glomerulonephritis, Henoch-Schönlein nephritis, polyarteritis nodosa, Goodpasture's syndrome, and various systemic or localized infections (staphylococci, enterococci, salmonella, pneumococci, *Treponema pallidum*, malaria, hepatitis B, infectious mononucleosis, variola, and others).

NEPHROTIC SYNDROME

Edema, hypoalbuminemia, proteinuria (over 3.5 g/1.73 m^2/day or, in children, 0.05–0.1 g/kg/day), hyperlipidemia, and lipiduria characterize the nephrotic syndrome. A variety of conditions have been implicated etiologically, with glomerulonephritis the most frequently involved (Tables 9-5 and 9-6), but no cause can be identified (idiopathic form) in three out of four cases. The degree of renal impairment is highly variable. Edema may be only periorbital or distributed widely with ascites. Evaluation should proceed as suggested for glomerulonephritis. Complement level may be a particularly useful test, being low in certain instances and not in others (Table 9-6).

Treatment is aimed at reducing protein loss, relieving edema without compromising the plasma volume, managing associated symptoms, and responding to the underlying cause. This may involve the use of steroids, thiazide diuretics, furosemide, ethacrynic acid, metolazone, antihypertensives, immunosuppressive drugs such as cyclophosphamide or chlorambucil, anticoagulants, and antiplatelet drugs. (Note: Cyclophosphamide may produce oligospermia in a pubertal or postpubertal male.) After an initial remission, chronic management often requires long-term steroid therapy, which creates its own problems: cushingoid appearance, exacerbation of acne, impairment of physical growth,

TABLE 9-6
DISORDERS ASSOCIATED WITH OR CAUSES OF NEPHROTIC SYNDROME

1. Idiopathic
2. Glomerulonephritis (acute poststreptococcal,* membranoproliferative*)
3. Systemic lupus erythematosus*
4. Polyarteritis nodosa
5. Amyloidosis
6. Henoch-Schönlein syndrome
7. Bacterial infections (including subacute bacterial endocarditis,* syphilis, tuberculosis)
8. Viral infections (including hepatitis B, cytomegalovirus, infectious mononucleosis)
9. Protozoan infections (including malaria,* toxoplasmosis)
10. Allergens (serum sickness, bee sting, inhalant pollen)
11. Neoplasms
12. Goodpasture's syndrome
13. Wegener's granulomatosis
14. Disseminated intravascular coagulopathy
15. Heroin abuse/addiction
16. Toxins (gold, mercurials, trimethadione, probenecid, etc.)
17. Diabetes mellitus
18. Mechanical obstruction (renal vein thrombosis, constrictive pericarditis, etc.)
19. Hemolytic uremic syndrome*

*Causes of nephrotic syndrome associated with reduced serum complement levels.

delayed puberty, and psychologic effects. Alternate-day therapy appears to obviate some of these problems and is the preferred schedule if the remisssion can be sustained. Current investigation with methylprednisolone pulse therapy may offer yet another alternative.

Complications of the nephrotic syndrome include protein malnutrition, thromboembolism, atherosclerosis, bacterial infections (particularly due to pneumococcal and gram-negative organisms with peritonitis a frequent form), the Fanconi syndrome, rickets, osteomalacia, and renal failure. Prognosis varies and depends on the underlying cause.

NEPHROLITHIASIS

Although nephrolithiasis is not a common condition among adolescents, it occurs with sufficient frequency to warrant its inclusion here. It also is a significant diagnostic consideration when a teenager presents with an acute abdominal condition or hematuria.

TABLE 9-7
NEPHROLITHIASIS

Type of stone	Description	Treatment
Calcium stones	Ca oxalate stones are radiopaque and may be due to hyperoxaluria (excess dietary intake of oxalate-containing foods, excessive intake of vitamin C, oxalosis, and others). Ca phosphate stones also are radiopaque and due to abnormal calcium metabolism. Together, Ca oxalate and phosphate stones are the most commonly encountered of all types.	Eliminate excess calcium intake; increase fluid intake (2500 ml/24 hours); administer thiazide diuretics, sodium phosphate, allopurinol, cellulose phosphate, and/or magnesium gluconate; treat underlying disorders of secondary hypercalcemia.
Cystine stones	Radiopaque; commonest cause of stone formation in young children and is an autosomal recessive with positive family history; accounts for 2%-5% of stones overall (including adults).	Increase water intake (over 3 L/day); alkalinize urine (15-25 g/day of oral sodium bicarbonate); penicillamine (1.5-2 g/day).
Uric acid stones	Slightly radiopaque; occur in hyperuricemic states (gout, neoplastic disease, diuretic treatment, diabetic ketoacidosis, renal failure, rapid weight loss, sickle cell anemia, lead poisoning, psoriasis, sarcoidosis, hyperparathyroidism, or hypoparathyroidism). Also can form with normal serum and uric acid levels. May be a history of frequent colic. Account for 5%-10% of stones overall.	Treat uric acid levels over 9 mg/ml with or without symptoms (probenecid; allopurinol, 300 mg/day); alkalinize urine, and restrict dietary proteins or purine; increase fluid intake.
Triple phosphate stones (struvite or infective stones)	Radiopaque; consist of calcium phosphate and magnesium-ammonium phosphate. Form in urine with pH over 6.5; often seen with ureteropelvic obstruction and urinary tract infections where gram-negative bacteria produce an alkaline urine and promote stone formation. May become exceptionally large filling renal pelvis (staghorn calculus). Accounts for 15% of stones overall.	Remove stone surgically; treat infection with antibiotics (acute and prophylactic), thiazide diuretics to decrease the urine calcium excretion; acetohydroxamic acid.

Crystals form in the urine when the concentration of a crystalline substance exceeds its solubility and precipitates out. This process usually begins in the collecting ducts and smaller calyces of the renal pelvis with progressively enlarging crystal deposits until a definitive stone is formed. The stone may vary in size from only a few millimeters to a large staghorn calculus filling the entire pelvis. The smallest stones tend to pass out in the urine unnoticed; slightly larger ones may appear as sand in the urine; still larger ones may lodge in the ureter and induce ureteral colic. Any stone that causes obstruction also predisposes the urinary tract to infection, one of the major causes of stones in the first place. Other contributing factors include urine stasis, a urinary pH that diminishes crystal solubility, deficiency of endogenous crystal inhibiting substances, and disorders that increase the concentration or amount of stone-forming substances in the urine.

The more important types of stones are summarized in Table 9-7 and the differential diagnosis in Table 9-8. Bladder dysfunction (particularly neurogenic bladder), chronic urinary tract infections, and exogenous steroids are among the more common contributory factors seen in adolescents, but a significant number of cases are idiopathic. Calcium oxalate and calcium phosphate stones are the most common types.

The presence of nephrolithiasis should be suspected in instances of acute and/or recurrent colicky abdominal (or flank) pain, hematuria, pyuria, recurrent urinary tract infections, or with a history of passing sand. A dietary history may reveal increased intake of calcium (excessive milk, cheese, ice cream, antacids) or oxalate (tea, oranges, cranberry juice, spinach, rhubarb). Large amounts of vitamins also may be contributory, as vitamin D promotes calcium absorption and vitamin C that of oxalate.

Evaluation depends somewhat on the type of stone. When available for chemical analysis, infrared spectroscopy is the preferred method. Stones frequently may be obtained by passing all urine through

TABLE 9-8
DISORDERS
ASSOCIATED WITH RENAL STONES

1. Urologic obstruction
2. Urinary tract infections (with stasis)
3. Medullary sponge kidney
4. Renal tubular acidosis
5. Alkaptonuria
6. Idiopathic
7. Primary hyperoxaluria
8. Cystinuria
9. Gout
10. Xanthinuria
11. Hypercalcemic states
    a. Hypercalciuria with hypercalcemia
       (1). Hyperparathyroidism
       (2). Sarcoidosis
       (3). Cushing's syndrome; steroid administration
       (4). Neoplasm
       (5). Immobilization
       (6). Hypervitaminosis D
       (7). Hyperthyroidism
       (8). Milk-alkali syndrome (due to increased intake of antacids with sodium bicarbonate)
       (9). Acromegaly
    b. Hypercalciuria with normal serum calcium
       (1). Idiopathic
       (2). Immobilization (casting, prolonged bed rest, acquired paraplegia/quadriplegia)
       (3). Exogenous corticosteroids
       (4). Some endocrine disorders
       (5). Distal renal tubular acidosis
    c. Normocalciuria with normal serum calcium and calcium stones
12. Others
    a. Munchausen syndrome
    b. Ethylene glycol ingestion
    c. Large amount of ascorbic acid ingestion
    d. Rhubarb overdose

a cloth sieve. Other laboratory tests include urinalysis, urine culture, the pH of a number of serial urine specimens, and a 24-hour collection for total calcium, uric acid, magnesium, oxalate, amino acids, and creatinine. Useful blood tests include serum calcium, phosphorus, alkaline phosphatase, uric acid, electrolytes, bicarbonate, urea nitrogen, creatinine, and protein. Radiologic studies include an abdominal flat plate, intravenous pyelogram, renal tomograms and, possibly, ultrasound or computerized tomography.

Treatment is based partly on the type of stone present (Table 9-7) and partly on the underlying cause. In addition, the pain of renal colic may be sufficiently severe to require narcotic analgesia; atropine or amyl nitrite can be used to reduce ureteral spasm. Surgical removal is necessary in some instances, but conservative management usually suffices, except in staghorn calculi. It is also possible to fragment bladder stones too large to pass through the urethra by the use of high-frequency sound waves through a cystoscope. Preventive measures (Table 9-7) should also be taken in patients at high risk of stones; in the adolescent age group this is most apt to be those with paraplegia or quadriplegia or a neurogenic bladder from some other cause, as well as those who may be immobilized for prolonged periods inducing calcium mobilization from bone and high urinary calcium output.

Enuresis

Enuresis, or the periodic involuntary passage of urine, is not an uncommon problem in adolescence, although frequently the young person will not reveal it unless directly asked due to embarrassment and humiliation. Approximately 4%-5% of young people have this condition at age 12, but only 1% or fewer by age 19, whether interventive steps are taken or not. In most instances (60%) the enuresis is primary, that is, has been present from early childhood without interruption. In 40% the condition is secondary —it appeared after at least 3-6 months total continence. Ninety percent of individuals with enuresis experience this problem only at night during sleep (nocturnal enuresis), but 10% experience it during the day as well (diurnal enuresis). More males than females are affected.

Most cases of primary nocturnal enuresis are idiopathic, but various constitutional and social factors have been implicated. These include a positive family history, low socioeconomic status, institutionalization, deep sleeping, and reduced bladder capacity. Psychogenic factors may be contributory but generally have been greatly overstated. An exception may be in secondary or diurnal enuresis without organic cause.

Organic causes of enuresis that should be considered include obstructive lesions of the urethra or bladder, other urinary tract abnormalities, urinary tract infection, diabetes mellitus, diabetes insipidus, psychogenic water intoxication, sickle cell disease, and mental retardation.

Patients with primary nocturnal enuresis demonstrating a normal physical examination, normal urinalysis, and negative urine cultures probably do not need any further evaluation. Secondary or diurnal enuresis is more likely to have an underlying organic cause; therefore an intravenous pyelogram, cystoscopy and, possibly a voiding cystourethrogram are indicated.

Treatment of idiopathic enuresis produces variable results; whether therapy or time is the critical factor is unknown in light of the high rate of spontaneous resolution. Two methods stand in favor today; tricyclic antidepressants and behavior modification conditioning devices. The latter are enjoying increasing favor. Some consider this the treatment of first choice because positive results are more probable and psychoactive drugs can be avoided. Whichever method is selected, the goal is to secure prompt relief from the humiliating symptoms. This is not a time for temporization and simple observation. Imipramine hydrochloride (Tofranil) may be given in the range of 25–75 mg at bedtime. An initial dose of 25 mg h.s. is gradually increased every 4–7 days until a therapeutic effect is achieved (with a maximum dose of 75 mg). This schedule continues for 1–2 months, then switches to every other night for 2–4 weeks, to every third night for a similar period and, finally, tapers to a total treatment time of from 4–6 months. If at any point enuresis recurs, the dosage and/or frequency of administration reverts to a previously effective level, continues for 2–4 weeks, and then is tapered again. Side effects of imipramine include restlessness, anxiety, poor concentration, weight loss, syncope, and constipation, although these tend to be less pronounced with a single bedtime dose than with divided doses during the day. Overdosage may be encountered when taken in an abusive manner or as a suicidal act; symptoms include coma, seizures, and cardiac arrhythmias.

If imipramine is ineffective, dextroamphetamine (15–20 mg) at bedtime can be tried, particularly in patients who sleep deeply. This has been somewhat less successful than imipramine but does offer an alternative. The problem of rapid tolerance and the possibility of abuse should be kept in mind; further, amphetamine is not approved for use in enuresis by the Federal Drug Administration and thus, is not available on Medicaid prescription.

A number of operant conditioning devices are available; the Enurotone is prototypical. A wired cotton absorbent pad is placed under the bottom sheet and connected to an alarm, which goes off when the pad is dampened by a small amount of urine, closing the circuit. The patient is awakened to the sensations of bladder fullness and micturition and rises to complete voiding on a voluntary basis. Bladder retention exercises have been employed with success on occasion; the patient is instructed to try to hold his or her urine for increasingly longer periods of time after experiencing the urge to micturate. Fluid restriction in the evening and rousing the patient to void when the last family member goes to bed may be helpful adjunctive measures but generally are futile in and of themselves. Counseling or psychotherapy can be tried, but have been minimally successful in ameliorating enuresis per se, although they may benefit emotional distress or coexistent emotional problems.

Male-Specific
Sexually Transmitted Diseases

Although most of the sexually transmitted diseases (STD) are dealt with in Chapter 17 and those which are general infections but commonly transmitted by sexual intimacy are covered in Chapter 15 (Table 9-9). We include here three disease syndromes of special relevance for males: nongonococcal urethritis, Reiter's syndrome, and Behçet's syndrome. In addition one should be familiar with the many STDs noted among homosexual individuals. Recent literature has implicated some unusual disorders, including cytomegalovirus infection, Pneumocystis pneumonia, and kaposi's sarcoma. Rectal and pharyngeal STDs are also noted in some homosexual youths.

NONSPECIFIC URETHRITIS

Nonspecific urethritis (nongonococcal urethritis, NSU, NGU) is a term used to describe symptoms similar to gonorrhea in males but without the presence of gonococcal organisms. This nomenclature simply reflects our ignorance and failure to isolate the causal agent, but, as discussed in the following sections, considerable progress has been made, and today NSU is recognized as a symptom complex that can be caused by any of a number of microorganisms, singly or in combination.

Chlamydia trachomatis seems to be the most common cause. *Ureaplasma urealyticum* is also implicated with some frequency and appears to be involved in balanitis and prostatitis as well. *Trichomonas vaginalis* is often asymptomatic in males but may be the responsible agent in 10%–15% of cases of chronic urethritis. *Neisseria meningitidis* urethritis can present with a white, mucoid urethral discharge and, sometimes epididymitis as well; a history of fellatio often is obtained, and the Gram stain is positive, but cultures for *N. gonorrhoeae* are negative. *Candida albicans* balanitis and urethritis may be a complication of broad-spectrum antibiotic use and/or coitus with an infected female; it usually resolves with local nystatin ointment and temporary sexual abstinence. *Hemophilus vaginalis* (Gardnerella vaginalis) may also cause male urethritis.

CHLAMYDIA
TRACHOMATIS URETHRITIS

The chlamydia (previously known as bedsonia) are obligate intracellular parasites that require tissue culture techniques such as McCoy's cells for isolation. Two species are recognized: *C. psittaci* (psittacosis) and *C. trachomatis. C. trachomatis* consists of a number of different subspecies that are immunologically and epidemiologically distinct and cause trachoma, lymphogranuloma venereum, cervicitis, or NSU.

C. trachomatis has now been identified as the causal organism in 30%–50% of cases of NSU and in 60%–70% of instances of postgonococcal urethritis (a symptom complex in which NSU appears 7–10 days or so after treatment of a gonococcal infection). It also has been found to coexist with gonococcus 30%–40% of the time. At least one-third of asymptomatic female partners of infected males have positive cervical cultures for *C. trachomatis*, but the incidence in asymptomatic males appears to be variable.

Symptoms of disease include dysuria with a clear, light, mucoid or heavier mucopurulent urethral discharge developing 1–3 weeks after coitus with an infected partner. There is a greater tendency for dysuria and a longer incubation period than with gonorrhea; differentiation, however, is not always possible solely on clinical grounds. *C. trachomatis* infection usually is a presumptive diagnosis based on the presence of urethritis without evidence of *N. gonorrhoeae*, unless McCoy's or other tissue culture techniques are available. This organism may also cause epididymitis, arthritis, proctitis, endocarditis, and others.

Treatment may be with tetracycline, doxycycline, erythromycin, or trimethoprim-sulfamethoxazole. Tetracycline, however, may be the preferred agent, as it is the one that also is most effective against *N. gonorrhoeae* and *U. urealyticum*. Recurrences are common.

REITER'S SYNDROME

Reiter's syndrome, a symptom complex predominating in males between 18–40 years of age (50:1-male to female ratio), consists of urethritis, conjunctivitis, arthritis, and mucocutaneous lesions in varying combination. Two epidemiologic forms have been recognized: one following bacillary, amebic, or nonspecific dysentery, the other related to sexual contact. The latter form is classified as a sexually transmitted disease and accounts for 1%–2% of all cases of NSU. *C. trachomatis* and the mycoplasmas have been implicated in some instances but not proven as causal. A strong association exists between Reiter's syn-

---

TABLE 9-9
SEXUALLY TRANSMITTED
DISEASES IN MALE ADOLESCENTS

1. Gonorrhea
2. *Chlamydia trachomatis* urethritis
3. Other causes of "nonspecific" urethritis (as *Ureaplasma urealyticum, Trichomonas vaginalis, Candida albicans, Hemophilus vaginalis*, and others)
4. Herpes simplex infections
5. Syphilis
6. Behçet's syndrome
7. Reiter's syndrome
8. Scabies
9. Pediculosis (*Phthirus pubis*)
10. Condylomata accuminata
11. Molluscum contagiosum
12. Chancroid
13. Lymphogranuloma venereum
14. Granuloma inguinale
15. Proctitis or other gastrointestinal infections due to *Shigella, Salmonella, Giardia, Entamoeba, Campylobacter*, and others.
16. Hepatitis
17. ? Cytomegalovirus infection
18. ? Kaposi's sarcoma
19. ? Pneumocystis carinii

---

drome and the histocompatibility antigen HLA-B27, this being present in 75% of affected individuals.

Urethral irritation and a mucoid or mucopurulent discharge are often, but not invariably, the first signs and develop several days to weeks after coital exposure. Urethral obstruction, prostatitis, or hemorrhagic cystitis (20%) also may occur. There is no satisfactory treatment of the urethritis, but it usually has been regarded as NSU and tetracycline administered. Thus a history of unresponsiveness to such treatment may be significant in the diagnosis.

Some 10–14 days later, the patient may experience an asymmetric, progressive arthritis, most commonly involving the knees and sacroiliac region. Achilles tendonitis and plantar fasciitis can be noted as well. Reiter's syndrome is one of the more common causes of arthritis in young adult males, with a differential diagnosis of ankylosing spondylitis, rheumatoid arthritis, psoriatic arthritis, and other forms of joint disease.

Other aspects of this disease emerge in a highly variable pattern over weeks to months. Possible manifestations include mild bilateral conjunctivitis (sometimes purulent) and acute unilateral uveitis. Cardiac lesions (conduction defects, pericarditis, myocarditis, and aortic valve disease) also may occur. Neuritis, transient hemiplegia, epistaxis, and pleurisy are other complications that have been noted in some cases. Various dermatologic lesions are encountered relatively frequently and include the following:

1. Keratodermia blennorrhagica (80% of cases): erythematous macules or erosions that become hyperkeratotic and involve the palms, soles, and/or nails.

2. Mouth lesions: asymptomatic, superficial, erythematous erosions on the buccal mucosa, palate, tongue, and gums.

3. Genital lesions: lesions similar to those encountered in the mouth but involving the glans penis (circinate balanitis), corona, and/or periurethral area.

Significant laboratory data include an elevated erythrocyte sedimentation rate, high complement levels in joint fluid, the presence of HLA-B27, and negative urethral cultures. Occasionally, normochromic anemia, leukocytosis, and/or positive stool cultures (shigella, amoeba, or other organisms) may be found.

There is no known cure, and treatment is limited to symptomatic measures with arthritis usually the most pressing complaint. In this instance indomethacin, phenylbutazone, and other nonsteroidal anti-inflammatory agents may be effective; aspirin is only minimally so. Uveitis may respond to steroid eye drops. The prognosis varies depending on the nature and severity of complications. Even though a remission can be expected, with symptoms subsiding spontaneously after 2-6 months, recurrences are common and occur in 60%-70% of cases.

BEHÇET'S SYNDROME

Behçet's syndrome is one of a group of arthritic disorders that are seronegative for rheumatoid factors (ulcerative colitis, Crohn's disease, ankylosing spondylitis, psoriatic arthritis, and Reiter's syndrome). An increased incidence of HLA-B5 has been reported. Behçet's syndrome is often regarded as a sexually transmitted disease of unknown etiology and is most commonly seen in males aged 15-40 years.

The hallmark of this disease is the appearance of single or multiple oral aphthous ulcers that are painful and resemble canker sores. Diverse genital lesions appear shortly thereafter in 80% of the cases and include erythematous macules, papules, pustules, aphthouslike ulcers (1-2 cm in diameter), or folliculitis. Oral and genital lesions heal spontaneously without scarring in 1-2 weeks but may recur at any time. Iritis or uveitis also appears in 80%. Other possible complications include polyarthritis (30%-60%), epididymitis, thrombophlebitis (33%), and central nervous system involvement. Blister formation or an inflammatory reaction may develop at the site of a venipuncture or scratch in some patients. Recurrent oral ulcers combined with two or more of the other possible manifestations are highly suggestive of this diagnosis.

There is no known effective therapy. Oral prednisone, cyclical hormone therapy (oral contraceptives), chlorambucil, cyclophosphamide, levamisol, and tetracycline have been tried with only limited success. Chronic eye disease or central nervous system involvement often bears a poor prognosis.

Scrotal Disorders

Various lesions may occur in the scrotum, the more common of which are discussed in this section. Table 9-10, however, indicates the full range of conditions that may be encountered and should be referred to in making a differential diagnosis.

HYDROCELE

A hydrocele is a cystic collection of clear or slightly yellow fluid within the tunica vaginalis or processus vaginalis. Most congenital, communicating types are detected in childhood. Occasionally scrotal trauma, epididymitis, or a testicular tumor is sufficiently irritating to produce an acquired hydrocele of the tunica vaginalis or spermatic cord.

Characteristic findings are a nontender, firm or tense, sometimes intermittent scrotal swelling, which transilluminates with a bright light. The testis on the affected side may or may not be palpable. Sometimes an inguinal hernia is present as well. Differential diagnosis includes a hernia, varicocele, trauma-induced hematocele, and testicular tumor.

Diagnosis is by clinical signs. Aspiration is contraindicated due to the risk of introducing infection or of bowel perforation if a hernia is present. No treatment is necessary if the hydrocele is asymptomatic and the youth is not distressed by its appearance. A hydrocelectomy is indicated for discomfort or cosmetic reasons and as an ancillary procedure in the course of repairing a coexistent hernia.

VARICOCELE

Varicocele is found in 15% of older adolescents and young adults. It consists of the tortuous dilation of pampiniform veins in the scrotum. A primary varicocele usually is left-sided and due to a faulty venous valve system allowing retrograde blood flow and pooling; the greater gravitational effect of a longer spermatic vein on the left may have something to do with this predilection. Secondary varicoceles usually are right-sided and due to mechanical venous obstruction in the lower abdomen or pelvic region, as may occur with a retroperitoneal tumor or kidney tumor. Varicoceles may be associated with infertility, but this is an infrequent event in the primary form of this disorder and most affected males are normally fertile.

Examination of the *standing* patient reveals dilated, wormlike cords running the scrotal length. A primary varicocele (usually left-sided) disappears in the recumbent position; a secondary varicocele (usually right-sided) does not disappear on lying down. This is an important distinction, as a secondary lesion requires a vigorous search for causal pathology, whereas the primary form needs no such investigation. In the latter instance no treatment is necessary unless warranted by oligospermia, physical discomfort, or psychologic distress. In such cases surgical excision may be done.

SPERMATOCELE

Spermatocele is a small, usually nontender cyst that develops from epididymal tubules. It transilluminates and contains milky, sperm-filled fluid. Evaluation should rule out a testicular tumor or other cause of a scrotal mass. Surgical excision may be done if discomfort or pain develops.

TESTICULAR TORSION

Improper containment of the testicle by the tunica vaginalis may result in a twisting of the spermatic cord with concomitant twisting and occlusion of the testicular and epididymal vasculature. This is a bilateral congenital defect, but the peak incidence of actual torsion does not occur until adolescence, when puberty undoubtedly introduces a facilitating effect. Usually, acute torsion is unilateral and only rarely bilateral. But even if only one side is involved, the patient is at risk for a similar episode occurring on the opposite side at a future time.

The patient with torsion classically experiences the sudden onset of acute scrotal pain accompanied by swelling and discoloration. Sometimes the onset is spontaneous; sometimes it is associated with exercise or trauma. Nausea and vomiting also may be present. Physical examination reveals the affected testicle to be very tender and lying in a transverse position high in the scrotal sac; the equally tender epididymis is in an anterioposterior rather than posterolateral (normal) position. Elevation of the testicle does not relieve the pain (negative Prehn's sign) and it does not transilluminate. There are no urethral symptoms, and the urinalysis is normal. A scrotal scan with technetium-99m demonstrates reduced perfusion.

TABLE 9-10
CAUSES OF SCROTAL PAIN AND SWELLING

1. Testicular torsion
2. Torsion of appendix testis (hydatid of Morgagni)
3. Torsion of appendix epididymis
4. Orchitis
5. Epididymitis
6. Acute idiopathic scrotal edema
7. Henoch-Schönlein purpura (with spermatic cord vasculitis)
8. Hernia
9. Hydrocele
10. Varicocele
11. Spermatocele
12. Hematocele
13. Testicular tumor
14. Generalized edema

Reference should be made to Table 9-10 for differential considerations. The most common problem is to distinguish between testicular torsion and epididymoorchitis. Such discrimination is urgent, and any case of even suspected torsion should be viewed as a potential surgical emergency. It is essential that the torsion be reduced and normal blood flow returned as quickly as possible. Irreversible infarction occurs in 5–6 hours and Leydig cell necrosis in 10–12 hours, although survival times up to 24 hours have been reported on occasion. When the testis can be salvaged, reduction of the torsion should be followed by fixation so that there will be no recurrence; a dead testicle should be removed with plans for a later prosthesis. In either instance, it should be kept in mind that the opposite testicle also is vulnerable to torsion; it, too, should be explored and fixed.

The appendix testis (hydatid of Morgagni) or the appendix epididymis also may develop torsion. Clinical signs may be indistinguishable from torsion of the entire testis or somewhat milder. If differentiation can be made, surgical intervention is not necessary and there is no damage to testicular function. If in doubt, surgical exploration is the treatment of choice.

ACUTE EPIDIDYMITIS

Inflammation of the epididymis can be precipitated by many factors, including urethritis, urinary tract infection, prostatitis, testicular tumor, urologic surgery, respiratory tract infection, genitourinary tuberculosis, mumps, other viral infections, and bacterial infections capable of hematogenous spread. Chlamydial or gonococcal urethritis and idiopathic disease (in 40%–60%) account for most cases in adolescents. Idiopathic epididymitis may be related to trauma or exercise-induced reflux of sterile urine through the vas deferens with a resultant chemical irritation. In some instances, inflammation involves the testicle as well, producing epididymoorchitis.

Epididymitis is marked by the gradual or sudden onset of epididymal pain, tenderness, and local swelling. Inflammation may be mild or severe. In contrast to torsion, elevation of the testicle and epididymis does relieve pain (positive Prehn's sign). Urethritis, symptoms simulating cystitis, fever, toxicity, pyuria, bacteriuria, and positive urethral cultures are variable findings. A scrotal scan with technetium-99m reveals increased vascularity (in torsion it is decreased). Persistence of inflammation for more than 14 days suggests a coexistent testicular tumor; this presents in conjunction with epididymitis 10% of the time. Table 9-11 outlines treatment. Surgical exploration is indicated if testicular torsion has not been ruled out promptly by clinical and laboratory findings.

TESTICULAR NEOPLASMS

The incidence of testicular tumors is 1.0 per 100,000 males in the 15–19 year age group. Although less common than lymphomas, leukemia, bone tumors, and tumors of the central nervous system, testicular neoplasms occur with sufficient frequency to mandate examination of the testes in all "routine" physical examinations and to educate the adolescent to palpate his gonads himself on a regular basis. Moreover, when the young male becomes an adult, testicular tumors will be the most common solid neoplasm he may encounter until over 39 years of age; inculcating self-examination habits early will have long-term benefits.

Two tumor types, both of germ cell origin, predominate: seminoma and embryonal carcinoma. Functional non-germ cell tumors, however, can be encountered on occasion (interstitial cell, Sertoli cell, or granulosa cell) and may be associated with precocious puberty, persistent gynecomastia, or feminization. Patients with ectopic or undescended testes are at greater risk for testicular tumors than the population at large; other predisposing factors are unknown.

A painless, firm, unilateral testicular mass should raise a high index of suspicion for this diagnosis. Evaluation includes a biopsy together with a thorough staging of the progression of the disease by means of a chest roentgenogram, intravenous pyelogram, skeletal survey, liver scan, lymphangio-

TABLE 9-11
TREATMENT OF EPIDIDYMITIS

1. Bedrest
2. Scrotal elevation (by means of a towel placed between the legs and an athletic supporter)
3. Analgesics
4. Infiltration of the spermatic cord with a local anesthetic
5. Antibiotics
    a. Tetracycline hydrochloride (500 mg q.i.d. for 10 days)*
    b. Doxycycline (100 mg b.i.d. for 10 days)*
    c. Ampicillin (500 mg q.i.d. for 10 days)
    d. Cephalothin (500 mg q.i.d. for 10 days)
6. Antiinflammatory drugs (oxyphenbutazone, steroids) for severe disease

*Preferred agents due to their broad-spectrum coverage, including gonococcus and chlamydia.

gram, 17 ketosteroids, gonadotropins, pregnancy test (chorionic gonadotropins), and alpha-fetoprotein. Unfortunately, by the time a first diagnosis has been made, 20% of the patients already will have metastases to the retroperitoneal lymph nodes, lungs, liver, and/or bones.

Treatment includes radical orchiectomy, chemotherapy, and/or radiotherapy. The survival rate depends on the tumor type and clinical staging. The best outlook is with a seminoma; it is highly radiosensitive and afflicted patients have a 90% 5-year survival rate.

Prostatitis

Infection of the prostate is less common in adolescents than in adults, but it can occur on occasion in the teenage years, usually as a complication of some other urogenital infection. Contributing factors include urethritis, urinary tract infections, sepsis, and urethral instrumentation. *E. coli* is the most commonly implicated organism, but gonococcus is not far behind. The prostate increasingly is recognized as the reservoir for gonococcus in asymptomatic male carriers; this condition may be accompanied by prostatic enlargement in some instances. A number of other cases are caused by *Staphylococcus* or *Streptococcus*. Recent literature also implicates *C. trachomatis*.

Acute prostatitis is variably characterized by fever, dysuria, frequency, painful erection or ejaculation, painful defecation, constipation, perineal discomfort and, sometimes, lower abdominal or lower back pain. Rectal examination reveals a large, tender, boggy prostate, but this also may be noted in some healthy individuals and is an equivocal finding. (Vigorous examination or massage should be avoided in *acute* disease to avoid precipitating hematogenous spread.)

Recurrent prostate infection is common and most often due to residual bacteria, this tissue being relatively resistant to penetration by antibiotics. Recurrent urinary tract infections may occur as well. Differentiation between prostatitis and cystitis is made by comparing bacterial colony counts of prostatic fluid (ejaculate) and urine; prostatic infection is indicated by a tenfold higher count.

Treatment is with antibiotics (ampicillin, tetracycline, cephalosporins, sulfas) for at least 10–14 days in acute cases and up to 28 days in chronic cases. A 6–12 week course has been used for some chronic cases. Trimethoprim-sulfamethoxazole (two tablets standard strength b.i.d. or q.i.d.) is the preferred drug if causal organisms are sensitive, as it appears to penetrate prostatic tissues in higher concentrations than other antimicrobial agents. Highly febrile and toxic patients should be hospitalized and treated intravenously. Chronic disease is particularly difficult to eradicate and has a high recurrence rate; weekly massage as an adjunctive measure to antibiotics may be helpful.

Miscellaneous Disorders

BALANOPOSTHITIS

Inflammation of the penile prepuce (posthitis), penile glans (balanitis), or both may be due to phimosis (inability to retract the prepuce), masturbation injury, urethritis or, on occasion, paraphimosis (inability to replace the retracted prepuce). Treatment involves oral antibiotics and antibiotic compresses. The role of circumcision in this condition is controversial, but probably it is not necessary in most cases.

HYPOSPADIAS

Ventral displacement of the urethral meatus is a congenital abnormality that should have been recognized and dealt with by surgical correction in childhood. Several aspects, however, have significance for the adolescent. First, recent evidence supports a possible association of hypospadias with diethylstilbestrol (DES) exposure in utero. Other recognized correlates are epididymal cysts and reduced sperm density. Thus the presence of hypospadias should lead to inquiries about DES exposure, which in turn should lead to evaluation of possible infer-

tility and counseling at an appropriate time. Second, a few males with this condition may also have a chordee (ventral bowing of the penis); it may not be particularly noticeable in the flaccid state but becomes readily apparent, and distressing, upon erection. Inquiries about a possible chordee are indicated in the pubertal male with hypospadias; surgical release should be carried out if the condition is present.

CRYPTORCHIDISM

Cryptorchidism is a genitourinary problem of childhood (which should be corrected by orchiopexy between the ages of 2–4 years) that also has significance for the adolescent. Causes of cryptorchidism include primary testicular defects or infarction before proper descent. Delayed surgery may also result in a permanently damaged gonad. A small, atrophic testis invariably prompts concern in the adolescent about his normalcy, sexual competence, and fertility. These matters should be responded to by evaluating hormonal levels (usually adequate), spermatogenesis (may be impaired in bilateral disease), and counseling. A single small atrophic testis, even if in a proper location, may warrant removal and replacement with a proper-sized prosthesis, matching the opposite and normal side.

Adolescents with intraabdominal testes that have not been removed face a significant risk of developing a seminoma at any time. Surgical removal should be carried out promptly on diagnosis and a prosthesis inserted in the scrotal sac.

PRIAPISM

Persistent painful erection is not a common event in adolescents except those with sickle cell disease, in whom it may be a complication of crisis. In this instance, failure to detumesce is thought due to occlusion of the venules draining the corpora cavernosa into the dorsal vein of the penis. In the rarer instances of idiopathic priapism, there may be a congenital faulty valve mechanism. An episode of priapism from any cause may last minutes to days. Twenty-four hours, however, is a critical point, as persistence beyond this time results in blood sludging, anoxia, and tissue damage. In turn, this frequently leads to fibrosis and impotence. Unfortunately, afflicted adolescents frequently present for medical attention quite late due to embarrassment about the awkwardness of this situation.

Male adolescents with sickle cell disease and those who have had an idiopathic episode (and thereby are at risk of recurrence) should be advised to seek prompt assistance for this condition. Any patient whose priapism lasts more than an hour or two should be hospitalized and a urologic consultation obtained. Conservative measures include bed rest, warm compresses, and sedation, together with appropriate measures for a sickle cell crisis if coexistent. Failing results with these methods, irrigation of the corpora cavernosa and surgical reestablishment of a venous pathway should be carried out.

Bibliography

Babb, R. R. 1980. Evaluation of acute proctitis. *J.A.M.A.* 244-358.

Bayer, A. S. 1980. Gonococcal arthritis syndrome. An update on diagnosis and management. *Postgrad. Med.* 67:200.

Berger, O. G. 1980. Varicocelled in adolescents. *Clin. Pediatr.* 19(12):810.

Bergstein, J. M. 1982. Hematuria, proteinuria and urinary tract infections. *Pediatr. Clin. North Am.* 29:55.

Calabro, J. J.; Garg, S. L.; Khoury, M. I.; et al. 1974. Reiter's syndrome. *Am. Family Phys.* 9:80.

Cassell, G. H., and Cole, B. C. 1981. Mycoplasmas as agents of human disease. *N. Engl. J. Med.* 304:80.

Cattran, D. C. 1978. Glomerulonephritis. *Primary Care* 5:21.

Corey, L. 1982. The diagnosis and treatment of genital herpes. *J.A.M.A.* 248:1041.

Cunha, B. A. 1981. Urinary tract infections. *Postgrad. Med.* 70:141.

Durack, D. T. 1981. Opportunistic infections and Kaposi's sarcoma in homosexual men. *N. Engl. J. Med.* 305:1465.

Felman, Y. M. 1980. Homosexual hazards. *Practitioner* 224:1151.

Fiumara, N. J. 1982. Scabies and genital herpes: a problem in management. *Am. Family Phys.* 25:125.

Fiumara, N. J. 1981. Treating gonorrhea. *Am. Family Phys.* 23:123.

Fraley, E. E.; Lange, P. H.; and Kennedy, B. J. 1979. Germ-cell testicular cancer in adults. *N. Engl. J. Med.* 301:1370.

Gonorrhea. C.D.C. recommended treatment schedules, 1979. 1979. *M.M.W.R.* 28(2):13.

Gott, L. J. 1977. Common scrotal pathology. *Am. Family Phys.* 15:164.

Govan, D. E., and Kessler, R. 1980. Urologic problems in the adolescent male. *Pediatr. Clin. North Am.* 27:109.

Greydanus, D. E., and McAnarney, E. R. 1979. Vulvovaginitis in the adolescent. *J. Curr. Adol. Med.* 1(1):56; 1(2):52; 1(4):40.

Greydanus, D. E., and McAnarney, E. R. 1980. Chlamydia trachomatis. An important sexually transmitted disease in adolescents and young adults. *J. Family Pract.* 10:611.

Greydanus, D. E., and Schaff, E. 1981. Gonococcal perihepatitis. (Fitz-Hugh-Curtis syndrome). *J. Curr. Adol. Med.* 3(2):9.

Handsfield, H. H. 1982. Sexually transmitted diseases. *Hosp. Pract.* 17:99.

Lynch, P. J. 1982. Therapy of sexually transmitted diseases. *Medical Clin. North Am.* 66:915.

Mearnes, E. M. 1980. Prostatitis and related diseases. *D.M.* 26(8):3-40.

Nagar, D., and Wathen, R. L. 1979. Nephrotic syndrome. *Primary Care* 6:541.

Nissenson, A. R.; Baroff, L. J.; Fine, R. N.; et al. 1979. Poststreptococcal acute glomerulonephritis: fact and controversy. *Ann. Intern. Med.* 91:76.

O'Duffy, J. D. 1978. Summary of international symposium on Behçet's disease. *J. Rheumatol.* 5(2):229.

Owen, W. F. 1980. Sexually transmitted diseases and traumatic problems in homosexual men. *Ann. Intern. Med.* 92:805.

Panwalker, A. P. 1981. Modern management of urinary tract infections. *Drug Ther.* 11(4):73.

Rambar, A. C., and MacKenzie, R. G. 1978. Urolithiasis in adolescents. *Am. J. Dis. Child.* 132:1117.

Rein, M. F., and McCormack, W. M., editors. 1981. Changing epidemiologic patterns in sexually transmitted diseases: therapeutic implications. *Sex. Trans. Dis.* 8(2):93-174.

Riff, L. J. M. 1978. Evaluation and treatment of urinary tract infection. *Med. Clin. North Am.* 62:1183.

Schmitt, B. D. 1982. Daytime wetting (diurnal enuresis) and nocturnal enuresis: an update on treatment. *Pediatr. Clin. North Am.* 29:9-36.

Sparling, P. F. 1979. Current problems in sexually transmitted diseases. *Adv. Intern. Med.* 24:203.

Tu, W. H. 1978. Work-up of the patient with suspected renal disease. *Primary Care* 5:1.

Ward, M. S. 1978. The office determination of proteinuria in adolescents. *Pediatr. Ann.* 7(9):97.

Wiesner, P. J., and Thompson, S. E. 1980. Gonococcal diseases. *D.M.* 26(5):3-44.

Zornow, D. H., and Landes, R. R. 1981. Scrotal palpation. *Am. Family Phys.* 23:150.

–10–
Neurologic Disorders

Seizure Disorders
Overview □ Classification □ Special considerations in drug treatment
Psychologic and social aspects
Headaches
Migraine headaches □ Classification
Tension headaches □ Other headache complexes
Papilledema
Benign intracranial hypertension □ Pseudopapilledema
Vertigo and Dizziness
Syncope
Vasovagal syncope □ Orthostatic hypotension
Postmicturition syndrome □ Narcolepsy □ Voluntary syncope
Coma and Semicoma
Meningitis
Brain abscess □ Bacterial meningitis □ Viral encephalitis
Multiple Sclerosis
Guillain-Barré Syndrome
Bell's Palsy
Miscellaneous Disorders
Muscular dystrophy □ Myotonic dystrophy □ Polymyositis
Peripheral neuropathy □ Cerebral palsy □ Neurocutaneous syndromes

Seizure Disorders

OVERVIEW

The annual incidence of a seizure disorder among 10–14 and 15–19 year old adolescents is 24.7 and 18.6 per 100,000 respectively. The disorders are therefore relatively common during the teenage years, either as a carryover from childhood or as a new event. A wide variety of underlying diseases may precipitate a seizure response (Table 10-1), but most cases are idiopathic, particularly in adolescents under 16 years of age. The probability of a causal space-occupying lesion increases with advancing age, but even though idiopathic forms gradually diminish in frequency, they still are commonly seen throughout the teenage years. Additional differential considerations include conditions that may mimic a seizure disorder such as hysteria, hyperventilation, vertigo, vasomotor syncope, migraine headaches,

narcolepsy, night terrors or nightmares, chorea, Gilles de la Tourette syndrome, and tardive dyskinesia, oculogyric crisis, or dystonia following phenothiazine ingestion.

Historical, physical, and laboratory evaluations focus on distinguishing between differential concerns and detecting possible precipitating factors (Table 10-1). Particular historic points of note are prenatal and perinatal events, family history, and past or present injuries, although it should be kept in mind that head trauma is ubiquitous in the life of children and the significance must be judiciously weighed. A careful description of the seizure itself and associated events will assist in classification and provide insight as to precipitating factors. Other points of note are directed by differential considerations. Dermatologic clues can be particularly important (see section on neurocutaneous syndromes). The electroencephalo-

TABLE 10-1
EVALUATION OF SEIZURES IN ADOLESCENTS

Differential diagnosis	Possible precipitating factors in idiopathic epilepsy seizures	Laboratory evaluation*
Infectious: bacterial/viral meningitis, encephalitis; systemic infection with fever, sepsis	1. Puberty	1. Complete blood count
	2. Menses	2. Urinalysis
	3. Trauma	3. Erythrocyte sedimentation rate
Congenital defects: AV malformations, porencephaly, etc.	4. Fever	
Trauma	5. Drugs (alcohol, phenothiazines, tricyclic antidepressants, antihistamines, others)	4. Calcium, phosphorous, electrolytes, urea nitrogen, creatinine
Neoplasms: CNS primary, metastatic		
Neurocutaneous syndromes: Sturge-Weber, tuberous sclerosis, neurofibromatosis	6. Psychologic stress	5. Blood glucose (fasting, tolerance test)
	7. Sleep/sleep deprivation	6. Toxic drug screen
Metabolic: hypoglycemia, hypocalcemia, hyponatremia, inborn errors of metabolism	8. Hyperventilation (with petit mal)	7. Amino acid screen
	9. Photic stimuli (flashing or flickering light, television)	8. Lumbar puncture†
Vasculitis		9. Skull
	10. Olfactory or tactile stimuli	10. Electroencephalogram
Cerebrovascular accident: ruptured aneurysm (congenital, mycotic), AV malformation, thrombocytopenia	11. Ingestion of certain foods	11. Computerized axial tomography (CAT)
	12. Reading	12. Brain scan
	13. Music	13. Arteriogram
Drug-related: withdrawal from anticonvulsant drugs, withdrawal from CNS depressant addiction (including alcohol), phencyclidine overdose	14. Laughter	14. Other as indicated by prior findings (blood culture, liver function tests, urine porphyrins, urinary VMA, etc.)
Hypertensive encephalopathy: primary, renal, coarctation		
Idiopathic		

*Perform those tests indicated by clinical judgment and clinical signs.

†Perform lumbar puncture only with great caution if cerebral bleed or increased pressure from other cause suspected. CAT may be safer as first procedure.

gram (EEG) should be performed while the patient is awake and, if possible, asleep, as well as during photic and hyperventilatory stimuli. The EEG, however, is only adjunctive to the diagnosis and may not be abnormal in every case.

CLASSIFICATION
Focal, psychomotor, grand mal, and petit mal epilepsy are the most common seizure patterns in adolescents. The majority of patients experience only one pattern, although mixed patterns of two or more types are common. The latter cases are more difficult to control.

Focal motor seizures. Focal motor (Jacksonian) seizures usually consist of a brief period of tonic and/or clonic movements beginning in a single body part and extending progressively to other muscle groups on the ipsilateral side. A more generalized convulsion sometimes is seen. Consciousness tends not to be impaired, although speech dysfunction or sensory symptomatology may occur. Previous trauma or CNS infection with residual scarring is often causally implicated; tumor, focal bleeding, or one of the neurodermatoses also must be considered in the differential diagnosis. Treatment usually is with phenytoin, phenobarbital, and/or carbamazepine (Table 10-2).

Temporal lobe or psychomotor epilepsy. Consequent to a temporal lobe focus, seizure pattern manifestations vary. Four stages are commonly seen. The prodrome is marked by irritability, confusion, headache, appetite changes, and/or pallor and can develop from hours to days before the aura. The aura itself is manifested in a few minutes of sensory disturbances (taste, smell, vision), psychologic aberrations (fear, rage, anxiety, depression, inappropriate laughter, mental confusion, hallucinations), abdominal discomfort, and/or lacrimation, among other symptoms. Ictus quickly follows with both motor and psychic components. Motor phenomena vary from simply staring to repetitive purposeless movements or complex automatisms (aimless walking, lip smacking, picking at clothes, picking at other objects, pulling at body parts), as well as aphasia, numbness, a choking sensation, headache, and gastrointestinal disturbances. Psychic components are similar to those experienced during the aura. The seizure (ictus) phase lasts from one to several minutes or longer and gradually abates, giving way to the postictal state with lethargy, hunger, and headache being the most common symptoms. Amnesia is often but not invariably present. There may be many episodes each day, or attacks may only occur at widely spaced intervals. Diagnosis can be difficult and requires a high index of suspicion, particularly in adolescents having bizarre or disturbed behavior. Misdiagnosis in ascribing a psychiatric cause is common. An EEG with an additional nasopharyngeal lead may demonstrate a temporal lobe focus, although this is not always the case, as the tracing can be normal during the seizure-free state. Response to antiseizure medication (phenytoin, carbamazepine, phenobarbital, and/or primidone) is diagnostic as well as therapeutic. Psychiatric disturbances will not benefit.

Major motor or grand mal epilepsy. Along with petit mal, grand mal epilepsy is the most common form of seizure disorder in adolescents. It begins with a brief aura (flashing lights, peculiar taste, buzzing or ringing ears, feelings of depression, premonitory anxiety) and rapidly progresses into generalized bilateral tonic and/or clonic movements, jerky respirations, tongue biting, and incontinence (fecal, urinary) with complete or partial loss of consciousness. The convulsions usually abate within 5 minutes or less and are followed by postictal somnolence lasting from a few minutes to several hours. Amnesia for the event is common. The frequency of grand mal seizures varies from several times a day to once or twice a year. Progression to status epilepticus is an infrequent complication (see section on status epilepticus). EEG abnormalities usually are present, but their nature varies. Treatment employs phenytoin, carbamazine, phenobarbital, and/or primidone.

Minor motor seizures. The simple "absence" or petit mal episode is the classic form of minor motor seizures. It often develops between 4–8 years of age and disappears by midadolescence. A typical attack consists of a brief moment (15–30 seconds or less) of staring or lapse of consciousness without any prodrome, aura, or postictal state. Clonic movements or automatism is uncommon but may be seen on occasion. Petit mal seizures tend to occur with greater frequency than other types, sometimes as often as 100 or more times a day. Hyperventilation is a frequent precipitant. The EEG characteristically demonstrates a three-per-second (range 2.5–4) spike and wave pattern and is a diagnostic finding. Treatment includes valproic acid, ethosuximide, or clonazepam. The prognosis is generally good, although some patients will develop grand mal epilepsy at a later date. While other forms of minor motor seizures have been identified, they are exceptionally rare in adolescence and are omitted here.

SPECIAL CONSIDERATIONS IN DRUG TREATMENT

Table 10-2 provides data relevant to the use of the more commonly employed anticonvulsant drugs. All have significant side effects requiring periodic monitoring and careful titration up to therapeutic levels. The precise dosage and combination of drugs required for control is a highly individualized matter. In addition, an increased dosage may be needed at certain times, such as during menstruation or infections. When it is evident that more than one agent is required for control, a new drug should not be started until full therapeutic dosages of preceding ones have been achieved and the patient stabilized. A new drug also should be introduced gradually with careful titration and attention to drug interactions (Table 10-2), whereas old drugs deemed ineffective should be tapered rather than abruptly discontinued. Phenytoin or phenobarbital usually is preferred initially for grand mal and focal seizures. These are less effective in petit mal, and therefore one of the drugs more specific for this type generally is preferred. Up to three agents ultimately may be required for the maximal possible control, which may take months or even years to achieve. Valproic acid is one of the newer anticonvulsant agents and seems useful in some generalized and myoclonic seizures.

Common practice is to initiate medication after even a single seizure, although this has been a matter of some debate. The decision to stop medication is equally debatable. An adolescent with idiopathic disease and only a single seizure or with a childhood onset who is wholly controlled by medication probably is a candidate for discontinuance after treatment for 2–4 years. Gradual tapering of the medication over 3–18 months is important to pre-

TABLE 10-2
DRUGS IN THE TREATMENT OF SEIZURE DISORDERS

Drug, indication,* and dose	Therapeutic serum levels and drug interactions	Side effects and comments
Phenobarbital: G, T, F; 2-5 mg/kg/day; 150-250 mg/day	10-25 or 35 μg/ml; increased by phenytoin, primidone, and valproic acid	Drowsiness, lethargy (tend to improve with continued administration), stupor, coma (with levels over 60 μg/ml), fever, nystagmus, and ataxia. Less commonly seen: osteomalacia with chronic use, hepatic dysfunction, leukopenia, lymphadenopathy, maculopapular or bullous rash, Stevens-Johnson syndrome.
Phenytoin (Dilantin): G, F, T; 4-8 mg/kg/day; 300-400 mg/day	10-20 μg/ml; increased by valproic acid and many other drugs; decreased by phenobarbital, primidone, carbamazepine	Gingival hyperplasia (can prevent with good oral hygiene), hypertrichosis, nystagmus (with levels over 25-30 μg/ml), ataxia, dysarthria, diplopia, choreoathetosis, lethargy, stupor, excitement, peripheral neuropathy, hepatic dysfunction, lymphadenopathy, hypocalcemia, osteomalacia, rickets, hyperglycemia, folic acid deficiency. Idiosyncratic reactions may occur (usually within first 1-4 weeks), including exfoliative dermatitis and other rashes, a lupuslike reaction, Stevens-Johnson syndrome. Overdose results in acute cerebellar symptoms, delirium, and coma.
Ethosuximide (Zarontin): P; 15-40 mg/kg/day; 750-1500 mg/day	40-100 μg/ml	Nausea, vomiting, lethargy, anorexia, hiccups, irritability, G.I. irritation, headaches, abdominal pain, skin rash, leukopenia, eosinophilia, ataxia, nystagmus, urticaria, bone marrow depression, lupuslike syndrome, dyskinesis, emotional reaction.
Carbamazepine (Tegretol): G, T, F; 10-25 mg/kg/day; 400-1200 mg/day	3-10 μg/ml; decreased by phenytoin, primidone, phenobarbital	Fatigue, malaise, dizziness, anorexia, lethargy, nausea, vomiting, diplopia, nystagmus, ataxia, hepatic dysfunction, bone marrow depression, cardiac arrhymias, inappropriate ADH secretion, leukopenia, skin rashes, eosinophilic myocarditis, Stevens-Johnson syndrome.
Primidone (Mysoline): G, T. F; 10-20 mg/kg/day; 500-1500 mg/day	5-12 μg/ml; increased by carbamazepine	Lethargy, dizziness, vertigo, nausea, vomiting, ataxia, nystagmus, diplopia, megaloblastic anemia (folic acid deficiency), behavioral changes, bone marrow depression, edema, lupuslike syndrome. Tolerance develops if previously on phenobarbital. Often used as adjunct to phenytoin and carbamazepine.
Trimethadione (Tridione): P; 10-25 mg/kg/day; 300-1500 mg/day	15-40 μg/ml	Lethargy, increased light glare, may precipitate tonic-clonic seizure in patients with combined petit mal–grand mal disorder, exfoliative dermatitis, other skin rashes, blood dyscrasia, hepatitis, nephrosis, neutropenia, aplastic anemia, lupuslike syndrome, myasthenic syndrome.
Valproic acid (Depakene): P; 15-40 mg/kg/day; 1000-3000 mg/day	40-100 μg/ml; increased by ethosuximide	Nausea, emesis, abdominal cramps, diarrhea, lethargy, transient alopecia, abnormal clotting, reduced platelets and platelet aggregation, hepatic dysfunction, weight changes, increased salivation, skin rashes, insomnia, headache. Take with meals to reduce G.I. side effects.

Continued

TABLE 10-2
DRUGS IN THE TREATMENT OF SEIZURE DISORDERS (CONTINUED)

Drug, indication,* and dose	Therapeutic serum levels and drug interactions	Side effects and comments
Clonazepam (Clonopin): P, other minor motor seizures; 0.03–0.1 mg/kg/day; 1.5–20 mg/day	13–72 nanograms/ml	Lethargy, irritability, belligerence, weight gain, ataxia, dysarthria. Tolerance can develop if given with valproic acid, as may be needed in petit mal.

*G, grand mal seizures; T, temporal lobe seizures; F, focal seizures; P, petit mal seizures.

vent recurrences. On the other hand, epilepsy with an adolescent onset and requiring 3 or more years to control or seizures stemming from an identifiable organic disorder tend to persist and often return when medication is stopped. Under these circumstances, treatment for life usually is indicated.

Forty percent of epileptics are not wholly controlled by medication. Factors contributing to incomplete control include mixed or complex seizure disorders, underlying diseases or metabolic processes that are difficult to manage in and of themselves (for example, cerebral edema, tumors, severe congenital or acquired brain damage, pubertal changes). Other issues that should be considered are poor compliance with the recommended regimen, the use of an inappropriate drug, subtherapeutic dosage, drug interference or interactions when two or more agents are combined, malabsorption, the development of physiologic drug tolerance, and incorrect diagnosis.

Status epilepticus, a state of continuous or rapidly sequential seizures (usually tonic-clonic type) without a return of consciousness, may occur with the precipitant removal of anticonvulsant medication (particularly phenobarbital), infection, metabolic dysfunction, alcohol, or other substance abuse, cerebral edema and trauma, among other causes. Although a favorable outcome with appropriate management usually is the expected course, death from exhaustion, anoxia, and cardiovascular collapse is possible. After establishing an airway and ensuring adequate ventilation, the following regimens can be tried singly or in combination:

1. Diazepam (Valium), 5–10 mg IV, to be repeated every 25 minutes but at a rate not to exceed 15 mg/minute, 30 mg/hour, and/or 100 mg/24 hours.

2. Phenytoin (Dilantin), 15 mg/kg IV, as a loading dose followed by 100–150 mg IV every 30 minutes but at a rate not to exceed 50 mg/minute and/or 1.5 g/24 hours.

3. Phenobarbital, 150–400 mg IV, as a loading dose followed by 120–240 mg every 20 minutes but at a rate not to exceed 40 mg/minute and/or 1 g/24 hours.

4. Paraldehyde (4% solution) 0.1 cc/kg IM or by slow IV push with a maximum dose of 5 ml.

Diazepam is the drug of choice with either phenobarbital or phenytoin added if the response is inadequate or as a transitional measure in reestablishing maintenance control with the oral form of either medication. Caution should be exercised against overdosage resulting in excessive central nervous depression to the point of apnea when diazepam and phenobarbital are used together. Phenytoin also poses risk of cardiovascular collapse and/or CNS depression if administered too rapidly (see preceding recommended rate). Paraldehyde may have particular advantage when the maximum rate of administration of other agents has been reached, but the patient still is not under satisfactory control and demonstrates significant respiratory depression. Paraldehyde is less likely to depress respiration further than the other CNS depressants. Sometimes even these measures are ineffective, and general anesthesia with or without a muscle relaxant (succinlycholine) may be required.

PSYCHOLOGIC AND SOCIAL ASPECTS

Attention to the psychosocial dimension of the adolescent with epilepsy also is critical to successful management in ensuring optimal developmental progress and minimizing compliance problems (see Chapter 21). Specific concerns of an epileptic youth include driving, vocation, genetic counseling, and childbearing. Well-controlled adolescents usually are eligible for a driver's license if seizure-free for 2 or more years even if on medication. In most states, however, the physician must report a person of driving age with epilepsy to the state motor vehicle office.

TABLE 10-3
DIFFERENTIAL DIAGNOSIS OF HEADACHES

A. Central nervous system disorders
  1. Infections: meningitis, encephalitis, brain abscess
  2. Subarachnoid or subdural hemorrhage: trauma, spontaneous rupture of aneurysm or arterio-venous fistula
  3. Thromboembolism
  4. Cerebral edema: pseudotumor cerebri, benign intracranial hypertension
  5. Brain tumor
  6. Hydrocephalus

B. Vascular disorders
  1. Migraine headaches
  2. As a component of tension headaches
  3. Primary hypertension or hypertension secondary to renal disease, pheochromocytoma, carcinoid tumors

C. Disorders of the eyes, ears, nose, and throat
  1. Eye disorders: eye strain, optic neuritis, glaucoma
  2. Referred otalgia (secondary to disorders of the teeth, nasopharynx, temporomandibular joint)
  3. Sinusitis
  4. Otitis (acute or chronic)

D. Systemic and metabolic disorders
  1. Endocrine dysfunction (hypoglycemia, diabetes mellitus)
  2. Collagen vascular disorders
  3. Acute and chronic infections other than CNS, particularly with fever and toxicity

E. Musculoskeletal disorders
  1. Tension headaches
  2. Cervical spine disorders

F. Food and drug related disorders
  1. Caffeine withdrawal (coffee, tea, cola beverages, cocoa)
  2. Ergotamine withdrawal (in relation to migraine treatment)
  3. Alcohol or other CNS depressant intoxication
  4. Nicotine use or withdrawal (cigarettes)
  5. Monosodium glutamate ingestion in susceptible persons
  6. Nitrate and nitrite food preservatives
  7. Foods that exacerbate migraine (see text)

G. Psychiatric disorders
  1. Psychosis
  2. Depression

H. Miscellaneous
  1. Exercise
  2. Temporal arteritis
  3. Trigeminal neuralgia

Adolescent females should be counseled to avoid pregnancy, as it may exacerbate seizures as well as raise a host of other problems; an effective contraceptive method should be provided if the patient is sexually active. If an unplanned pregnancy does occur, possible teratogenic effects of the seizure medications should be evaluated and taken into consideration when deciding what to do about the pregnancy. Teratogenicity must also be considered in older adolescents and young adults on antiseizure drugs who are contemplating becoming pregnant. Most adolescents, both male and female, also will be concerned for the possible genetic transmission of epilepsy to future offspring. Unless there is a strong family history for seizure disorders, they should be appropriately reassured.

Lastly, reality dictates that certain vocations will be closed to the epileptic individual. It certainly would be ill advised for teenagers with uncertain control to contemplate any job that places them or others at physical risk should they have a seizure (operating certain types of machines, working at high altitudes in the contruction business, and so on). Even those with full control will encounter difficulty in enlisting in the armed forces or obtaining acceptance into police or fire departments.

Headaches

Headache is one of the most common of adolescent complaints. They can be classified as to whether they reflect (a) spasm of the external musculature of the head, face, and neck with or without involvement of the external vasculature (tension headaches); (b) alteration of the intracranial vasculature (migraine headaches); or (c) an intracranial lesion. Although many conditions can cause headache (Table 10-3), most cases in adolescents are of the tension type. Migraine is commonly encountered, but intracranial pathology is a relatively rare cause.

Specific points to be noted in evaluation include the duration and frequency of acute episodes, a description of the pain, the degree of disability experienced, any associated symptomatology (weight loss, visual impairment, fever, vomiting, recent personality changes, neurologic deficits), and a detailed neurologic as well as general examination. Table 10-4 cites various laboratory procedures that may be useful in further evaluation, although just how many to employ and their sequence is a matter of judgment based on data already obtained. Both migraine and tension headaches often are readily diagnosed on the basis of the history and physical examination alone. These are often classic symptoms with no physical findings of note.

MIGRAINE HEADACHES

Migraine affects 3%–15% of the population. It predominates in females (male–female ratio = 1:3.5) and has a strong association with a positive family history (60%–90%). In approximately one-third of all cases migraine begins in childhood. The incidence gradually increases at the time of puberty, peaks during late adolescence, and thereafter declines. Childhood-onset migraine commonly abates during puberty, but initiation at the time of adolescence often presages the continuation of attacks into adulthood.

A wide variety of manifestations and symptoms has been described (see following section), but the most common complaints among adolescents are of recurrent, unilateral or bilateral, pounding headache associated with photophobia, pallor, nausea, vomiting, and anorexia. Diarrhea, constipation, diuresis, edema, fever, and blood pressure changes also have been described. Twenty-five percent of patients with migraine headaches experience an antecedent aura variably consisting of sensory phenomena (flashing lights, peculiar smell or taste, ringing or buzzing in ears), autonomic signs (pallor, syncope, hyperhidrosis, nausea, vomiting), psychic manifestations (apprehension, anxiety, mood change), and/or motor abnormalities (from localized weakness to hemiparesis).

The etiology of migraine is unclear beyond a strong familial factor, although a wide variety of precipitating events has been implicated in the vulnerable individual. These include fatigue, stress, menses, ovulation, flickering lights, barometric or humidity changes, missed meals, changes in sleep patterns (too much, too little), hypertension, allergens, exercise, coitus, and various ingestants or drugs such as oral contraceptives, caffeine, alcohol, reserpine, vasodilator drugs, tyramine, nitrate preservatives, citrus fruits, and monosodium glutamate.

Pathophysiologic mechanisms involve the intracranial vasculature with an initial vasoconstrictive phase lasting several minutes to half an hour (the aura) followed by an extended period of vasodilation (the headache). Vasoconstriction may affect any part of the brain or brain stem, the precise vessels involved determining whether the aura is predominantly one of nausea and emesis (medulla), fever, edema, and irritability (hypothalamus), sensory changes relating to light, taste, sound, or motor function (cortex), or a combination of these. Vasodilation manifested in the typical headache appears closely related to the increased accumulation in the perivascular region of various pain sensitizors such as serotonin, catecholamines, histamine,

---

TABLE 10-4
**CLINICAL AND LABORATORY
EVALUATION OF HEADACHES**

1. History: Location, description, duration, frequency, time of day, precipitating events, how obtains relief, associated symptoms and signs, other health and mental health issues, including use of drugs, alcohol, cigarettes, oral contraceptives

2. Physical examination: Particular attention to blood pressure, eyes (including fundi and visual acuity), ears (including Weber and Rinne tests and auditory acuity), nose, sinuses, throat, cardiovascular system, neurologic system

3. Laboratory tests (to be performed according to clinical judgment as suggested by prior findings and clinical course):
   a. Routine: complete blood count, urinalysis, VDRL
   b. Erythrocyte sedimentation rate
   c. Blood values: urea nitrogen, creatinine, glucose (fasting or tolerance test)
   d. Roentgenograms: skull, cervical spine, sinuses, ear and mastoid, temporomandibular joint
   e. Other imaging procedures: computerized axial tomography, angiogram, arteriogram, myelogram, tomography
   f. Lumbar puncture
   g. Electroencephalogram
   h. Visual fields, intraocular pressure
   i. Specialized neurologic and neuroendocrine procedures
   j. Therapeutic trial with ergotamine tartrate in migraine suspects
   k. Psychologic and/or psychiatric evaluation

---

bradykinin, angiotensin, and prostaglandins. Increased vessel permeability to these substances also may play a role. The precise mechanisms for the release of these substances is not entirely clear but in part may be due to increased platelet aggregation during the vasoconstrictive phase.

CLASSIFICATION

Classic migraine: Approximately 10% of migraine headaches are of the "classic type" with an abrupt, sharply defined aura lasting 10–30 minutes followed by a 4–6 hour unilateral, pounding headache with nausea, emesis, and anorexia.

Common migraine: Occurring in 80%–85% of all vascular headache complexes, this is the most frequent form. The aura is less well defined and merges into the vasodilatory phase. The headache itself lasts hours to days and, while usually unilateral, is bilateral one-third of the time. Withdrawal from caffeine, changes in sleep patterns (for example, excessive sleep on weekends), and stress appear to be significant precipitants. Although any of the factors discussed in the overview may be implicated, "letdown" migraine is a variant sometimes seen with the relief of stress such as during weekends, vacations, or holidays. The frequency of attacks varies from daily episodes to ones separated by wide time intervals.

Rare and unusual forms: Cluster migraine usually affects older males between 30–60 years and accounts for 4%–5% of all vascular headaches. There is an abrupt onset of unilateral headache, facial pain, flushing, lacrimation, conjunctival injection, and hyperhidrosis of the affected side. One out of five patients also demonstrates an ipsilateral Horner's syndrome. Episodes tend to be nocturnal, last ½–1½ hours, and recur over a period of 8–12 weeks with subsequent remission. Ophthalmoplegic migraine consists of a typical headache and oculomotor paralysis lasting 3–5 days. Spontaneous clearing is the general rule, but permanent nerve injury has been noted. Hemiplegic migraine is similar to opthalmoplegic migraine but with hemiplegia, aphasia, or hemisensory deficits replacing eye signs. The differential diagnosis in either case includes intracranial tumor, cerebrovascular accident, other space-occupying lesions, multiple sclerosis, encephalomyelitis, and others. All laboratory evaluation in either ophthalmoplegic or hemiplegic migraine, including cerebrospinal fluid, is negative. Basilar artery migraine is primarily noted in females and appears to be closely related to menses. It is characterized by a 20–40 minute aura with loss of vision, emesis, vertigo, ataxia, dysarthria, parathesias, weakness, tinnitus, and/or alteration of consciousness followed by a throbbing headache in the occipital region.

Treatment. Migraine may occur in conjunction with other disorders such as sinus, dental, or ear infections, or with tension headaches; attention should first be directed at isolating any such coexisting matters. A careful search of the patient's history for possible factors triggering the migraine itself (see overview) will suggest modifications in the patient's lifestyle, habits, foods, or medications that may help to decrease the frequency of attacks.

Specific drug treatment for an acute episode largely relies on ergotamine tartrate (Table 10-5) due to its vasoconstrictive properties; it usually is effective in aborting an attack if given early in the cycle, preferably at the first signs of an aura. Responsiveness to a clinical trial also is diagnostic in that other forms of headache are not alleviated.

Ergotamine, however, should not be prescribed for patients with prolonged aura (it will intensify the vasoconstrictive effects), those who are pregnant, and those who have peripheral vascular occlusive disease, hypertension, or other conditions that could be exacerbated by increased vascular resistance. Side effects include nausea, vomiting, muscle aches, paresthesias, habituation (in relation to use for headaches), rebound vascular headaches, ischemia of coronary or cerebral vessels, thrombophlebitis, and chronic ergotism (peripheral circulatory insufficiency, fatigue, depression, persistent nausea, and vomiting). Failure of a response to ergotamine may be due to taking it too late in the migraine cycle, malabsorption, the coexistence of tension headaches, misdiagnosis, and, in some patients, individual idiosyncratic resistance.

Various combinations of analgesics, antinauseants, and sedatives or tranquilizers (Table 10-5) may be used to replace ergotamine entirely when it is ineffective or when side effects require discontinuance or as a supplement when only partially effective. In the latter instance, ergotamine, an analgesic, and an antinauseant can be a helpful combination. Prednisone has produced dramatic results in severe, persistent cases, and chlorpromazine has been found beneficial on occasion, although both these drugs should be limited in their use if resorted to at all. Unremitting cases have been treated with some success by means of a "deep sleep" regimen using intravenous sedative and tranquilizer combinations.

Prophylaxis. Patients with frequent episodes of migraine headaches (two or more per month) warrant a preventive regimen with particular attention to precipitating causes plus medication and/or education of the patient undergoing an alternative pain control technique (operant conditioning, self-hypnosis, behavior modification, biofeedback techniques, meditation, body relaxation exercises). A wide variety of agents has been employed in medicational prophylaxis (Table 10-6). Propranolol is commonly given to adults with frequent migraines. Unfortunately, those which are most effective (methysergide, propranolol, steroids) also have major side effects, and their use in adolescents with migraine requires extreme caution. Propranolol is preferred by many clinicians.

TENSION HEADACHES
Sustained contraction or spasm of the muscles about the head and neck with or without vascular involvement identifies the tension headache and is an exceptionally common complaint among adolescents.

TABLE 10-5
DRUGS IN TREATING ACUTE MIGRAINE HEADACHES

Drug	Dosage
ERGOTAMINE TARTRATE	
1. Cafergot tablets (1 mg ergotamine tartrate plus 100 mg caffeine; available as suppository in different dose)	Do not give more than 6 mg/24 hr or 10 mg/week; 1-2 tab p.o. stat, then 1 tab 1 30 min if necessary; maximum dose, 6 tabs/24 hr, 10 tabs/week
2. Ergomar sublingual tablets (2 mg ergotamine tartrate)	1 sublingual tab stat, then 1 tab q 30 min if necessary; maximum dose, 3 tabs/24 hr, 5 tabs/week
3. Cafergot P-B suppositories (2 mg ergotamine tartrate, 100 mg caffeine, 0.25 mg Bellafoline, 60 mg pentolbarbital sodium; available as p.o. tablet in different dose)	1 suppository stat, then 1 suppository in one hour if necessary; maximum dose, 2 suppositories/24 hr, 5 suppositories/week
4. Wigraine suppositories (1.0 mg ergotamine tartrate, 100 mg caffeine, 0.1 mg belladonna alkaloids, 130 mg phenacetin; also available as p.o. tablets)	1-2 suppositories stat, then 1-2 suppositories q 15-30 min if necessary; maximum dose, 6 suppositories/24 hr, 12 suppositories/week
5. Ergotamine tartrate medihaler	1 inhalation stat, then 1 inhalation q 5 min if necessary; maximum dose, 6 inhalations/24 hr
6. Others: Migral, Ergostat, Oxoids	
D.H.E. 45 (dihydroergotamine mesylate injection)	1 ml IM stat, then 1 ml q 60 min if necessary; maximum dose, 3 ml/24 hr
ANALGESICS	
Weak analgesics	
1. Acetylsalicylic acid (aspirin)	650 mg p.o. q 4 hr p.r.n.
2. Acetaminophen (Tylenol, Datril)	650 mg p.o. q 4 hr p.r.n.
3. Fiorinal; (50 mg butalbital, 200 mg aspirin, 130 mg phenacetin, 40 mg caffeine; as tablets or capsules; also available with codeine	1-2 tabs or caps q 4-6 hr; maximum dose, 6 tabs or caps/24 hr
4. Midrin (65 mg isometheptene mucate, 100 mg dichloralphenazone, 325 mg acetaminophen)	1-2 capsules q 4 hr; maximum dose, 8 caps/24 hr
Narcotics	
1. Codeine	30-100 mg p.o./24 hr
2. Popropoxyphene (Darvon)	65 mg p.o. q 4 hr
3. Oxycodone (Percodan)	4.5 mg p.o. q 6 hr
4. Meperioine (Demerol)	50-100 mg IM q 3-4 hr
Nonsteroidal antiinflammatory drugs (mefenamic acid, naproxen, indomethacin)	
ANTINAUSEANTS	
1. Cyclizine (Marezine; available as tablet, suppository, or injectable)	a. 1 tab q 4-6 hr for nausea; maximum dose, 4/24 hr b. 1 ml (50 mg) q 4-6 hr; maximum dose, 200 mg/24 hr (IM) c. 1 suppository (100 mg) q 4-6 hr; maximum dose, 4/24 hr
2. Promethazine hydrochloride (Phenergan; available as tablet, suppository, or injectable)	12.5-25 mg p.o. or rectally q 4-6 hr; adjust IM dose as needed. Demerol and Phenergan are often used together for relief of severe episodes.
SEDATIVES, TRANQUILIZERS	
1. Chloral hydrate	250 mg t.i.d.-q.i.d. p.o.; maximum dose, 2 g/24 hr
2. Diazepam (Valium; also available as injectable)	2-10 mg b.i.d.-q.i.d. p.o.
3. Chlorpromazine (Thorazine; also available as injectable)	50 mg p.o. or IM stat, then 50 mg q 30-60 min if necessary; maximum dose 300 mg first 4 hr, 1000 mg/24 hr; ergotamine tartrate may be added
STEROIDS, PREDNISONE	30-60 mg/24 hr X 3-5 days; taper to discontinuance over 1 week

TABLE 10-6
DRUGS IN MIGRAINE PREVENTION

Drug	Comment
Methylsergide maleate (Sansert)	Dose, 2-6 mg/day. Serotonin antagonist with many side effects, including nausea, vomiting, peripheral circulatory insufficiency, edema, depression, angina, and fibrosis of retroperitoneal, pulmonary, and cardiac regions. A respite for 2 months of every 6 months is recommended to reduce incidence of fibrosis.
Propranolol hydrochloride (Inderal)	Dose, 80 mg/day initially, up to 160-240 mg/day. Beta-adrenergic blocker with many side effects, including rebound headaches on withdrawal; if maximum dose not effective within 4-6 weeks, withdraw slowly over 2 weeks. Do not use in conjunction with ergotamine or in patients with sinus bradycardia, bronchial asthma, or congestive heart failure.
Cyproheptadine hydrochloride (Periactin)	Dose, 4-8 mg t.i.d. Serotonin and histamine antagonist sometimes effective alone or with other medications. Side effects include lethargy, inappropriate appetite, weight gain.
Bellergal, Bellergal-S	Dose, one standard tablet t.i.d. or q.i.d.; one S tablet b.i.d. (sustained time release). Can be used with other medications.
Anticonvulsants	May be beneficial if EEG abnormal (Table 10-2).
Antidepressants, other psychotherapeutic drugs	Useful when depression underlies migraine. Chlorpromazine (50-150 mg/day), imipramine have been tried with some success. Lithium carbonate under investigation.
Steroids	Prednisone; 30-60 mg/day or q.o.d.
Minor tranquilizers and sedatives	Diazepam, chloral hydrate, others.
Weak analgesics	As per Table 10-5.

The etiology is unclear, although emotional tension and stress appear to be involved. Symptomatology varies greatly, but the pain frequently is described as a dull, constant ache over the entire head or as a sensation of tightness (bandlike, viselike) about the forehead, head, and neck. Other common features are insidious onset, bilateral involvement, increase in discomfort as the day progresses, and onset or exacerbation with exposure to stress. Tenderness of neck or scalp muscles may be present as well. An aura is notably absent, as are autonomic signs, and the pain is less likely to be pounding or unilateral, differentiating tension from migraine etiologies. On the other hand, a middle ground exists where it may be difficult to differentiate common migraine from tension headaches, and, to further confuse matters, both may coexist.

Diagnosis usually can be made on clinical grounds alone. Visual acuity deficits and chronic sinusitis should not be difficult to rule out in that the pain and discomfort from these conditions usually are limited to the periorbital or sinus areas with associated visual difficulties in the one instance and tenderness to pressure or percussion over the frontal region in the other. Headaches due to intracranial lesions tend to be much more severe, well defined, and accompanied by neurologic deficits. Further evaluation (Table 10-4) may be indicated when signs and symptoms are more ambiguous or severe than commonly encountered.

Treatment of tension headaches employs weak analgesics alone or in combination with other agents (aspirin, phenacetin, Fiorinal, Midrin; see Table 10-5), although increasing favor is being given to body relaxation techniques and helping the patient to deal with stress more effectively as an alternative to drug-mediated solutions. Reassurance also is an important measure, many adolescents believing their symptoms to be much more serious than they are. Psychiatric or social intervention may be indicated in cases where psychogenic factors clearly are involved.

OTHER HEADACHE COMPLEXES
The history and physical examination alone usually distinguish headaches other than those due to migraine and tension (Table 10-3) and give direction for further evaluation (Table 10-4). A cerebrovascular accident due to a ruptured congenital aneurysm or arteriovenous malformation can be a particularly

TABLE 10-7
DIFFERENTIAL FEATURES OF PAPILLEDEMA AND PSEUDOPAPILLEDEMA

	Papilledema	Pseudopapilledema
DEFINITION	Noninflammatory swelling and edema of optic nerve head with elevation of optic disk due to increased intracranial pressure.	Indistinct disk margins due to localized cause, generally a benign finding
DISK APPEARANCE	Disk elevated; may be hyperemic; margins obliterated	Disk not elevated; margins only blurred
RETINAL VESSELS	Dilated and tortuous veins with deflection and compression of all vessels over disk edge	No abnormality
RETINAL PATHOLOGY	Hemorrhages, exudates, and edema may be seen	None
VISUAL FIELDS	Progressively enlarging blind spot	May have enlarged blind spot but not progressive

serious cause of severe headache in adolescence and constitutes a medical emergency. The onset tends to be sudden and commonly is occipital, with associated nuchal rigidity, confusion, lethargy, irritability, emesis, pyrexia and, in 15%, convulsions. There may or may not be a history of antecedent trauma. The finding of blood in the cerebrospinal fluid is diagnostic, but a lumbar puncture should only be done with the greatest of caution to avoid brain stem herniation. Emergency computerized axial tomography is now considered the diagnostic procedure of initial choice. Further definition as to the site and nature of the causal defect may be obtained through angiography. Treatment includes bed rest, analgesics, oxygen, antifibrinolytics (Amicar), anticonvulsants, and/or surgery. If the patient survives the initial insult, the severity of the pain usually abates in 2–7 days, but full resolution may take several months. Additional neurosurgical evaluation is indicated in assessing the risk of a recurrence and what further intervention is required.

Brain tumor (Chapter 13) headaches vary in location, depending on the tumor's site. Pain tends to be severe and consistent in manifestations. Vomiting *without* nausea, often in the early morning, may be a particular clue. Papilledema also is present when the lesion is supratentorial but may be absent if infratentorial (for example, of the cerebellum or brain stem). In most instances, additional localizing neurologic signs are noted; particular attention should be given to examination of cranial nerves, visual fields, and cerebellar function. Some tumor patients may have headache with major emotional or behavioral changes but minimal neurologic signs.

A psychiatric etiology for sudden alteration in personality or mood should be one of exclusion following careful investigation for an underlying organic cause.

Papilledema
BENIGN INTRACRANIAL HYPERTENSION

Headache, visual disturbances and, sometimes, syncopal attacks with papilledema and increased spinal fluid pressure but without other signs of neurologic disorder comprise benign intracranial hypertension, or pseudotumor cerebri. In many respects this is a diagnosis of exclusion; other causes of papilledema—primarily space-occupying lesions— must be thoroughly ruled out (Table 10-4).

Some cases of benign intracranial hypertension are idiopathic. Others may be seen in association with a wide variety of disorders, including obesity, menstrual disorders, vitamin A intoxication, hypoparathyroidism, adrenal insufficiency, pregnancy, systemic lupus erythematosus, iron deficiency anemia, polycythemia, thrombocytosis, lateral sinus occlusion, and the administration of oral contraceptives, steroids, or tetracycline, although in most cases cause and effect relationship is unclear.

Treatment includes repeated lumbar punctures with the removal of up to 50 ml of spinal fluid each time to reduce pressure, oral steroids, and attention to any coexisting related factors as noted above. Rarely, surgical decompression may be required. The prognosis generally is good, but it may take up to 3 months for headaches, papilledema, and other symptoms to improve and up to 12 months for headaches to disappear altogether. Ten percent of all patients experience a recurrence, and a few may have permanent visual impairment.

PSEUDOPAPILLEDEMA

Not all instances of blurred optic discs reflect true papilledema. Some cases simply reflect a localized process of the optic nerve head and do not signify increased intracranial pressure. Table 10-7 provides differential points.

Vertigo and Dizziness

Vertigo describes the sensation of spinning in the environment or, alternatively, that the environment is spinning instead. The feeling of motion is integral. Dizziness defines lightheadedness or giddiness but without the perception of motion. The latter is a common complaint among adolescents, whereas vertigo is rare. The conditions producing dizziness are usually relatively benign, often being related to standing up too quickly (orthostatic hypotension), hyperventilation, or a prodrome of vasovagal syncope. More significant but less common causes include peripheral vestibular disorders, peripheral neuropathy, visual disorders, hypertension, anemia, cerebral hypoxia due to cardiovascular disease, or carotid sinus hypersensitivity and other neurologic or emotional disorders. Vertigo also may be due to a variety of conditions, generally of a more serious nature (Table 10-8), and sometimes coexistent with dizziness.

The history is directed at differentiating between these two symptoms and the elucidation of possible underlying causes, including trauma, tinnitus, unilateral hearing loss and other evidences of ear disease. Physical examination is particularly directed to the eyes, ears, heart, and neurologic system. A lateral jerk nystagmus (Chapter 4) often is noted with vertigo but not with dizziness. The Weber and Rinne tests, audiometry, Barony response, caloric testing, electronystagmography, and other procedures as indicated also facilitate diagnosis.

Among three primary vestibular disorders, benign positional vertigo is an idiopathic, self-limiting condition in which there are frequent, transient episodes of vertigo occurring in 1-6 week cycles with gradually diminishing severity and ultimate clearing over a 6-12 month period. Labyrinthitis (vestibular neuronitis) is characterized by the sudden onset of vertigo that increases in severity over 8-12 hours and then gradually clears from 4 days to 3 weeks. The etiology is unknown, but toxin exposure, drug ingestants, and infections of the ear or upper respiratory tract are thought to be contributing fac-

TABLE 10-8
DIFFERENTIAL DIAGNOSIS OF VERTIGO

DISORDERS OF THE EAR
Ceruminosis
Otitis media
Deafness
Labyrinthine disease, benign positional vertigo, labthitis, Meniere's disease
Other ENT disorders

CENTRAL NERVOUS SYSTEM DISORDERS
Acoustic neuroma
Vertiginous seizure disorder
Migraine headache
Space-occupying lesions: subarachnoid hemorrhage (spontaneous, traumatic), posterior fossa tumor
Transient ischemic attacks
CNS infections: meningitis, encephalitis, abscess
Multiple sclerosis

SYNCOPE (see Table 10-9)

MISCELLANEOUS
Drug toxicity (licit, illicit); aminoglycosides, aspirin, phenothiazines, alcohol, other CNS depressants
Metabolic disorders: diabetes mellitus, hypoglycemia, hypothyroidism, hyperthyroidism
Temporomandibular joint syndrome

tors. Meniere's syndrome is a rare chronic condition characterized by recurrent episodes of vertigo, fluctuating hearing loss, and tinnitus. Attacks tend to last several hours at a time and occur every 4-8 weeks. The etiology is unknown.

Treatment of any of the labyrinthine disorders (or vertigo from any cause) is symptomatic and employs the following antinauseant drugs alone or in combination with a weak tranquilizer (diazepam).

- Meclizine hydrochloride (Antivert, Bonine), 25 mg b.i.d. or q.i.d. p.o.
- Nylidrin hydrochloride (Arlidin), 3-10 mg t.i.d. or q.i.d. p.o.
- Dimenhydrinate (Dramamine), 25-50 mg q.i.d. p.o.
- Ru-vert (pentylenetetrazol, pheniramine maleate, plus nictinic acid), 1-2 tablets t.i.d. p.o.

Drug treatment is not always effective in Meniere's disease, and labyrinthectomy may be necessary in particularly resistant and dysfunctional states.

Syncope

Syncope, or fainting, is the transient loss of consciousness due to a diminished cerebral blood flow with resultant anoxia. Faintness, also referred to as dizziness, defines the presyncopal period with a sense of impending consciousness loss. Vasovagal syncope is most common, but other possible causes of fainting are listed in Table 10-9. The history, physical examination, and laboratory evaluation are primarily directed at the eyes, ears, heart, neurologic system, and psychosocial factors. The more significant of these disorders are discussed in the following sections.

VASOVAGAL SYNCOPE

Vasovagal syncope (simple faint) is a common adolescent phenomenon, particularly in females. Precipitating factors include any set of circumstances that can induce autonomic dysfunction; intense emotion, stress, traumatic injury, pain or threat of pain, sight of blood, fasting, intrauterine device insertion, other medical procedures, fatigue, and sudden exposure to cold. Signs and symptoms are dizziness, weakness, nausea, diaphoresis, blurred vision, salivation, and tachycardia shortly followed by bradycardia. If the individual is sitting or standing, the sudden decrease in cerebral perfusion attendant to the bradycardia results in cerebral anoxia and loss of consciousness for 10 seconds up to several minutes. During this time, the patient is limp, pale, diaphoretic, and unresponsive with flaccid musculature, bradycardia, and mydriatic but light-reactive pupils. Infrequently, tonic-clonic movements or opisthotonus are noted as well, but in these circumstances the diagnosis of vasovagal syncope can only be made after careful exclusion of other possible causes. On return to consciousness, the patient is fully alert without evidencing a postictal state, although symptoms of continued autonomic dysfunction may persist from 5–20 minutes; if the patient stands up during this time, syncope may recur. Syncope itself may be aborted in the presyncopal phase if the head is placed at or below heart level. This is accomplished by lying the patient down or, if sitting, by placing the head between the knees. During an actual syncopal episode, the patient should be placed on his or her back with legs elevated and the airway cleared.

ORTHOSTATIC HYPOTENSION

Orthostatic (postural) hypotension is a particularly common complaint in adolescents of either sex. Dizziness and lightheadedness, with or without actual loss of consciousness, are experienced on standing up rapidly from a sitting or lying position. Although many predisposing factors have been iden-

TABLE 10-9
DIFFERENTIAL DIAGNOSIS OF SYNCOPE
(SUDDEN LOSS OF CONSCIOUSNESS)

VASOMOTOR DISORDERS
1. Simple faint (vasovagal syncope)
2. Orthostatic hypotension
3. Hyperventilation (exercise, anxiety)
4. Miscellaneous: postmicturition and posttussive syncope syndromes, voluntary syncope

CENTRAL NERVOUS SYSTEM DISORDERS
1. Seizure disorder
2. Subarachnoid or subdural hemorrhage (spontaneous, traumatic)
3. Brain stem or spinal cord lesion (paralytic syncope)
4. Migraine headache
5. Narcolepsy
6. Glossopharyngeal neuralgia
7. Other cerebrovascular disease

CARDIOVASCULAR DISORDERS
1. Stokes-Adams syncope (third-degree heart block with asystole)
2. Tachyarrhythmias
3. Aortic stenosis
4. Takayasu's disease

MISCELLANEOUS
1. Hysteria
2. ENT disorders: Meniere's disease, swallow syncope due to esophageal dysfunction
3. Endocrine dysfunction: hypoglycemia, hypocalcemia
4. Heat stroke
5. Anemia (severe)
6. Pulmonary hypertension
7. Pulmonary embolism

tified, a lag in the adjustment of carotid sinus sensitivity in relation to pubertal growth with its rapidly rising center of gravity and expanding blood volume may be a uniquely adolescent phenomenon. Other common associations are prolonged motionless standing, anemia, pregnancy, alcohol or other central nervous system depressants, and the administration of some antihypertensive agents or phenothiazines. More serious related conditions are rare in adolescents and, if present, give other indications and are not cited here. Treatment is by reassurance, instructions to rise more slowly from the lying or sitting state, and attention to underlying pathologic conditions. Vulnerable adolescents who must stand for long periods may attenuate their problem by isometric exercises of the legs and thighs.

POSTMICTURITION SYNDROME

The postmicturition syndrome occasionally is seen among males who consume large amounts of alcohol, fall asleep, rise to urinate, and then faint. This appears to be due to the effects of vasodilation from alcohol and the warmth of the bed in combination with a sudden reflex reduction in peripheral vascular resistance following bladder emptying.

NARCOLEPSY

Narcolepsy, although not strictly a syncopal disorder, is sufficiently similar to warrant consideration in the differential diagnosis, even though relatively rare in the adolescent population. It is characterized by an intermittent, irresistable urge to sleep for periods lasting from minutes to several hours and without discrimination as to time, place, or circumstances. Some patients also experience an inability to move their extremities for several seconds just before or after falling asleep (sleep paralysis). Hypnagogic hallucinations and daytime cataplexy also may occur. The electroencephalogram may demonstrate a rapid eye movement (REM) sleep disorder.

VOLUNTARY SYNCOPE

Voluntary syncope sometimes is induced by adolescents seeking an altered mental state. This may be accomplished by the sequence of squatting, hyperventilating, standing up rapidly, and performing a Valsalva maneuver. Syncope also may be induced by having a confederate compress the chest with a sustained bear-hug squeeze from behind.

Coma and Semicoma

Coma refers to sustained unconsciousness with unresponsiveness to any stimuli. Stupor, or semicoma, defines a less profound, sleeplike state from which the patient can be aroused, but only by constant stimulation. This section provides direction for the initial management of such states in the adolescent. Although many conditions may produce coma given the right set of circumstances, this event usually occurs late in the course of a disease and symptoms suggesting the cause commonly occur long before reaching this stage. Even if coma is the presenting sign, there usually are sufficient clues in the physical examination and history pointing to the underlying cause. Here the discussion focuses on those situations likely to be encountered during the second decade that tend to alter consciousness as a major and early sign posing a diagnostic dilemma.

The most common causes of coma or semicoma in the adolescent age group are drug overdose and

TABLE 10-10
DIFFERENTIAL DIAGNOSIS OF
COMA AND SEMICOMA IN ADOLESCENCE*

DRUG OVERDOSE (see Chapter 20)
Unintentional secondary to abuse
  CNS depressants (barbituates, tranquilizers, alcohol)
  Narcotics
  Phencyclidine
  Atropine, scopolamine (rare)
Suicidal act
  CNS depressants
  Aspirin
  Anything else in medicine cabinet

TRAUMA
Intracranial space-occupying lesion
Tumor
Cerebrovascular accident
  Ruptured aneurysm, AV malformation, etc.
  Thrombocytopenia, other bleeding disorders (rare)

METABOLIC
Diabetes mellitus
  Ketoacidosis
  Hypoglycemia secondary to insulin overdose
Primary hypoglycemia (rare)
Adrenal insufficiency (rare)
Uremic encephalopathy (rare)
Hepatic coma (rare)

INFECTIOUS DISEASES
Bacterial meningitis
Viral encephalitis
Herpes encephalitis (rare)

MISCELLANEOUS
Hypertensive encephalopathy (rare)
Reyes syndrome
Status asthmaticus (rare)
Status epilepticus (rare)
Catatonic schizophrenia (rare)

*See also Table 10-9.

trauma. If overdose is due to miscalculation during drug abuse, central nervous system depressants, narcotics, or phencyclidine are most likely to be involved (see Chapter 20). If coma is consequent to a suicidal act, virtually anything in the family medicine cabinet may be involved. Trauma should be evident on examination or by history, although other possible causes should be considered if the patient is found unconscious on the street, even if scalp contusions or abrasions are present.

On a statistical basis, the next most frequent cause of coma is a cerebrovascular accident due to a ruptured congenital aneurysm, arteriovenous malformation, or hemangioma. Classically, loss of consciousness is anteceded by an excruciating headache.

Persons with thrombocytopenia and some other bleeding disorders also are at risk of cerebrovascular accidents, but this fact usually is known already, as coma is an unusual initial presentation.

Diabetic ketoacidosis, bacterial meningitis, and viral encephalitis are more frequently encountered in adolescents than a cerebrovascular accident but are less likely to produce coma. Nonetheless, these are all reasonable contenders in the comatose adolescent. Hypoglycemia due to insulin overdose should also be considered in the already diagnosed diabetic receiving insulin treatment. Brain tumors also fit in this category but far more often are evident in other signs and symptoms of a space-occupying lesion, such as alteration of cerebellar function, cranial nerve palsies, headache, or vomiting.

Coma can be associated with a wide variety of other symptoms and signs that contribute to more specific diagnostic considerations. When seen in combination with hyperventilation or Cheyne-Stokes respirations, metabolic acidosis or encephalopathy is suggested, whereas irregular breathing with periods of apnea is more characteristic of brain stem damage. Coma with hypertension may indicate uremic encephalopathy, but an association with hypotension points to septicemia, severe dehydration, adrenal insufficiency, or cerebral hypoxia. Stupor and meningismus occur with meningitis, meningoencephalitis, subarachnoid hemorrhage, or posterior fossa tumor. The comatose patient with bilateral dilated pupils failing to react to light may be experiencing anoxia secondary to a CNS depressant overdose, whereas a narcotic overdose produces miosis. Phencyclidine overdose may be characterized by rotatory nystagmus, coma, and a strychninelike response to external stimuli. Midbrain disease results in irregular, nonreactive pupils, whereas herniation or damage to the third cranial nerve nucleus tends to be manifested in a unilateral, fixed, and dilated pupil.

Coma or stupor comprise a medical emergency. A protocol for immediate management is proposed in Table 10-11. Two cardinal rules must be observed regardless of other issues. The first is the signal importance of maintaining or restoring oxygenation. The second is to proceed with *extreme caution* in performing a lumbar puncture if a cerebrovascular accident or other space-occupying lesion is suspected to *any* degree; herniation of the brain stem through the foramen magnum with sudden death is a real possibility. It can be far safer to first proceed with computerized axial tomography.

TABLE 10-11
EMERGENCY MANAGEMENT OF COMA

1. Ensure adequate oxygenation; intubate and ventilate if necessary.
2. Establish intravenous line.
3. Obtain blood for stat studies.
   a. Barbituates, alcohol; start screen for other drugs.
   b. Glucose (Dextrostix may be done at bedside; if hypoglycemic, treat immediately with 50% glucose solution by IV push).
   c. Electrolytes.
   d. Blood gases, pH.
   e. Others as indicated (e.g., blood culture for suspected meningitis, urea nitrogen if hypertensive, ammonia levels for possible liver involvement, etc.).
4. Physical examination in more detail than initial observations while carrying out previous steps. (Note that there may be increased intracranial pressure in the posterior fossa without manifesting papilledema.)
5. Obtain history from accompanying persons; check for medical ID cards, bracelets, etc. if parents not available.
6. Evaluate for intracranial pathology.
   a. Stat computerized axial tomography procedure of first choice.
   b. Lumbar puncture, but only with *extreme caution* (see text).
7. Proceed with further diagnostic, consultative, and treatment measures as indicated by the preceding.

Meningitis

Meningitis (inflammation of the meninges and spinal fluid) may be caused by a wide variety of microbial agents with pneumococci, *Hemophilus influenzae*, and *Neisseria meningitidis* the most commonly implicated organisms in adolescence. Symptoms and signs include fever, headache, irritability, confusion, lethargy, meningismus (nuchal rigidity, positive Brudzinski and Kernig signs), cranial nerve palsies, convulsions, and petechiae, among others.

The cerebrospinal fluid characteristically contains an increased number of white blood cells, increased protein, and decreased glucose in relation to the blood glucose. A Gram stain often reveals intracellular and extracellular bacteria. A positive spinal fluid culture is definitive; the blood culture may be positive as well. Counterimmune electrophoresis (CIE) antigen in either blood or spinal fluid may be an important diagnostic aid when the Gram stain or culture is unrevealing (as may occur if the patient already has been given antibiotics). Conditions that may be particularly difficult to distinguish from each other include partially treated bacterial meningitis, viral meningitis, or meningoencephalitis, tuberculous meningitis, vasculitis, neoplasm, and brain abscess.

BRAIN ABSCESS

A brain abscess should be suspected in the face of meningitis symptoms with negative cerebrospinal fluid cultures, an elevated erythrocyte sedimentation rate, and/or neurologic deficits. Various causes of such an abcess are sepsis, bacterial endocarditis, mycotic aneurysm, chronic sinus or ear infections, pulmonary infections, or the systemic use of contaminated illicit drugs. A brain scan, computerized axial tomography, and/or angiography are helpful in the diagnosis.

BACTERIAL MENINGITIS

Treatment of bacterial meningitis depends on prompt antibiotic administration. Unless specific direction is provided by culture and sensitivity results, a combination of intravenous chloramphenicol (100 mg/kg/day) and ampicillin (200 mg/kg/day) may be employed if a gram-negative organism is suspect, or intravenous penicillin G (12–20 million U/day) if pneumococcus is suspect. Treatment should *not* be withheld pending culture results, although modification of an existing schedule may be indicated at this time. Antibiotics should be continued for 10 days or more, depending on clinical response and spinal fluid clearing. Bone marrow suppression is a rare complication from a single course of chloramphenicol and is more commonly seen with chronic or repetitive administration. Blood counts, however, should be carefully monitored in any circumstance. Prompt and adequate treatment minimizes the possibility of meningitis complications, which include cerebral edema, herniation, toxic encephalopathy, cranial nerve palsies, inappropriate antidiuretic hormone secretion (avoid fluid overloading), seizures, subdural effusion, residual motor deficits, chronic hydrocephalus, recurrent meningitis, and permanent deafness, among others.

VIRAL ENCEPHALITIS

Viral encephalitis is more likely to be accompanied by an alteration in mental status than by meningeal signs, although this is not an invariable finding and bacterial and viral forms may have identical presentations. The cerebrospinal fluid in viral infections tends to have fewer white blood cells (10–200/mm^3) in contrast to bacterial forms ($>$ 200/mm^3), and lymphocytes rather than polymorphonuclear cells predominate. Although the spinal fluid protein may be elevated in both, the glucose usually remains normal in viral infections and decreases in bacterial infections. Many viruses have been causally implicated, including enteroviruses, mumps, herpes simplex, lymphocytic choriomeningitis virus, arthropod-borne agents, adenovirus, and rubeola. A postinfectious encephalitis may be seen with measles, vaccinia, chickenpox, and mumps. Treatment of the fulminant form of herpes hominis encephalitis with cytosine arabinoside (ara C) is one of the newer advances in managing severe viral infections. The usual recommended daily dosage is 40 mg/m^2 given intravenously for 5 days. Intrathecal administration of 10 mg/m^2 for 3–5 days has been used in conjunction. This agent does have serious side effects, as well as being potentially mutagenic. Its use is not to be undertaken lightly and a confirmed diagnosis, only obtainable by brain biopsy, is an essential precondition.

Multiple Sclerosis

Multiple sclerosis is the commonest chronic degenerative neurologic disorder affecting young female adults (female to male ratio = 10:1). The peak age of onset is in the fourth decade, but it is not uncommon for multiple sclerosis to begin in adolescence. It is characterized by episodic patchy inflammation with resultant destruction of central nervous system white matter in the spinal cord and brain occurring in a series of periodic relapses and remissions over years and decades with significant, but gradually lessening, degrees of recovery each time. Ten percent of these patients, however, have a much more rapid, unremitting course without intercurrent improvement. The actual sites of involvement are highly variable and unpredictable.

The etiology is unknown, although measles virus, parainfluenza-1 virus, and a "multiple sclerosis-associated agent" have all been implicated. Genetic factors also seem to contribute in that 10% of close family members already have or will develop this disease.

Symptoms and signs vary and depend on the particular areas of the nervous system affected. In general, both motor and sensory deficits with muscular weakness, spasticity, paresthesias, and loss of cutaneous sensation are seen. The deficits tend to be distributed symmetrically, are particularly likely to involve the extremities, and, even if improved during remission, often reappear in conjunction with new areas of involvement at each relapse. Relapses are inconsistent in duration, lasting from minutes to days or longer. Remissions are equally inconsistent varying from only a few days to many years. Transient blindness from optic nerve involvement often is a premonitory or herald sign anteceding other neurologic symptoms by days to years. Lethargy, malaise, and/or headaches often precede an exacerbation.

Physical findings parallel the degree of neurologic deficits present at the time but may include nystagmus, optic disc pallor (with or without optic neuritis), ataxia, spastic paraplegia, intention tremor, scanning speech, and inappropriate affect (predominantly euphoria). Retrobulbar neuritis, variable degrees of limb paralysis, and paresthesias predominate.

Characteristic spinal fluid findings demonstrate a normal or slightly increased protein, normal glucose, increased mononuclear cells (5-50/mm^3), an abnormal gold curve (with a negative VDRL), and elevated IgG. Other sometimes positive laboratory tests include reduced erythrocyte electrophoretic mobility, adherence of peripheral blood lymphocytes to measles virus–infected tissue culture cells, and delayed visually evoked electropotentials. But none of these is specific to the diagnosis of multiple sclerosis. A definitive pathologic diagnosis can only be made at autopsy.

The differential diagnosis includes virtually any other progressive degenerative disease of the central nervous system or any condition, acute or chronic, that can produce neurologic deficits. However, the index of suspicion should be high in an adolescent female evidencing a central nervous system disease manifested in multiple, unpredictable lesions with a patchy distribution and relapsing-remitting course.

There is no effective treatment. Steroids may help induce a remission but do not seem to alter the course overall. Impaired breathing may require ventilatory assistance with a respirator. Physiotherapy and rehabilitative measures are important in maintaining maximal function. Psychologic counseling or specific psychotherapy is a desirable adjunct in helping the adolescent deal with the life-long implications of this disease. The prognosis is not entirely predictable. Although some patients may experience a rapid downhill course over only a year or two, others will have a normal life expectancy, or one only modestly curtailed but with slowly increasing motor disability and sensory and sphincter disturbances. Involvement of the muscles of respiration is

a particularly serious sign and, if persistent, predisposes the patient to recurrent lung infections. Death ultimately occurs from such an event.

Guillain-Barré Syndrome

Guillain-Barré syndrome is characterized by an acute inflammation of the peripheral nerves and is manifested by a symmetric and rapidly ascending paralysis with variable sensory loss. It has an incidence of 1.6-1.9/100,000 in the general population with a slight predominance in males. The etiology is unknown, but hypersensitivity reactions, toxins, vaccines, and various viral and bacterial infections have all been implicated at times; the onset often occurs 10-21 days after an upper respiratory or gastrointestinal tract infection.

An initial, peripheral neuritis of the lower extremities with tender muscles and reduced deep tendon reflexes is soon followed by flaccid paralysis. Involvement quickly progresses upward over several hours or days to affect the abdominal, thoracic, and upper extremity musculature to a variable degree. Paresthesias, myalgias, mild meningeal signs, bulbar symptoms, sensory loss, and cranial nerve palsies may be evident as well. The cerebrospinal fluid characteristically reveals a normal pressure, normal glucose, elevated protein, and no pleocytosis. The differential diagnosis includes any condition that also manifests an acute peripheral neuritis or generalized muscular weakness, such as poliomyelitis (in unimmunized individuals), multiple sclerosis, acute transverse myelopathy, spinal cord tumor, tethered cord, and myasthenia gravis. The prognosis generally is favorable, with symptoms often beginning to reverse after a few days or several weeks; full recovery, however, may take from 2-18 months. Complications include pneumonia, paralysis of the muscles of respiration, inappropriate antidiuretic hormone secretion and, uncommonly, death. Treatment is nonspecific, including ventilatory support, high quality nursing care, and physiotherapy. Steroids have been used but are without a clearly beneficial role.

Bell's Palsy

Bell's palsy is marked by the acute onset of facial weakness due to inflammation and compression of the seventh cranial nerve as it passes through the temporal bone. No clear etiology has been identified and although acute otitis media or herpes zoster have been implicated, these associations are inconsistent. The appearance of weakness takes place rapidly over several hours and usually is without other symptoms or signs excepting possible ear pain on the affected side. Characteristic findings include the loss of the nasolabial fold, a drooping mouth corner, inability to shut the eyelid with upward deviation of the eye itself, and a pulling of the mouth to the normal side on smiling or grimacing. Loss of taste over the anterior two-thirds of the tongue, hyperacusis, and other auditory symptoms also may be evident, depending on the precise location and extent of the inflammation. Most patients recover spontaneously within a few weeks or months, but 10%–20% sustain permanent injury.

The differential diagnosis includes any other lesion that may cause facial nerve palsy such as brain tumor, skull fracture, or meningitis. The Melkersson syndrome is a rare idiopathic condition marked by recurrent episodes of seventh nerve weakness and edema of the lips.

Treatment is first directed at protecting the cornea on the involved side by periodic irrigation with cellulose eye drops and keeping the eye patched or taped shut. Steroids are commonly used at the first signs of disease in an attempt to reduce the degree of nerve swelling and avoid permanent damage, but the results vary greatly. Prednisone, 40 mg/day × 3, may be given, then tapered over 1 week. Newer therapeutic considerations involve surgical decompression of the nerve itself when indicated by deteriorating electropotentials as measured by electromyography. Referral to an appropriate specialist for such an assessment may well be indicated, but it must be early in the course. If delayed until it becomes evident that function is not returning, permanent irreversible nerve injury already has taken place.

Miscellaneous Disorders

MUSCULAR DYSTROPHY

Muscular dystrophy encompasses a group of disorders characterized by progressive muscular weakness and muscular degeneration. Duchenne's muscular dystrophy is the classic type. It is an X-linked recessive disease often beginning at age 2–3 years with rapid progression of proximal muscle weakness. Usually this condition has been diagnosed by puberty; its significance for adolescence rests in the severe limitations on function usually present by this time and the prospect that death is a probable event within the next few years. Congenital muscular dystrophy is a variant with an even earlier age onset.

Becker's muscular dystrophy also is an X-linked disorder but with onset during adolescence. It is characterized by proximal muscle weakness, pseudohypertrophy, cardiac disorders, and impaired intelligence. Limb-girdle muscular dystrophy is another type that may begin in adolescence and is marked by a slow progression in muscle weakness of the pelvic or shoulder girdle or both. Facioscapulohumeral dystrophy may present at any time during the first three decades of life and manifests in gradually increasing weakness of the shoulder, neck, facial, and peroneal musculature; kyposcoliosis and lumbar lordosis can develop. Diagnosis of any of the muscular dystrophies is based on the clinical course in conjunction with characteristic findings on electromyography and muscle biopsy. Treatment is supportive with attention focused on rehabilitative measures to ensure attainment of maximum function.

MYOTONIC DYSTROPHY

Myotonic dystrophy is an autosomal dominant disorder manifested by myotonia or the abnormal persistence of voluntary muscular contractions, or both; for example, the patient is unable to clench and unclench his or her fist in rapid sequence. It may appear in adolescence as an isolated disease or in combination with hypothyroidism or polymyositis. Further characteristics include the slow progression of muscular weakness involving the face, neck, flexor groups, and distal legs. Frontal alopecia, cataracts, testicular atrophy, and cardiac abnormalities also have been seen. The electromyogram and muscle biopsy aid in the diagnosis. Treatment with phenytoin seems to stabilize the disorder and inhibits progression to some extent.

POLYMYOSITIS

Polymyositis is an inflammatory disease of the muscles evident in proximal, symmetric weakness of various muscle groups. Those of the arms, legs, neck flexors, and posterior pharyngeal area are most likely to be involved. Serum CPK is elevated, and the electromyogram is similar to that seen with Duchenne's muscular dystrophy; a muscle biopsy aids in diagnosis. Polymyositis may be an isolated condition or occur in combination with dermatitis, Raynaud's phenomenon, and malignant tumors, among other conditions. It should be differentiated from Charcot-Marie-Tooth disease, a polyneuropathy that presents with progressive peroneal atrophy, partial paralysis of the legs and, sometimes, partial paralysis of the forearms.

PERIPHERAL NEUROPATHY

A generalized term for inflammation of peripheral nerves, peripheral neuropathy manifestations include sensory and lower motor neuron symptoms. Symmetric or asymmetric weakness and wasting of distal muscles with muscular cramps and pain are often seen. Other findings include reduced or absent deep tendon reflexes, absent Babinski signs, and variable sensory deficits. Poliomyelitis is the prototypical cause but an uncommon one today. Various other viruses also may be involved, particularly the coxsackie virus. Peripheral neuropathy also is a common late manifestation of diabetes mellitus.

CEREBRAL PALSY

Cerebral palsy is a collective term applied to variable upper motor neuron dysfunctions stemming from prenatal or perinatal injury. Usually it has been diagnosed in early childhood and primarily poses therapeutic rather than diagnostic problems in the adolescent with all the considerations raised by a chronic illness of any type (Chapter 21). Mild degrees of cerebral palsy, however, may be missed until adolescence, when limb size disparity is magnified by pubertal growth, earlier "clumsiness" is not outgrown, or the increased demands for coordination and athletic competence bring formerly modest, compensated deficits to greater light. Cerebral palsy is characterized by increased deep tendon reflexes, positive Babinski signs, clonus, and spastic diplegia together with a tendency toward contracture of involved muscle groups. Puberty tends to increase the disproportion between affected and nonaffected extremities consequent to the former's restricted growth. Treatment is rehabilitative and psychotherapeutic. Muscle relaxers are used, as diazepam, baclofen, and dantrolene.

NEUROCUTANEOUS SYNDROMES

Neurocutaneous syndromes are characterized by a congenital ectodermal dysplasia evident in various lesions of the skin and central nervous system. In each case, treatment is supportive and symptomatic and the prognosis highly variable.

Tuberous sclerosis. Tuberous sclerosis (Bourneville's disease) is a major cause of mental retardation with severe epilepsy. It is characterized by adenoma sebaceum of the nose and cheeks with tubers (sclerotic patches) or dysplastic lesions in the brain, heart, kidneys, bones, lungs, or virtually any other organ. Intracerebral calcifications can develop and may be a useful diagnostic finding. Other skin lesions include pigmented nevi, hypopigmented macules, café au lait spots, shagreen patches (raised, indurated skin lesions commonly found on the back), lipomas, and fibromas. Mesodermal tumors of the kidney, rhabdomyoma of the heart, retinal phakomas, sclerosis of

various bones, and other lesions also may be seen. Status epilepticus and renal failure are major complications.

Neurofibromatosis. Neurofibromatosis (von Recklinghausen's disease) is an autosomal dominant disorder characterized by congenital café au lait spots and the progressive but variable development of multiple fibrous tumors of the skin, subcutaneous tissues, peripheral and cranial nerves, and other organs. Intraspinal tumors, optic gliomas, acoustic neuromas, meningiomas, pheochromocytomas, as well as sarcomatous degeneration and intracranial calcification may occur. Optic atrophy, scoliosis, hemihypertrophy, other gross visible deformity, precocious puberty, seizure disorders, and mental retardation have been seen. Despite the multiplicity of possible complications, the course in a given individual is unpredictable. The patient may never evidence any symptoms of this disorder, whereas others may develop severe complications related to the location and type of tumors at any time in life. The diagnosis is based on clinical grounds with or without a subcutaneous nodule biopsy. The presence of six or more café au lait spots alone, if all are more than 2 cm in diameter, is presumptive evidence of this disease even in the absence of other findings.

Sturge - Weber - Dimitri syndrome. Sturge - Weber - Dimitri syndrome (encephalotrigeminal angiomatosis) is characterized by a large facial capillary hemangioma, or "port wine stain," which usually is unilateral and tends to follow the trigeminal nerve distribution. Angiomas of the neck, mucous membranes, ocular choroid, and meninges are common. Meningeal angiomatosis often leads to seizures, mental retardation, and/or progressive contralateral hemiparesis. Eye involvement may result in buphthalmos, exophthalmos, and/or glaucoma. Intracranial calcifications and angiomas of the gastrointestinal tract, bladder, or other organs may occur on occasion.

Von Hippel-Lindau disease. Von Hippel-Lindau disease is an autosomal dominant familial disorder characterized by the gradual appearance of retinal angiomas, cerebellar hemangioblastomas, and/or spinal cord hemangiomas. Visual loss with cerebellar, spinal cord dysfunction, or both may present in late adolescence. Other possible lesions are hypernephroma, cystic adenomas of the pancreas, as well as tumors and angiomas of other organs. There are no characteristic skin lesions.

Ataxia-telangiectasis. Ataxia-telangiectasis (Louis-Bar syndrome) is an autosomal recessive disease with an early childhood onset and progressive cerebellar ataxia and/or choreoathetosis. Telangiectasia appear on the skin somewhat later, often in adolescence, and are particularly likely to be located about the conjunctivae, malar region of the cheeks, elbows, and knees. Mental retardation, sinusitis, bronchiectasis, and low IgA and IgE levels are the more frequent complications seen with time.

Bibliography

SEIZURE DISORDERS
Conomy, J. P. 1978. Long-term use of major anticonvulsant drugs. *Am. Family Phys.* 18:107.

Livingston, S. 1979. The medical treatment of epilepsy: maintenance of drug therapy. *Pediatr. Ann.* 8:232.

Morris, H. H. 1981. Current treatment of status epilepticus. *J. Family Pract.* 13:987.

Penry, J. K., and Newmark, M. E. 1979. The use of antiepileptic drugs. *Ann. Intern. Med.* 90:207.

Penry, J. K., and Porter, R. J. 1979. Epilepsy: mechanisms and therapy. *Med. Clin. North Am.* 63:801.

Rothner, A. D., and Erenberg, G. 1980. Status epilepticus. *Pediatr. Clin. North Am.* 27:592.

Singer, H. S., and Freeman, J. M. 1975. Seizures in adolescents. *Med. Clin. North Am.* 59:1461.

Williams, D. T.; Spiegel, H.; and Mostofsky, D. 1978. Neurogenic and hysterical seizures in children and adolescents: differential diagnosis and therapeutic considerations. *Am. J. Psychiatr.* 135:82.

HEADACHES
Caviness, V. S., and O'Brien, P. 1980. Headache. *N. Engl. J. Med.* 302:446.

Friedman, A. P., editor. 1978. Symposium on headache and related pain syndromes. *Med. Clin. North Am.* 62:427.

Greydanus, D. E. 1981. Alternatives to adolescent pregnancy. *Semin. Perinatol.* 5:62.

Lapkin, M. L., and Golden, G. S. 1978. Basilar artery migraine. *Am. J. Dis. Child.* 132:278.

Millac, P. A. H. 1980. Headache. *Practitioner* 224:705.

Peterson, H. 1981. Headaches in teenagers: a common problem. *Drug Therapy* 11(9):87.

Saper, J. R. 1978. Migraine I and II. *J.A.M.A.* 239:2380; 2480.

Shimar, S., and D'Souza, B. J. 1982. The diagnosis and management of headaches in children. *Pediatr. Clin. North Am.* 29:79.

VERTIGO
Branch, W. T., and Funkenstein, H. 1977. Clinical evaluation of vertigo. *Primary Care* 4:267.

Dobie, R. A. 1980. Vertigo: a physiological approach. *J. Family Pract.* 11:623.

Eviatar, L., and Eviatar, A. 1977. Vertigo in children: differential diagnosis and treatment. *Pediatrics* 59:833.

Warlow, C. P. 1980. Blackouts. *Practitioner* 224:711.

ALTERED STATES OF CONSCIOUSNESS
Anders, T. F.; Causkadon, M. A.; and Dement, W. C. 1980. Sleep and sleepiness in children and adolescents. *Pediatr. Clin. North Am.* 27:29.

Margolis, L. H., and Shaywitz, B. A. 1980. Prolonged coma in childhood. *Pediatrics* 65:477.

O'Connor, P. J. 1976. Syncope. *Practitioner.* 216:276.

Sabin, T. D. 1981. Coma and the acute confusional state in the emergency room. *Med. Clin. North Am.* 65(1):15.

Thomas, J. E.; Schirger, A.; Fealey, R. D.; et al. 1981. Orthostatic hypotension. *Mayo Clin. Proc.* 56:117.

Treiman, D. M., and Delgado-Escueta, A. V. 1980. How to evaluate and treat episodic loss of consciousness. *Drug Therapy* 10(11):112.

INTRACRANIAL HEMORRHAGE
Crowell, R. M., and Zervas, N. T. 1979. Management of intracranial aneurysm. *Med. Clin. North Am.* 63:695.

Eyster, E. F. 1980. Spontaneous subarachnoid hemorrhage. *Contin. Educ. Family Phys.* 12:21.

Tarlov, E. 1979. Subarachnoid hemorrhage. *Primary Care* 6:791.

CENTRAL NERVOUS SYSTEM INFECTIONS
Butler, I. J., and Johnson, R. T. 1974. Central nervous system infections. *Pediatr. Clin. North Am.* 21:649.

Feigin, R. D., and Dodge, P. R. 1976. Bacterial meningitis: newer concepts of pathophysiology and neurologic sequelae. *Pediatr. Clin. North Am.* 23:541.

Oppenheimer, E. Y., and Rosmin, N. P. 1976. Bacterial meningitis in childhood: neurological complications and their management. *Pediatr. Ann.* 5:10.

MULTIPLE SCLEROSIS

Arnason, B. G. W. 1982. Multiple sclerosis: current concepts and management. *Hosp. Pract.* 17:81.

Hart, R. G., and Sherman, D. G. 1982. The diagnosis of multiple sclerosis. *J.A.M.A.* 247:498.

Poser, C. M. 1979. Multiple sclerosis: a critical update. *Med. Clin. North Am.* 63:729.

MISCELLANEOUS

Appel, S. H. 1978. The muscular dystrophies. Clinical update on two major types. *Postgrad. Med.* 64:93.

Barone, D. A. 1979. Neurofibromatosis: a clinical overview. *Postgrad. Med.* 66:73.

Chalhub, E. G. 1976. Neurocutaneous syndromes in children. *Pediatr. Clin. North Am.* 23:499.

Furukawa, T., and Peter, J. B. 1978. The muscular dystrophies and related disorders. I and II. *J.A.M.A.* 239:1537; 1654.

Kennedy, R. H.; Danielson, M. A.; Mulder, D. W.; et al. 1978. Guillaine-Barré syndrome. A 42-year epidemiological and clinical study. *Mayo Clin. Proc.* 53:93.

Marguis, P. 1979. Therapies for cerebral palsy. *Am. Family Phys.* 19:101.

Riccardi, W. M. 1981. Von Recklinghausen neurofibromatosis. *N. Engl. J. Med.* 305:1617.

Sibley, W. A. 1972. Polyneuritis. *Med. Clin. North Am.* 56:1299.

Slater, G. E., and Swaiman, K. F. Muscular dystrophies in childhood. *Pediatr. Ann.* 6:50.

Taft, L. T., editor. 1979. Symposium on new insights in cerebral palsy. *Pediatr. Ann.* 8:14–68.

Watson, W. 1978. Selected genodermatoses. *Pediatr. Clin. North Am.* 25:263.

–11–
The Musculoskeletal System

Specific Spine and Joint Disorders
Neck: Torticollis □ Spine □ The hip: slipped femoral epiphysis
Knee □ Leg aches □ Ankle and foot
Benign Bone Tumors: Osteoid Osteoma
Miscellaneous Orthopedic Disorders
Pectus excavatum □ Pectus carinatum
Congenital absence of the pectoralis muscles □ Epicondylitis
Arthritis
Juvenile rheumatoid arthritis □ Infectious arthritis
Viral arthritis □ Miscellaneous arthropathies
Osteomyelitis
Marfan Syndrome
Pilonidal Cyst and Sinus

Specific Spine and Joint Disorders*
NECK: TORTICOLLIS

Torticollis, or wryneck, refers to restricted neck motion with abnormal head posturing, usually involving the sternocleidomastoid, trapezius, and/or scalenus muscles. It is often bilateral and sustained for varying lengths of time. A slow, twisting, tilting head motion occurring intermittently is called spasmodic torticollis. Retrocollis refers to forceful neck extension, and antecollis implies forward flexion. Chronic torticollis can result in muscular hypertrophy or atrophy; it usually affects the sternocleidomastoid, but facial muscles can be involved as well.

Table 11-1 lists causes of torticollis. Most commonly, it is due to a congenital muscle anomaly, trauma, and/or rotary (atlantoaxial) subluxation. Often, the patient awakens with a tilted head and painful unilateral spasm of the neck muscles. There may be a history of recent neck strain, sleeping near a draft, or edema caused by acute pharyngitis, tonsillitis, or regional adenitis. Cervical roentgenograms (anterioposterior, lateral, and open-mouth odontoid)

*See also Chapter 18 for athletic injuries.

are indicated if persistent or chronic intermittent tilting develops.

Treatment varies and depends on etiology. Analgesics, moist heat, cervical traction, and/or a cervical collar may be helpful. Prompt resolution in 7-10 days usually occurs. Diphenhydramine hydrochloride (Benadryl), 2 mg/kg IV, may reverse the torticollis sometimes seen with phenothiazine toxicity. Chronic disease may necessitate surgical excision of anterior cervical root, spinal accessory nerve, or muscle insertions. Eye patching, antiparkinsonian medications, or psychiatric intervention may help in appropriate situations.

SPINE

Scoliosis. A lateral deviation and rotation of adjacent vertebrae from the normal midline axis is called scoliosis. Table 11-2 outlines the many different types that have been described. Eighty percent or more of adolescents with this deformity have idiopathic adolescent scoliosis, which usually consists of a painless right thoracic curve beginning at puberty and rapidly progressing during maximum spinal growth (average: Tanner stage 2-3 in females and stage 3-4 in males). It occurs eight times more fre-

TABLE 11-1
CAUSES OF TORTICOLLIS

1. Osseous or ligamentous
   a. Odontoid process defects
   b. Congenital vertebral anomalies (Klippel-Feil Syndrome [fusion of cervical vertebra with short neck, low posterior hair line, and limited neck motion]; scoliosis, renal anomalies, or Sprengel's scapulae elevation may also be noted)
   c. Juvenile rheumatoid arthritis
   d. Osteoid osteoma
   e. Eosinophilic granuloma
   f. Rotary subluxation (may follow upper respiratory tract infections, wrestling trauma, or edema secondary to pharyngitis, tonsillitis, poliomyelitis, syphilis, tuberculosis)
2. Muscular
   a. Congenital sternocleidomastoid or other muscle anomaly
   b. Dystonia musculorum deformans
3. Neurologic
   a. Posterior fossa tumor
   b. Phenothiazine toxicity (with extrapyramidal signs due to haloperidol, chlorpromazine, and others)
   c. Myasthenia gravis
   d. Syringomyelia
   e. Postencephalitic extrapyramidal involvement
4. Ocular
   a. Fourth cranial nerve palsy
   b. Congenital nystagmus
5. Functional (psychogenic disorder)

TABLE 11-2
TYPES OF SCOLIOSIS

1. Infantile idiopathic scoliosis (ages 0–3; left thoracic curve; mostly males; 20% are progressive)
2. Juvenile idiopathic scoliosis (ages 3–10; equal male/female ratio)
3. Adolescent idiopathic scoliosis (see text)
4. Functional scoliosis (compensatory spinal curve due to structural defect other than in the spine; e.g., a shortened leg)
5. Congenital scoliosis (congenital vertebral anomalies; hemivertebrae, failure of segmentation; 25%–50% also have renal anomalies; cardiac anomalies also noted)
6. Neuromuscular scoliosis (cerebral palsy, poliomyelitis, spinal muscle atrophy, muscular dystrophy, childhood paraplegia, arthrogryposis, amyotonia congenita, others)
7. Neurofibromatosis (short, angular thoracic scoliosis that may produce paraplegia)
8. Miscellaneous
   a. Spinal cord tumor
   b. Marfan's syndrome
   c. Morquio's disease
   d. Ehlers-Danlos syndrome
   e. Juvenile rheumatoid arthritis
   f. Fractured vertebra
   g. Post irradiation
   h. Post burns

quently in females than in males and appears to be transmitted as an autosomal dominant trait in some families. Estimates of the incidence of scoliosis among adolescents vary widely (1.5%–10%), but most studies indicate that 3%–4% of all teenage girls will be affected; to some degree 15% of these will have serious enough disease to require treatment.

Careful screening of all teenagers for scoliosis is important, particularly during early adolescence and the period of rapid growth. Indicative findings include spinal curvature in combination with a compensatory pelvic tilt and asymmetry of the flanks, scapulae, shoulders, and rib cage. An important aspect of the examination is the forward-bending test: the patient stands up with feet together and hands held (palms together) directly downward in front with elbows extended; he or she bends over 90 degrees or more while the examiner observes for any deviation of the spine from the midline and evidence of thoracic asymmetry. Curves under 25 degrees are difficult to detect unless a careful inspection is performed. Findings of café au lait spots, nerve root irritation, muscle spasms, other evidence of a painful curvature, and/or unequal leg length suggest scoliosis other than the idiopathic type. Spinal roentgenograms (including a standing anteroposterior film) in idiopathic adolescent scoliosis usually reveal a right thoracic curvature from T-5 or T-6 to T-11, or T-12, or L-1 and a left lumbar curve from T-11 or T-12 to L-4. Left thoracic or right lumbar curves are unusual and often indicate some other etiology. In the latter instance, a myelogram or intravenous pyelogram may be indicated to detect renal and other spinal anomalies seen in association with some forms of congenital scoliosis.

Treatment of idiopathic adolescent scoliosis depends upon the degree of curvature, the rate of curvature change, associated symptomatology, and the ability of the patient to comply with treatment regimens (Table 11-3). The use of back exercises, Milwaukee or other braces, and surgery must be planned by an orthopedic surgeon skilled in the correction of spinal defects. Surgery is indicated in advanced cases or in those refractory to conservative measures. Following a several-day period of traction, the spine is surgically stabilized with a Harrington

TABLE 11-3
TREATMENT OF
ADOLESCENT IDIOPATHIC SCOLIOSIS

Degree of curvature	Action and comment
Under 20 degrees (Cobb method of measurement, see references on scoliosis)	Check every 3–6 months with a single AP standing roentgenogram and photographs. See patient more frequently if rate of change is rapid.
20–40 degrees	Use Milwaukee brace for 23 of 24 hours. Back exercises without the brace are useless.
45 degrees or more	Surgery (Table 11-4). Exact timing of surgery varies.
Over 55 degrees	Respiratory compromise develops with increased residual volume, increased dead space, and decreased vital capacity. The higher the scoliosis and the more the curvature, the greater are the pulmonary (and cardiac) difficulties due to compression.

TABLE 11-4
STRUCTURAL DEFECTS OF THE LOWER SPINE

1. Spondylolysis
2. Spondylolisthesis
3. Structural scoliosis or kyphosis involving the lower spine
4. Lumbarization (six instead of five lumbar vertebrae)
5. Sacralization (four lumbar vertebrae with the fifth being part of the sacrum)
6. Spina bifida occulta
7. Lumbar sclerotic pedicle (benign sclerosis of a lumbar pedicle with bony hypertrophy opposite a defect of the pars interarticularis)

rod. A corrective body spica cast is then applied and kept on for 8–9 months. This usually results in good correction with only little if any loss of mobility. The primary care physician may notice complications of surgical correction such as cranial and other nerve injuries, wound or pin sepsis, immobilization hypercalcemia, thrombophlebitis, anxiety reactions, and body image distress secondary to the procedure and prolonged casting. Failure to detect scoliosis early or inadequate treatment may result in serious back deformity with a poor adolescent self-image and long-term possibilities for degenerative arthritis, chronic back pain and, in advanced cases, serious cardiorespiratory consequences. Untreated severe scoliosis will continue to progress in adulthood, leading to impaired respiration with resultant alveolar hypoventilation, polycythemia, increased pulmonary vascular resistance, pulmonary hypertension, and congestive heart failure. Future treatment for scoliosis may involve correction of the back deformity by using electrical stimulation of back muscles. This promising method may reduce the number of scoliotic youth needing surgery.

Kyphosis. Kyphosis is a malalignment of the spine in the sagittal plane that increases the posterior convex curvature. Two main types occur in adolescence: postural kyphosis and Scheuermann's disease.

Postural kyphosis accounts for 95% or more of cases observed in teenagers and is seen in individuals who chronically slouch to a marked degree. Slouching may be to hide developing breasts, because of habit, or for other reasons. Postural lordosis (lumbar anterior convexity) with exaggerated protrusion of sacrum and buttocks is a frequent concomitant. These curvatures may become chronic if not corrected, resulting in a protuberant abdomen and, possibly, degenerative changes in the spine. Congenital spinal deformities manifesting in kyphosis should be ruled out by roentgenograms. Treatment involves attention to proper positioning while sitting and standing and an exercise program to strengthen back muscles and promote good posture (weight lifting, track, ballet, modern dancing). Primary or secondary contributing psychologic factors also must be dealt with through counseling. The physician must differentiate, however, between the relatively rare instance of true postural kyphosis and the far more common casual slouch exhibited by many adolescents, particularly at times of rapid growth.

Scheuermann's disease, dorsum rotundum, is characterized by a thoracic deformity developing in the young teenager and often progressing to a painful "round back." This structural kyphosis may be confused with the postural type. Spinal roentgenograms are required for differentiation. Hyperextension exercises are helpful for mild disease, but bracing or occasionally surgery may be necessary for progressive deformity of over 45 degrees. Chronic low back pain can develop in adulthood if the curvature extends to the lumbar spine.

Spondylolisthesis. Spondylolisthesis, a structural defect of the lower spine, refers to the anterior displacement (subluxation) of a lumbar vertebra (usually L-5 or S-1), most commonly associated with a bilateral defect in the pars interarticularis (spondylolysis). Low back pain, with or without trauma or degenerative joint disease as a precipitating factor, usually is the first sign. Complications include increasing lumbar lordosis and sciatica (sharp, lower back pain radiating along the sciatic nerve to one or both lower extremities due to inflammation or pressure on lumbosacral nerve roots). The patient often feels better leaning forward. Table 11-4 lists this and other structural defects causing back pain.

Examination may reveal a "step-off" spinal deformity caused by forward vertebral displacement as well as hamstring spasm and limited straight-leg raising ability. An oblique lower spine roentgenogram often demonstrates a translucent defect in the pars interarticularis (spondylolysis), whereas a lateral film reveals vertebral subluxation. Most individuals have mild pain, and no treatment is needed except exercises to achieve good posture and improve paravertebral muscular tone. Spinal fusion may be required in the rare patient with severe intractable back pain.

Ankylosing spondylitis. Ankylosing spondylitis (Marie-Strümpell spondylitis), a chronic inflammatory disease of unknown etiology, is characterized by sacroiliitis with subsequent ascending vertebral arthritis and peripheral joint inflammation (hip, knee, shoulder, others). Nearly all cases are associated with the presence of the histocompatibility antigen HLA B27. Symptoms begin insidiously with low back pain, usually (but not exclusively) occurring in males between the ages of 15–30 years. The pain often is associated with morning stiffness or low-grade nocturnal lower back ache, which characteristically is relieved for 15–30 minutes by getting up and walking around. A positive family history is common. Table 11-5 lists many of the features and complications seen in patients with this disorder. Bilateral symmetric sacroiliitis on roentgenogram is crucial to the diagnosis.

Peripheral joint disease or anterior uveitis may antedate the development of a stiff, painful spine. Fever, fatigue, weight loss, anorexia, hypochromic anemia, and an increased erythrocyte sedimentation rate also may be noted. Other spondylarthropathies involving sacroiliitis, including inflammatory bowel disease, rheumatoid arthritis, psoriatic arthritis, and Reiter's syndrome, should be ruled out. Rheumatoid arthritis may involve the spine but without sacroiliitis.

Treatment includes the use of a firm mattress, exercise (especially swimming), antiinflammatory medication (Table 11-6), intraarticular steroid injec-

TABLE 11-5
FEATURES OF ANKYLOSING SPONDYLITIS

1. Bony ankylosis of the posterior intervertebral, costovertebral, and sacroiliac joints.
2. Ossification of the spinal ligaments and intervertebral disk margins.
3. Rigid, immobile, bony thoracic cage. (Chest pain develops due to involvement of the manubrosternal joint.)
4. Peripheral joint swelling, tenderness, and motion restriction of various joints including hip, shoulder, knee, wrists, metacarpophalangeal joints, metatarsophalangeal joints, and others. Joint damage is especially noted in the hips and shoulders.
5. Achilles tendonitis.
6. Nongranulomatous anterior uveitis (25%).
7. Cardiac defects
   a. Aortic insufficiency (root of aorta and aortic valve affected)
   b. Conduction defects noted on ECG: increased PR interval, bundle branch block, complete AV dissociation, and others.
8. Apical pulmonary fibrosis (a late complication characterized by bronchiectasis, cavity formation, fibrosis, and aspergilloma).
9. Cauda equina syndrome (urinary incontinence, muscle wasting, pain, and sensory loss due to involvement of the cauda equina).
10. Secondary renal amyloidosis.

tion, and surgery. Some patients benefit by taking their total 24-hour medication at bedtime to relieve nocturnal or early morning pain. Most individuals with this disease live a normal life span.

Low back pain syndrome. Complaints of pain in the lower back are commonly encountered in the adolescent. All of the foregoing conditions may cause low back pain, as well as those listed in Table 11-7. Persistent or recurrent complaints require full evaluation of the spine and associated nerve roots by examination and roentgenogram. Frequently this evaluation is revealing. In particular, early signs of slipped intervertebral disk may be difficult to detect with absent or only fleeting sciatic pain; as this is not an uncommon condition in adolescence, it should be considered in the differential diagnosis. Various exogenous factors also should be investigated; these may include a recent change from high- to low-heeled shoes or vice versa, the wearing of new fad shoes (Earth shoes and platform shoes), cramped study or working conditions, and/or a poorly supporting bed. Participation in sports or other activi-

TABLE 11-6
DRUG THERAPY IN
ANKYLOSING SPONDYLITIS

1. Salicylates (see Table 11-15).
2. Indomethacin, 25 mg b.i.d., up to q.i.d. (headaches, giddiness, nausea, emesis, peptic ulcer, depression, psychosis, and other side effects reported).
3. Phenylbutazone, up to 300–400 mg/day (agranulocytosis, salt, and water retention, dermatitis, peptic ulcer, and other side effects reported).
4. Naprosyn (naproxen), 250 mg b.i.d.; see text on arthritis.
5. Steroid injection into the joint.
6. Topical steroids for anterior uveitis (systemic steroids may be needed).

TABLE 11-7
CAUSES OF LOW BACK PAIN

1. Idiopathic
2. Trauma
   a. Paravertebral muscle strain
      Acute (often in athletics or sudden lifting/moving of heavy objects)
      Chronic (exogenous stress factors, such as improper shoes, poor preathletic conditioning, too small school desk or chair, sagging bed, etc.)
   b. Slipped or ruptured intervertebral disk
   c. Compression fracture
3. Scoliosis
4. Spondylolisthesis
5. Spinal arthritis
   a. Ankylosing spondylitis
   b. Rheumatoid arthritis
   c. Other
6. Congenital bony defects of the spine
7. Tumors
   a. Osteoid osteoma
   b. Primary bone neoplasms
   c. Metastatic neoplastic lesions
8. Infections: osteomyelitis and disk space
9. Psychogenic

ties involving stress to the back without prior proper conditioning, lifting or pushing heavy weights, and so forth are possible causes of chronic muscular strain and spasm. Other instances may be psychogenic and should be considered, particularly if the patient presents with various ill-defined complaints in other parts of the body as well.

THE HIP: SLIPPED
CAPITAL FEMORAL EPIPHYSIS

A slipped capital femoral epiphysis usually occurs in an obese, early pubertal adolescent (Tanner stage II–III) or preadolescent. It also may occur in somewhat older, thin teenagers at the peak of their growth spurt. It more commonly occurs in males (2–3:1 male/female ratio), tends to be chronic rather than acute (80%), and is unilateral more often than bilateral (3:1 unilateral/bilateral ratio), although a number of patients presenting with unilateral disease may develop slippage on the opposite side at a later time. More blacks are affected than Caucasians and the peak incidence is in spring or summer months. Its cause is unknown, but increased stress on a wide and rapidly growing epiphyseal plate has been postulated. Rarely, this condition has been associated with hypothyroidism or hypopituitarism.

The patient often first notes an aching sensation in the groin, buttocks, lateral hip, or knee, which may or may not increase in severity with time. In some instances, mild discomfort over several weeks or months may be followed by the acute onset of marked pain when a slight degree of slippage suddenly becomes severe. Sometimes knee pain is the only manifestation and a slipped capital femoral epiphysis should not be overlooked in the diagnosis of this complaint.

Examination varies from being relatively unrevealing to demonstrating a limp with an externally rotated foot and limited internal rotation, abduction, and flexion of the hip. Occasionally, the patient's only complaint may be of a painless limitation of hip rotation or an externally rotated leg and foot.

Table 11-8 cites differential considerations, but hip roentgenograms (lateral as well as anteroposterior views) are diagnostic. Early in the course, *lateral* films reveal displacement of the femoral head posteriorly and medially. An increased width of the epiphyseal plate with irregular margins also may be seen. In more advanced cases, anteroposterior views show the femoral head to be displaced superiorly and laterally in relation to the femoral neck. A technetium bone scan demonstrates increased uptake at the epiphyseal plate.

Early diagnosis is essential so that surgical pinning can stabilize the femoral head, preventing further displacement. Treatment at this stage offers an excellent prognosis in most cases. Delayed treatment with significant slippage may require a corrective osteotomy in returning the femoral head to a more normal weight-bearing position. Unfortunately, the outcome of surgery in severe cases often is unsatisfactory. Occasionally the adolescent or the parents refuse surgical correction; in these instances a bilateral leg cast with cross bars or spica cast is an

TABLE 11-8
DIFFERENTIAL DIAGNOSIS
OF HIP PAIN IN TEENAGERS

1. Trauma strain
2. Slipped capital femoral epiphysis
3. Transient synovitis
4. Monarticular arthritis
5. Septic hip arthritis
6. Avascular necrosis
7. Osteochondritis dissecans
8. Idiopathic chondrolysis
9. Late-onset Legg-Perthes disease
10. Osteoid osteoma
11. Sickle cell anemia
12. Collagen vascular disorders
13. Knee disorders

TABLE 11-9
CAUSES OF KNEE PAIN IN TEENAGERS

1. Osgood-Schlatter disease
2. Chondromalacia patellae
3. Osteochondritis dissecans
4. Menisci injuries
5. Ligamentous instability
6. Patellar dislocation or subluxation
7. Popliteal cyst
8. Arthritis
9. Hemophilia
10. Synovial tumors (pigmented villonodular synovitis or synovial chondromatosis)
11. Leg aches

alternative. If adequate surgical correction is not possible, the patient faces the probability of chronic hip pain, stiffness, and limp due to articular cartilage thinning (chondrolysis) and traumatic arthritis. Hip fusion or total hip replacement may be required.

All patients also should be x-rayed periodically on the noninvolved side during their growth spurt to detect possible delayed involvement.

KNEE

Osgood-Schlatter disease. Osgood-Schlatter disease (tibial tuberosity apophysitis) is a common disorder that classically occurs in Tanner II or III adolescent males and, less commonly, in females who are very active physically and frequently involved in sports requiring repeated torsional knee movements (basketball and football). It consists of a partial avulsion of the patellar tendon, presumptively due to repeated stress in a rapidly growing individual. The patient usually presents with a history of increasing unilateral knee pain. Finding an enlarged tender tibial tubercle is virtually diagnostic, although roentgenograms should be taken to rule out the rare possibility of other disorders. Table 11-9 cites the differential diagnosis of knee pain in adolescents.

It is important to note that this is a self-limited aseptic, nonneoplastic disorder, and overtreatment should be avoided. Although avulsion of the tibial tuberosity may be a rare complication, in most instances the only indicated treatment is limitation of activities that cause pain. All other activities may be pursued and should be encouraged. On occasion, marked discomfort may require cylinder casting for a few weeks. Steroid injections are not beneficial. Even without any treatment the prognosis is excellent. The process generally resolves spontaneously

in 1–2 years with the completion of growth and, at most, leaves the individual with residual painless enlarged tibial tubercles.

Chondromalacia patellae. Chondromalacia patellae (patellar instability syndrome) is most commonly seen in rapidly growing, athletic adolescent females. This disorder only recently has been recognized as the cause of obscure knee pain, and was formerly often thought to be psychosomatic. It is believed due to an instability of the patella resulting in maltracking within the femoral groove and an irritation, softening, and erosion of the patellar cartilage consequent to constant friction between the articular surfaces. Causes include congenital abnormalities in patellar-femoral groove relationships, malinsertion of the vastus medialis, trauma, stress, or strenuous exercise. Symptoms include unilateral or bilateral chronic knee pain exacerbated after prolonged running, climbing, walking, or bicycle riding. There is a characteristic inability to sit for prolonged periods of time with the knee in a flexed position, as in a car, at a movie or at a desk. Some patients give a history of the knee giving way on climbing stairs, crepitus with knee motion, joint effusion, and/or quadriceps atrophy.

Findings on examination usually are limited to the patella, with pain experienced while the knee is in a flexed position or when the patella is moved from side to side with the knee extended. Pain also is elicited by palpating and exerting pressure on the articular margins of the patella while displacing it medially or laterally. Isometric quadriceps contraction with the leg extended may reveal a subtle lateral patellar deviation. This is best detected by placing a row of three dots in a straight line while the knee is relaxed (one several inches above the

**TABLE 11-10
TREATMENT OF
CHONDROMALACIA PATELLAE**

1. Limit activity that worsens knee pain (jogging, jumping, climbing).
2. Encourage isometric exercises such as straight leg raising against resistance.
3. Encourage other activity such as swimming.
4. Cast or splint.
5. Surgical correction of associated patellar malalignment.
6. Patellar drilling to stimulate formation of new fibrocartilage in degenerated areas.
7. Patellectomy.

knee in the mid-line, one several inches below and one at the mid patella point) and observing for an lateral displacement of the patellar dot on isometric quadriceps contraction. Table 11-9 lists differential considerations.

Standard knee roentgenograms generally are unrevealing, but special "sunset" views taken horizontally through the patellar-femoral groove area with the knee bent at 90 degrees may demonstrate abnormal relationships. Arthroscopy, articular biopsy, or both show a thinned, irregular cartilage. Varying degrees of erosion may be noted as well in advanced cases. Table 11-10 outlines treatment. Careful orthopedic evaluation and followup are indicated, as chronic, disabling knee pain may result.

Osteochondritis dissecans. Osteochondritis dissecans is a condition characterized by the gradual separation of a fragment of bone and associated cartilage from the medial femoral condyle. It most commonly appears in males during late childhood or adolescence and is unilateral in 90%. Sometimes the lateral femoral condyle, the femoral head, or even the patella may be involved. The patient commonly presents with an aching sensation over the affected knee after exercising. Examination reveals local condylar tenderness, particularly when the knee is flexed. Knee roentgenograms reveal the separation. Treatment requires the application of a long leg cast for several weeks or longer.

If the condition is not diagnosed early, full separation of the fragment may occur with dislocation into the joint space; this is demonstrable on roentgenogram. Limp, swelling, limited knee motion and locking episodes suggest this possibility. Surgical treatment is required with removal of the fragment or fixing the fragment back into its proper place

with screws. Osteochondritis dissecans also can be seen in the hip, elbow, and ankle.

Blount's disease. Growth disturbance of the posterior and medial portions of the proximal tibia may result in a severe bow leg deformity in childhood known as Blount's disease, or tibia vara. Occasionally a mild unilateral form occurs in early adolescence during growth. Consequent shortening of leg length on the involved side may necessitate surgical correction.

Popliteal cyst. Popliteal cyst (Baker's cyst) is a painless, benign cystic mass of variable size (pea to golfball) arising from the gastrocnemiotsemimembranous bursa, which communicates with the knee joint. It is a smooth, firm, nonpulsatile, slow-growing lesion in back of the knee, rarely causing symptoms unless it becomes very large. Rupture of the cyst into the calf may produce symptoms mimicking thrombophlebitis. Pain or motion restriction, as well as pressure on sciatic nerve branches, also have been seen. Aspiration reveals gelatinous fluid similar to a wrist ganglion cyst. Differential diagnosis includes muscle tears, vascular aneurysms, and benign tumors. Though treatment usually is not necessary, surgical excision may be done if symptomatic. Postoperative recurrences or occurrence on the opposite side are not usual.

LEG ACHES

Intermittent aches or pains in the lower leg or thigh muscles are usually easily distinguished from specific knee or hip disorders. Occasionally, pain in other areas is noted as well, including the groin and in or behind the knees. There is no known etiology, and this condition has been linked to such diverse causes as puberty, rapid growth, overexertion with lactic acid buildup, excessive caffeine intake, and even acne! Typically, the pain is bilateral, occurs in the late afternoon or early evening, or awakens the patient from sleep. Older children and young teenagers seem particularly prone to this complaint, which has been called idiopathic myalgia or, simply, leg aches. No specific disorder is found. Roentgenograms and laboratory tests, including erythrocyte sedimentation rate, creatine, phosphokinase are normal. Heat, massage, salicylates, and reassurance are recommended. Resolution occurs over several months or years, and there are no sequelae.

ANKLE AND FOOT

Ankle pain. One of the most common causes of ankle pain is a sprain of the lateral collateral liga-

TABLE 11-11
CAUSES OF FOOT AND ANKLE PAIN IN TEENAGERS

1. Ill-fitting shoes
2. Ankle sprain, strain
3. Occult fracture (ankle or foot) due to specific trauma or chronic stress
4. Achilles tendonitis (with or without hypermobile flat feet)
5. Pes cavus (high arched feet)
6. Ingrown toe nails
7. Ganglion cyst
8. Osteomyelitis (including Brodie's abscess)
9. Infection from accidental puncture wound of the plantar surface with or without retained foreign body
10. Accessory navicular bone
11. Tarsal coalition
12. Osteochondroses
    a. Sever's disease
    b. Freiberg's disease
    c. Köhler's disease
13. Tumors
    a. Synovial sarcoma
    b. Ewing's sarcoma

TABLE 11-12
DIFFERENTIAL DIAGNOSIS OF OSTEOID OSTEOMA

1. Osteoid osteoma
2. Fibrous dysplasia
3. Aneurysmal bone cyst
4. Giant cell tumor
5. Osteochondroma
6. Malignant tumors
    a. Osteogenic sarcoma
    b. Ewing's tumor
    c. Soft tissue sarcoma
    d. Leukemia

ment due to trauma (see Chapter 18). Table 11-11 lists other causes. The location of the pain, x-ray findings, laboratory data (WBC, ESR), and other tests (bone scan) often aid in the correct diagnosis.

Miscellaneous ankle conditions. Achilles tendonitis sometimes occurs in the athletic adolescent subject to repeated stress. Small tears develop in the Achilles tendon, causing a variable amount of heel pain and limping. Treatment consists of avoiding stretching activity; casting may be needed in serious cases.

Brodie's abscess, a subacute form of osteomyelitis involving the distal fibula, small foot bones, or both, is most often noted in males. Antibiotic penetrance into these areas is poor, and surgical excision may be necessary.

Occult fractures are especially apt to occur in the second metatarsal or at the base of the fifth metatarsal in improperly conditioned youths during the start of a sport season. They also have been noted among those of the Hari Krishna sect as a stress fracture due to continual dancing and among joggers. X-ray evidence of callus formation may take 10 days to appear.

Accessory navicular bone is usually asymptomatic.

A tarsal coalition may present with a rigid spastic foot and peroneal muscle spasm. Tomograms may be needed to identify the diagnostic features of subtle bone ridges between the calcaneus and navicular bones.

Occurring chiefly on the dorsum or lateral aspect of the foot, ganglion cysts have the same characteristics as a popliteal cyst (see section on the knee). They arise from any of the tendon sheaths of tarsal or metatarsal joints and frequently follow regional trauma. Aspiration reveals a gelatinous material and affords temporary relief when painful. Surgical excision is required for a permanent cure, but spontaneous resolution is seen occasionally. The cysts are benign and without significant consequence except if uncomfortable. Many instances are quite asymptomatic. Ganglion cysts also frequently occur in the wrist.

Osteochondrosis, an idiopathic aseptic necrosis, may occur in several foot bones:

□ Sever's disease—necrosis of the apophysis of the os calcis.
□ Köhler's disease; necrosis of the tarsal navicular bone.
□ Freiberg's disease; necrosis of the second metatarsal. Treatment is symptomatic.

Benign Bone Tumors: Osteoid Osteoma

A relatively common benign bone tumor,* osteoid osteoma is seen in older children, adolescents, and young adults. It should be suspected when pain localized to a bone or joint worsens during rest and at night and lessens with exercise and aspirin administration. The pain varies in intensity but often is exquisitely severe. Most tumors are single and located in the femur or tibia, but almost any bone may be a site. Multiple tumors have been reported

*Note: Malignant bone tumors are covered in Chapter 13.

on rare occasion. Physical symptoms and signs vary from none to localized swelling, muscle atrophy, favoring of the affected extremity, or degenerative joint changes, depending on the tumor's location. Osteoid osteoma of the spine may cause a painful scoliosis due to paravertebral muscle spasm.

Roentgenograms classically reveal a small radiolucent, rounded nidus, usually less than a centimeter in diameter and sometimes only 2–3 mm, surrounded by reactive sclerotic bone. Calcium deposits may or may not be noted within the central area. Diagnosis is by history and x-ray findings. Sometimes, however, the tumor is not readily visible on standard films, as the lesion can be easily obscured by normal, overlying dense bone. This is particularly apt to occur in the spine. If the patient history suggests a tumor but one is not evident initially, tomograms, lateral films, or both may be helpful. Table 11-12 cites other lesions that should be considered in the differential diagnosis.

Simple surgical excision results in a full cure, although recurrences are possible if removal is not complete.

Miscellaneous Orthopedic Disorders

PECTUS EXCAVATUM

Pectus excavatum or funnel chest is a congenital sternal depression that can be an isolated defect or associated with weak chest and abdominal muscles. The depression is commonly noted over the xiphisternal junction and may be due to an abnormality of the diaphragmatic attachment. Pectus excavatum may be noticed at birth or take years to develop, becoming particularly pronounced during adolescent growth. The major consequences are cosmetic with significant psychologic sequelae. Particularly marked deformities, however, with a sharply reduced anteroposterior diameter may result in cardiac compression, shortness of breath, dizziness, chest pain, arrhythmias and, rarely, congestive heart failure. Sometimes a benign parasternal systolic murmur may be heard. Anteroposterior roentgenograms may demonstrate an "enlarged" displaced heart, whereas lateral films will reveal the true state of affairs. Surgical correction is indicated for significant degrees of deformity and is best carried out in childhood.

PECTUS CARINATUM

Pectus carinatum, or pidgeon breast is a relatively rare defect characterized by the forward protrusion of the sternum with everted ribs. It, like pectus excavatum, varies in time of onset and degree of deformity but may worsen during the adolescent growth spurt. It is an isolated and asymptomatic

defect, but the deformity may have significant psychologic impact. Repair in childhood is indicated in noticeable cases. Mild deformity in female children may become hidden by pubertal breast development, and assessment for possible surgery is best deferred until this time.

CONGENITAL ABSENCE OF THE PECTORALIS MUSCLES

Congenital absence of the pectoralis muscles results in a flat chest with high nipples and the absence of well-developed anterior axillary folds. It may be associated with scoliosis or other abnormalities. Poland's syndrome is pectus carinatum together with hypoplasia and syndactyly of an upper extremity.

EPICONDYLITIS

Epicondylitis, overuse of the elbow in sports, particularly tennis or baseball, may produce tenderness over the lateral epicondyle at the point of the extensor tendon insertion (epicondylitis, or tennis elbow). This condition usually responds well to rest, local steroid injection, and a proper program of reconditioning before the patient resumes full activity. Two other painful disorders of the upper extremity are: the carpal tunnel syndrome and DeQuervain's tenosynovitis.

Arthritis

Arthritis is characterized by synovial inflammation evidenced in joint swelling, pain, redness, increased warmth, loss of motion, and/or stiffness. Arthralgia defines joint pain or discomfort without objective findings. The causes of arthritis and arthralgia in the adolescent are legion (Table 11-13). Discussion here is limited to the more commonly seen forms.

JUVENILE RHEUMATOID ARTHRITIS

Rheumatic arthritis (Still's disease) occurring in children or adolescents under age 16 is termed juvenile rheumatoid arthritis (JRA). Current classification divides JRA into five groups (Table 11-14).

Fever is a characteristic symptom of the systemic type with spikes up to 102–106 F in the later afternoon or early evening. The rheumatoid rash, characterized by fleeting nonpruritic, salmon-colored macules with central clearing, often appears in concert with temperature elevations. Polyarticular forms most commonly occur in females and pauciarticular disease in males, whereas the distribution of systemic JRA is divided equally between both sexes.

Polyarthritis in the older adolescent does not always conform to the juvenile form, often behaving more like adult rheumatoid arthritis with symmetric involvement of small joints, morning stiffness, low-

TABLE 11-13
DIFFERENTIAL DIAGNOSIS
OF ARTHRITIS IN ADOLESCENCE

1. Rheumatoid arthritis: juvenile or adult form
2. Rheumatic fever
3. Ankylosing spondylitis
4. Infectious joint disease
   a. Septic arthritis
   b. Viral arthropathy
   c. Complication of osteomyelitis
   d. Venereal disease arthritis
5. Collagen disorder
   a. Systemic lupus erythematosus
   b. Dermatomyositis
   c. Scleroderma
6. Vasculitis
   a. Henoch-Schönlein syndrome
   b. Polyarteritis nodosa
   c. Mucocutaneous lymph node syndrome
   d. Sjögren's syndrome
7. Generalized disorders commonly complicated by arthritis
   a. Hemophilia
   b. Sickle cell disease
   c. Serum sickness
   d. Secondary gout and pseudogout
   e. Chondrocalcinosis
   f. Lyme arthritis
   g. Polychondritis
   h. Hypertrophic osteoarthropathy
8. Diseases sometimes complicated by arthritis
   a. Psoriasis
   b. Inflammatory bowel disease
   c. Acne fulminans
   d. Hyperlipidemia
   e. Acromegaly
   f. Hyperparathyroidism
   g. Hemochromatosis
   h. Sarcoidosis
   i. Alkaptonuria
   j. Whipple's disease
   k. Familial Mediterranean fever
   l. Hypogammaglobulinemia
9. Traumatic arthritis
   a. Slipped femoral epiphysis
   b. Legg-Perthe's disease
   c. Chrondromalacia patellae
   d. Congenital dislocation of the hip
   e. Any poorly healing fracture, inadequately treated infection, etc.

grade fever, anemia, subcutaneous nodules, and a positive rheumatoid factor. Complications of juvenile or adult types include destructive joint inflammation, carditis, iridocyclitis, secondary amyloidosis, and growth retardation.

Diagnosis should rule out all other causes of arthritis. Laboratory testing should include a complete blood count, erythrocyte sedimentation rate, rheumatoid factor, antinuclear antibody test, and other tests as indicated by symptoms and differential considerations. The antinuclear antibody test results may be positive but is nonspecific in reaction. Arthrocentesis can be helpful in differentiating rheumatoid from other forms of arthritis and usually reveals a leukocytosis (at least $200/mm^3$ and often up to $10,000–100,000/mm^3$), normal glucose and complement levels, normal mucin clot, no crystals, and sterile cultures. Roentgenograms are not diagnostic in early disease, demonstrating nonspecific inflammation only. Evidence of joint destruction accompanies more advanced states.

Table 11-15 outlines various treatment modalities. General measures include physiotherapy, hot baths, isometric muscle exercises, and night splints. It is important to maintain as full a range of motion as possible as well as minimizing painful muscle spasms and contractures. Prolonged immobilization, however, should be avoided. Frequent slit-lamp examinations of the eye are indicated to detect complicating uveitis, particularly if the patient is in the high-risk, pauciarticular group. Synovectomy may be required to prevent severe joint damage, and corrective surgery may be indicated in cases with severe contractures.

The prognosis is highly variable. Polyarticular forms with a positive rheumatoid factor have the poorest outlook, with 50% of patients developing severe chronic arthritis. Patients with other types may have anything from minimal involvement with periodic exacerbations, easily controllable with anti-inflammatory drugs, to an unremitting course with progressive disability. Cases with prepubertal onset may improve considerably during adolescence if permanent joint damage has not already occurred. Mild disease has a tendency to "burn out" with time, regardless of the age of onset.

INFECTIOUS ARTHRITIS

Septic arthritis. Bacterial infection of the synovial space should be suspected when there is rapid onset of joint pain, with swelling, tenderness, and limited motion in the absence of trauma. Usually it is accompanied by fever, malaise, and other systemic signs. Septic arthritis should be high on the list of diagnostic contenders in any instance of acute joint disease, particularly if it involves the knee, hip, wrist, or elbow. To miss this diagnosis for even a relatively brief period may result in irreversible joint damage. Predisposing factors include bacteremia, septicemia, penetrating wounds and, possibly, local cellulitis.

TABLE 11-14
TYPES OF JUVENILE RHEUMATOID ARTHRITIS

Type	Description	Treatment*
Systemic JRA	Fever, rash, anorexia, weight loss, pericarditis, pleurisy, hepato-splenomegaly, generalized lymphadenopathy, and other evidence of a systemic disease developed. Arthritis develops within several weeks or months. Any joint can be involved, and 25% develop severe disabling arthritis. Lab tests: normochromic anemia, leuko-cytosis, elevated ESR, negative RF,[†] negative ANA;[‡] arthrocentesis differentiates from other causes of joint effusion (see text).	Salicylates Other antiinflam-matory drugs Gold therapy Steroids
Polyarticular (negative RF test)	Main feature is the involvement of several joints (over 4 or 5) in which the RF is negative and ANA is positive in only 1 of 4 patients. Generally a good prognosis. Approximately 10% develop disabling arthritis. Any joint can be involved. Features of systemic type can occur but often are not as severe.	Salicylates Other antiinflam-matory drugs
Polyarticular (positive RF test)	Any joint can be involved. The RF and ANA tests are positive. This has a worse prognosis—50% develop severe arthritis. Rheumatoid nodules may develop, as well as other features of systemic disease.	As above
Pauciarticular with eye involvement	Limited number (under 4 or 5) of joints affected, usually the knees, ankles, and/or elbows. Small joints sometimes affected such as the toes or fingers. Half of the patients develop chronic iridocyclitis, but severe arthritis is uncommon. The RF is often negative, but half develop a positive ANA.	Salicylates Topical steroids and ophthalmologic dilating agents for iridocyclitis
Pauciarticular with sacroiliitis	Knees, ankles, hips are affected along with sacroiliitis. Ankylosing spondylitis develops in some; negative RF and ANA. The HLA B27 antigen is also present in many cases.	Salicylates Indomethacin Phenylbutazone

*See also Table 11-15.

[†]RF, rheumatoid factor test.

[‡]ANA, antinuclear antibody test.

Hemophilus influenzae is a common causal agent in young children while *S. aureus* is most common in older children. *Neisseria gonorrhoeae*, however, predominates in adolescence. Gonococcal septic arthritis should be considered in any sexually active teenager (suspected as well as confirmed) and may involve one or several hot, painful joints. Although males frequently also have a history of the purulent, painful penile discharge seen with gonorrhea, females may have no genital signs. Spread is presumed to be hematogenous. Some patients with gonococcal arthritis also may demonstrate a few purpuric spots varying from 1–5 mm in diameter anywhere on the body. Diagnosis is established by the finding of gram-negative intracellular diplococci in joint fluid aspirates with confirmation by appropriate cultures. A high probability exists when septic arthritis closely follows genital gonorrhea or, in females, positive endocervical cultures for gonococcus are found. Other features of gonococcal arthritis and differential considerations between this and Reiter's syndrome or Behçet's syndrome, both of which also may be associated with genital infections, are given in Table 11-16.

Gram-negative organisms other than *Neisseria gonorrhoeae* may be causal in patients with diabetes or other chronic illnesses interfering with host defense mechanisms. Heroin addicts may develop staphylococcal arthritis of the sternoclavicular or sacroiliac joints. Tuberculosis and atypical mycobacteria, *Brucella* species, and a wide variety of fungi also have been implicated on occasion.

In addition to clinical findings indicating acute joint pathology, laboratory tests usually reveal a leukocytosis with shift to the left and an elevated erythrocyte sedimentation rate. Arthrocentesis may demonstrate opaque, thick synovial fluid with marked leukocytosis ($20,000-200,000/mm^3$; 75% polymorphonuclear cells), friable mucin clot, low glucose (compared to blood glucose), no crystals, intracellular bacteria on Gram stain, and positive cultures. As joint fluid cultures are not always positive, repeat blood cultures should be obtained to enhance the likelihood of recovering the causal

TABLE 11-15
DRUGS USED FOR JUVENILE RHEUMATOID ARTHRITIS

Drug	Dosage	Comments about administration	Side effects
Salicylates (aspirin)	90–130 mg/kg/day (3.6–6.0 g/day)	Therapeutic serum level: 20–25 mg/100 ml. Give in four divided doses with meals and at h.s. with milk. Obtain serum levels 2–3 hours after a dose. Use for 3–6 weeks before trying other drugs.	Gastritis, GI upset, inhibits platelet aggregation, increases serum transaminases, salicylism (nausea, tinnitus, hearing difficulty). May worsen asthma (aspirin-nasal polyps-asthma syndrome).
Indomethacin (Indocin)	25–50 mg q.i.d.	Use with care in adolescents; not recommended for patient under age 14. May be helpful for sacroiliitis. May give half the daily dose with milk.	Nausea, peptic ulcer, headaches, depression, vertigo, mental confusion, hypertension, edema, bone marrow depression, hematuria, asthma.
Phenylbutazone (Butazolidin)	50 mg q.i.d. (400 mg/day maximum)	Not recommended for patients under 14 years of age. May be helpful for sacroiliitis.	Agranulocytosis, aplastic anemia, CNS or GI bleeding, blurred vision, optic neuritis, hearing loss, edema, hepatitis, dermatitis, hypertension, hyperglycemia, glomerulonephritis.
Tolmetin (Tolectin)	400 mg t.i.d. (2000 mg/day maximum)	May use as aspirin substitute. One of several new nonsteroidal, antiinflammatory drugs developed for the treatment of arthritis. Others include naproxen (250 mg b.i.d. up to 750–1000 mg/day maximum); ibuprofen (400 mg q.i.d. up to 2400 mg/day maximum); and fenoprofen calcium (600 mg q.i.d. up to 3200 mg/day).	GI bleeding, anaphylactic reaction, blurred vision, edema. Avoid if the patient has aspirin-asthma sensitivity, as it worsens the asthma.
Antimalarials	Variable	Chloroquine or hydroxychloroquine. Used by some rheumatologists for severe arthritis.	Dermatitis, GI toxicity, macular (retinal) degeneration.
Steroids (prednisone)	Variable; daily, alternative day, or intermittent; 1–3 mg/kg/day	Used for severe pericarditis, severe systemic JRA, and iridocyclitis (topical steroids may be enough; systemic steroids for severe eye disease).	Cushingoid appearance, peptic ulcer, hypertension, sodium and fluid retention, osteoporosis, muscle weakness, thinning of connective tissue, pseudotumor cerebri, growth suppression, latent diabetes mellitus, adrenocortical and pituitary suppression, emotional disturbances.
Gold salts (gold sodium thiomalate, aurothioglucose, others)	Variable	Used by some for severe arthritis not responding to other medications. Use for a 20-week trial period. Some respond very well. Use with caution.	Exfoliative dermatitis, kidney or liver toxicity, blood dyscrasia
Others: Immunosuppressive drugs, penicillamine, Levamisole	Variable	Experimental drugs for severe disease.	Variable.

TABLE 11-16
ARTHRITIS ASSOCIATED WITH GENITAL INFECTIONS

Disease	Description	Type of arthritis
Gonococcal arthritis	*Neisseria gonorrhoeae* produces a urethritis in males or cervicitis in females with the possibility of many complications. Transmission usually is by sexual contact. Arthritis is part of the gonococcal septicemia, seen in 1%–3% patients with urethral or cervical disease. Dermatitis may also be seen: pustule with a necrotic, umbilicated center; other lesions also seen.	Two types reported: 1. Polyarthritis (with tenosynovitis) develops with fever, chills and dermatitis. The joints are swollen, painful, and warm. Blood cultures are positive. Joint cultures may be negative. May develop 2 weeks after venereal exposure. 2. Monarthritis (often the knee or wrist) with minimal effusion, no dermatitis, negative blood culture, and often positive joint culture. The arthritis resolves with penicillin therapy.
Reiter's syndrome (see text)	Triad of urethritis, conjunctivitis (iritis), and arthritis, which can follow dysentery (as shigellosis) or can be venereally acquired. Balanitis circinata, keratoderma blennorrhagicum, Achilles tendonitis, increased ESR and HLA B27 also noted. Most cases occur in males.	Variable arthritis picture. Often acute, self-limiting involvement of the lower extremity joints that develops 10–14 days after the urethritis. Severe destruction of joints seen in only a few. Sacroiliitis seen in a few, resembling ankylosing spondylitis. Treat with aspirin, indomethacin, or phenylbutazone.
Behçet's syndrome (see text)	Triad of recurrent aphthous, genital ulcerations and iritis in association with many other features, including polyarthritis. Also: thrombophlebitis, meningoencephalitis, erythema multiforme, vasculitis, pyodermas, epididymitis, and others. Seen especially in Japan and Mediterranean countries. Increased HLA B5 reported. Placed in a group of spondarthroses seronegative for RF with peripheral arthritis and sacroiliitis.	Variable pattern. Transient arthritis of various joints that resolves without sequelae. Aspirin used as treatment.

organism; associated bacteremia may be present. Appropriate endocervical or penile cultures also should be taken in sexually active youths. Joint roentgenograms are not helpful, revealing nonspecific changes with widening of the synovial space.

Treatment consists of antibiotics, symptomatic therapy and, in some cases, drainage by periodic joint aspiration (wrist or knee) or open drainage (hip). Gonococcal arthritis is treated with a daily dose of 10 million units of penicillin given intravenously for 3 days, followed by oral ampicillin or tetracycline at a dosage of 2 g/day for 7 days. Intravenous penicillin for the full 10 days may be a desirable alternative in adolescents with particularly severe disease or in those likely to be poorly compliant with oral therapy. Tetracycline or erythromycin may be used for the entire treatment course in patients allergic to penicillin. Gram-positive arthritis usually responds to methicillin or nafcillin, 8–12 g/day intravenously, with a cephalosporin as an alternative. Gram-negative organisms usually respond to intravenous gentamicin (5 mg/kg/day) and carbenicillin (25–30 g/day). Culture results (aerobic-anerobic, acid-fast, and fungal) determine what antibiotics should be used in resistant cases. Septic arthritis due to tuberculosis should not be overlooked and presents as monarticular disease in 85% of the cases.

VIRAL ARTHRITIS
Certain generalized viral illnesses may manifest synovial inflammation in addition to their other signs. Deposition of immune complexes may be responsible. Rubella and hepatitis B are the most

TABLE 11-17
REVIEW OF MISCELLANEOUS ARTHRITIS (RHEUMATOID FACTOR NEGATIVE)

Type	Description	Treatment
Psoriatic arthritis	About 5% of the patients with psoriasis develop a variable arthritis, particularly likely to involve the upper extremity. Some develop a chronic form resembling rheumatoid arthritis. Others develop asymmetric involvement of the interphalangeal joints of the hands and feet, while a few (5%) develop an ankylosing spondylitislike picture. Psoriatic arthritis has been described after recurrent attacks of Reiter's syndrome. RF is negative.	Physical therapy, salicylates, steroids. Avoid antimalarials as severe exfoliative dermative arthritis can develop.
Inflammatory bowel disease	About 10% of the patients with Crohn's disease or ulcerative colitis develop peripheral arthritis involving a few enlarged joints (ankles and the knees especially), which can precede the bowel manifestations by months or years. Most episodes of joint inflammation are transient and resolve with damage. Severe joint disease (hips, shoulders) has been described. There may be an increased incidence of erythema nodosum and acute uveitis in the arthritic group. Growth retardation can be profound. Ankylosing spondylitis has also been described in 2%–6% of all patients.	Control the bowel disease, as arthritis may parallel the course of GI manifestation. Specific treatment of the arthritis may be necessary and is as described in Table 11-15.
Lyme arthritis	A recently described arthritis reported from Lyme, Connecticut, involving various ages (more males) during the summer and early fall. Characterized by fever, headaches, myalgia, and monarticular inflammation (often the knee) for up to 7 days. An erythematous, elevated annular rash (erythema chronicum migrans) may precede the joint involvement. Recurrent attacks and polyarthritis may develop. Joint damage is not usually noted The etiology may be an arthropod (tick)-borne virus.	Symptomatic.
Acne fulminans	Also called acute febrile ulcerative conglobate acne with polyarthralgia. A rare disorder, described mostly in men with generalized acne conglobate (acne nodules, cysts, sinus tracts) manifested in episodes of fever and swollen joints (hips, knees, hands). Recurrent attacks common.	See treatment of acne vulgaris. Salicylates. (See Table 11-15.)
Malignant joint disease	Infiltration of the joint with malignant cells may produce synovial inflammation resembling arthritis. Severe bone pain and joint destruction develop. May also be transient or recurrent. Osteolytic areas may be seen on roentgenogram. Peripheral smear, bone marrow aspiration, joint aspiration, or biopsy establishes the diagnosis. Hodgkin's disease, other lymphoma, leukemia, rhabdomyosarcoma, and others have been implicated. Primary synovial tumors also seen.	As indicated by nature of neoplasm.

commonly encountered causes of viral arthropathy in adolescents. Epstein-Barr virus (mononucleosis), mumps, chickenpox, adenovirus, and coxsackievirus have been implicated on occasion. Regardless of etiology, most cases involve only one or two joints, are self-limiting, and resolve in 2-5 days without sequelae. An exception sometimes is seen with hepatitis B arthritis, which may present with a more severe polyarticular involvement resembling rheumatoid arthritis. Treatment of viral arthritis is symptomatic.

MISCELLANEOUS ARTHROPATHIES
Table 11-17 reviews several other forms of arthritis with significance for the adolescent. Rarer arthritic diseases include the following:

Jaccoud's arthritis: Noted in some patients with recurrent episodes of acute rheumatic fever and characterized by progressive and deforming but painless periarticular fibrosis of the joints of the hands and feet.

Felty's syndrome: A form of rheumatoid arthritis associated with ulcers, keratoconjunctivitis, splenomegaly, and neutropenia.

Polychondritis: Inflammation and destruction of the cartilage of the face, trachea, pharynx, costochondral joints, peripheral and other joints, combined with fever, iritis, cataracts, and aortitis.

Palindromic rheumatism: Recurrent transient episodes of polyarthritis without constitutional symptoms, each attack resolving in 2–4 days without permanent joint injury; may progress to rheumatoid arthritis in some cases.

Intermittent hydrarthrosis: Recurrent joint effusions (particularly of the knee) often associated with menses but without other symptoms or signs; rarely, this condition progresses to chronic synovitis.

Reactive arthritis: A sterile joint effusion associated with proximate bacterial infections or infections of more distant sites, usually the gastrointestinal tract. *Salmonella*, *Shigella*, and *Yersinia* enterocolitis have been implicated.

Secondary gout: Abnormal purine metabolism with hyperuricemia and urate crystal deposition in cartilage or joints resulting in arthritis. Gout essentially is a disease of older adults. Secondary gout, however, can occur in adolescents with blood dyscrasias and neoplasms or in those receiving certain drugs for the treatment of renal or neoplastic disease; concurrent rapid cellular destruction produces marked elevation of blood urate levels with crystalline urate depositions as in true gout.

Chondrocalcinosis: A form of pseudogout with the deposition of calcium pyrophosphate dihydrate crystals in joints (particularly hips and knees) seen in a variety of disorders, including hemochromatosis, hyperparathyroidism, Wilson's disease, and acromegaly. X-ray evidence of calcium deposits may be noted, and crystals may be detected by examining joint fluid aspirates under polarized light microscopy.

Alkaptonuria: Abnormal metabolism of homogentisic acid resulting in its accumulation in the body; joint space deposition may result in degenerative arthritis.

Sarcoidosis: Transient, acute polyarthritis of the lower extremities and erythema nodosum sometimes are seen along with the more characteristic features of hilar adenopathy.

Whipple's disease: A migrating polyarthritis or arthralgia may occur, along with the classic signs of malabsorption, fever, and anemia.

Other diseases that commonly or occasionally have joint manifestations as a part of a broader picture are cited in Table 11-13 and discussed elsewhere (see Index).

Osteomyelitis

Bacterial infection of the metaphysis often is due to hematogenous spread from other foci in the body (as furunculosis). Trauma, sickle cell disease, hemodialysis, and heroin addiction may serve as precipitants. The resultant metaphyseal abscess ruptures and spreads along the bone shaft under the periosteum and then penetrates the bone marrow. Any bone can be involved, especially the humerus, femur, and tibia. Septic arthritis may eventually develop, especially if the proximal femur or proximal humerus is involved, since these joint capsules insert distal to the metaphysis, allowing for direct extension from the metaphysis to the joint. "Sympathetic" effusions due to the osteomyelitis may occur, producing increased synovial fluid.

The patient often presents with a high fever, toxic appearance, and a very swollen, tender metaphysis with or without adjacent joint effusion. The erythrocyte sedimentation rate is elevated. Blood cultures are positive in over 50% of patients. Repeat blood cultures are recommended to maximize the chances of establishing the etiology, which includes *Staphylococcus aureus* (the main one), *Streptococcus*, *Pneumococcus*, *Hemophilus influenzae*, *Salmonella*, other gram-negative organisms, and anaerobic bacteria. The differential diagnosis includes osteitis, osteomyelitis (with or without sterile sympathetic joint effusions), septic arthritis, soft tissue abscess with or without cellulitis, and cellulitis with ascending lymphadenitis. Although the role of aspiration is controversial, the use of bone scans is considered very useful, especially to identify subacute or chronic forms that present with signs much more subtle than acute osteomyelitis. Bone roentgenograms are normal until 10–14 days after onset. At this time erosion and radiolucency of the affected site become evident with periosteal new bone formation noted after 2 weeks. Technetium scans, however, can be helpful. Increased uptake by involved bone is evident early in the course. This procedure also assists in diagnosing subacute or chronic forms that may be much more subtle and ill defined in presentation.

Recommended treatment regimens vary. Initial high doses of intravenous antibiotics followed by oral antibiotics to complete a total of 4-6 weeks therapy is one recommendation. For example, 8–12 g/day of nafcillin given intravenously for 2–4 weeks followed by 1–2 g/day by mouth for a total treatment period of 6–8 weeks.

Other recommended regimens employ the intravenous or oral route exclusively but for the same length of time. Antibiotic selection is based on culture results; the duration of therapy is correlated with signs of clinical and laboratory improvement. Treatment often needs to be initiated before culture results are available and, in a good number of cases, cultures remain sterile. In these instances antibiotic treatment should employ multiple agents and be sufficiently broad to cover all organisms associated with acute disease. More prolonged courses of antibiotic therapy are indicated for chronic osteomyelitis in combination with surgical drainage and removal of infected bone.

Marfan Syndrome

Marfan syndrome (arachnodactyly) is a generalized congenital connective tissue disorder characterized by many features (Table 11-18). The youth typically is tall and slender with a general elongation of the extremities, especially the fingers. Other findings vary and may include eye defects, cardiac defects, scoliosis, and/or hyperextensible lax joints. Evaluation should include a careful family history (since this is an autosomal dominant disorder with variable genetic penetrance), body measurements (trunk versus extremities), slit lamp examination of the eyes, scoliosis screen, and cardiac evaluation (chest roentgenogram, electrocardiogram, and echocardiography). Diagnosis is based on the typical teen appearance with one or more associated abnormal findings.

It should be remembered that persons with Marfan's syndrome are of completely normal intelligence. Similar features with mental retardation have been noted in patients with homocystinuria, an autosomal recessive metabolic disease associated with marfanoid skeletal changes, ectopia lentis (with a downward displacement), renovascular thrombosis, and osteoporosis.

Management of Marfan's syndrome consists of appropriate treatment for existent defects and continuing surveillance for progression in eye, skeletal, and/or cardiac problems. All can worsen during the teenage years and young adulthood. Genetic counseling is necessary. Psychosocial counseling and special measures required for chronic illness (Chapter 21) may be indicated, depending on the severity of complications.

TABLE 11-18
FEATURES OF THE MARFAN SYNDROME

1. Tall, slender individual whose extremities are very long (limbs versus trunk)—the midfinger tip span greater than height
2. Long, slender fingers (spider fingers)
3. Long, narrow skull with high-arched palate
4. Eye defects
   a. Ectopia lentis: upward lens subluxation
   b. Myopia with retinal detachment
   c. Strabismus, nystagmus, cataracts, megalocornea, coloboma, iris tremor
5. Cardiac defects
   a. Valvular heart disease (mitral disease, aortic regurgitation)
   b. Aortic aneurysm (can be dissecting and cause of early death)
   c. Aorticocystic medionecrosis
   d. Resultant chamber hypertrophy
6. Scoliosis or kyphosis
7. Chest wall deformity
   a. Pectus excavatum
   b. Pectus carinatum
8. Loose joints (hyperextensible), including joint dislocations (especially hip)
9. Renal ectopy
10. Recurrent inguinal hernias
11. Pes planus
12. Others

Pilonidal Cyst and Sinus

Pilonidal cyst and sinus, a common embryonic defect represents failure of the distal end of the neurenteric canal to close completely. Although present at birth as an asymptomatic sinus tract, the sinus often becomes infected in adolescence or adulthood. In the noninfected state the only evidence of the sinus is a small dimple located at the upper end of the gluteal crease over or just below the coccygeal region. Sometimes it may be further marked by a small tuft of hair. (In this instance spina bifida occulta also should be ruled out.) Infectious complications include local pain, erythema, and swelling progressing to a variably sized chronic or recurring cyst or abscess with or without a draining sinus tract. The patient often presents with a history of infection cycles alternating with the asymptomatic state. Possible contributing factors include recurrent trauma from activities such as horseback riding, trail riding on a motorcycle or jeep, or foreign body irritation from the tuft of hair. Rupture of the cyst into the cerebrospinal fluid with resultant meningitis is a rare complication.

Treatment consists of antibiotics, local hot soaks, attention to hygiene, and incision and drainage when indicated. Severe or recurrent symptoms may require surgical excision of the sinus tract.

Bibliography

Banks, H. H., editor. 1980. Symposium on sports injuries. *Orthoped. Clin. North Am.* 11:685.

Barnes, C. G. 1980. Less common forms of arthritis. *Practitioner* 224:45.

Bartholomew, L. E.; Rynes, R. I.; Hedbery, S. A., et al. 1976. Management of rheumatoid arthritis. *Am Family Phys.* 13:116.

Baum, J. 1981. Juvenile arthritis. *Am. J. Dis. Child.* 135:557.

Bradford, D. S., editor. 1979. Symposium on scoliosis and related spinal disorders. *Orthoped. Clin. North Am.* 10:749.

Capello, W. N., and Pierce, R. O. 1977. Soft tissue injuries to the ankle. *Am. Family Phys.* 15:152.

Clark, R. N. 1976. Diagnosis and management of torticollis, *Pediatr. Ann.* 5:43.

DeHaven, K. E.; Dolan, W. A.; and Mayer, P. J. 1980. Chondromalacia patellae and the painful knee. *Am. Family Phys.* 21:117.

Doherty, S. M., and Yates, D. A. H. 1980. Ankylosing spondylitis. *Practitioner* 224:34.

Engleman, E. G., and Engleman, E. P. 1977. Ankylosing spondylitis. Recent advances in diagnosis and treatment. *Med. Clin. North Am.* 61:347.

Franklin, E. C. 1978. Arthralgias and arthritis in viral infection. *Am. Family Phys.* 17:161.

Griffin, P. P.; Green, N. E.; and Beauchamp, R. D. 1980. Legg-Calvé-Perthes disease: treatment and prognosis. *Orthoped. Clin. North Am.* 11:127.

Kalenak, A. 1979. The swollen knee. I. Noninfectious causes. *Consultant* 19(2):108.

Kummel, B. M. 1980. The diagnosis and treatment of patellofemoral problems. *Primary Care* 7:195.

Laskin, R. S., editor. 1979. Symposium on disorders of the knee joint. *Orthoped. Clin. North Am.* 10:1–280.

Lindsley, C. B. 1981. Pharmacotherapy of juvenile rheumatoid arthritis. *Pediatr. Clin. North Am.* 28:161.

Lockshin, M. D., and Brause, B. D. 1982. Infectious arthritis. *D.M.* 28:3–51.

Marino, C. T., and Greenwald, R. A. 1981. Acute arthritis. *Med. Clin. North Am.* 65:177.

Orlowski, J. P., and Mercer, R. D. 1977. Osteoid osteoma in children and young adults. *Pediatrics* 59:526.

Passo, M. H. 1982. Aches and limb pain. *Pediatr. Clin. North Am.* 29(1):209–229.

Pyeritz, R. E., and McKusick, V. A. 1979. The marfan syndrome: diagnosis and management. *N. Engl. J. Med.* 300:772.

Seifert, M. H. 1978. The arthritis of venereal disease. *Practitioner* 220:103.

Staheli, L. T. 1980. Spinal deformity. *J. Family Pract.* 10:1071.

Staheli, L. T., editor. 1977. Symposium on common orthopedic problems. *Pediatr. Clin. North Am.* 24:663–918.

Stoeber, E. 1981. Prognosis in juvenile chronic arthritis. *Europ. J. Pediatr.* 135:225.

Ward, J. R., and Atcheson, S. G. 1977. Infectious arthritis. *Med. Clin. North Am.* 61:313.

Weierman, R. J.; Lowell, H. A.; Nadel, C. I.; et al. 1980. Scoliosis: to refer or not to refer. *Primary Care* 7:287.

Weinstein, A. J. 1981. Osteomyelitis: microbiologic, clinical and therapeutic considerations. *Primary Care* 8:557.

West, R. J. 1976. Acute polyarthritis: *Clin. Rheumatol. Dis.* 2:305.

Wofsy, D. 1981. Seronegative spondylarthritis. *West. J. Med.* 134:134.

–12–
Endocrine Disorders

Diabetes Mellitus
Overview and diagnosis □ Diabetic ketoacidosis □ Chronic management
Brittle diabetes □ Long-term complications □ Other management considerations
Hypoglycemia
Reactive hypoglycemia □ Fasting hypoglycemia
Thyroid Disorders
Hypothyroidism □ Euthyroid goiters □ Hyperthyroidism □ Thyroid tumors
Growth Disorders
Short stature □ Excessive height
Pubertal Disorders
Precocious puberty □ Pubertal delay
Hermaphroditism
Male pseudohermaphroditism □ Female Pseudohermaphroditism
True hermaphroditism
Adrenal Dysfunction
Cushing's syndrome □ Adrenal insufficiency
Parathyroid Dysfunction
Hyperparathyroidism □ Hypoparathyroidism
Syndrome of Inappropriate Antidiuretic Hormone Secretion

Diabetes Mellitus

OVERVIEW AND DIAGNOSIS

Diabetes mellitus affects some 100,000 individuals under age 20 in the United States and is one of the most common endocrine disorders in children and youth. It has an incidence of 5.8–10.0 per 100,000 in the population at large. Two forms have been identified. Type I, or insulin-dependent disease (formerly known as juvenile diabetes mellitus), is the more frequent form in adolescence. It is associated with certain HLA antigens (B8, BW15, DW3, D4), a higher incidence of certain autoimmune disorders such as Addison's disease, and chronic lymphocytic thyroiditis (Hashimoto's) and with circulating antibodies to pancreatic islet cells. Although heredity appears to play a role, type I diabetes often appears in only one member of a generation; a sibling or offspring of an affected individual has only a 5% chance of also developing the disease during younger years, although the risk is somewhat greater after age 40. This form most commonly appears in normal-weighted youths between ages 11–14 years and is more often diagnosed in the fall or winter months. Type II, or non-insulin-dependent diabetes mellitus—classically seen in the older individual—occasionally is noted in older adolescents; disease onset is insidious, and the patients often are obese and may resist the development of ketosis. These individuals can secrete C-peptide (which is a marker for endogenous insulin) when challenged by a glucose load.

The basic defect in either type I or II diabetes is dysfunction of the pancreatic islet beta cells with reduced or absent insulin secretion. Alpha cell dysfunction probably also exists with elevated glucagon levels. Other hormonal abnormalities also have been noted, including elevated levels of growth hormone, cortisol, epinephrine, and norepinephrine; these are

TABLE 12-1
DIFFERENTIAL
DIAGNOSIS OF HYPERGLYCEMIA

1. Diabetes mellitus
2. Salicylate poisoning
3. Hyperthyroidism
4. Cushing's syndrome
5. Stress glycosuria with or without abnormal renal glucose threshold
6. Hypernatremia
7. Nonketotic hyperosmolar coma
8. Meningitis
9. Cerebrovascular accidents
10. Intracranial neoplasm

TABLE 12-2
DIFFERENTIAL
DIAGNOSIS OF KETOACIDOSIS

1. Diabetes mellitus
2. Renal glycosuria
3. Lactic acidosis
4. Salicylate intoxication and certain other drug overdoses
5. Uremic poisoning
6. Cerebrovascular accidents
7. Any acute situation resulting in glucose depletion and gluconeogenesis from fats (acute gastrointestinal disease, acute abdominal conditions, illness-induced anorexia, others)
8. Voluntary or involuntary starvation

probably secondary to the basic pancreatic abnormality. The fundamental cause of diabetes is thought to be autoimmune islet cell destruction facilitated by hereditary factors (possibly an allele located on chromosome 6 that contains the associated HLA antigens) and induced by environmental factors. Viral infections may play a role. It has been observed that mumps epidemics are followed by an increased incidence of diabetes mellitus in the succeeding 4 years. Patients with congenital rubella syndrome also have an increased risk for developing this disease. Coxsackie and other viruses also may contribute to the pathogenesis. Other causes may include production of abnormal insulin or defects in insulin receptors.

Prediabetes defines the asymptomatic state in an individual who later develops disease. Latent or chemical diabetes refers to a situation in which there are abnormal glucose tolerance test results and increased basal insulin levels but no clinical signs. Overt diabetes describes clinically manifest disease.

In adolescence, overt diabetes usually develops abruptly over days or several weeks and is characterized by the three classic "polys"; polydipsia, polyuria, and polyphagia. Weight loss is also a classic sign. Occasionally vaginitis due to *Candida albicans* may be the presenting complaint. Laboratory studies reveal hyperglycemia and glycosuria. Other conditions that also may present with hyperglycemia are considerably less common during the adolescent years but should be considered in the differential diagnosis (Table 12-1).

An elevated fasting or 2-hour postprandial blood glucose (over 200 mg/dl) with significant historic features and a negative physical examination, except for evidence of recent weight loss, usually is sufficient for the diagnosis. An oral glucose tolerance test demonstrating persistent high blood glucose levels is confirmatory, as are reduced blood insulin levels. An intravenous or cortisone-stressed glucose tolerance test may be done but usually is unnecessary.

DIABETIC KETOACIDOSIS

Approximately 15% of individuals with type I diabetes initially present with ketoacidosis. This also is one of the major intercurrent complications seen in adolescents and can lead to an emergency metabolic state. Ketoacidosis is due to prolonged hypoinsulinism and inability to utilize glucose for cellular energy; fats and proteins are used instead, and the result is hyperglycemia, proteolysis, and a rise in fatty acid metabolites, or ketones. Signs and symptoms are highly variable and may include an altered sensorium (lethargy, semicoma, or coma), Kussmaul respirations with "fruity" breath, emesis, dehydration (10% or more), abdominal pain, hyperglycemia (average blood glucose in ketoacidosis being 600 mg/dl with a range of 150–2000 mg/dl), glycosuria, ketonemia (beta-hydroxybutyric acid, acetoacetic acid, and acetone), ketonuria, acidosis (pH under 7.30 and serum bicarbonate under 15–20 mEq/L), leukocytosis, hyperamylasemia, and others. Ketonemia may be noted as either strongly positive at over 1:2 serum dilution or directly measured as over 7 mM/L. Table 12-2 lists differential considerations.

Proteolysis, acidosis, and polyuria also produce a reduced total body potassium. The *serum* potassium is usually normal, reflecting an acidosis-mediated intracellular to extracellular transfer. A patient in ketoacidosis with a low serum potassium has a

TABLE 12-3
MANAGEMENT OF DIABETIC KETOACIDOSIS

A. Correction of dehydration and electrolyte imbalance
  1. Assume 10% dehydration or use formula of 2500 ml/m^2/day; use normal saline solution initially.
  2. Give 50% of estimated fluid deficit in first 6-8 hours and balance (plus maintenance) over next 16 hours. Thereafter give daily maintenance plus calculated and actual losses.
  3. Add glucose (as 5% dextrose) when blood glucose is less than 300 mg/dl.
  4. Replace electrolytes
    a. Sodium: 3 mEq/kg/day
    b. Chloride: 2 mEq/kg/day
    c. Potassium: 3-5 mEq/kg/day (half as KCl and half as K phosphate to raise lowered DPG* levels and improve oxygen release from hemoglobin).
  5. Give bicarbonate *only* when pH is less than 7.1-7.2 and serum bicarbonate is under 12 mEq/L. The following formula will raise bicarbonate levels up to 12 mEq/L:

$$(12 - \text{serum HCO}_3^-) \times 0.6 \times \text{kg}$$

B. Regulation of glucose metabolism (alternate methods)
  1. Continuous regular (crystalline) insulin infusion; give 0.1 U/kg IV as a bolus, then 0.1 U/kg/hour.

*2.3-diphosphoglycerate

  2. Intermittent subcutaneous insulin; give 0.25-2 U/kg/ of regular (crystalline) insulin SQ every 2-4 hours depending on the degree of blood glucose elevation. Half of this calculated dose is sometimes given as an initial IV bolus.

C. Measures after metabolic stabilization
  1. Institute oral feedings when tolerated.
  2. Switch to NPH insulin given SQ; use one-half the previous day's total of regular insulin. Adjust over the next several days for optimum glucose control using blood levels and urine ketones as guides. A few patients will require a combination of regular (peak action in 4-6 hr) and NPH or lente insulin (peak action in 10-12 hr). After the honeymoon period (see text), growing adolescents usually need between 0.8-1.2 U/kg/day and those who have completed growth between 0.5-1.0 U/kg/day for a total somewhere between 40-60 U/day.
  3. Diabetic education program
  4. Appropriate diet
    a. 1000 calories plus 100 calories per year of age per day up to 2700 cal for an 18-year-old male or 2500 cal for a 15-year-old female plus adjustments for unusual degrees of exercise.
    b. Divide into 45% carbohydrate (limiting concentrated sweets), 15%-20% protein, and 30%-40% fats (including polyunsaturated fatty acids).

---

dangerously low total body level (noted in 10%-15%). Sodium, chloride, phosphorus, magnesium, nitrogen, and calcium also may be reduced. A factitious hyponatremia, however, can occur in the presence of severe hypertriglyceridemia.

Table 12-3 outlines therapeutic principles for diabetic ketoacidosis. Properly paced rehydration (not too rapidly), electrolyte and nutrient replacement, and insulin administration are important. A fluid deficit of 6-10 L is often noted. Continuous low doses of intravenous insulin (2-4 units regular insulin per hour) is now preferred by many authorities over intermittent subcutaneous insulin administration. It is thought to be more physiologic, to permit a more gradual and titrated drop in glucose values (75-100 mg/dl/hour), and to avoid overshooting the mark, thus producing hypoglycemia. The use of bicarbonate to raise serum pH requires caution; it may increase cerebrospinal acidosis, produce alkalotic impairment of oxygen dissociation, or worsen hypokalemia. Only partial correc-

tion with bicarbonate is recommended. Additional buffer action is provided by the elevated ketones.

Table 12-4 lists major complications that may be encountered in managing ketoacidosis. Careful treatment, however, should result in a very low mortality rate, less than 1%-2%. Poor prognostic factors include a very low serum pH, low potassium levels, coexistent severe infection, elevated lactic acid levels, and prolonged coma. Diabetic ketoacidosis during pregnancy may result in fetal death in 50% of the cases.

CHRONIC MANAGEMENT

The chronic management of an adolescent with type I diabetes mellitus may be a very difficult task with many complications. The following points may be helpful in minimizing such problems.

Once the diabetes is diagnosed and stabilized, insulin requirements progressively drop to 0.3 units per kilogram or less in more than half the patients. This "honeymoon period" may last from several

TABLE 12-4
COMPLICATIONS OF DIABETIC
KETOACIDOSIS AND ITS MANAGEMENT

Complication	Comment
Hypoglycemia	Due to overcorrecting of the hypo-insulin state.
Hypokalemia	Failure to provide enough potassium supplementation.
Severe acidosis	
Alkalosis	Too much bicarbonate given.
Cerebral edema	This develops within 4–14 hours of treatment: too-rapid reduction of blood glucose levels may be a factor.
Renal failure	
Cardiac failure	Sudden death may occur due to cardiac failure or other complications.

weeks up to 2 years and is related to basal insulin reserves. During this time, maintenance requires only small amounts of insulin to avoid hypoglycemic reactions. Many patients and parents interpret this interim period as evidence of a cure and thus tend to deny the diagnosis and to develop compliance problems. Sooner or later, however, insulin requirements increase to between 40–80 units of insulin per day depending on basal and activity requirements. A new type of therapy may involve the use of somatostatin, which is a potent inhibitor of the secretion of insulin, glucagon, and growth hormone. Since diabetes involves excess glucagon secretion, a somatostatin analog may be shown to be useful for some diabetics. More research is needed.

Because of shifting requirements caused by the honeymoon period and by rapid growth and shifting activity levels, hypoglycemic reactions are common, particularly in the first several years and/or during the deceleration phase of the growth spurt. Such reactions occur when the blood glucose falls below 60 mg/dl. (Table 12-7 describes symptoms.) Immediate treatment of hypoglycemia is aimed at raising the blood glucose level as quickly as possible. In mild instances this may be by the ingestion of sucrose-containing foods such as orange juice, candy, or plain sugar. More severe cases require intravenous glucose. Alternative treatments include epinephrine (0.25 ml of 1:1000 aqueous solution given subcutaneously) or glucagon (0.5–1.0 mg intramuscularly).

After stabilization, the reason for the hypoglycemia should be determined and alterations in diet, insulin dose or form, and exercise made accordingly. Exercise, however, should not be curtailed, and adolescent diabetics should be encouraged to participate in the full range of athletics. Parenthetically, it is wise to avoid the use of muscle groups important to the performance of favored sports as sites for insulin injection. Simple or split insulin regimens are used for most youths, depending on the youth's acceptance and the clinician's preference. The decade of the 1980s may allow the development of a reliable insulin pump, which will slowly infuse insulin at a constant or intermittent rate. This will more closely simulate a normal pancreas and allow for better diabetic control. Early models of such a pump already exist.

Continued monitoring of the adolescent diabetic's metabolic status is important, whether through frequent checks of urine glucose or blood sugars (including self-administered Dextrostix testing). Quantitative glucose determinations of fractionated 24-hour urine collections (for example, collection in four separate aliquots from 8 AM to noon, noon to 4 PM, 4 PM to 8 PM, and 8 PM to 8 AM) are useful in instances of unstable control to determine patterns of glucose spillage and to indicate modifications in the time, type, and amount of insulin or other aspects of management. The patient should be taught to carry out most of the testing and to make minor adjustments on his or her own. Spillage of less than 20–40 g of glucose per day is desirable. Hemoglobin AlC (glycosylated hemoglobin) levels are useful in monitoring the degree of control over time in that elevation (two to three. times normal) indicates poor control over the previous several months. Mechanical devices are now available to monitor blood glucose levels at home, thus making urine tests unnecessary for these youths. This relatively painless procedure is well accepted by many teenagers.

Careful patient education and psychologic management is as critical as attention to glucose metabolism. The most commonly encountered problem in adolescent diabetics is poor compliance stemming from various emotional responses to this disease by the patient or parents. Chapter 2 details management of chronic illness using diabetes as the prototype.

Ideal management goals seek minimal glycosuria while ensuring the patient is not teetering on the brink of hypoglycemia, a 2-hour postprandial blood glucose under 200 mg/dl, no ketones in blood and urine, normal serum lipids, no episodes of ketoacidosis or hyperglycemia, normal growth and development, and good psychosocial adjustment, including adequate school performance, rewarding interpersonal relationships, and progress toward emancipation.

BRITTLE DIABETES

The previously stated goals are not always easy to achieve. Poor metabolic control, or a "brittle" diabetic state, is not uncommon in adolescents with this disease. Table 12-5 cites factors that should be considered. The more significant are considered in the following sections.

The Somogyi phenomenon. The Somogyi phenomenon consists of cyclical hypoglycemic-hyperglycemic episodes in combination with headaches, lethargy, moodiness, irritability, dizziness, and sleeplessness often in association with nightmares. Other symptoms and signs include constipation, visual difficulty, hepatomegaly, abdominal pain, growth failure, and/or amenorrhea. Wide fluctuations in blood glucose levels occur over several hours with hypoglycemia and negative urine sugars shortly followed by moderate or severe hyperglycemia and glycosuria. Although the hypoglycemic phase can occur at any time of day, it is more common at night; when the patient presents to the physician's office during daytime hours, hyperglycemia erroneously suggests the need for more insulin, but an increase fails to alter the patient's symptoms. A diabetic who has any of the symptoms just described should be suspected of having this phenomenon. Those receiving more than 2 units/kg/day of insulin are particularly prone to this condition and probably are receiving too much. A fractionated 24-hour urine study will help detect this process. The cause of the Somogyi reaction is an excess of exogenous insulin and consequent hypoglycemia, which precipitates the secondary rebound of antiinsulin hormones (for example, corticosteroids, growth hormone, epinephrine, glucagon) and resultant hyperglycemia. Treatment consists of gradually reducing the insulin dose and attention to other factors contributing to poor control (Table 12-5).

Insulin resistance. Currently available insulin preparations may precipitate the development of antibodies to foreign protein contaminants and render the entire product relatively or totally ineffective. Treatment consists of a change in the type of insulin (substituting a pure beef or pure pork form for a combined beef-pork insulin). An almost completely pure form of insulin has been tested and is available

TABLE 12-5
FACTORS CONTRIBUTING
TO BRITTLE DIABETIC STATUS

1. Psychosocial factors pertaining to adolescent developmental concerns.
2. Management errors
   a. Unintentional patient or physician mistakes in estimating insulin dose, diet, or exercise pattern.
   b. Faulty urine collection with incomplete bladder emptying and/or faulty urine testing procedures.
   c. Wrong estimate of insulin action and duration.
3. Singularly high or low renal threshold for glucose.
4. Somogyi phenomenon.
5. Infections, other acute or chronic illnesses, trauma, surgery.
6. Unrecognized associated endocrine disorders (hyperthyroidism, Cushing's syndrome, Addison's disease, hypopituitarism, others).
7. Use of oral contraceptives.
8. Pregnancy.
9. Alcohol or other drug abuse, including cigarettes.
10. Certain medications (corticosteroids, diuretics, adrenergic blockers, others).
11. Excessive carbohydrate intake (uncertain).
12. Insulin resistance
    a. Insulin antibodies.
    b. Abnormal insulin or C-peptide metabolism.
13. Changes in rate of growth (acceleration or deceleration in the growth spurt); changes in weight when growth complete.
14. Marked change in exercise pattern.

in European markets; prolonged use has not produced antibodies and may offer a solution to this dilemma in the United States when approved for use by the Federal Drug Administration. Recently, insulin has been synthesized by *Escherichia coli* microorganisms. This example of modern recombinant DNA technology may provide large amounts of pure insulin.

Infections. Acute infections of any nature are common precipitants of diabetic ketoacidosis, particularly in patients already in poor metabolic control. Treatment of the ketoacidosis may be more problematic in this instance in that concomitant infection slows the rate of lowering blood glucose values even during continuous insulin therapy. Rates may be as low as 40–50 mg/dl/hour in contrast to the usual rate of 75–100 mg/dl/hour.

Psychologic factors. When presented with an adolescent with brittle diabetes who requires repeated hospitalizations for ketoacidosis or hypoglycemia or both without apparent organic cause, psychologic factors should be suspected and a careful psychosocial history carried out (Chapter 23). Denial, rebellion, acting-out, or unconscious manipulation for secondary gain may all be encountered. It should also be noted that the relatively existential orientation of the young and midadolescent makes it particularly difficult for him or her to appreciate the need for careful control when the worst that seems to happen is a few days' hospitalization every now and then. Nor can the adolescent appreciate the significance of the disease for the future. These factors coupled with the impact of chronic illness for adolescent developmental concerns (Chapter 21) make compliance particularly difficult during these years. Often a team approach with a generalist, psychiatrist or psychologist, social worker, endocrinologist, nutritionist, and others working together is helpful. It is essential to prevent the diabetes from becoming a focus for power struggles between the youth and his or her parents. This is best accomplished by giving the patient full responsibility for managing the disease in collaboration with the physician as early in the teen years as possible.

LONG-TERM COMPLICATIONS

Many type I diabetics begin to experience long-term complications about 10 years after the onset of their disease and face a life span shortened by about 20 years. Other patients initiate complications either sooner or later and some never encounter them at all. Although the cause of these problems has been controversial, the best current evidence suggests that there is a significant correlation with the degree of blood glucose control. Most diabetologists now agree that strict control of blood glucose does prevent or reduce the incidence of these complications.

Specific complications are legion (Table 12-6) and have a complex, heterogeneous expression. The development of microangiopathy, for instance, occurs in many organ systems and may result in blindness, renal failure, severe neuropathy, or any combination of these. It may take years to develop or not develop at all. Approximately 25% of all patients escape significant arteriosclerotic vascular complications. On the other hand, 90% develop some degree of neuropathy after 25–30 years. Dialysis, renal transplantation, laser-beam photo coagulation, vitrectomy, penile implants, and other measures may be needed.

It is difficult for adolescents to apply concepts of good control in anticipation of possible complications three decades in the future, particularly when they feel well. Those who encounter more immedi-

TABLE 12-6
COMPLICATIONS OF DIABETES MELLITUS

1. Ketoacidosis
2. Hypoglycemic episodes
3. Retinopathy (microaneurysms)
4. Neuropathy (peripheral neuritis)
5. Nephropathy (Kimmelstiel-Wilson's disease)
6. Psychologic reactions
7. Atherosclerosis
8. Insulin-induced lipoatrophy (at or distant from injection site; more common with combined than single forms of insulin)
9. Dermatologic disorders (in 30%)
  a. Rubeosis (rosy face; sometimes hands and feet)
  b. Necrobiosis lipoidica diabeticorum (1–3 mm scaly, erythematous patches progressing to atrophic, shiny plaques in association with telangiectasia; may antecede clinical diabetes)
  c. Bullous diabeticorum
  d. Benign acanthosis nigricans
  e. Vitiligo
  f. Granuloma annulare
  g. Scleroderma
  h. Carotenemia
  i. Xerosis
  j. Pruritus
10. Anhydrosis or oligohydrosis
11. Infections: bacterial and fungal, including tuberculosis
12. Chronic gastritis; steatorrhea
13. Sexual dysfunction (male impotence, retrograde ejaculation)
14. Growth failure and/or delayed puberty (rare)

ate problems such as growth failure, pubertal delay, or compromised sexual function in association with poor control may be motivated to do better. (Note: Impotence or retrograde ejaculation occurs in 0.9% of 15–19 year old diabetic males and increases in incidence with age.)

OTHER
MANAGEMENT CONSIDERATIONS

Genetic and personal counseling are important in helping the young person make future plans. He or she should be encouraged to pursue whatever life plans would have been pursued had diabetes not intervened. Examples of successful diabetics in all careers from the most rigorous of athletics to the most demanding of professions abound. Neither the youth nor his or her parents should be dissuaded from fulfilling all potentials. On the other hand, beginning with late adolescence patients should be aware of the long-range implications for them-

TABLE 12-7
CLINICAL SIGNS AND SYMPTOMS OF HYPOGLYCEMIA

ADRENERGIC SIGNS AND SYMPTOMS
1. Anxiety
2. Tremulousness
3. Palpitations
4. Increased perspiration
5. Tachycardia
6. Tachypnea
7. Widened pulse pressure
8. Pallor
9. Hunger (bulimia)

CLASSIC HYPOGLYCEMIC
(NEUROGLYCOPENIC) SIGNS AND SYMPTOMS
1. Headache
2. Changes in sensorium (mental dullness, confusion, coma)
3. Lethargy
4. Amnesia
5. Hypothermia
6. Visual difficulties
7. Dizziness (vertigo)
8. Seizures

TABLE 12-8
DIFFERENTIAL DIAGNOSIS OF SYMPTOMATIC HYPOGLYCEMIA

1. Reactive hypoglycemia
   a. Functional (reactive, simple, or relative hypoglycemia)
   b. Early diabetes mellitus
   c. Following gastrectomy, gastrojejunostomy, vagotomy, or pyloroplasty
2. Insulinoma
3. Nonpancreatic tumor (carcinoma, particularly of adrenal, liver and GI tract; mesothelioma; others)
4. Endocrine hypofunction (pituitary, adrenal cortex or medulla, glucagon insufficiency)
5. Malabsorption
6. Severe liver disease
7. Reye's syndrome
8. Idiopathic hypoglycemia of childhood
9. Prolonged muscular exercise
10. Inborn errors of metabolism (glycogen storage, fructosemia, galactosemia, and so on)
11. Drugs (insulin, oral antidiabetic agents, propranolol, sulfonylureas, haloperidol, large amounts of salicylates, acetaminophen, MAO inhibitors, INH, PAS
12. Hypoglycine ingestion (ackee nut)—Jamaican vomiting sickness
13. Hemodialysis
14. Sudden cessation of intravenous glucose solution

selves—the need for continued good control and medical supervision. If care has been rendered by an adolescent medicine specialist or pediatrician, specific plans should be made to transfer care to a knowledgeable internist or family practitioner. Adolescents approaching adulthood will also want to know the implications of their disease for any children they may have; the low inheritance risk (5%) for their offspring, at least up to age 40, should be reassuring.

Finally, it is important to note exciting new therapeutic possibilities. Current research on glycosylated hemoglobins (HgAlc), somatostatin (produced by pancreatic delta cells; inhibits insulin and glucagon release), continuous self-monitoring microdose insulin pumps, pancreatic transplantation, and an artificial pancreas all hold promise of better diabetic management and the potential for a healthier, longer life span.

Hypoglycemia

Normal blood glucose levels are maintained by the interplay of multiple factors, including glucose intake, insulin secretion, hepatic glycogenolysis and gluconeogenesis, and various hormone levels (insulin, glucagon, catecholamines, growth hormone, glucocorticoids). Abnormalities in any of these factors may result in symptomatic hypoglycemia when circulating blood glucose drops below 40–50 mg/100 dl. Clinical manifestations (Table 12-7) take two forms: those related to reactive catecholamine secretion in attempting to raise blood sugar to normal values and those due to the effects of glucose deprivation on the central nervous system. It is obvious that many of these signs and symptoms are nonspecific and may occur in a wide variety of other conditions, both organic and psychogenic. It is easy to overdiagnose hypoglycemia and desirable to document two episodes with the finding of low blood sugar levels before it is established.

The differential diagnosis must include multiple underlying causes (Table 12-8). Particular historic points to be noted are age of onset, relation of symptoms to meals (fasting versus postprandial), family history of hypoglycemia, diet habits, previous surgery, and ingestion of drugs (licit and illicit) or toxins. Physical findings of significance are indications of endocrine dysfunction or liver disease. Pertinent laboratory data include urinalysis (for glucose, nonglucose sugars, ketones) and blood levels of glucose, insulin, ketones, free fatty acids, and lactate. A 5-hour glucose tolerance test, with a 50–100 g dose of glucose p.o., is often used to evaluate possible postprandial hypoglycemia. Results are highly variable on a number of factors including sex, weight, rate of gastric emptying, absorptions, and others. An intravenous glucose tolerance test obviates a number of variables but should be done only under carefully controlled circumstances, as it may precipitate severe hypoglycemia in vulnerable individuals. A 24-hour fast is used to evaluate "fasting" hypoglycemia; the normal individual with normal glucose stores will maintain blood sugar well above the hypoglycemic range, although he or she may develop a rise in ketones and free fatty acids along with a drop in insulin levels.

REACTIVE HYPOGLYCEMIA

A hypoglycemic rebound of a modest degree is a normal physiologic reaction to a large carbohydrate load. This response may be exaggerated in some essentially healthy individuals and accounts for a significant percent of those persons diagnosed as hypoglycemic. Symptoms tend to occur 3–4 hours postprandially and rarely last beyond 30 minutes or result in syncope. Otherwise the patient is well. Plasma insulin levels are normal. An underlying emotional basis may contribute to this condition in that those with perfectionistic or impulsive personalities seem more prone than others. A common modality of treatment is a low-carbohydrate, high-protein diet (1.5–2 g/kg) divided into five or six small meals per day; it is not always helpful and attention may be needed for underlying psychologic problems. Table 12-8, item 10, lists other causes of reactive hypoglycemia.

FASTING HYPOGLYCEMIA

Most other types of hypoglycemia are in the fasting category. They are unrelated to meals, and symptoms occur upon starvation. Drug-induced episodes are the most common form seen in adolescents, primarily insulin overdose in diabetics. Hypoglycemia due to alcoholism and poor diet or salicylate overdose may be seen rarely. Other etiologies (Table 12-8) should be ruled out, but few occur in adolescents except under unusual circumstances. Inborn errors of metabolism usually are diagnosed well before the second decade.

Thyroid Disorders
HYPOTHYROIDISM

Hypothyroidism, or thyroid deficiency of any degree, may result from any of a variety of etiologies (Table 12-9). The most common cause in adolescents is chronic lymphocytic thyroiditis and affects

TABLE 12-9
CAUSES OF HYPOTHYROIDISM

1. Primary thyroid disease
   a. Idiopathic
   b. Chronic lymphocytic thyroiditis (Hashimoto's thyroiditis)
   c. Following treatment of hyperthyroidism (medical or surgical)
   d. Congenital
   e. Iodide administration
   f. Goitrogen ingestion
   g. Infectious granulomatosis
   h. Infiltrative disease (cystinosis, oxalosis)
   i. Transient reactive, following discontinuation of long-term thyroid medication
2. Secondary thyroid disease (TSH* deficiency)
   a. Pituitary tumors (most common is craniopharyngioma)
   b. Sheehan syndrome (postpartum pituitary hemorrhage)
   c. Idiopathic
   d. Postsurgical (for pituitary tumor, in connection with cancer therapy, and so on)
3. Tertiary thyroid disease (TRF† deficiency)
   a. Hypothalamic tumor
   b. Idiopathic
   c. Postencephalitis
   d. Posttrauma
4. Sick euthyroid syndrome (clinical hypothyroidism) without confirmatory laboratory findings
5. Schmidt's syndrome (primary hypothyroidism plus primary adrenal insufficiency and/or other endocrine dysfunction)

*TSH, thyroid-stimulating hormone.
†TRF, thyroid-releasing factor.

females predominantly (see next section), but even such cases are relatively rare until later years. Table 12-10 lists signs and symptoms of this condition, but manifestations are apt to be poorly defined and thus missed. On the other hand, any degree of lethargy, overweight, or sluggishness may be attributed to hypothyroidism erroneously.

Confirmatory laboratory findings for primary hypothyroidism (thyroid gland malfunction) include a low serum thyroxine (T_4), low serum triiodothyronine (T_3), elevated thyroid-stimulating hormone (TSH), normal or low serum resin uptake, elevated cholesterol levels, and no response to TSH stimulation. Secondary hypothyroidism due to pituitary disease is indicated by low levels of serum thyroid hormones coupled with a low TSH level and a positive response to TSH stimulation but without response to thyrotropin-releasing hormone (TRH).

Tertiary of hypothalamic-derived hypothyroidism produces similar results but a positive response to TRH stimulation with a rise in TSH.

Hypothyroidism that has been present for a number of months or several years may have concomitant x-ray findings of epiphyseal dysgenesis and delayed bone age. This finding would also be manifested in delayed growth and maintenance of childhood upper-lower body segment ratios. Skull roentgenograms may reveal an enlarged sella turcica with pituitary disease, commonly craniopharyngioma. Enlargement may also be noted with primary hypothyroidism due to the hypertrophy of TSH-secreting cells.

Treatment of any form of hypothyroidism is with thyroid hormone replacement and attention to underlying factors. Thyroid USP, 90–180 mg/day; levothyroxine (Synthroid), 0.15–0.40 mg/day; liothyronine (Cytomel), 0.025–0.075 mg/day; or liotrix (Euthroid), 1 tablet per day, may be used. Thyroid USP is cheap and effective but may take several weeks before achieving replacement levels. Other forms act more rapidly. Control may be induced with a short-acting form for quick results and thyroid USP substituted at a later date. Patients usually begin with the lower dosage of the chosen drug and increase dosage every 2 weeks or so until a euthyroid state is achieved. Some recommend raising the level just to toxicity as indicated by signs of hyperthyroidism (see section on hyperthyroidism) and then cutting back to the maximum dose tolerated while remaining euthyroid. If the patient with secondary hypothyroidism has adrenocorticotropic hormone (ACTH) deficiency as well, giving thyroid hormone without ACTH or corticosteroid replacement may precipitate an addisonian crisis.

EUTHYROID GOITERS

Chronic lymphocytic thyroiditis. Chronic lymphocytic thyroiditis (Hashimoto's thyroiditis, Hashimoto's struma, autoimmune thyroiditis), an autoimmune disorder, is the most common thyroid disease in adolescence, particularly in females, and comprises a major cause (80%) of euthyroid goiter in this age group. It sometimes is associated with other autoimmune disorders of the endocrine glands. A positive family history is common as well.

The patient often presents with a sense of pressure or fullness in the neck that has existed for several weeks or months. She usually is clinically euthyroid, although hyperthyroidism or hypothyroidism may rarely be present. Examination reveals a moderately and diffusely enlarged thyroid gland that is somewhat firm, pebbly, and nontender. Thirty per-

TABLE 12-10
SIGNS AND SYMPTOMS OF HYPOTHYROIDISM

1. Neurologic
   a. Poor coordination; may be ataxic
   b. Lethargy, laconic speech
   c. Reduced intellectual function, poor or deteriorating school function, reduced attention span
   d. Impaired mental status
   e. Delayed relaxation time of deep tendon reflexes (use Achilles tendon)
2. Dermatologic
   a. Puffiness (myxedema); eyelids may be particularly noticeable
   b. Coarse dry skin and hair; cool skin
   c. Alopecia
   d. Carotenemia
   e. Easy bruisability
3. Cardiovascular
   a. Bradycardia
   b. Hypotension
   c. Low pulse pressure
   d. Enlarged heart
   e. Low voltage on ECG
4. Growth and puberty
   a. Delayed puberty, delayed dentition
   b. Slow growth rate with immature upper-lower segment ratio
   c. Menorrhagia or amenorrhea
   d. Hirsuitism
   e. Galactorrhea
   f. Weight gain
5. Miscellaneous
   a. Anemia (macrocytic or microcytic)
   b. Constipation, bloating
   c. Cold intolerance
   d. Hoarse voice, thick tongue
   e. Flabby, aching muscles; myxedema
   f. Anorexia
   g. Depression
   h. Hyponatremia
   i. Carpal tunnel syndrome
   j. Goiter (iodine deficiency)
   k. Increased respiratory depression with opiates and sedatives
6. Rare syndromes associated with hypothyroidism
   a. Pendred syndrome (hypothyroidism and neurosensory deafness)
   b. Debré-Sémélaigne syndrome (hypothyroidism, and pseudomuscular hypertrophy)

cent of these patients also evidence nontender cervical adenopathy. Sixty percent have antithyroglobulin and/or thyroid microsomal antibody titers of 1:4 or greater. Thyroid function studies are quite variable; the more commonly seen abnormalities include an elevated TSH, a positive perchlorate discharge test, and a protein-bound iodine (PBI) level that exceeds that of T_4 by 2 μg per 100 ml or more. A thyroid scan (scintiscan) may show irregular radioiodine distribution. A fine needle biopsy is diagnostic but rarely indicated in the face of typical historic, physical, and laboratory findings. Major differential considerations include simple colloid goiter, hyperthyroidism (toxic goiter), and thyroid cancer. Iodine-deficient colloid goiters are rarely encountered today due to the widespread use of iodinated salt.

The clinical course is unpredictable. There may be an uneventful recovery after a number of months (although some fullness may persist indefinitely) or a slow progression to hypothyroidism over a number of years. Replacement therapy with one of the thyroid hormone preparations mentioned above (see section on hypothyroidism) is usually recommended. This at least tends to shrink an unsightly goiter; it also may inhibit the later development of hypothyroidism by placing the thyroid gland at rest during the active phase, although this is purely hypothetical. When treatment is instituted, it should be maintained for a number of months to a year (or longer) and then slowly tapered to discontinuance if there is no evidence of the goiter's recurrence.

Simple goiter. Simple goiter is also a common cause of euthyroid goiter in adolescence, especially in females. Except for neck fullness, the patient with simple goiter is completely asymptomatic. Physical examination reveals a diffusely enlarged thyroid, variably soft to firm in consistency. Significant features that differentiate it from chronic lymphocytic thyroiditis include a greater likelihood of being soft and smooth in contrast to firm and pebbly; a lower incidence of a family history of thyroid disease; significantly fewer clinical symptoms, and being predominantly related to local pressure. Etiology is due to hyperplasia probably consequent to relative or absolute iodine deficiency. Evaluation is similar to that for chronic lymphocytic thyroiditis, the primary differential consideration. Thyroid tests generally fall within the normal range; low iodine levels may be encountered on occasion. Treatment is indicated only if iodine deficiency is documented (with iodine replacement) or if the goiter is cosmetically distressing or causes pressure symptoms; in the latter instances treatment is thyroid hormone replacement (according to previously cited schedules) for prolonged periods.

Other causes. Other forms of euthyroid goiters are rare in adolescence, although they should be considered in the differential diagnosis. These include

---

TABLE 12-11
SYMPTOMS AND SIGNS OF
DIFFUSE TOXIC GOITER (GRAVES' DISEASE)

1. Nervousness with tremor
2. Goiter; may have thyroid bruit
3. Exophthalmos (proptosis, lid lag, stare)
4. Tachycardia with wide pulse pressure at rest
5. Irritability, restlessness, personality change
6. Muscle weakness; may have myopathy
7. Heat intolerance
8. Hyperhidrosis, smooth, moist, warm skin
9. Weight loss of 5–15 pounds or more
10. Palpitations
11. School problems, shortened attention span
12. Disturbed sleep
13. Easy fatigability
14. Amenorrhea
15. Increased appetite
16. Increased deep tendon reflexes
17. Cardiac enlargement; may have flow murmur; may progress to failure
18. Diarrhea
19. Uncommon but sometimes seen; ocular pruritus and lacrimation, pretibial myxedema, paradoxical lethargy, onycholysis, clubbing, increased growth rate and bone maturation

---

chronic fibrous thyroiditis, multinodular colloid goiter, primary thyroid neoplasms, secondary neoplasms (lymphoma), partial congenital defects in hormone synthesis, acute suppurative and acute nonsuppurative thyroiditis, and goitrogen-induced (iodine excess, drugs, foods) conditions.

HYPERTHYROIDISM

Hyperthyroidism, or thyrotoxicosis, is characterized by an excess of one or more thyroid hormones. Although a variety of causes exists in the population at large (diffuse toxic goiter or Graves' disease, toxic adenoma, toxic multinodular goiter, functional thyroid neoplasms, McCune-Albright syndrome and others), all but diffuse toxic goiter are rare in adolescence. Diffuse toxic goiter, however, is seen with some frequency primarily in adolescent girls and is an autoimmune disorder associated with the presence in the blood of long-acting thyroid stimulator (LATS). Table 12-11 cites signs and symptoms. Physical findings include a firm, smooth, enlarged, and nontender thyroid gland with well-demarcated borders. A bruit also may often be heard. Abnormal eye findings indicative of some degree of exophthalmos occur in most patients at some point; these include proptosis, lid lag on upward gaze, lid retraction with a rim of sclera visible between the upper lid and iris, and a staring appearance. The size of the goiter, degree of exophthalmos, and degree of toxicity bear no relationship to each other.

Supportive laboratory data include elevated serum levels of thyroxine (T_4), free T_4 and triiodothyronine (T_3); increased T_3 resin uptake; increased but nonsuppressable radioactive iodine uptake; and low levels of thyroid-stimulating hormone (TSH). A thyroid scan with technetium reveals diffuse enlargement.

The use of antithyroid medications is considered by many the treatment of first choice; either propylthiouracil, 100 mg t.i.d., or methimazole, 10 mg t.i.d. Therapy continues for a number of months to a year. Monitoring for drug side effects, including agranulocytosis, is indicated. Some experts recommend a subtotal thyroidectomy initially; it will be necessary in the event that drug treatment fails or unacceptable degrees of drug toxicity are encountered. The use of therapeutic amounts of radioactive iodine in adolescents is controversial due to the long-range potential for radiation-induced neoplasms.

THYROID TUMORS

Although a nodular form of chronic lymphocytic thyroiditis, thyroid cysts, or adenomas and ectopic thyroid masses may occur in adolescents, these are exceptionally rare. Although thyroid neoplasms also are uncommon in this age group, they remain the leading cause of a nodular, asymmetric or irregularly enlarged gland. Radiation to the neck or mediastinum in childhood may be a predisposing factor to the development of papillary or follicular carcinoma. Metastatic lesions, particularly lymphomas, also may occur.

Diagnostic aids include ultrasonography, thyroid scan (revealing "cold" nodules), thyroid function studies, and tissue biopsy. An elevated serum calcitonin may be encountered in the rare syndrome of multiple endocrine neoplasia. Treatment is by total thyroidectomy and excision of regional lymph nodes. Radioactive iodine therapy may be a useful adjunct in tumors possessing hormonal activity. Thyroid replacement is necessary as well. The prognosis varies, being good for the more differentiated forms (papillary or follicular) and less optimistic for those that are anaplastic.

Growth Disorders

SHORT STATURE

Although many factors interfere with the aquisition of normal height (Table 12-12), the most common reasons are constitutional delay in growth (and puberty), genetic (familial) short stature, and chronic

---

TABLE 12-12
CAUSES OF
SHORT STATURE IN ADOLESCENCE

1. Familial or genetic (primordial dwarfism)
2. Constitutional delay in growth
3. Growth hormone deficiency (isolated or panhypopituitarism)
4. Hypothalamic disorders
5. Skeletal dysplasias (achondroplasia, osteogenesis imperfecta, Morquio's syndrome, others)
6. Turner's syndrome and other chromosomal abnormalities
7. Excess cortisol (Cushing's syndrome, exogenous)
8. Inflammatory bowel disease with malabsorption and debility
9. Hypothyroidism
10. Chronic illness (infections; collagen diseases; hematologic, renal, cardiac, pulmonary, liver disorders; malignancy)
11. Hypogonadism (primary, secondary)
12. Infancy and childhood conditions with possible carry-over into adolescence
    a. Intrauterine growth retardation (small for gestational age)
    b. Psychosocial dwarfism (emotional deprivation)
    c. Nutritional deficiency (starvation)
13. Syndromes (Russell-Silver syndrome, pseudohypoparathyroidism [Albright's hereditary osteodystrophy])

---

debilitating illness. Evaluation includes a history of growth and pubertal patterns of parents and siblings (age onset of growth spurt, age onset of sexual maturation, menarche, final adult height), the patient's prenatal and perinatal history, birth weight and height and ages of childhood and adolescent developmental milestones, including sexual maturation if it has occurred (see Chapter 2). Plotting the patient's childhood and adolescent heights and weights on a standard growth chart is helpful. When these data are not available, some assessment of chronologic progress may be gleaned from group photographs including the patient, reports of changes in shoe and clothing size, and other such indicators.

A normal growth rate of 5 cm per year is characteristic from age 2 until the onset of the pubertal growth spurt. It then increases in rate to an average peak of 9 cm per year in Tanner stage II–III females and 10.2 in Tanner stage III–IV males (see Appendix I). The wide range in the normal ages of pubertal events from one individual to another, however, should always be kept in mind. The potential for additional growth after achieving full sexual maturity (Tanner stage IV–V) is limited; staging correlates well with epiphyseal closure. Males, however, can expect to gain approximately 2 cm between the completion of sexual maturation and age 21. Considerable growth potential remains for the short adolescent who has not yet entered puberty or still is early in its progress. Definitive assessment of remaining growth potential is forthcoming from a bone age roentgenogram (left hand and wrist as per Greulich and Pyle or Tanner-Whitehouse standards). Data obtained up to this point will suggest additional diagnostic studies, including hormonal evaluations and assessment for chronic illnesses and metabolic conditions that interfere with growth. Differential considerations cited in Table 12-12 provide direction.

All adolescents with short stature also need evaluation and attention to their psychosocial status. Psychologic problems often are present. Society has generally responded to the appearance of these young people rather than their cognitive maturity. A 16-year-old who appears no more than 11 or 12 inevitably is set apart from peers and is inappropriately treated as a child. Short-statured children often come into adolescence with poor self-esteem and emotional immaturity. It is as important to deal with these factors as it is to carry out an organic assessment. At all points, the physician should relate to these adolescents in terms of their intellectual capacity and not physical size and appearance. Others should be encouraged to do the same.

Familial or genetic short stature. Individuals with this situation are short at birth and grow throughout childhood at a rate below but parallel to the third percentile. They enter puberty at an average age, remain short in relation to their peers throughout adolescence, and end up as short adults. Characteristically, the parents of these patients also tend to be short relative to their ethnic background. There is no effective treatment. Counseling is important and focuses on body image concerns, finding compensatory methods for achieving self-esteem, ensuring socialization, and planning for a vocation and career compatible with the projected adult height.

Constitutional delay in growth. The most common cause of short stature first presenting in adolescence is constitutional delay in growth. The patient usually is male (there appears to be a greater incidence in this sex as well as more concern than in short-statured females) and gives a history of normal height and weight at birth. Growth often is below the mean for the first few years, with a more normal rate during the rest of childhood and a tendency to remain at or slightly under the third percentile. Pubertal onset is late, and the growth spurt occurs well after that of average peers; when it does occur, the total period of growth may be more prolonged. These adolescents ultimately catch up with peers and end up with an adult stature in the normal range. Sixty percent of individuals with constitutional delay of the growth spurt and puberty also have members in their immediate family with similar patterns.

Differentiation from genetic short stature or from pituitary or gonadal failure may not always be easy. Consultation with an endocrinologist is indicated when there are no signs of puberty by age 15 in females or age 16 in males. Measurement of serum gonadotropins and testosterone or estrogen may be helpful. Additional information may be obtained from a luteinizing-releasing hormone (LRH) stimulation test, buccal smear for Barr bodies, a definitive karyotype, and other tests for endocrine dysfunction. Debilitating chronic conditions impairing growth also must be ruled out. Medical treatment is usually unnecessary. Adolescents with significant delay, however, may be seriously compromised on a psychologic basis, and intervention to produce some evidence of the true growth potential and puberty may be indicated from an emotional perspective. Oxandrolone has been used to promote growth in some instances. Others have used a brief 3-month course of testosterone, which induces visible pubertal changes without compromising inherent growth potential to any significant degree. A 3–6 month course of chorionic gonadotropin injections has been used by some in an effort to induce puberty; results are inconclusive and some evidence suggests this may produce antitesticular antibodies at some future time.

Growth hormone deficiency. Deficiency in growth hormone (HGH) seriously impedes childhood and adolescent growth and results in marked dwarfism; height is 3–4 or more standard deviations below the mean. Although there are a variety of causes (Table 12-13), pituitary dysgenesis is most common. Classically, the patient's birth weight and length are normal, as is growth during the first year or two of life. Growth failure makes its appearance at about age 2 and persists until (or unless) medical intervention occurs. Physical signs include a baby face, infantile features and body proportions, a weight age greater than height age, and delayed puberty. Half of these patients have an isolated growth hormone defect;

TABLE 12-13
PITUITARY DEFECTS THAT MAY
RESULT IN GROWTH HORMONE DEFICIENCY

1. Pituitary dysgenesis (aplasia, hypoplasia)
2. Septo-optic dysplasia
3. Craniopharyngioma and other pituitary tumors
4. Aneurysms
5. Sarcoidosis
6. Tuberculosis
7. Hand-Schüller-Christian disease
8. Toxoplasmosis
9. Basilar skull fractures
10. Complications of radiation therapy
11. Following meningitis or encephalitis

TABLE 12-14
CAUSES OF EXCESSIVE HEIGHT

1. Constitutional tall stature
2. Excessive HGH (pituitary tumor)
3. Cerebral gigantism (Soto's syndrome)
4. Precocious puberty
5. Hyperthyroidism
6. Primary hypogonadism (male)
   a. Klinefelter's syndrome
   b. Kallmann's syndrome
7. Marfan's syndrome
8. Homocystinuria
9. Testicular feminization syndrome
10. Neurofibromatosis

the remainder have deficiencies of the other pituitary hormones to a variable degree. Short stature in this instance may be further complicated by diabetes insipidus, hypoadrenalism, hypothyroidism, and/or hypogonadism. Thus an adolescent with growth hormone deficiency only ultimately will enter puberty; those with deficiency of gonadotropins as well will not.

Management by an endocrinologist at a center approved for receiving and distributing human growth hormone from the national collection center is essential; this substance is in low supply and carefully regulated to ensure that the diagnosis is well founded. Evaluation includes assessment of HGH levels and responsiveness to various stimuli such as arginine and insulin together with the functioning of other hormonal and body systems regulated by the pituitary.

Treatment consists of HGH replacement: 0.05–0.1 IU/kg given intramuscularly two or three times a week over a prolonged period. The best response occurs within the first year of treatment. Anabolic steroids (oxandrolone) may be added thereafter in maximizing the growth spurt. Replacement with other hormones may be necessary when multiple pituitary deficiencies exist. A normal adult stature is rarely achieved, but it is possible to achieve a stature that does not relegate the individual to a life of isolating dwarfism.

Miscellaneous causes. A teenage female with growth retardation and sexual immaturity may have ovarian dysgenesis (Turner's syndrome) as discussed further in the section on pubertal delay. Various skeletal dysplasias may produce an upper to lower body segment greater than the normal adult ratio of 1:1. Chronic hypothyroidism results in short lower extremities relative to the trunk and short stature.

Psychosocial dwarfism (emotional deprivation) may occur in an infant or child with carry-over effects into adolescence. Prolonged steroid administration in the range of 4.0 mg/m^2 or more of prednisone a day also may inhibit normal growth. A wide variety of various syndrome states also are associated with short stature with or without pubertal delay (Table 12-12).

EXCESSIVE HEIGHT

Various conditions may cause excess height (Table 12-14), but in most instances it is familial or constitutional in origin. Excessive height is without medical significance, and the implications are primarily psychosocial depending on the degree to which the patient, usually female, perceives her height as isolating from her peers and experiences diminished self-esteem. There usually is a positive family history for tall stature, and the girl has grown in a normal manner but at or above the ninety-fifth percentile. The onset and sequencing of pubertal events usually is at the upper end of the normal range. Bone age, Tanner staging, age at menarche, and parents' heights can be used to roughly predict ultimate height. More precise evaluation is needed if hormonal intervention is contemplated; this is best carried out by an endocrinologist.

Treatment is highly controversial in terms of appropriateness and effectiveness. It consists of estrogen administration to induce earlier and/or more rapid puberty with earlier epiphyseal closure and termination of the growth potential at an earlier age than might naturally occur. Consideration of whether to carry out such therapy is a prepubertal or early pubertal matter; once past Tanner stage III the patient is already decelerating growth and initiating epiphyseal closure; estrogen therapy has little effect (documented by the failure of oral contraceptives to interfere with growth following menarche). On the average, girls have reached an untreatable point in pubertal advance by age 13 or 14 years at the latest.

Psychologic intervention usually is the course of choice. Counseling and helping a girl to deal with arbitrary societal dictates of what is a proper female height can be helpful. Those who have particular difficulty in adaptation may benefit by consultation with a mental health professional.

Pituitary tumors (eosinophilic adenomas or chromophobe adenomas) may induce rapid and excessive growth during childhood due to increased secretion of growth hormone. High levels after epiphyseal closure can only affect those portions of the skeleton capable of growth at any time in life (hands, feet, ears, and mandible). Excessive growth of these body parts due to increased growth hormone constitutes acromegaly. Other possible symptoms of a pituitary tumor include visual impairment, papilledema, and headaches. Neuroradiologic studies are indicated (skull roentgenograms, computerized tomography, angiogram, others). Treatment is by surgical removal.

Pubertal Disorders

The association of sexual maturation with skeletal growth makes it almost impossible to separate this category of problems from those relating to too tall or too short height. In making the discrimination as to categorization, the most likely presenting complaint was the determining one. On the other hand, some conditions producing variations or abnormalities in puberty are independent of growth.

PRECOCIOUS PUBERTY

By definition, precocious puberty cannot be diagnosed unless sexual maturation occurs before minus 2½ SD of the normal range or before age 8 in females and age 9 in males. Precocious puberty, then, is not a disease of the adolescent years, but affected children bring their precocity into adolescence with associated psychosocial problems. Some may need to deal with the fact that while exceptionally tall as children, their full growth potential is limited with early epiphyseal closure and they may end up as short adults. Occasionally precocious puberty is not diagnosed until a pubertal history reveals it in adolescence.

Although many causes of precocious puberty exist (Table 12-15), 85%–90% of cases in females are idiopathic. In contrast, 50%–60% of premature sexual development in males is due to a demon-

---

TABLE 12-15
CAUSES OF PRECOCIOUS PUBERTY

TRUE OR COMPLETE SEXUAL PRECOCITY
1. Idiopathic
2. Central nervous system lesions (congenital hypothalamic or pituitary defects, tumors, postinfectious sequellae, hydrocephalus, posttrauma)
3. McCune-Albright syndrome (café au lait spots, fibrous dysplasia, and cysts of skull and long bones)
4. Neurofibromatosis
5. Tuberous sclerosis
6. Hypothyroidism with growth failure, hyperprolactinemia, and galactorrhea (Grumback-van Wyk syndrome)
7. Gonadotropin-secreting tumors
   a. Hepatoblastoma
   b. Teratoma (intracranial)
   c. Chorioepithelioma
   d. Retropleural polyembryoma
8. Russell-Silver syndrome

INCOMPLETE OR
PSEUDOPRECOCIOUS PUBERTY
1. Exogenous estrogen administration (feminization)
2. Exogenous administration of anabolic steroids or androgens (virilization)
3. Adrenal abnormalities
   a. Adrenal tumor (virilizing or feminizing)
   b. Congenital adrenal hyperplasia (virilization)
4. Gonadal tumors
   a. Ovarian
      (1) Benign ovarian cyst (feminization)
      (2) Granulosa-theca cell tumor (feminization)
      (3) Dysgerminoma (feminization)
      (4) Arrhenoblastoma (masculinization)
   b. Testicular
      (1) Leydig cell tumor (masculinization)
      (2) Seminoma (feminization)

---

strable etiology. Complete, or true, precocious puberty refers to central nervous system stimulation and elevated gonadotropin levels relative to age with resultant full sexual maturation or its potential. Incomplete or pseudoprecocious puberty refers to an infrapituitary disorder with stimulation of testosterone or estrogen production independent of gonadotropin levels; pubertal development is only partial and gonadotropins are at preadolescent levels. Development appropriate to the patient's gender is termed isosexual precocious puberty; opposite gender change is termed heterosexual change.

Females may demonstrate either premature thelarche (breast development and, sometimes, estrogenization of vaginal mucosa) or premature adrenarche (development of pubic and, sometimes, axillary hair) as well as a more complete picture. Premature thelarche is most often noted in females between ages 2–4 years. Idiopathic in origin, it is benign and nonprogressing in most instances; normal puberty ensues at an appropriate time. It is thought possibly due to unusual end organ sensitivity to low levels of circulating estrogen or to intermittent gonatotropin elevation. Exogenous estrogens may be implicated in some cases. Premature adrenarche, due to a rise in adrenal androgens (dihydroandrosterone and sulfated forms), is most commonly noted between ages 6 and 8 years. Growth rate and bone age are normal or only slightly increased. Onset and growth in idiopathic precocious adrenarche in males resembles that in premature adrenarche in females. Penile enlargement to a modest degree may or may not occur, although full precocious puberty demonstrates testicular and definitive penile enlargement as well as body hair. In both males and females, 17 keto-steroid levels (a measure of androgen production) are higher than normal based on chronologic age but consistent with gender and degree of sexual maturation (Appendix I).

In establishing the diagnosis (Table 12-15), examination should include neurologic evaluation with funduscopic and visual field assessment of genitalia, rectal, and pelvic structures. When other than idiopathic isosexual precocious puberty is suspected, a sonogram may be particularly helpful in defining pelvic structures. Laparoscopy today is a safe and simple procedure in skilled hands and permits a biopsy as well as direct visualization.

Most instances of previously undiagnosed precocious puberty, premature thelarche, or premature adrenarche first uncovered in adolescence are idiopathic and among females. More serious causes should have been manifested at a far earlier date. The one condition that may have been missed is precocious puberty caused by a central nervous system lesion. Exogenous estrogens or androgens and ovarian tumors may have been missed on rare occasion.

PUBERTAL DELAY

Some healthy and normal adolescents do not begin puberty until after 14–15 years of age and will present before this time out of concern that something is wrong. Provided all else is normal in the history and physical examination, particularly with a familial history of late puberty and provided the patient has been growing at a consistent rate (even if at the lower end of the percentile range), there is no

TABLE 12-16
CAUSES OF DELAYED PUBERTY

1. See causes of short stature (Table 12-12)
2. Hypogonadotropic hypogonadism (secondary)
   a. Pituitary tumor or congenital defects
   b. Anorexia nervosa
   c. Laurence-Moon-Biedl syndrome (mental retardation, obesity, retinitis pigmentosa, polydactyly, hypogonadism)
   d. Prader-Willi syndrome (mental retardation, obesity, orthopedic abnormalities, insulin-resistant diabetes, hypogonadism)
   e. Fertile eunuch syndrome (isolated defect of luteinizing hormone)
   f. Kallmann syndrome (olfactory-genital syndrome; anosmia and isolated gonadotropin deficiency)
   g. Friedreich's ataxia
3. Hypergonadotropic hypogonadism (primary)
   a. Turner's syndrome (46 XO)
   b. Klinefelter's syndrome (47 XXY)
   c. Autoimmume oophoritis
   d. Orchitis (as in mumps)
   e. Male Turner syndrome
   f. Turner syndrome mosaics
   g. Bilateral torsion of the ovarian pedicle or testes
   h. Following surgery, radiation, and trauma
   i. Drug effect (cyclophosphamide)
   j. Ovarian cyst or neoplasm
   k. Myotonic dystrophy
   l. Reifenstein's syndrome
   m. Del Castillo syndrome (germinal cell aplasia with normal luteinizing hormone and high follicle-stimulating hormone levels)

reason for medical concern unless the delay is more than 2.5 standard deviations from the norm (Appendix I, Tables 1 and 2). The concern of some teenagers, however, is so great that more than simple physical and historic evaluation is needed to reassure them.

Table 12-16 cites differential considerations, and Figure 12-1 presents a flow chart for evaluation. Elevated gonadotropin levels will be noted in primary hypogonadism but not in secondary forms due to pituitary deficiency. Various androgenic and estrogenic substances also may be measured to further define the nature of the problem when indicated (Appendix I; Tables 7A, 7B). Determination of karyotype also can be helpful. In most instances such an evaluation requires an endocrinologic consultation, but it is the responsibility of the primary care physician to ensure that some other cause such as chronic illness has not been overlooked.

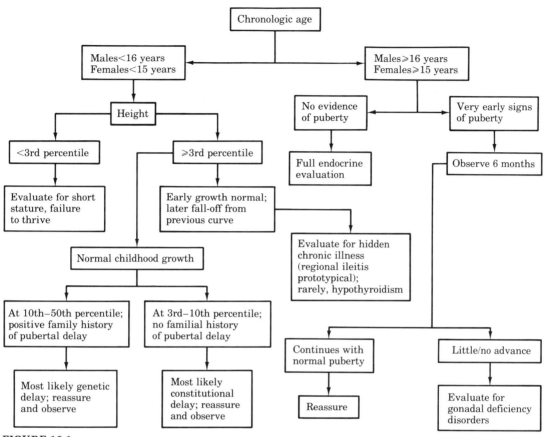

FIGURE 12-1
FLOW CHART FOR THE EVALUATION OF PUBERTAL DELAY

Notes:

1. Effective Tanner staging (Chapter 2) often obviates the need to obtain bone-age roentgenograms and other endocrine studies as part of initial assessment. Nothing more than clinical evaluation usually is needed in instances of familial or constitutional delay.

2. Be sure there indeed are no signs of puberty if this is the complaint. Early breast buds, early testicular enlargement may well be overlooked by the patient.

3. The growth spurt may antecede sexual development in some individuals and is predictive of puberty. If data available, plot annual growth rate velocities.

4. In some cases of constitutional or familial delay, additional studies may be necessary to allay the concerns of singularly anxious adolescents and their parents. Modify clinical evaluation plan accordingly.

Turner's syndrome. Also known as ovarian dysgenesis, Turner's syndrome, occurring in one in 2000 female births, is characterized by short stature, persistent sexual infantilism (although a small amount of pubic hair may appear at the time of anticipated puberty), 45 XO karyotype, and a variable number of other signs (Table 12-17). Mental retardation is not a common feature but may occur to a mild or moderate degree in some.

The major endocrine defect stems from failure of the ovarian development and persistence of the gonadal streak, resulting in hypergonadotropic hypogonadism; estrogen levels are low or absent with elevated follicle-stimulating hormone (FSH) and

TABLE 12-17
FEATURES THAT MAY BE SEEN
IN CLASSIC TURNER'S SYNDROME

1. Short stature (growth usually does not exceed 142 cm)
2. Sexual infantilism with streak ovaries (may have slight amount of pubic hair)
3. Turner facies (fish mouth, low-set ears, malformed ear lobes, epicanthic folds, micrognathia)
4. Short, webbed neck with low hair line
5. Cubitus valgus (wide carrying angle of forearms)
6. Finger or digit anomalies
7. Shield chest with broadly spaced, hypoplastic nipples
8. Abnormal hearing and vision, including color blindness
9. Cardiovascular disorders (hypertension, coarctation of the aorta, aortic stenosis, bicuspid aortic valve)
10. Multiple renal anomalies
11. Multiple pigmented nevi
12. Association with recurrent otitis media, diabetes mellitus, chronic lymphocytic thyroiditis
13. Features in infancy: short birth length, lymphedema of hands and feet, loose posterior neck folds

leuteinizing hormone (LH). The bone age usually is delayed and buccal smear negative for Barr bodies. The karyotype is diagnostic.

Estrogen replacement therapy should be initiated in adolescence to induce and maintain secondary sexual maturation and delay the aging processes associated with an estrogen-deprived state. The possible long-range development of endometrial carcinoma in patients on chronic estrogen therapy may be a concern, but current experience with oral contraceptives does not suggest the risk is great, at least through the fourth decade. Once satisfactory development has been achieved, cyclical hormone therapy may be introduced (Chapter 17) to allow for menstruation. Anavar may be used in conjunction with estrogen (or estrogen-progesterone cycling) to stimulate vertical growth. Psychologic support in general and counseling the patient about her sexuality and infertility are essential companion measures.

Many variants of the Turner syndrome have been described, including mosaicism (46 XO/46 XX), isochromosome X, pure gonadal dysgenesis (46 XX or 46 XY), and the pseudo-Turner syndrome (Noonan, or Ullrich, syndrome). Mosaic forms have highly variable stigmata and may even demonstrate a normal buccal smear (presence of Barr bodies); pregnancy has occurred in some instances. Patients with pure gonadal dysgenesis have a normal female habitus without Turner stigmata and a normal karyotype but streak ovaries resulting in elevation of LH and FSH, primary amenorrhea, minimal secondary sexual development, and normal or above average height. Gonadal dysgenesis with a 46 XY karyotype is associated with increased incidence of gonadoblastomas.

The pseudo-Turner syndrome describes persons with some of the Turner stigmata but normal karyotypes. This terminology is more often applied to males but may be used to describe females as well. This condition has also been called Ullrich syndrome, Noonan syndrome, and the male Turner syndrome. The more common findings include triangular facies, pectus excavatum, webbed neck, ptosis, cubitus valgus, pulmonary stenosis or atrial septal defect, short stature, and mental retardation.

Klinefelter's syndrome. Occurring in 1 out of every 600 male births, Klinefelter's syndrome is manifested in hypergonadotropic hypogonadism due to a 47 XXY karyotype and testicular dysfunction. The individual usually appears normal throughout childhood, with a problem first manifesting at adolescence when pubertal failure is associated with a variable number of other features (Table 12-18). The testes usually are small and may not exceed an infantile size (2.0 cm) with azoospermia. The penis, although normal in size, also remains immature. Gynecomastia is noted in 40%-50% of the cases and bears a somewhat increased risk of breast cancer. Treatment consists of testosterone administration for life, testicular prostheses, and surgical correction of gynecomastia. Counseling about sexual and reproductive issues plus psychologic support in the emotional dimensions of this disorder are also important.

Many variants of this syndrome are described; some may manifest only some of the stigmata such as entering puberty at a normal or delayed time with normal or only moderately reduced Leydig cell function but dysfunctional spermatogenesis and oligospermia or aspermia. Occasionally a patient is noted with Klinefelter's features but a normal 46 XY karyotype. Table 12-16 cites other causes of hypogonadism.

Hermaphroditism
MALE PSEUDOHERMAPHRODITISM
Manifesting in a male karyotype and female phenotype, the testicular feminization syndrome (TFS) is the classic example of male pseudohermaphroditism. Due to the insensitivity of end organs to androgens, characteristic findings include a female phenotype

TABLE 12-18
FEATURES OF KLINEFELTER'S SYNDROME

1. Delayed puberty and/or incomplete sexual maturation
2. 47 XXY karyotype with positive buccal smear for Barr bodies
3. Height over fiftieth percentile
4. Arm span exceeds height by 2.5 cm or more
5. Decreased upper to lower body segment ratio
6. Eunuchoid fat distribution
7. Gynecomastia
8. Small, firm testes; pubic hair and penile development are greater than testicular development
9. Elevated gonadotropins
10. Azoospermia
11. Association with lung disease, varicose veins, breast cancer

with abnormal internal structures (for example, mature breast development but with small pale nipples); scant pubic and axillary hair; normal or hypoplastic vulva with normal clitoris; short, blind vagina and absent uterus; primary amenorrhea (may be the presenting complaint); gonads comprised of testicular tissue located intraabdominally or within a hernia or the labia majora, 46 XY karyotype, and adult male levels of serum testosterone with elevated LH and normal FSH. These patients also have an increased incidence of inguinal hernias and gonadoblastomas. Incomplete forms of TFS also are described with an enlarged clitoris and deep voice in addition to the female phenotype. Stein-Leventhal syndrome and pure gonadal dysgenesis (46 XX) sometimes may be confused with this condition.

Treatment involves postpubertal gonadectomy because of the high risk of cancer, continuation with a female gender assignment, and estrogen replacement therapy. Surgical correction of an incompetent vagina, an enlarged clitoris, or both (in incomplete forms) is indicated to provide for optimal sexual performance. Tact and sensitivity in counseling is essential. Prophylactic psychiatric consultation can be beneficial in helping the adolescent adjust to an exceptionally confusing and upsetting revelation.

Reifenstein syndrome denotes an individual with a 46 XY karyotype and evidence of defective androgen action in perineal hypospadius, small testis with or without cryptorchidism, and a normal phallus. Gynecomastia, hypogonadism, female pubic hair escutcheon, a small penis, and infertility become evident in adolescence. Treatment consists of surgical correction of the hypospadius, androgen therapy, and the later removal of testes with prosthetic replacement to prevent development of gonadoblastomas.

In the syndrome of pseudovaginal perinoscrotal hypospadius, the patient presents with a pseudovagina, a phallus with a ventral urethral groove and perineal urethral meatus, and a cleft scrotum resembling labia majora. Müllerian duct structures are absent. When the condition is not diagnosed in infancy, the patient is usually reared as a female, but puberty brings androgenic rather than estrogenic effects. This condition is due to a deficiency in 5 alpha-reductase. The karyotype is that of a normal male; 46 XY and plasma testosterone levels are normal. In most instances the individual is best managed by retaining the gender of rearing and undergoing appropriate surgical and hormonal treatment.

FEMALE PSEUDOHERMAPHRODITISM

Virilization of an individual with a female karyotype (46 XX) is most often due to congenital adrenal hyperplasia with either 21-hydroxylase deficiency (seen in 90%) or 11-hydroxylase enzyme deficiency with a rise in 17-ketosteroids and consequent masculinization. These females are born with ambiguous genitalia comprised of an enlarged clitoris and fused labia, sometimes mistaken for a hypospadic, cryptorchid male. Precocious virilization occurs early in childhood. Deficiency of 11-hydroxylase is also accompanied by hyperaldosteronism (compound S) and the salt-losing syndrome presenting as a neonatal emergency. This diagnosis is rarely missed today, and appropriate therapy with cortisone administration obviates many of the consequences of this disease. Reconstructive surgery in separating the fused labia should be done in childhood. Most specialists in gender ambiguity prefer to defer correction of the enlarged phallus until adolescence and to accomplish this by reimplantation up under the pubic fat pad rather than by amputation, thus preserving clitoral eroticism. Although cortisone replacement is necessary for life, many of these young women grow well, enter a normal puberty and menarche, and are able to bear children. As this is an inherited disorder (autosomal recessive), genetic counseling is in order.

TRUE HERMAPHRODITISM

True hermaphroditism is an exceptionally rare phenomenon in which both ovarian and testicular tissue is present in the same individual. Karyotypes may be 46 XX, 46 XY, or mosaics. Variable pubertal features appear. Treatment consists of selecting a gender of rearing in infancy, surgical genital reconstruction, hormone replacement consistent with the chosen phenotype, and removal of the gonads at some point before young adulthood to prevent later malignancy. It generally is far more satisfactory for these individuals to be raised as females; it is not too difficult to reconstruct a functional vagina and provide the option of a satisfactory sexual relationship. It is impossible to reconstruct a satisfactory, functional penis.

Adrenal Dysfunction

CUSHING'S SYNDROME

Chronic elevation in plasma glucocorticoids produces a constellation of clinical manifestations comprising Cushing's syndrome (Table 12-19). The etiology in adolescents is most commonly exogenous steroid administration for some other disease. Other causes include pituitary tumors and excessive ACTH production, an adrenal tumor (malignant or benign), or adrenal hyperplasia (Cushing's disease). In rare instances, a bronchogenic or thymic tumor may produce a polypeptide with ACTH-like effects.

Laboratory studies reveal polycythemia, lymphopenia, eosinophilia, hyperglycemia, hypokalemia, increased plasma glucocorticoids, and 17-ketosteroids, absence of the cortisol diurnal pattern, and an enlarged sella turcica when of pituitary origin. Differentiation between hyperplasia and tumor may be difficult, and the dexamethasone suppression test is helpful here; marked reduction of 17-hydroxycorticosteroids with moderate doses of dexamethasone is characteristic with hyperplasia and a minimal response with tumor. It should be kept in mind, however, that marked reduction of 17-hydroxycorticosteroids also may occur with low doses of dexamethasone in persons who are simply exogenously obese; this observation should not confuse the diagnosis of those with Cushing's disease.

Treatment varies depending on the cause. Exogenous steroids should be eliminated or reduced to the lowest effective dose. Alternate-day or three-times-a-week treatment schedules may obviate cushingoid effects. Bilateral total or subtotal adrenalectomy, hypophysectomy, or pituitary radiation are among the procedures employed for primary adrenal or primary pituitary disease.

ADRENAL INSUFFICIENCY

Table 12-20 cites the differential diagnosis of adrenal insufficiency. Clinical symptoms and signs include lethargy, anorexia, weight loss, hypotension, abdominal pain, hyperpigmentation, eosinophilia,

TABLE 12-19
CLINICAL FEATURES OF CUSHING'S DISEASE

1. Pseudoobesity (with moon facies and increased fat distribution around the girdle areas; buffalo hump)
2. Thin extremities
3. Hirsutism
4. Hypertension
5. Fatigue and weakness
6. Easy bruisability
7. Amenorrhea
8. Osteoporosis
9. Purple or brown striae
10. Reduced growth rate
11. Abnormal glucose tolerance test
12. Increased susceptibility to infections
13. Acne
14. Deepening of the voice
15. Clitoral hypertrophy

seizures, and hypoglycemia. An acute addisonian crisis may present as shock and coma. Treatment with steroid replacement usually is necessary.

Parathyroid Dysfunction

HYPERPARATHYROIDISM

Hyperparathyroidism may be due to a parathyroid adenoma (single or multiple), carcinoma, or hyperplasia. Clinical features include lethargy, polydipsia, polyuria, nocturia, osteoporosis, bone deformities such as scoliosis, nephrolithiasis, pancreatitis and parotid duct stones. Laboratory data reveal hypercalcemia, hypercalciuria, hypophosphatemia and, in some cases, elevated phosphatase levels. (Note, however, that normal adolescents during rapid growth may have high phosphatase levels, particularly if male.) Treatment is by surgical removal of a parathyroid adenoma or subtotal parathyroidectomy for hyperplasia. Hypoparathyroidism may be a surgical complication requiring chronic calciferol administration.

Other causes of hypercalcemia include vitamin D intoxication, prolonged immobilization, sarcoidosis, thyrotoxicosis, bony neoplastic metastases, leukemia, and idiopathic causes.

HYPOPARATHYROIDISM

Low parathormone levels are usually due to an autoimmune disorder of the parathyroid glands, which may be associated with other autoimmune phenomena (ovarian failure, Addison's disease, mucocutaneous candidiasis). Symptoms include multiple cramps and muscle pain, tetany, carpopedal spasm,

TABLE 12-20
CAUSES OF ADRENAL INSUFFICIENCY

1. Hypothalamic or pituitary disease
2. Primary adrenal insufficiency (isolated Addison's disease or in association with other autoimmune disorders—Schmidt's syndrome)
3. Inborn defect of steroid production (congenital adrenal hyperplasia)
4. Tuberculosis of adrenal gland
5. Waterhouse-Friderichsen syndrome (adrenal hemorrhage associated with bacterial infection; usually *Neisseria meningitidis* sepsis)
6. Postadrenalectomy
7. Mitotane-O, P'-DDD administration
8. Sudden withdrawal of exogenous steroids or ACTH (relative insufficiency with stress for up to 1 year following administration of steroids for more than 2 weeks even if tapered before discontinuing)
9. Overwhelming physical stress, particularly sepsis

TABLE 12-21
DISEASES IN WHICH INAPPROPRIATE ANTIDIURETIC HORMONE SECRETION MAY OCCUR

1. Central nervous system disorders
   a. Infection (meningitis, encephalitis, abscess)
   b. Intracranial tumor
   c. Trauma
2. Pulmonary disorders
   a. Bacterial or viral pneumonia
   b. Tuberculous pneumonia
   c. Status asthmaticus
   d. Patients with respiratory assistance (on ventilators)
3. Hypothyroidism
4. Guillain-Barré syndrome
5. Miscellaneous tumors
   a. Pancreas
   b. Pulmonary
   c. Thymus
   d. Duodenum
6. Miscellaneous drugs
   a. Chlorpropamide
   b. Cyclophosphamide
   c. Vincristine

laryngeal stridor or spasm, and convulsions. Physical signs include positive Trousseau and Chvostek signs (for example, induction of carpopedal spasm by maintaining a blood pressure cuff midway between diastolic and systolic pressures for 5 minutes; induction of a facial tic by percussing the masseter muscle tendon in the region of the temporomandibular joint) and any of the previously mentioned symptoms. Treatment is directed at maintaining normal serum calcium levels with either vitamin D or dihydrotachysterol (calciferol). True hypoparathyroidism should not be confused with pseudohypoparathyroidism (Albright's hereditary osteodystrophy).

Syndrome of Inappropriate Antidiuretic Hormone Secretion

Syndrome of inappropriate antidiuretic hormone secretion (SIADH) refers to inappropriately increased levels of antidiuretic hormone, which results in low serum sodium and serum hypoosmolality with increased urine sodium and urinary hyperosmolality in the presence of normal renal and adrenal function. Serum sodium may fall below 110 mEq/L, causing water intoxication with convulsions and coma. SIADH is a potential complication of many disease states (Table 12-21). Treatment involves fluid restriction and correction of the underlying etiology.

Bibliography

Bailey, J. D., editor. 1982. Symposium on paediatric endocrinology. *Clinics Endocrinol. Metabol.* 11(1):1-265.

Barnes, H. V. 1975. The problem of delayed puberty. *Med. Clin. North Am.* 59:1337.

Baruch, S.; Sherman, L.; and Markowitz, S. 1981. Diabetic ketoacidosis and coma. *Med. Clin. North Am.* 65:117.

Bennett, D. L. 1978. The adolescent with diabetes mellitus. *Pediatr. Ann.* 7(9):81.

Bierich, J. R., editor. 1975. Disorders of puberty. *Clin. Endocrinol. Metabol.* 4:3-222.

Boutros, A. R.; Esfandiari, S.; Orlowski, J.; et al. 1980. Reye syndrome: a predictably curable disease. *Pediatr. Clin. North Am.* 27:539.

Clark, F. 1982. Thyrotoxicosis. *Practitioner.* 226:197.

Colwell, M. A. 1977. Hypoglycemia. *Primary Care* 4:681.

Crawford, J. D. 1981. Hyperthyroidism in childhood. *Am. J. Dis. Child.* 135:109.

Ehrlich, R. M. 1982. Diabetes mellitus in childhood. *Clinics Endocrinol. Metabol.* 11(1):195-210.

Finkelstein, J. W. 1980. The endocrinology of adolescence. *Pediatr. Clin. North Am.* 27:53.

Gouterman, I. H., and Sibrack, L. A. 1980. Cutaneous manifestations of diabetes. *Cutis* 25:45.

Greydanus, D. E., and Hofmann, A. D. 1979. Psychological factors in diabetes mellitus. A review of the literature with emphasis on adolescence. *Am. J. Dis. Child.* 133:1061.

Greydanus, D. E., and McAnarney, E. R. 1979. The value of the Tanner staging. *J. Curr. Adol. Med.* 2(2):21.

Howard, C. P., and Hayles, A. B. 1978. Hyperthyroidism in childhood. *Clin. Endocrinol. Metabol.* 7:127.

Grumbach, M. M. 1980. The neuroendocrinology of puberty. *Hosp. Pract.* 15:51.

Havel, R. J., editor. 1982. Symposium on lipid disorders. *Med. Clin. North Am.* 66(2):317–550.

Henrichs, S. A., and Lippe, B. M. 1979. Short stature in children: finding the cause. *Consultant* 19(9):23.

Johnson, D. D. 1980. Reactive hypoglycemia. *J.A.M.A.* 243:1151.

Kaplan, S. A., editor. 1979. Symposium on pediatric endocrinology. *Pediatr. Clin. North Am.* 26:1–256.

Kappy, M. S. 1980. A diagnostic approach to metabolic acidosis in children. *Pediatrics* 65:351.

Marshall, R. N. 1982. Juvenile diabetes mellitus. *Am. Family Phys.* 25:192.

Medvei, V. L., editor. 1980. Symposium on endocrinology. *Practitioner.* 224:129.

Perlman, K., and Ehrlich, R. M. 1982. Steroid diabetes in childhood. *Am. J. Dis. Child.* 136:64.

Ratcliffe, S. G. 1982. Klinefelter's syndrome in adolescence. *Arch. Dis. Child.* 57:6.

Raskin, P., editor. 1982. Symposium on diabetes mellitus. *Med. Clin. North Am.* 66:750.

Rimoin, D. A., and Horton, W. A. 1979. Short stature. I and II. *J. Pediatr.* 92:523; 697.

Rupp, W. M., Barbosa, J. J., Blackshear, P. J., et al. 1982. The use of an implantable insulin pump in the treatment of type II diabetes. *N. Engl. J. Med.* 307:265–270.

Salans, L. B. 1982. Diabetes mellitus. *J.A.M.A.* 247:590.

Shenker, I. R.; Nussbaum, M.; and Kaplan, E. 1979. Delayed puberty and short stature in adolescents. *Pediatr. Ann.* 7(9):56.

Spaulding, S. W. 1977. Hypothyroidism. Early diagnosis and treatment. *Primary Care* 4:79.

Tattersall, R. 1977. Brittle diabetes. *Clin. Endocrinol. Metabol.* 6(2):403.

Temple, T. E.; Miller, M. B.; Charlton, J.; et al. 1981. The complicated insulin-dependent juvenile diabetic. *J. Family Pract.* 12:745.

Thompson, R. G. 1975. The management of diabetes mellitus in the adolescent. *Med. Clin. North Am.* 59:1349.

Wabrek, A. J. 1979. Sexual dysfunction associated with diabetes mellitus. *J. Family Pract.* 8:735.

Warner, A., and Vaziri, N. D. 1981. Treatment of lactic acidosis. *South Med. J.* 74:841.

Wheat, L. J. 1980. Infections and diabetes mellitus. *Diabetes Care* 3:187.

–13–
Hematology and Oncology

Anemia
Iron deficiency anemia □ Hemolytic anemias
Sickle cell disorders □ Thalassemia syndromes
Bleeding Disorders Due to Coagulation Factor Deficiencies
The hemophilias □ Von Willebrand's disease
Thrombocytopenia
Decreased platelet production □ Decreased platelet survival
Leukopenia
Oncology
Leukemia
Hodgkin's Disease
Non-Hodgkin's Lymphomas
Malignant Bone Tumors
Central Nervous System Tumors
Radiation and Chemotherapy

Anemia

Serious symptomatic anemia is relatively uncommon in adolescence. When it does occur, the range of diagnostic considerations is similar to that for children. Genetic recessive disorders in their homozygous form manifest long before the teenage years, and medical management protocols will already have been established. New medical concerns, however, may be introduced by menstruation, contraception, and pregnancy in females or by pubertal delay in those of either sex who have been chronically ill. Management also must focus on the psychosocial dimension and the critical need to respond to the impact of chronic disease on adolescent developmental issues as reviewed in Chapter 21; failure to respond can seriously impair the young person's present and future quality of life.

Heterozygous forms of genetic disorders may well escape detection during earlier years and only come to light during adolescence through screening programs, as for sickle cell trait. This introduces the need for genetic counseling; reaching maturity and searching for a life partner with whom to establish a family may create complex psychologic problems under these circumstances.

Mild-to-moderate degrees of anemia may occur with chronic occult blood loss or chronic infection, but fortunately these conditions also are relatively uncommon. Far more frequent are mild, asymptomatic degrees of anemia due to inadequate iron intake.

Table 13-1 offers a differential diagnosis of the congenital and acquired anemias that may be seen during the teenage years.

IRON DEFICIENCY ANEMIA

Iron deficiency is the most common cause of anemia in adolescence. Rapid expansion of blood volume in conjunction with the growth spurt increases requirements for dietary iron in puberty. Additional amounts are required by postmenarchial females to make up for menstrual loss, but the diet of the average adolescent in the United States tends to be inadequate in meeting these demands (Chapter 19).

TABLE 13-1
CAUSES OF ANEMIA IN ADOLESCENTS

A. Decreased production of hemoglobin and/or red blood cells
   1. Nutritional anemia
      a. Iron deficiency
      b. Folic acid deficiency
      c. Vitamin B_{12} deficiency (megaloblastic anemia)
   2. Secondary anemias
      a. Chronic infections or inflammatory diseases
      b. Chemotherapy
   3. Marrow failure
      a. Aplastic anemia
      b. Leukemic or tumor cell infiltration
B. Increased loss or destruction of red blood cells
   1. Acute or chronic blood loss
   2. Hereditary hemolytic anemias
      a. Membrane defects (congenital spherocytosis, stomatocytosis, or elliptocytosis)
      b. Hemoglobinopathies (sickle cell disease, thalassemia)
      c. Enzyme defects (pyruvate kinase deficiency or glucose-6-phosphate dehydrogenase deficiency)
   3. Acquired hemolytic anemias
      a. Coombs'-positive autoimmune anemia
      b. Paroxysmal nocturnal hemoglobinuria
      c. Transfusion reaction
      d. Lead poisoning
      e. Heart valve prosthesis effect
      f. Diffuse intravascular coagulation
      g. Hemolytic uremic syndrome
      h. Splenic sequestration or hypersplenism
      i. Acquired membrane alterations due to drugs, venoms (spider, snake), malaria, metabolic consequences of kidney or liver failure

TABLE 13-2
LABORATORY CHARACTERISTICS OF IRON DEFICIENCY ANEMIA IN TEENAGERS

Test	Value
Hemoglobin	< 11.5 g/dl; 12-year-old males or females < 12.0 g/dl; 12–18-year-old females < 12.5–13.0 g/dl; 12–18-year-old males
Hematocrit	< 35%; 12-year-old males or females < 36%; 12–18-year-old females < 38%; 12–18-year-old males
Mean corpuscular volume (MCV)	< 76 fl in 12-year-old < 78 fl in mid- and older adolescents
Serum ferritin	< 10 (normal, 100)
Serum iron/total iron-binding capacity (TIBC) ratio	< 16% (normal, 35%–40%)
Serum iron	< 40 mg/100 ml (normal, 50–140 mg/100 ml)
TIBC (total iron-binding capacity)	350–500 mg/100 ml (normal, 250–380 mg/100 ml)
FEP (free erythrocyte protoporphyrin)	≥ 150–200 µg/100 ml red blood cells (normal, 54 ± 20)

Symptoms and signs. Iron deficiency develops in three stages. First is a decrease in iron stores with a low serum ferritin. This is followed by a drop in serum iron with a parallel increase in total iron-binding capacity. Overt microcytic, hypochromic anemia is last to appear. Clinical *symptoms* are not usually noted until significant anemia develops. Although fatigue, irritability, and poor school performance have been attributed to a drop in hemoglobin of only 1–2 g/dl, this is difficult to prove and chronic anemia in the range of 6–9 g/dl has been noted to have remarkably few symptoms. Clinical *signs* of anemia may appear when the hemoglobin is under 8 g/dl and can include paresthesias, glossitis, stomatitis, angular cheilitis, pica (in children), and "spoon nails." If the hemoglobin falls below 5–6 g/dl, tachy-cardia, hypotension, retinal hemorrhage, shock, and/or congestive heart failure may develop. Most iron-deficient adolescents, however, only have mild, asymptomatic degrees of anemia.

Diagnosis. As iron deficiency anemia may occur in virtually any adolescent, male or female, all teenagers should be checked periodically for hemoglobin or hematocrit values (Chapter 3; Appendix I). Diagnosis is based on the finding of a microcytic, hypochromic anemia and other laboratory values as given in Table 13-2 and differentiated from other mild-to-moderate microcytic anemias (Table 13-3). Sources of unusual blood loss should be ruled out before attributing iron deficiency anemia to dietary inadequacies alone.

Treatment. A two-pronged approach includes oral iron therapy and encouragement of an iron-rich diet. Oral therapy may be with ferrous succinate, ferrous gluconate, or ferrous sulfate. The succinate

TABLE 13-3
DIFFERENTIAL DIAGNOSIS OF MILD-TO-MODERATE HYPOCHROMIC-MICROCYTIC ANEMIA

	Hg (g/dl) and Hct (%)	MCV* (fl)	Plasma iron (mg/100 ml)	TIBC† (mg/100 ml)	FEP‡ (μg/100 ml RBC)	Hemoglobin electrophoresis
IRON DEFICIENCY	Low	Low	5–40	350–500	30–200	Normal (may have decreased hemoglobin A_2)
THALASSEMIA MINOR	Low	Low	60–160	150–350	Normal	Increased hemoglobin A_2 or F with beta trait
CHRONIC INFECTION	Low	Low	25–125	Normal	Normal	Normal
LEAD POISONING	Low	Low	Normal (50–140)	250–380	> 200	Normal

*Mean corpuscular volume.
†Total iron-binding capacity.
‡Free erythrocyte protoporphyrin.

form is best absorbed but has the greatest gastrointestinal side effects. Ferrous sulfate is cheapest. Enteric coated tablets or timed release capsules are not recommended, as they may carry the iron beyond the duodenum and upper jejunum, the best sites for absorption.

Although recommended dosage varies, 2–3 mg/kg/day of elemental iron in two or three divided doses is often used. One 300 mg tablet of hydrated ferrous sulfate contains 60 mg of elemental iron. A rise in reticulocytes will be noted within 5–10 days unless the anemia is very mild, in which case no notable increase occurs. A rise in hemoglobin or hematocrit occurs in 2–3 weeks in most instances, but the rate of increase depends on the initial degree of anemia, being more rapid in those with greater levels of iron deficiency. Lack of improvement generally is due to poor compliance; the reasons for the patient's difficulty need to be reviewed in an understanding and empathic manner.

Major side effects of iron therapy include nausea, gastritis, vomiting, diarrhea, constipation, and greenish black stools. A slow buildup of the total calculated dose may minimize these problems. This is accomplished by starting with one tablet a day and increasing by one additional tablet every 2–3 days until the full dose is achieved. Taking the iron with meals further minimizes gastrointestinal distress, although it should be kept in mind that absorption will be inhibited by cereals and eggs. In addition, antacids, magnesium trisilicate, and tetracycline also inhibit absorption; increased amounts of iron may be needed when these medications are being taken.

Conversely, oral contraceptives, vitamin C, and allopurinol increase iron absorption. Therapy should continue for 4–6 months after normal hemoglobin levels have been reached to ensure adequate body iron stores.

Dietary change to enhance iron intake from nutrient sources should look to fish, meats, and fortified cereals and breads. Iron may also be obtained from eggs, spinach, and other green vegetables but is less well absorbed due to the formation of phytate or phosphate salts.

Failure of oral iron therapy to correct the anemia may be due to continued blood loss, misdiagnosis, malabsorption, or poor compliance—the last being most common in adolescence. When assured of the diagnosis and unable to achieve improvement in instances of significant and symptomatic anemia, parenteral iron therapy may be used. Two milliliters of iron dextran (Imferon), containing 50 mg elemental iron per milliliter, is given intramuscularly in the gluteal region once a day until the total amount required is administered as determined by the following formula;

$$\text{Total mg iron} = \frac{(1 - \text{Hg (in g/100 dl)})}{15} \times 30 \times \text{weight}$$

in pounds

Side effects of parenteral iron may include painful injection and injection site, local skin reactions, permanent skin staining, sterile abscess, anaphylaxis, myalgia, hypotension, lymphadenopathy, urticaria, abdominal pain, bradycardia, and/or pleural effusion.

TABLE 13-4

OUTLINE OF THE MORE COMMON HEMOLYTIC ANEMIA DISORDERS

Name	Defect	Clinical features	Diagnosis	Treatment
Hereditary spherocytosis (congenital hemolytic anemia)	Abnormal RBC membrane that is very permeable to sodium	Congenital autosomal dominant, familial hemolytic anemia of variable severity; especially noted in individuals of North European ancestry. Characterized by spherocytosis and splenomegaly. Cholelithiasis and leg ulcers may occur in untreated cases. Aplastic crises have been reported.	Anemia Hyperbilirubinemia Spherocytes in blood smear Positive osmotic fragility tests Positive autohemolysis test Negative Coomb's test	Splenectomy by age 4–6 years prevents complications of chronic anemia hemolysis and allows for normal hemoglobin levels. Postsplenectomy infection risk occurs and requires pneumococcal vaccine and antibiotic prophylaxis for life. No treatment necessary for the mild form.
Hereditary elliptocytosis	RBC membrane defect	Usually very mild or no anemia; 10% have severe disease with anemia, hyperbilirubinemia, spenomegaly, aplastic crisis, gallstones.	Elliptical cells, spherocytes, microcytes, reticulocytes, anemia.	Splenectomy diminishes the hemolytic process in severe cases (with same precautions as above).
Sickle cell disease	See text.	See text.	See text.	See text.
Thalassemia disorder	See text.	See text.	See text.	See text.
Glucose-6-phosphate dehydrogenase deficiency (G-6PD)	Sex-linked disorder in which RBCs are unable to produce enough reducing compounds within the cells, due to partial or full absence of this enzyme.	Episodic hemolytic anemia precipitated by infections or certain drugs. Enzyme deficiency noted in 10% of American black males. Also noted in some caucasian, Mediterranean African and Oriental populations. The hemolytic process begins 2–3 days post oxidant drug ingestion and lasts 7–12 days. A severe, spontaneous hemolytic anemia can develop in individuals with very low or absent enzyme levels.	History of episode Positive methylene blue test Positive methemoglobulin test Reduced G-6PD enzyme activity in old RBCs	Drug withdrawal, symptomatic. Many episodes resolve without treatment and even if drug is continued. Screen individuals at risk (as black males in the military).
Pyruvate kinase deficiency	RBC deficiency of pyruvate kinase.	Congenital hemolytic anemia with jaundice and splenomegaly.	Anemia Reticulocytosis Negative osmotic fragility tests (nonincubated) Positive autohemolysis test Spectrophotometric assay: reduced pyruvic kinase enzyme in RBCs	Transfusions, splenectomy (with postsplenectomy precautions as in treatment of hereditary spherocytosis above).

Disease	Mechanism	Clinical Features	Diagnostic Tests	Treatment
PNH (paroxysmal nocturnal hemoglobinuria)	Abnormal RBC; highly susceptible to complement-induced lysis	Chronic hemolytic anemia with hemoglobinuria during sleep with infections. Dark brown urine can last several days. Pattern of severity variable; anywhere from 1%–90% of RBCs may be affected. Hemosiderinuria, abdominal pain, pyelonephritis, dysphagia, pancytopenia, hepatic or cerebral vein thromboses, and even death can occur in severe forms. (Rule out march hemoglobinuria due to RBC trauma as may occur with running, karate, etc.)	History of urine color change during sleep. Positive Ham test (acid hemolysis test). Positive thrombin test. Reduced RBC acetylcholinesterase activity	Transfusions, anticoagulation, supplemental iron and folic acid, androgens, prednisone.
Autoimmune hemolytic anemia (associated with "warm" antibodies)	Complex autoimmune mechanisms	Variable severity of hemolytic anemia. May be secondary to an underlying disease (as chronic lymphatic leukemia, lymphoma, systemic lupus erythematosus, ulcerative colitis, rheumatoid arthritis, Wiskott-Aldrich syndrome, others. Splenomegaly and lymphadenopathy can develop; spontaneous remission may occur.	Anemia. Positive Coomb's test. Hyperbilirubinemia. Presence of antibodies active at 37 C. Spherocytosis in blood smear	Transfusions, prednisone, other immunosuppressive drugs, splenectomy (with postsplenectomy precautions as in treatment of hereditary spherocytosis noted above).

HEMOLYTIC ANEMIAS

Hemolytic anemia is characterized by an increased rate of red blood cell (RBC) destruction and a shortened RBC life span. Other findings include reticulocytosis, abnormal peripheral smear, hyperbilirubinemia (indirect form), increased plasma hemoglobin, decreased haptoglobin and hemopexin, bone marrow hyperplasia, splenomegaly, and cholelithiasis. Table 13-4 reviews differential considerations of the more common causes of hemolytic anemia, except for sickle cell disease and the thalassemias, which are discussed in the text. Most of these conditions are noted in childhood and continue with various degrees of severity into adolescence and young adulthood. Mild forms, however (spherocytosis, sickle cell trait, drug-induced glucose-6-phosphate dehydrogenase deficiency) may not be noted until the teenage years. Autoimmune hemolytic anemia can develop at any time.

SICKLE CELL DISORDERS

Over 180 defects in hemoglobin synthesis have been identified. The most common is the abnormal production of hemoglobin S (in which valine is substituted for glutamic acid on the sixth position of the hemoglobin molecule beta chain) manifesting in sickle cell trait or disease. Approximately 8% of black Americans and 0.5%–3% of Spanish Americans carry this autosomal recessive gene. Twenty-five percent of the offspring of two parents with trait (heterozygous) will have sickle cell disease (homozygous).

Sickle cell anemia. The hemoglobin of a person with disease is comprised of up to 90% Hg S and contains no Hg A. Clinical manifestations usually first appear after the newborn period, when Hg S replaces Hg F as the major hemoglobin type. Laboratory data confirming the diagnosis demonstrate a normocytic anemia in the range of 5-10 g/dl; an elevated reticulocyte count ($\geq$ 10%); marked sickling of RBCs with sodium metabisulfite; hemoglobin electrophoresis with 80%–90% Hg S, 2%–10% Hg F, 2%–3% Hg A_2 and no Hg A; positive solubility tests; and an abnormal peripheral blood smear with polychromatophilia, stippling, target cells, Howell-Jolly bodies; and nucleated red blood cells. The leukocyte count may be elevated in the range of 15,000-25,000/mm^3 with an increased platelet count. It should be noted, however, that standard hemoglobin electrophoresis has its limitations and cannot distinguish related disorders such as sickle cell–thalassemia disease or sickle cell–Hg D disease. These should be suspected if there is persistent splenomegaly combined with only mild anemia.

The presence of large amounts of Hg S tends to cause sickling of the red blood cells under reduced oxygen tension. This increases the viscosity of the blood, causing sludging and plugging of small blood vessels. Episodic painful vasoocclusive crises occur throughout life and may be generalized or localized to various organ systems and are variably comprised of capillary stasis (predominantly abdominal organs, lower spine, and extremities), venous thromboses (extremities, pelvis, liver, spleen, meninges), and pulmonary arterial emboli. Although the frequency, severity, and form of crises may vary from patient to patient, they tend to follow a consistent pattern in any one individual from late childhood on. Factors that may precipitate a crisis include infection, reduced temperature, dehydration, acidosis, anesthesia, and strenuous physical exercise, but many attacks are idiopathic. Signs and symptoms of a crisis include localized pain, fever, acidosis, and dehydration. Table 13-5 outlines treatment.

An aplastic crisis also can occur in which bone marrow erythropoietic activity is reduced or absent (leukocyte and platelet production remain normal). Infection or folic acid deficiency may be precipitants. Some episodes occur independently, and others follow on the heels of a hemolytic phase. These episodes are marked by a sudden drop in hematocrit, reticulocyte count, and bilirubin and may result in a life-threatening situation. Treatment is by transfusion and general support.

Splenic sequestration and splenomegaly, usually developing in the young child, can sometimes be seen in the adolescent or adult, particularly those with a variant of sickle cell anemia such as Hg S-C disease. Treatment is supportive, although splenectomy is indicated for a particularly enlarged organ with recurrent sequestration episodes.

The adolescent with sickle cell anemia may be relatively well between crises, although growth in height and weight may be diminished, puberty delayed, and fertility impaired. He or she, however, is subject to any of a myriad of complications (Table 13-6). Osteomyelitis may be particularly difficult to differentiate from bone pain due to a crisis; a technetium bone scan and an absolute polymorphonuclear band cell count may be helpful.

Although the life span often is curtailed, many individuals with sickle cell disease survive well into the fifties with careful treatment; infection is the major cause of death. Some amelioration of the severity of crises appears to occur with age. All in-

TABLE 13-5
TREATMENT OF VASOOCCLUSIVE CRISIS AND SICKLE CELL ANEMIA

A. Preventive
1. Avoid precipitating factors (see text)
2. Early treatment of infections
3. Well-balanced diet with iron and folic acid supplementation
4. Avoidance of tight clothes and any other causes of venous stasis (as tourniquets)
5. Evaluate for associated disorders, as G-6PD deficiency, hereditary spherocytosis
6. Psychologic support to patient and family

B. Supportive*
1. Bed rest and sedation
2. Analgesics
   a. Aspirin, 1 g q 4 hours
   b. Acetaminophen, 600 mg or more q 4 hours
   c. Codeine, 20–30 mg q 4 hours
   d. Meperidine HCl, 50–75 mg q 4 hours
3. Adequate hydration
   a. 2500 ml/m^2/24 hours
   b. Maintain urine output at 2.5–3.0 L/day
   c. Use 0.45 normal saline and 5% glucose
4. Eliminate acidosis (may need to add sodium bicarbonate [1 ampule/L] to IV fluids)
5. Oxygen: 2–4 L/min (as needed for respiratory infection or low arterial PO$_2$)
6. Treat infections vigorously (high risk of *Salmonella, Pneumococcus, Hemophilus influenzae,* and *Mycoplasma pneumoniae* infections)
7. Partial exchange blood transfusion (reduce hemoglobin S to 40% or less of total hemoglobin content; avoid overloading the patient with fluid; repeat in 2–3 weeks, if necessary) May be useful in:
   a. Prolonged painful vasoocclusion crisis
   b. Pregnancy complications
   c. Priapism
   d. Elective surgery preparation (1–2 days before surgery, reducing hemoglobin S to under 20%)
   e. Cerebrovascular acidosis
   f. Congestive heart failure
   g. Chronic severe leg ulcerations
   h. Aseptic necrosis of the bone
   i. Marked liver or kidney disease

*Note: There is no evidence that alkali, hyperbaric oxygen, or intravenous urea are helpful.

dividuals with sickle cell disease should receive pneumococcal vaccine for prophylaxis.

Sickle cell trait. Persons who are heterozygous for the sickle cell gene have only 25%–45% Hg S and 55%–75% Hg A. Although sickling occurs with sodi-

TABLE 13-6
COMPLICATIONS OF SICKLE CELL ANEMIA

1. *Orthopedic:* joint effusions with painful crises; osteomyelitis; aseptic necrosis; septic arthritis
2. *Pulmonary:* pneumonia; pulmonary emboli and infarctions
3. *Genitourinary:* hematuria; hyposthenuria; nephrotic syndrome; priapism; gonadal atrophy
4. *Liver:* hepatitislike picture; cholelithiasis with complications
5. *Cardiac:* enlargement; congestive heart failure
6. *Central nervous system:* infarctions or cerebral vein thrombosis; cerebrovascular accidents; enhanced neuropathy in coexisting lead poisoning
7. *Spleen:* hypersplenism; infarction with autosplenectomy and consequent increased risk of pneumococcal infections
8. *Dermatologic:* chronic leg ulcers
9. *Eye:* retinal vascular disease
10. *Pregnancy:* increased incidence of maternal and fetal death; 50% probability of offspring having disease if father has trait and mother has disease

um metabisulfite or solubility tests, the patient is asymptomatic and without clinical or laboratory signs of anemia. Whether there are significant risks in having sickle cell trait is a matter of controversy. In any event, longevity and fertility are not affected. In light of current knowledge, encouragement of a normal, active life without restriction is an appropriate course for an adolescent with sickle cell trait. Genetic counseling, however, is essential for the older youth who anticipates having children.

THALASSEMIA SYNDROMES
Thalassemia is a hereditary hemolytic anemia with two forms characterized by impaired synthesis of either the beta or alpha chain of the globin moiety.

Beta-thalassemia. Beta chain involvement is the most common type with 0.8% of black Americans and 1%–10% of those with Mediterranean ancestry carrying this autosomal recessive gene. Three clinical subgroups have been identified; thalassemia minor, intermedia, and major—or Cooley's anemia. Each is distinguished by the degree of anemia. The minor form is heterozygous and produces little or no anemia. Splenomegaly may or may not be present. Laboratory studies demonstrate microcytic red blood cells with target cells and, on hemoglobin electrophoresis, a predominance of Hg A, a slight increase in Hg A$_2$ and, sometimes, a slight increase in Hg F. There is no effect upon longevity or fertility

TABLE 13-7
CORRELATION OF
PLASMA FACTOR VIII LEVELS AND
DEGREE OF BLEEDING IN HEMOPHILIA A

Factor VIII level (IU/100 ml)	Degree of bleeding
50+	None
25–50	Only occurs with trauma or surgery
5–25	Various degrees of excess bleeding with *minor* trauma or surgery
1–5	Occasional spontaneous bleeding
0–1	Frequent spontaneous bleeding

and treatment is not necessary, but genetic counseling is important. The differential diagnosis includes iron deficiency anemia and lead poisoning.

Thalassemia intermedia may be heterozygous or homozygous and produces a moderate anemia, hepatosplenomegaly, and bone marrow hyperplasia, but usually the anemia is not severe enough to require transfusions. Laboratory data also reflect a transitional state between minor and major forms.

Thalassemia major, or Cooley's anemia, is homozygous, and is characterized by severe anemia, massive hepatosplenomegaly, and bone marrow hyperplasia with hyperplastic changes in lamellar bone reflected in a characteristic facies and widening of the skull on roentgenogram. A blood smear reveals abnormal RBCs as in thalassemia minor, but electrophoresis demonstrates Hg F to be the dominant form of hemoglobin with variable amounts of Hg A and normal or increased levels of Hg A_2. A rare type of thalassemia major may be encountered with 100% Hg F.

Frequent transfusions are required and hemosiderosis is a major complication, often resulting in death during childhood or adolescence. New treatment methods, however, employing frequent transfusions to maintain the hemoglobin at a functional level in combination with the daily administration of chelating agents to remove excess iron, diminish the degree of hemosiderosis and improve growth, physical function, and life expectancy. Referral to a hematology center for such management is indicated.

Alpha-thalassemia. Alpha-thalassemia occurs with some frequency among the Oriental population. It also is seen in persons of Mediterranean and African ancestry. The heterozygous form usually is asymptomatic and difficult to detect after the newborn period, when cord blood demonstrates 5%–20% Hg H. Homozygous alpha-thalassemia, however, is a rare but severe hemolytic anemia occurring predominantly in Orientals; 80% Hg H is common and in utero death likely. Lesser percentages of Hg H produce a chronic hemolytic disorder of lesser severity and is found in other ethnic groups as well as Orientals, including northern Europeans. Splenomegaly may be present.

Bleeding Disorders Due to Coagulation Factor Deficiencies
THE HEMOPHILIAS

Classic hemophilia (hemophilia A) is caused by factor VIII deficiency, whereas Christmas disease (hemophilia B) is a deficiency of factor IX. Classic disease occurs in 1 of 25,000 births and is five times more common than Christmas disease. Both forms are sex-linked recessive disorders in which the male is affected and the female an asymptomatic carrier. The degree of factor deficiency varies from one individual to another but is the determinant of bleeding severity (Table 13-7). All but the mildest of cases manifest before adolescence.

Bleeding into joints and muscles, either spontaneously or following trauma, is the most consistent symptom of hemophilia A. Painful hemarthroses are common, and permanent crippling may occur unless each bleeding episode is properly treated. Knee involvement is most common in young adolescents (10–14 years), with elbows the more frequent site in older teens (15–17 years). Muscle bleeding also can occur and may produce a variety of other symptoms in addition to local pain and swelling, such as femoral nerve compression or an acute abdominal condition. Spontaneous or posttraumatic hematuria of renal origin is common and may last for days or weeks. Clots may obstruct the renal pelvis or ureter. Epistaxis, gastrointestinal bleeding, and bleeding after dental extraction or surgery are other complications. The most common cause of death is intracranial hemorrhage following trauma. The clinical features of hemophilia B are similar. Diagnosis is based on the history of excessive bleeding in association with a normal platelet count, normal prothrombin, prolonged partial thromboplastin time, and low levels of plasma factor VIII or IX. Table 13-8 compares interpretation of basic screening tests in various bleeding disorders.

Management of an acute episode of bleeding consists of replacement therapy with factor VIII or IX and general supportive measures. Various factor VIII preparations are available, including fresh-frozen plasma, cryoprecipitate, freeze-dried factor

TABLE 13-8
INTERPRETATION OF SCREENING
TESTS IN BLEEDING DISORDERS*†

	Plate-lets	BT	PTT	PT	TT
Hemophilia, type A, B, or C	N	N	↑	N	N
von Willebrand's disease	N	↑	↑ or N	N	N
Thrombocytopenia	↓	↑	N	N	N
Disseminated intravascular coagulation	↓	↑	↑	↑	↑
Hemolytic uremic syndrome	↓↓	↑	N or ↓	N	↑

*Abbreviations: ↑, increased; ↓, decreased; ↓↓, greater decrease; N, normal; BT, bleeding time; PT, prothrombin time; PTT, partial prothrombin time; TT, thrombin time.

†Note: A wide variety of other blood dyscrasias may be manifested in a bleeding disorder. They are exceptionally rare and uncommonly encountered in adolescents. Focus has been limited to those conditions of major concern in this category. An excellent overview is provided by Montgomery, R. R., and Hathaway, W. E. 1980. Acute bleeding emergencies. *Pediatr. Clin. North Am.* 27:327.

VIII concentrate, commercial products, and bovine or porcine factor VIII concentrates. Acute bleeding requires between 5–20 IU/kg of factor VIII. The chronic use of somewhat lesser amounts given in a preventive home therapy program has been found particularly helpful in those with frequent bleeding episodes. Factor IX concentrates are also available for the management of hemophilia B; these contain factors II, VII, and X in addition. Potential side effects in using any of these preparations include hypervolemia, acute pulmonary congestion, acute allergic reactions, hepatitis, hemolytic anemia, and the development of factor antibodies. Antibody production sooner or later occurs in 5%–21% of all hemophilia patients treated with factor replacement and creates a particularly difficult situation, since factor infusion becomes ineffective. In this instance, prothrombin complex concentrates, porcine or bovine factor concentrates, steroids, immunosuppressive drugs, and/or antifibrinolytic agents have been tried with variable success.

Supportive measures include the relief of pain with analgesics, but salicylates should be avoided because they inhibit platelet aggregation. Pentazocine, Zomepirac sodium, and mefenamic acid may be used safely, as may even the stronger narcotics when

pain is severe. Involved joints should be immobilized during the acute episode to alleviate pain and minimize further bleeding. Following the cessation of bleeding, physical therapy should be instituted to prevent joint stiffness, promote rehabilitation, and maintain optimal physical conditioning. Orthopedic correction of knee or hip deformities may be necessary. Psychosocial counseling also is required, as for any significant chronic illness (Chapter 21). Genetic counseling is indicated in older adolescents.

Patients requiring surgery should have their serum levels of factor VIII or IX raised to 50 IU/100 dl for dental procedures and to 80 IU or more for major procedures.

VON WILLEBRAND'S DISEASE

Von Willebrand's disease (vascular hemophilia) is a relatively rare autosomal dominant hemorrhagic disorder predominantly seen in females. Gingival bleeding, epistaxis, excessive bleeding of superficial cuts, and menorrhagia are common. Gastrointestinal bleeding and hemarthrosis also may occur in severer forms. Diagnosis is based on history, the patient's sex, and confirmatory laboratory data consisting of a normal platelet count, normal prothrombin time, normal partial thromboplastin time, prolonged bleeding time, abnormal platelet adhesiveness (failure of aggregation with ristocetin), low factor VIII, and low factor VIII antigen levels.

Treatment is replacement with factor VIII as for hemophilia A. Recurrent menorrhagia may require suppression of ovulation and the maintenance of a less vascular secretory endometrium through cyclical hormone therapy using oral contraceptives (Chapter 17) or suppression of menstruation entirely by the continuous administration of estrogen without respite. Medroxyprogesterone (Depo-Provera) could be used in this situation to good advantage. Pregnancy and delivery (or abortion) present special problems for these young women, and they should be under the combined care of an experienced gynecologist and hematologist. Aspirin and related compounds must be avoided at any time.

Thrombocytopenia

Low platelets and the attendant risk or actuality of excess bleeding may be consequent to either reduced production or increased destruction. Characteristic clinical signs include petechiae, ecchymoses, purpura, increased bruisability, and the potential for serious internal hemorrhage. The most disastrous complication is a spontaneous or posttraumatic cerebral vascular accident. Bleeding into the spinal

---
TABLE 13-9
CAUSES OF APLASTIC ANEMIA

---

1. Idiopathic
2. Drug induced
   a. Analgesics (aspirin, indomethacin, phenylbutazone)
   b. Anticonvulsants (phenytoin, carbamazepine)
   c. Methimazole
   d. Antimicrobials (chloramphenicol, sulfonamides, streptomycin sulfate, tetracyclines)
   e. Psychotropics (chlordiazepoxide, chlorpromazine, glutethimide)
   f. Cancer chemotherapy
   g. Miscellaneous (probenecid, industrial chemicals such as benzene, toxins)
3. Radiation
4. Complications of hepatitis and other infections
5. Other
   a. Familial
   b. Fanconi's anemia
   c. Leukemia, preleukemic states, bone marrow metastases

---

cord also can occur. Bruising and petechiae may occur with platelet counts only a little under 100,000/mm^3. Serious bleeding, however, generally does not appear until the count is 20,000/mm^3 or less (normal platelet count, 150,000–450,000/mm^3). See Table 13-8 for interpretation of basic screening tests.

DECREASED PLATELET PRODUCTION
Inhibition of platelet formation usually is seen as a component of aplastic anemia. Agranulocytosis and failure of erythropoiesis also present, posing a serious medical crisis of many dimensions. Table 13-9 cites causes of aplastic anemia. Treatment is both supportive and directed at the underlying cause.

DECREASED PLATELET SURVIVAL
Idiopathic thrombocytopenic purpura. Idiopathic thrombocytopenic purpura (ITP) is one of the more common causes of thrombocytopenia and is due to the production of IgG autoantibodies, which destroy platelets. An acute form is seen in children (and an occasional adolescent) following a viral infection (rubella, rubeola, influenza). Few of these patients require treatment; three-quarters fully recover spontaneously within 3 months and 90% within 12 months. A chronic form appears in older children and adolescents. A wide variety of drugs and a number of diseases have been implicated as causal agents (Table 13-10), but, as the name suggests, no etiology can be found in many instances.

TABLE 13-10
CAUSES OF CHRONIC
IDIOPATHIC THROMBOCYTOPENIC PURPURA

---

1. Idiopathic
2. Chronic lymphocytic leukemia
3. Lymphoma
4. Systemic lupus erythematosus
5. Drugs: idiosyncratic or predictable toxic response to many drugs; examples follow.
   a. Antiinflammatory analgesics (aspirin, phenylbutazone)
   b. Antithyroid medications (thiouracil)
   c. Antimicrobials
      Cephalothin sodium
      Clindamycin
      Erythromycins
      Oxytetracycline HCl
      Penicillins
      Quinine sulfate
      Streptomycin sulfate
      Sulfonamides
   d. Psychotropics
      Dextroamphetamines
      Meprobamate
      Phenobarbital
      Tricyclic antidepressants
   e. Miscellaneous
      Estrogens
      Heparin sodium
      Quinidine salts
      Quinine salts
      Thiazide diuretics

Treatment includes withdrawal of any associated drugs, attention to any underlying disease, and prednisone therapy (1–2 mg/kg/day) as long as needed to maintain the platelet count in the 75,000/mm^3 range (or at least above the danger point for serious hemorrhage of 25,000/mm^3). Contact sports or other activities with significant risk of even modest trauma should be avoided with counts below 100,000/mm^3. Aspirin is contraindicated and may precipitate serious hemorrhage in any individual with compromised platelets.

If prednisone is required for more than 2 weeks, alternate-day administration should be tried. If successful, this obviates many of the complications of steroid therapy and minimizes the relative hypoadrenal state and increased susceptibility to stress seen in some individuals for up to a year following chronic steroid administration.

Splenectomy, immunosuppressive drugs, or both may be required in refractory cases. It should, however, be kept in mind that splenectomy for any reason poses a life-long risk of overwhelming sepsis, particularly from pneumococcal organisms. These patients should both be immunized with pneumococcal vaccine (if over 2 years of age) and placed on penicillin prophylaxis, as current vaccines do not protect against all strains that may be involved.

Thrombotic thrombocytopenic purpura. Also known as the hemolytic-uremic syndrome, this relatively rare disease is manifested in the triad of microangiopathic hemolytic anemia, nephropathy with uremia, and thrombocytopenia. It is most commonly noted in pre-school-age children following various viral infections or immunizations (mumps, smallpox). Improvement often occurs within 2 weeks and portends a good prognosis. An adult form (Gasser's syndrome) may occur in older adolescents and bears a poorer outlook. Thrombocytopenia together with thrombotic occlusions in the capillaries and arterioles of the brain and kidneys are dominant aspects. Treatment is empirical; corticosteroids, antiplatelet agents (aspirin, dipyridamole), anticoagulants, splenectomy, dextran, exchange transfusions, and plasmaphoresis have been tried with limited success. Death occurs in 80% within 3 months after onset due to neurologic complications.

Disseminated intravascular coagulation (DIC). Disseminated intravascular coagulation (DIC) may occur in the acute phase of any serious illness or injury or in patients with cavernous hemangiomas. Significant thrombocytopenia may occur due to a consumptive coagulopathy in which platelets are destroyed in a generalized process of thrombin and thrombi formation. Laboratory data vary greatly, depending on the course. The more characteristic findings are a platelet count less than $100,000/mm^3$; low factors I, II, V, and VIII; prolonged thrombin, prothrombin, and partial thromboplastin times; reduced fibrinogen; and the presence of fibrin split products due to fibrinolysis. Overt bleeding and/or clinical shock may occur. Treatment is directed at the underlying process together with replacement of depleted coagulation factors. Steroids, heparinization, antiplatelet medications (aspirin, dipyridamole), fibrinolytic inhibitors (aminocaproic acid, tranexamic acid), and fibrinolytic activators (streptokinase, urokinase) also may be useful.

Other forms. Reduced platelets may be encountered in hypersplenism when splenomegaly, due to some other disease, prompts sequestration and platelet destruction. Qualitative platelet dysfunction also may be encountered; platelets are not reduced in

TABLE 13-11
ETIOLOGY OF ACQUIRED LEUKOPENIA

1. Viral infections (rubella, influenza, infectious mononucleosis, infectious hepatitis)
2. *Severe* bacterial infections with septicemia
3. Other infections (typhoid, paratyphoid, rickettsia, malaria, brucellosis, tuberculosis)
4. Rheumatoid arthritis
5. Systemic lupus erythematosus
6. Aplastic anemia
7. Leukemia
8. Hypersplenism (anemia, leukopenia, thrombocytopenia often in association with an enlarged spleen)
9. Cancer chemotherapy
10. Radiation
11. Cyclic neutropenia (fever, oral ulcers plus neutropenia for 5-10 days in cycles of 2-7 weeks)
12. Drugs (phenothiazines, sulfonamides, thiouracil, phenylbutazone, and many others)

number and clotting factors are present in normal amounts, but the bleeding time is prolonged up to 7 minutes or more. This situation may be induced by such drugs as aspirin, indomethacin, or phenylbutazone. It also has been seen in association with a variety of diseases. Treatment is directed at the primary process; supportive measures are as required to prevent serious bleeding.

Leukopenia
Table 13-11 cites the differential diagnosis of acquired leukopenia. Mildly depressed white blood cell counts of $4000-4500/mm^3$ are commonly encountered in viral infections and with the administration of some drugs. Leukopenia of this degree rarely poses a problem and resolves spontaneously with clearing of the illness or discontinuance of the drug. In severer situations, the risk of secondary infection becomes a serious consideration when the leukocyte count reaches $500-1000/mm^3$; $200/mm^3$ is a point of critical risk. Treatment is aimed at protecting the patient against secondary infection with broad-spectrum antibiotics (both gram-positive and gram-negative organisms) and reverse isolation together with appropriate attention to the underlying cause.

Oncology
Cancer is the second leading cause of death among 5-14 year olds (5.0/100,000) and fourth among those between 15 and 24 (6.5/100,000), exceeded

TABLE 13-12
MAJOR CAUSES OF
OF CANCER IN ADOLESCENTS

1. Leukemia: 2.2/100,000 in 15–19 year old age group
   a. Acute lymphoblastic leukemia
   b. Acute myelogenous leukemia
2. Central nervous system tumors: 1.2/100,000 in 15–19 year old age group (see Table 13-15)
3. Hodgkin's disease: 1.1/100,000 in 15–19 year old age group
4. Bone tumors: 1.3/100,000 in 15–19 age group
   a. Osteogenic sarcoma
   b. Ewing's tumor
5. Non-Hodgkin's lymphomas: 0.6/100,000 in 15–19 year old age group
6. Other
   a. DES-related adenocarcinoma (Chapter 17)
   b. Gonadal (Chapter 17) and other endocrine tumors (Chapter 12)
   c. Multiple endocrine neoplasia (Sipple syndrome —combination of medullary thyroid cancer, pheochromocytoma, parathyroid tumors)

TABLE 13-13
DIFFERENTIAL DIAGNOSIS OF
EARLY ACUTE LYMPHOBLASTIC LEUKEMIA

1. Leukemoid reactions (secondary to infections, drugs, collagen disorders, others)
2. ITP (idiopathic thrombocytopenia purpura)
3. Aplastic anemia
4. Infectious mononucleosis
5. Infectious lymphocytosis
6. Rheumatoid arthritis
7. Rheumatic fever
8. Other malignancies

only by accidents, homicide, and suicide. The overall incidence of neoplastic disease among 15–19 year olds is 16.2/100,000. Table 13-12 lists the major types encountered and their frequencies.

Current methods of treating cancer are highly complex and require an integrated team approach. Although most of these young people are treated at a tertiary care facility, the primary care physician may well see the patient between visits to specialists, during remission, or after a "cure." The parent or youth may also seek a trusted primary physician's opinion about various aspects of cancer treatment. More importantly, the primary care physician usually is the first to discover a possible malignancy and, as treatment inevitably has a better outlook if discovered early, the physician must be alert to this possibility.

Leukemia

Leukemia is the most common malignancy seen in the adolescent age group. Approximately 85% of cases are acute lymphoblastic and 15% acute myelogenous; the chronic form of either variety is rare. Acute lymphoblastic leukemia may involve either T, B, or null cells. T cell disease in association with a mediastinal mass is most likely to be noted in adolescent males; otherwise there is little predilection for one sex. The etiology is unknown, but an increased incidence has been noted in Down's syndrome,

Fanconi's anemia, Bloom's syndrome, and after exposure to ionizing radiation or certain chemicals.

Symptomatology varies, depending on which organ systems are involved and the degree of infiltration. Fever, bleeding (purpura, epistaxis), anemia, lymphadenopathy, and hepatosplenomegaly are among the more common signs. Fatigue, anorexia, pain (bone, joint, abdomen), and weight loss also are often noted. Differential diagnosis early in the course poses the classic dilemma of distinguishing between malignancy, systemic infections, collagen vascular diseases and, other autoimmune disorders (Table 13-13).

Laboratory data usually reveal thrombocytopenia, normocytic anemia, and a variable white count. Blast cells are present in both the peripheral smear and bone marrow. Additional diagnostic evidence may include a decreased alkaline phosphatase and the presence of the Philadelphia chromosome.

Therapy consists of three stages: *induction*, or initial treatment aimed at putting the patient into remission; *sanctuary*, or treatment aimed at eradicating reservoirs in the central nervous system and, possibly, the testes; and *maintenance*, or periodic treatment to keep the patient in a disease-free state. A wide variety of chemotherapeutic agents is used (Table 13-17) and administered by various routes: oral, intravenous and intrathecal. These include vincristine, prednisone, L-asparginase and doxorubicin. Cranial radiation also is important. Supportive therapy includes treatment of anemia and infections as well as palliation of drug and radiation side effects (Tables 13-16 and 13-17). Allopurinol is used for hyperuricemia encountered when large numbers of blast cells are destroyed within a short period.

At least 90% of patients with lymphoblastic leukemia enter remission within 4–8 weeks. The longer it can be maintained, the better the outlook. A wide variety of other factors, however, also enters

TABLE 13-14
CRITERIA FOR STAGING OF
HODGKIN'S DISEASE (ANN ARBOR)

STAGE I: Involvement of a single lymph node region (I) or of a single extralymphatic organ or site (Ie)

STAGE II: Involvement of two or more lymph node regions on the same side of the diaphragm (II) or localized involvement (by direct extension) of an extralymphatic organ or site and one or more lymph node regions on the same side of the diaphragm (IIe)

STAGE III: Involvement of lymph node regions on both sides of the diaphragm (III), which may also be accompanied by localized involvement (by direct extension) of an extralymphatic organ or site (IIIe) or by the involvement of the spleen (IIIs) or both (IIIse)

STAGE IV: Diffuse or disseminated involvement of one or more extralymphatic organs or tissues with or without associated lymph node enlargement

All stages are subclassified as A or B to indicate the absence or presence, respectively, of one or more systemic symptoms, such as unexplained fever, night sweats, or weight loss greater than 10% of normal body weight.

in. A high initial white count (over 30,000/mm³), central nervous system involvement, and massive hepatosplenomegaly usually bear a poorer prognosis, as does acute myeloid leukemia or the T cell form of acute lymphoblastic leukemia. Relapses involving the testes or central nervous system also are grave signs.

HODGKIN'S DISEASE

Hodgkin's disease, a lymphoid tissue malignancy, most commonly presents as an enlarging, firm, painless cervical lymph node. It is the most common neoplasm in young adults, affecting 7000 Americans annually. Mediastinal, inguinal, axillary, and other lymph node sites also may be involved. Thirty-three percent of the cases have constitutional symptoms, including fever, night sweats, malaise, weight loss, or pruritus. Biopsy is diagnostic in revealing Sternberg-Reed cells. Various pathologic types have been identified and are of prognostic significance; lymphocyte-predominant forms have the best prognosis, lymphocyte-depletion types have the poorest prognosis; nodular sclerosing and mixed cellular forms are

somewhere in between. Treatment and prognosis depend not only on the particular cell type but also on the stage of the disease as determined by established criteria (Table 13-14). Staging is a critical aspect of management and includes CBC, ESR, SMA-12, bone marrow biopsy, chest roentgenograms and tomograms, computerized axial tomography, intravenous pyelogram, bone survey, lymphangiogram, gallium scan, and laparotomy with splenectomy, liver biopsy, and ovariopexy.

Radiotherapy and chemotherapy result in an excellent 5-year survival rate, particularly if introduced before the advent of stage IV disease (the 5-year survival rate is 90% at stage I or II, 80% at stage III, and 40% at stage IV). Current chemotherapy involves the traditional MOPP plan: mechlorethamine (nitrogen mustard), vincristine, procarbazine, and prednisone. Advanced disease may respond to newer regimens involving such drugs as doxorubicin, bleomycin, vinblastine, and dacarbazine (Imidazole carboxamide). Treatment side effects of baldness, aspermia, and gynecomastia are psychologic assaults that some youths may perceive as worse than the disease itself and must be dealt with in a highly sensitive and supportive manner. Treatment of children with Hodgkin's disease usually does not interfere with later pubertal development. Splenectomized patients of any age, even when in good health, are always at increased risk for overwhelming sepsis with pneumococci or streptococci and should receive pneumococcal vaccine and antibiotic prophylaxis.

NON-HODGKIN'S LYMPHOMAS

Many different types of non-Hodgkin's lymphomas have been identified, including lymphocytic (well or poorly differentiated), histiocytic, mixed, undifferentiated (as in Burkitt's lymphoma, African or American type), and unclassified. The African variety of Burkitt's lymphoma is one of the few tumors with a recognized cause in being associated with high titers of the Epstein-Barr virus. Non-Hodgkin's lymphomas, as well as acute lymphocytic leukemia, are sometimes seen secondarily a number of years after therapy for Hodgkin's disease. These tumors are staged and treated in a manner similar to Hodgkin's disease, but the prognosis generally is poor.

MALIGNANT BONE TUMORS

Malignant bone tumors comprise the fourth most common group of malignancies seen in adolescents; only leukemia and brain tumors occur more frequently. Osteogenic sarcoma is more common than Ewing's tumor.

Osteogenic sarcoma. Osteogenic sarcoma is predominantly an adolescent disease with the majority of cases occurring between 10 and 20 years of age. Males are affected from two to five times more often than females. The metaphyseal ends of long bones are most frequently involved, particularly the distal femur or proximal tibia. It also may appear in the proximal humerus, distal radius, distal tibia, and other sites. The etiology is unknown; frequently there is a history of trauma, but no clear association has been found.

Pain and swelling are the usual presenting symptoms and may be ascribed by the patient to a traumatic event. Sometimes osteogenic sarcoma is seen in association with a pathologic fracture. In other instances, pain may precede swelling by several weeks. Systemic symptoms are usually absent until the disease is quite advanced.

Roentgenograms of the affected area are highly suggestive, revealing a metaphyseal sclerotic lesion with ill-defined margins located in the medullary cavity, periosteal elevation, cortical destruction, and a calcified soft tissue mass. Ewing's tumor, osteomyelitis, lymphoma, and a benign cortical fibrous defect comprise the differential diagnosis. Biopsy confirms radiologic suspicion with the finding of a large spindle cell type sarcoma. Metastases to the lung are frequent; bone metastases are uncommon but occur occasionally. Chest roentgenograms and tomograms with bone scans are important for full evaluation. Serum alkaline phosphatase may be elevated beyond that normally seen during the growth spurt (see Appendix I).

Treatment consists of surgery (amputation or wide excision with an endoprosthesis replacing removed bone) and chemotherapy. High doses of methotrexate with citrovorum rescue and adriamycin are commonly used. The prognosis is often, but not invariably, poor. Other drugs include doxorubicin, cyclophosphamide, vincristine, and phenylalanine mustard.

Ewing's tumor. Ewing's tumor, a small cell sarcoma, commonly is located in the mid shaft of long bones, particularly the femoral diaphysis, or in flat bones including ribs, pelvis, and scapulae. Pain, swelling, fever, and leukocytosis are frequent presenting signs. Roentgenograms reveal a diffuse lytic lesion with erosion of the cortex, periosteal elevation, and, often a large soft tissue mass extending outward from the bone. This mass may have a layered "onion skin" appearance. The differential diagnosis includes a bone abscess, osteomyelitis, osteogenic sarcoma, lymphoma, and fibrous cortical defect. Although

---

TABLE 13-15
TYPES OF CENTRAL NERVOUS SYSTEM TUMORS SEEN IN ADOLESCENTS

1. Medulloblastoma (posterior fossa)
2. Astrocytomas (cerebral or cerebellar areas)
3. Ependymomas (posterior fossa or cerebellar)
4. Brain stem gliomas (posterior fossa)
5. Craniopharyngioma (cystic or solid)
6. Pineal tumors
7. Spinal cord tumors (low-grade astrocytomas, gliomas, ependymomas)
8. Metastatic from primary at another site (leukemia, lymphoma, etc.)

---

biopsy is the definitive diagnostic procedure, chest roentgenograms, chest tomograms, and total body scans are part of the initial evaluation to detect metastases. Ewing's tumor is more radiosensitive than osteogenic sarcoma; treatment combines radiotherapy, chemotherapy, and surgical excision of the mass and secondary metastases when feasible (for example, from the lung). Chemotherapy may include vincristine, cyclophosphamide, actinomycin D, and/or doxorubicin. The prognosis is guarded.

CENTRAL NERVOUS SYSTEM TUMORS

A wide variety of brain tumors, both malignant and benign, may occur in adolescents (Table 13-15). Evidence of increasing pressure is common and includes dull early morning headaches increasing in severity with time, emesis (also commonly occurring in the early morning, often without nausea), lethargy, irritability, diplopia (sixth nerve palsy), blurred vision, sleep or eating pattern disturbances, and/or papilledema. A stiff neck or torticollis also may be noted. Sometimes a seizure is the only presenting sign; it should be kept in mind that central nervous system tumors outdistance idiopathic epilepsy as the cause of seizures beginning around age 16. Other signs depend upon location (Table 13-16). Extracranial metastases are rare, but local spread is common.

Skull roentgenograms may be helpful if they demonstrate areas of calcification (craniopharyngioma, ependymoma) or signs of chronic increased intracranial pressure (erosion of posterior clinoids, thinning of sphenoid wings, or increased convolutions of the inner skull, sometimes referred to as a "beaten metal" appearance). Computerized axial tomography has revolutionized diagnosis and today is a mandatory procedure. Angiograms are indicated in situations where blood vessel malformations or

TABLE 13-16
SYMPTOMS, SIGNS, AND TYPES OF BRAIN TUMORS SEEN IN ADOLESCENTS

Tumor location	Clinical evidence
Cerebral hemispheres	Increased intracranial pressure (IIP); epilepsy (all types); paresis, spasticity; visual defects
Brain stem tumor	Cranial nerve palsies (V, VI, VII, IX, X); cerebellar signs (nystagmus, ataxia)
Cerebellum and fourth ventricle	Increased intracranial pressure; nystagmus; ataxia; personality changes; emaciation (characteristic of a diencephalon tumor)
Pituitary or hypothalamic tumor	Visual field defects; pituitary hormone deficiencies; hyperphagia; temperature regulation abnormalities; hypersomnia; diabetes insipidus

TABLE 13-17
EFFECTS OF RADIOTHERAPY

1. Growth retardation
2. Scoliosis
3. Radiation hepatitis
4. Radiation pneumonitis and pulmonary fibrosis
5. Pericardial fibrosis
6. Thyroid dysfunction
7. Amenorrhea
8. Aspermia
9. Secondary oncogenesis
10. Increased bone marrow depressive effect of chemotherapy
11. Transient encephalopathy
12. Chemical arachnoiditis and paraplegia (with intrathecal methotrexate)

tissue vascularity are important differential or therapeutic considerations. Pneumoencephalograms have little place in the contemporary diagnostic armamentarium. Technetium brain scans are helpful in a provisional and preliminary manner when computerized tomography is not immediately available.

Treatment employs a combination of surgery, radiotherapy, and chemotherapy. Medulloblastomas are highly sensitive to radiation and chemotherapy, ependymomas are variably so, and low-grade gliomas are minimally responsive. Effectiveness of chemotherapy also is modified by the ability to penetrate the blood-brain barrier. Additional treatment includes steroids to reduce cerebral edema, antiepileptic drugs, and hormonal replacement when the hypothalamus or pituitary is involved. The overall prognosis varies, but many even malignant tumors are slow growing, and the patient can be maintained in a reasonably functional state over prolonged periods of time even when the tumors cannot be removed.

RADIATION AND CHEMOTHERAPY

Early diagnosis and new forms of treatment (primarily extended and cyclical treatment schedules) provide a far more optimistic outlook for patients with some forms of cancer than was true a decade ago. But both radiation and chemotherapy treatment often pose their own problems in significant and serious side effects (Tables 13-17 and 13-18). Nausea, emesis, and bone marrow suppression are common to the use of many of these agents. It should be noted that tetrahydrocannabinol (marijuana) is the most potent antiemetic yet known in countering the nauseant effects of cancer chemotherapy. Self-hypnosis has also benefitted those with hyperemetic reactions or who are singularly fearful of treatments. Alopecia is another frequent side effect. This has a devastating impact on the adolescent and many will wish to plan for a wig in advance.

Factors complicating the choice of a chemotherapeutic agent include concurrent infection, pregnancy, bone marrow depression, recent radiotherapy, and impaired liver or renal function.

Secondary infection is a major complication of therapy and a significant cause of morbidity and mortality. Virtually any organism can be involved: bacterial, viral, fungal, or protozoan (*Toxoplasma gondii*, *Pneumocystis carinii*). Patients in need of frequent transfusion of blood or blood products are additionally at risk for hepatitis and other transfusion transmitted infections. Zoster immune globulin is indicated in those who are immunosuppressed and exposed to varicella as in gamma globulin for measles exposure. Amphotericin B is used for disseminated fungal infection, whereas pentamidine or trimethoprim-sulfamethoxazole is effective against *Pneumocystis carinii*. A fever of unknown origin may be treated with the triple combination of gentamicin, carbenicillin, and cephalothin until cultures identify the organism involved or some infectious cause is detected.

TABLE 13-18
AGENTS FOR CHEMOTHERAPY

Drug	Classification	Side effects
Adriamycin (doxorubicin)	Antibiotic	Alopecia, leukopenia, nausea, emesis, cardiotoxicity (in doses over 550 mg/m^2), bone marrow depression, red urine, hyperpigmentation
Asparaginase (L)	Enzyme derived from *Escherichia coli*	Nausea, emesis, coagulopathies, hypersensitivity reactions, pancytopenia, fatty liver metamorphosis
Bischlorethyl-nitrosourea (BiCNU; carmustine)	Nitrosourea, which is an alkylating agent	Nausea, emesis, hepatic dysfunction, bone marrow depression
Bleomycin (Blenoxane)	Antibiotic	Nausea, emesis, stomatitis, edema, dermatitis, hyperpigmentation, alopecia, pneumonia, cumulative pulmonary fibrosis (in doses over 360 units)
Busulfan (Myleran)	Alkylating agent	Bullous dermatitis, stomatitis, cataracts, hyperpigmentation, pulmonary fibrosis, adrenal insufficiency—like syndrome, menstrual irregularities, bone marrow depression
Corticosteroids (Prednisone)	Steroids	See index
Cyclohexylchloroethyl nitrosourea (CeeNU; Lomustine	Alkylating agent	Nausea, emesis, hepatic dysfunction, bone marrow depression
Cyclophosphamide (Cytoxan)	Alkylating agent	Bone marrow depression, alopecia, hemorrhagic cystitis, hyperpigmentation, transient azospermia, menstrual irregularity
Cytosine arabinoside (Cytosar-U)	Cytotoxic agent	Nausea, emesis, bone marrow depression, stomatitis, diarrhea, hepatic dysfunction, thrombophlebitis
Dactinomycin (Cosmegen)	Antibiotic	Nausea, emesis, stomatitis, alopecia, diarrhea, bone marrow depression
Daunorubicin (Cerubidin)	Antibiotic	Bone marrow depression, cardiotoxicity (in doses over 500 mg/m^2), alopecia, nausea, vomiting
Fluorouracil (5-FU)	Antimetabolite	Nausea, stomatitis, dermatitis, cerebellar ataxia, bone marrow depression
Mercaptopurine (6-MP) (Purinethol)	Purine antagonist antimetabolite	Bone marrow depression, stomatitis, hepatitis, hematuria, crystalluria
Methotrexate	Antimetabolite (folic acid antagonist)	Nausea, emesis, stomatitis, gastrointestinal ulcers, hepatitis, osteoporosis, bone marrow depression, acne
Procarbazine (Matulane)	Probably an antimitotic agent	Nausea, emesis, stomatitis, bone marrow depression, mental depression, constipation or diarrhea, myalgias, dermatitis, ataxia
Vinblastine (Velban)	Antimitotic (alkaloid)	Nausea, emesis, alopecia, areflexia, stomatitis, constipation, bone marrow depression, menstrual irregularities
Vincristine (Oncovin)	Antimitotic (alkaloid)	Neurotoxicity (peripheral neuropathy), foot drop, muscle weakness, paralytic ileus, hoarseness, bladder atony, dysuria, various pains in the abdomen or jaw, cranial nerve palsies, decreased reflexes, mild bone marrow depression

Bibliography

Aronstam, A. 1979. Patterns of bleeding in adolescents with severe haemophilia A. *Br. Med. J.* 1:469.

Baehner, R. L., editor. 1980. Symposium on pediatric hematology. *Pediatr. Clin. North Am.* 27:215–486.

Binder, R. A., and Kales, A. N. 1979. Evaluation of anemia. *Primary Care* 6:633.

Binder, R. A., editor. 1980. Hematology update. *Primary Care* 7:345.

Binder, R. A., and Kales, A. N. 1980. Leukemia: a spectrum of diseases. *Primary Care* 7:395.

Bloom, A. L. 1977. Factor VIII and its inherited disorders. *Br. Med. Bull.* 33:219.

Camitta, B. M., and Nathan, D. G. 1975. Anemia in adolescence. *Postgrad. Med.* 57:143;151.

Canale, V. C. 1974. Beta-thalassemia: a clinical review. *Pediatr. Ann.* 3:6.

Cancer chemotherapy. 1978. *Med. Let. Drug Therapy* 20(19):81.

Dallman, P. R. 1977. New approaches to screening for iron deficiency. *J. Pediatr.* 90:678.

Dallman, P. R. 1982. Manifestations of iron deficiency. *Semin. Hematol.* 19:19.

Daniel, W. A., Jr.; Gaines, E. G.; and Bennett, D. L. 1975. Iron intake and transferrin saturation in adolescence. *J. Pediatr.* 86:288.

Desforges, J. R.; Rutherford, C. J.; and Piro, A. 1979. Hodgkin's disease. *N. Engl. J. Med.* 301:1212.

Ertel, I. J. 1980. Brain tumors in children. *CA* 30:306.

Evans, A. E.; D'Angio, G. J.; and Koop, C. E.; editors. 1976. Symposium on pediatric oncology. *Pediatr. Clin. North Am.* 23:3–244.

Gilman, P. A., and Miller, R. W. 1981. Cancer after acute lymphocytic leukemia. *Am. J. Dis. Child.* 135:311.

Hardisty, R. M. 1977. Disorders of platelet function. *Br. Med. Bull.* 33:209.

Headings, V., and Fieldings, J. 1975. Guidelines for counseling young adults with sickle cell trait. *Am. J. Publ. Health* 65:819.

Herbert, V. 1980. The nutritional anemias. *Hosp. Pract.* 15:65.

Holleb, A. I. 1981. Smoking: the ticking time-bomb for teenage girls. *CA* 31:44.

Hoots, W. K. 1981. Bruising and recurrent bleeding in children. *Am. Family Phys.* 24:190.

Jagathambal, K.; Grunwald, H. W.; and Rosner, F. 1981. Evaluation and management of the bleeding patient. *Med. Clin. North Am.* 65:133.

Jenkin, R. D. T., and Berry, M. P. 1980. Hodgkin's disease in children. *Semin. Oncol.* 7:202.

Jones, P. 1977. Developments and problems in the management of hemophilia. *Semin. Hematol.* 14:375.

Kiely, J. M. 1981. Antineoplastic agents. *Mayo Clin. Proc.* 56:384.

Koller, C. A. 1980. Immune thrombocytopenic purpura. *Med. Clin. North Am.* 64:761.

Lukens, J. N. 1981. Sickle cell disease. *D.M.* 27(5):3–56.

1982. Lung cancer and smoking. *M.M.W.R.* 31(7):77.

Mayer, R. J. 1982. More than MOPP for advanced Hodgkin's disease? *N. Engl. J. Med.* 306:800.

Peterson, C. M. 1979. Managing iron deficiency. *Drug Therapy* 9(2):65.

Pochedly, C., editor. 1978. Symposium on childhood cancer: the leukemias and lymphomas. *Pediatr. Ann.* 7(7):15–92.

Riddoch, E.; Cotter, K. P.; and Penrose, J. H. 1977. Neoplasia in adolescence. *Practitioner* 218:249.

Rizza, C. R. 1977. Clinical management of haemophilia. *Br. Med. Bull.* 33:225.

Rosen, G. 1978. Malignant bone tumors. *Pediatr. Ann.* 7(8):8–51.

Sharp, A. A. 1977. Diagnosis and management of disseminated intravascular coagulation. *Br. Med. Bull.* 33:265.

Sheehy, T. W., and Plumb, V. J. 1977. Treatment of sickle cell disease. *Arch. Intern. Med.* 137:779.

Silverberg, E. 1982. Cancer statistics, 1982. *CA* 32:15.

Silverberg, E. 1982. Cancer in young adults (ages 15–34). *CA* 32:32.

Smith, S. D. 1981. Advances in the pharmacology of cancer chemotherapy. *Pediatr. Clin. North Am.* 28:145.

Smithson, W. A.; Gilchrist, G. S.; and Burgert, E. O. 1980. Childhood acute lymphocytic leukemia. *CA* 30:158.

Villee, C. A. 1976. Puberty and chemotherapy. *N. Engl. J. Med.* 294:1177.

Wolfe, L. C., and Lux, S. E. 1979. Nutritional anemias of childhood. *Pediatr. Ann* 8(7):38.

Woo, S. Y., and Sinks, L. F. 1979. Leukemia, Hodgkin's disease, Non-Hodgkin's lymphoma, and central nervous system tumors in the adolescent. *J. Curr. Adol. Med.* 1(1):42; 1(2):21; 1(3):28.

–14–
Disorders of the Skin

Acanthosis Nigricans

Bilateral, symmetric, hyperpigmented areas in association with epidermal hypertrophy and a verrucal appearance are apparent on the posterior neck, axillae, groin, or genital regions of patients with acanthosis nigricans. The color of these areas may be dark brown, light brown, yellow, or black. Both benign and malignant forms have been described in association with many disorders (Table 14-1). The most common form is benign acanthosis in obese individuals. Treatment focuses on the underlying cause. Lubricating ointments such as Vaseline Intensive Care Lotion, Lubriderm, or Keri Lotion may be used if the skin is very dry.

Acne Vulgaris

Acne vulgaris is a disorder of the sebaceous gland, sebaceous duct, and hair follicle in areas of high sebaceous density (the face, back, chest, and upper arms). It most commonly initiates in mid-adolescence and affects 90% of males and 80% of females in variable degrees. Rising plasma testosterone levels contribute to its development; testosterone is converted in the skin by 5-alpha-reductase to dihydrotestosterone, which directly stimulates sebaceous gland enlargement and activity through a cyclic AMP mechanism.

PATHOGENESIS

Three key elements in the pathogenesis of acne are sebum, keratin, and microbial skin flora. Sebum, the product of the sebaceous glands, consists of two-thirds triglycerides and one-third a mixture of wax esters, squalene, and steroid esters. Keratin consists of shed epithelial cells from the sebaceous gland mixed with sebum and bacteria. The most significant skin organism is *Propionibacterium acnes* (formerly known as *Corynebacterium acnes*), an anaerobic gram-positive diphtheroid. Coagulase-negative *Staphylococcus epidermidis* and the yeast *Pityrosporum ovale* also may be involved.

The basic acne process begins by altering the follicular epithelium and the production of horny cells, which stick together forming solid keratin impactions, or comedones. Closed comedones are called whiteheads; open comedones with pigmented epithelial cells (due to oxidation of sulfur radicals) are termed blackheads. Whether open or closed, the comedo obstructs the follicle duct and sebum outflow, resulting in distention of the follicle itself. Progressive distention causes local tissue damage, which is further exacerbated by the conversion of sebum triglycerides to irritating free fatty acids. Ultimate rupture of the follicle permits bacterial invasion and subsequent infection of the follicle and surrounding tissues. Erythematous papules, pustules, nodules, and/or cysts mark the phase of inflammatory acne vulgaris. At this point, healing may result in permanent scarring. Table 14-2 classifies variations in this process.

TREATMENT

Traditional treatment does not cure acne once and for all, and the condition follows a highly individual

TABLE 14-1
ASSOCIATIONS OF BENIGN
AND MALIGNANT ACANTHOSIS NIGRICANS

BENIGN ACANTHOSIS
1. Exogenous obesity
2. Diabetes mellitus
3. Epilepsy
4. Mental retardation
5. Adrenal disorders (Addison's disease; adrenal hyperplasia)
6. Stein-Leventhal syndrome
7. Neurofibromatosis

MALIGNANT ACANTHOSIS
1. Adenocarcinoma (various sites)
2. Epidermoid carcinoma
3. Osteogenic sarcoma
4. Malignant lymphoma
5. Pituitary tumor (acromegaly)

course. Some adolescents have only relatively circumscribed comedonal acne, lasting no more than a year or two. Others have extensive disease involving all potential areas with pustules and cysts and lasting 5–6 years. In some cases it continues on into young adulthood.

Treatment is aimed at controlling the condition; primary goals are immediate improvement in appearance and prevention of permanent scarring. To this end, varying combinations of local hygienic measures (face washing), bacteriostatic and peeling topical agents and, in severer inflammatory forms, topical or systemic antibiotics are employed.

Simple grade I acne sometimes may be treated by only washing the affected area two to three times a day with a mild soap containing a wetting agent to remove sebum from the skin and dislodge comedones. Such agents include acetone, dioctyl sodium sulfosuccinate, sodium nonoxyl-1-sulfate, sodium lauryl sulfoacetate, benzalkonium chloride, and polyoxyethylene lauryl ether. The frequency of use should be titrated according to individual tolerance. Insufficient use fails to improve the situation, but excessive use may cause unacceptable degrees of dryness or even acne mechanica. Adolescents unable to wash during the school day may use alcohol wipes or similar products designed especially for acne (Stridex pads); these come in individual foil-wrapped packets and can be tucked unobtrusively in pocket or purse. Adolescents should avoid squeezing the comedones, as this only increases tissue damage; however, a comedo extractor can be used to good advantage.

TABLE 14-2
CLASSIFICATION OF ACNE VULGARIS AND VARIANTS

Type	Comment
ACNE VULGARIS (GROUP I)	
Comedonal acne vulgaris	Disorder of sebaceous follicles with horny impactions. Graded according to percent of face involved; I = 10%; II = 10%–25%; III = 25%–50%; IV = more than 50%.
Papulopustular acne (inflammatory acne)	Rupture of the distended sebaceous gland with varying degrees of inflammation. Graded V–VIII.
Acne conglobata	Severe inflammatory acne vulgaris.
Acne tropicalis	Severe inflammatory acne vulgaris seen in young adult men exposed to tropical conditions.
Acne fulminans (acute febrile ulcerative conglobate acne)	Rare variant described in males characterized by large nodules, fever, ulcers, polyarthritis/arthralgia, and leukocytosis.
Back acne	Inflammatory acne limited to the backs of adult males.
ACNE VULGARIS VARIANTS (GROUP II)	
Infantile acne (acne neonatorum)	Comedonal acne of malar region of males during first few weeks to year of life. Occasionally noted in either sex from 1–2 years of age.
Premenstrual acne	Cyclical microcomedonal acne developing before the menstrual period.
Gram-negative folliculitis	Associated with long-term broad-spectrum antibiotic use. Variable patterns of facial nodules due to *Proteus*, *Pseudomonas*, *Klebsiella*, or *Enterobacter* organisms.
Excessive androgen acne	Severe acne related to high androgen levels (e.g., Stein-Leventhal syndrome).
Acne varioliformis (folliculitis decalvans)	Chronic, recurrent low-grade pustular dermatitis of the occipital and posterior neck regions. May result in scarring, keloid formation, and alopecia. Most commonly noted in black males. Treat with povidone-iodine shampoos and oral antibiotics.
Acne mechanica	Exacerbation of acne vulgaris by excessive rubbing to cause friction, as with over-zealous face washing.
Chemical acne	Exacerbation of acne vulgaris by cosmetics, detergents, hair creams/oils, chlorinated hydrocarbons, tars, emollient skin or bath oils.
Acne due to physical agents	Exacerbation of acne vulgaris by sunlight, ionizing radiation; Mallorca acne (acne aestivalis) a sunlight-induced, winter variant with papular folliculitis of arms, shoulders, and trunk; no comedones, nodules, or scarring.
Drug-induced acneform rashes	Iodides, bromides, isonicotinic acid, barbiturates, rifampin, others may be associated. Steroid acne a predictable complication and responds poorly to antibiotics. Patients with acne should be screened for medications and foods that might contain high levels of "acnegenic" substances.
NONACNE ACNEFORM RASHES (DIFFERENTIAL DIAGNOSIS)	
Pyoderma faciale	Progressive facial inflammatory lesions (nodules, hypertrophic scars and absence of comedones) occurring in adult females 20–40 years of age.
Acne rosacea	Facial papules and pustules associated with dilated blood vessels in the nasolabial area in adults age 30–50.
Hidradenitis suppurativa	Keratin obstruction of apocrine ducts with secondary infection of apocrine glands in axillae, areolae, labiae, scrotum, or perineum. Fluctuant nodules with purulent drainage and sinus tract formation. Associated with obesity, severe acne vulgaris, tropical climates, poor hygiene. Treatment is as for abscesses in general; intralesional steroid injection, exteriorization of sinus tracts, or excision of involved tissue may be required.

Continued

TABLE 14-2
CLASSIFICATION OF ACNE VULGARIS AND VARIANTS (CONTINUED)

Type	Comment
Folliculitis-associated immuno-logic defects	Example: Chronic granulomatous disease.
Perifolliculitis capitis abscendens et suffodiens	Diffuse, explosive scalp cellulitis associated with severe acne and hidradenitis suppurativa. Treat with antibiotics and retinoic acid.
Folliculitis barbae	Chronic folliculitis in beard area aggravated by shaving. Treat by growing a beard or frequent razor changes, antibiotic ointments, keratolytic agents, and systemic antibiotics if pronounced. Multiple small keloids may form in persons predisposed to keloid formation.
Trichostasis spinulosa	Facial eruption resembling blackheads but comprised of follicular papules containing vellus hairs, keratin, and melanin and distributed over the nose and malar regions. Treat with retinoic acid.
Adenoma sebaceum	Pinkish yellow sebaceous papules on face; commonly clustered in groups around the nose. One of the classic stigmata of tuberous sclerosis.
Also see molluscum contagiosum and verrucae	

Moderate grade II–III acne usually requires the treatment just described plus one of the myriad of drying and peeling agents currently available on the market. These usually depend on combinations of sulfur, rescorcinol, salicylic acid, and/or other agents that peel the skin and thereby remove surface keratin and inhibit the buildup of keratin plugs. The currently most favored preparation is benzoyl peroxide in a 5% or 10% concentration. This is available as Benoxyl lotion, Benzagel, Desquam-X gel, PanOxyl gel, PersaGel acne cream or lotion, and Vanoxide lotion. Benzoyl peroxide causes dehiscence of keratin with desquamation, reduces the local free fatty acid level, and is bacteriostatic. The frequency of use should be individualized to avoid the complications of erythema and dryness, especially in fair-skinned or atopic adolescents. A preliminary patch test is advisable to detect the 2%–3% of the population who may respond with a contact dermatitis. If the patch test is negative, the patient should begin benzoyl treatment with a thin layer of a 5% preparation for a few hours each day and gradually build up to, first, an overnight application and then an application twice a day. This should take days to weeks and should progress at a pace that produces some drying and peeling but avoids erythema, cracking, chapping, or discomfort. If tolerated, a 10% concentration can be gradually introduced for further improvement if needed. Variation can also be introduced by the use of the lotion or gel form, since gel is more highly absorbed.

Tretinoin (Retin-A) is another topical product for acne that has received considerable recent attention. It increases the rate of cell turnover in the follicular epithelium, decreases epithelial cell cohesiveness, thins the horny layer and, in consequence, reduces comedo formation. It also enhances antibiotic action. It is a highly effective agent in acne but can easily produce marked skin erythema and irritation, particularly during its initial use and on exposure to sun at any time. Caution and slow buildup is important. Protection with paraaminobenzoic acid (PABA) sunscreens should always be used in summer or on tropical vacations. The patient should also be warned about the possibility of transient irritation of formed comedones and a temporary pustular rash that occurs after 2–3 weeks use in one out of two individuals. Tretinoin is available as a 0.025% gel, 0.05% or 0.1% cream, and 0.05% liquid. Treatment should start with a less concentrated form applied once every second or third day, slowly building up to once or twice a day application. Face washing should employ only a very mild soap (Nutrogena, Purpose, Emulave) used for cleansing purposes only as needed. An effective regimen for severe inflammatory disease is the use of benzoyl peroxide in the morning and tretinoin at night together with systemic or topical antibiotics.

Antibiotics are indicated in cases with a significant number of inflammatory or cystic lesions or both. Efficacy seems related to suppression of *P. acnes*, inhibition of bacterial lipase, and possible improvement of local chemotaxis. Tetracycline hydrochloride (250–3000 mg/day) and erythromycin (250–1500 mg/day) are the most widely used agents. Minocycline (50–300 mg/day), clindamycin (150–600 mg/day), demeclocycline and trimethoprim-sulfamethoxazol have been used on occasion as well. Antibiotics are *not* indicated in mild disease and are always used in conjunction with topical treatment. Prototypically, tetracycline is initiated with a full therapeutic dose of 250 mg q.i.d. for 7–10 days; this is then gradually tapered to the lowest effective dose, which may be as little as 250 mg once a day or once every other day. On the other hand, 2–3 g/day are needed by some patients for effective control. Optimum absorption occurs when antibiotics are taken on an empty stomach (1 hour before or 2 hours after á meal), although compromise may be needed if the drug is not tolerated at this time. It may take up to 2–4 weeks before any improvement is noted.

Tetracycline has a wide margin of safety and can be used for years in many individuals. Side effects are directly related to dose and are most likely to occur when the daily intake exceeds 500 mg; these include gastrointestinal irritation, monilial vaginitis, allergic reactions, transient liver enzyme elevation, transient blood urea nitrogen elevation, transient leukopenia, inhibition of leukocytosis during acute infections, headache, and pseudotumor cerebri. Periodic screening with a complete blood count, blood urea nitrogen, creatinine, and liver enzymes should be done. Monilial vaginitis usually can be treated adequately without discontinuing tetracycline but may require a reduction in dose. It also should be noted that tetracycline can cause enamel defects in unerupted teeth or may be deposited in the bones and teeth of a fetus if the patient is pregnant. Erythromycin is the preferred alternative when tetracycline cannot be used for any reason. Reasons for failure to improve with antibiotic treatment include compliance or absorption problems, the presence of deep nodular lesions, persistent irritation due to excessive use of topical treatments, and misdiagnosis.

Recent promising studies suggest that topical antibiotic preparations are highly effective and may come to replace systemic use. Either erythromycin (1.5%), clindamycin (1%–2%), or tetracycline (1%–2%) in a lotion base is effective. Erythromycin or clindamycin may be preferred, as tetracycline is fluorescent under black "disco" light and also may cause a yellowish brown discoloration of the skin visible in daylight. The use of topical antibiotics may replace the need for oral antibiotics in most patients.

A wide variety of other measures has been employed in the treatment of acne. Intralesional steroid injection and/or incision and drainage can be an important adjunct in managing severe cystic acne. The proper use of a comedo extractor is advantageous in all forms. Diet is of no significance unless specific food items are clearly identified by the patient as exacerbating the acne; this is not common and in most instances diet is irrelevant to the course of disease. Estrogen administration is controversial; 80–100 μg/day is needed to improve acne, but the use of more than 50 μg (as determined by observations in contraceptive use) increases the risk of thromboembolic complications. Estrogens should not be used. Lastly, there is no place for x-ray treatment in modern regimens.

An interesting drug recently made available is 13-cis-retinoic acid (Isotretinoin). It reduces sebum production and shrinks sebaceous glands. Preliminary reports of patients with severe cystic disease given this drug orally (0.02–2.0 mg/kg/day) indicate a significant and sustained effect can be achieved even when given for a limited period of time (such as 8–16 weeks). This drug raises serum triglyceride levels in 25% of patients and is classified as a teratogenic agent. Cheilitis, dry skin, conjunctivitis, and other side effects are noted. Isotretinoin is a main advance for those with severe acne.

Treatment of acne must be individualized based on the severity of the condition, the life circumstances of the patient, and the degree of motivation. It should be kept in mind that treatment is likely to be sustained if the patient perceives his or her condition as worth treating and if the prescribed regimen produces visible results. Noncompliance is likely when the patient is not troubled by the lesions or when there is no readily observable benefit from treatment. This has particular significance in acne, as all therapeutic modalities take several weeks of diligent attention to achieve results and may well cause seeming exacerbation in the process. Considerable support for continuation is needed and considerable empathy when the patient has problems with compliance.

Referral to a dermatologist is indicated in most instances of severe cystic acne and in other cases in which a well-conceived and well-implemented treatment plan has failed.

Alopecia

The loss of scalp hair (alopecia, or baldness) to the point of partial or total baldness can be caused by a wide variety of conditions (Table 14-3). The following sections describe the more common causes encountered in adolescence.

PREMATURE BALDNESS

Genetically determined premature baldness with frontolateral thinning may be noted by males during late adolescence. The hair usually is thin and fine with a beaded (monilethrix) or twisted (pili torti) appearance. Female pattern baldness, with diffuse thinning, particularly near the hair part, also can occur but is rare. More commonly, adolescent girls (or boys) present with the complaint of losing more than customary amounts of hair on brushing and a modest thinning of childhood luxuriance. This is a normal physiologic event that does not presage baldness. A cosmetic approach with a wig or hair transplants is the only treatment for baldness.

TELOGEN EFFLUVIUM

Normally, 85%–90% of scalp hairs are in a growth (anagen) phase and 10%–15% are in a resting (telogen) phase at any one time. When a hair follicle converts from a resting to an active phase, a corresponding growing follicle reciprocates by entering a resting phase and sheds its hair. A major stress may suddenly increase the percentage of resting follicles up to 50% or more of the total. Inciting factors include severe illness, crash dieting, pregnancy, delivery, discontinuation of oral contraceptives, anemia, malnutrition, and others. Two to 4 months or more following such an episode these dormant follicles again become active with an equal number of other follicles shedding. This acute, diffuse hair loss is termed telogen effluvium. New hair growth eventually occurs at a rate corresponding to the general health of the patient. Treatment should be directed at the underlying cause; none is necessary for the hair loss itself.

ALOPECIA AREATA

Well-demarcated, round or oval patches of hair lost from the scalp without apparent abnormality of the underlying skin may develop suddenly in children or adolescents. Microscopic examination reveals proximal narrowing of the hair shaft referred to as an "exclamation point" hair. Eyebrows and eyelashes also may be lost (alopecia totalis); less commonly, the condition involves all body hair (alopecia universalis). Nail pitting may be a secondary sign. The principal differential considerations are tinea capitis and trichotillomania. In both of these conditions the hair is broken off at the base of the shaft, leaving a stubble; in alopecia areata the entire hair is lost and the skin is smooth.

The etiology is obscure. Although sometimes seen in chronic thyroiditis, vitiligo, collagen disorders, and atopic dermatitis, most cases are idiopathic. Frequently, emotional stress seems to be involved.

TABLE 14-3
CAUSES OF ALOPECIA

A. Genetic or premature baldness (male pattern)
B. Telogen effluvium
C. Alopecia areata
D. Trichotillomania
E. Fungal alopecia
F. Drug- or radiation-induced alopecia (anticoagulants, cancer chemotherapy, androgens, vitamin A, allopurinol, lithium carbonate, propranolol, trimethadione, colchicone methysergide)
G. Traction alopecia
H. Miscellaneous
  1. Iron deficiency
  2. Psoriasis
  3. Seborrheic dermatitis
  4. Acne varioliformis (folliculitis decalvans)
  5. Thyroid disorders (hyperthyroidism, hypothyroidism)
  6. Systemic or discoid lupus erythematosus
  7. Lichen planus
  8. Syphilis (secondary or tertiary)
  9. Herpes zoster

The course is unpredictable with remissions and exacerbations occurring in a variable manner. No matter what treatment is invoked, some patients get full hair return after only a brief episode; others recover after months or even years of hair loss and some remain partially or totally bald for life.

Treatment generally is unsatisfactory. Intradermal or systemic steroids, dinitrochlorobenzene applications, or both have produced variable success. Dermatologic consultation usually is indicated in persistent cases. Associated medical conditions or psychologic stress factors should be looked for and treated appropriately. Secondary emotional distress can be profound. Hair loss is devastating to an adolescent, for whom hair and hair style is such an important determinant of attractiveness. A hairpiece can be an important therapeutic measure and should be recommended early in the course if the alopecia is obvious and pronounced.

TRICHOTILLOMANIA

Irregularly shaped bald patches with stubby hairshafts broken off at different lengths and without any exclamation point hairs, as in alopecia areata, are usually caused by trichotillomania, or the patient's pulling out his or her own hair. This may be voluntary in some disturbed individuals; more commonly it is due to the unconscious habit of twisting and pulling on a lock of hair. Differentiation should be made between this condition, alopecia areata, and tinea capitis. Treatment is directed at identifying the circumstances of hair pulling and responding accordingly. Behavioral modification is usually sufficient in a normal adolescent with a simple habit pattern; psychiatric evaluation is indicated in those for whom this is a manifestation of a more serious emotional disturbance.

FUNGAL ALOPECIA
See tinea capitis.

DRUG-INDUCED ALOPECIA
Many drugs can cause hair loss of a variable degree; sometimes the effect is not noted for 6-8 weeks. Cancer chemotherapy, androgens, anticoagulants, vitamin A, methysergide maleate, allopurinol, lithium carbonate, propranolol, trimethadione, colchicine, and quinacrine are some of the agents that have been implicated. Causal mechanisms include destruction or damage to the growing hair and shortening or lengthening of hair growth cycles. High dose x-ray can destroy hair follicles; low dosage injures them. Regrowth usually, but not invariably, occurs once the offending agent is discontinued.

MISCELLANEOUS CAUSES
Traction alopecia may occur secondary to excessive tension on the hair due to frequent use of hair curlers, strenuous brushing, braiding, or other practices. These measures tend to damage and break hair shafts off or to pull the entire hair out. The patient must alter these practices before irreversible damage occurs. Alopecia with scarring may be noted in discoid lupus erythematosus, lichen planus, acne varioliformis, and other scalp conditions. Diffuse hair thinning may be noted in psoriasis and seborrheic dermatitis. Treatment in any of these instances is directed at the underlying condition; when thinning is severe, a hair piece should be considered.

Atopic Dermatitis
Atopic dermatitis (eczema) is an acute or chronic hypersensitivity reaction of the skin to inhalants, topical agents, or both. In adolescence, it most commonly is a continuation or recurrence of the childhood form and is characterized by pruritic papules and plaques that tend to be dry and variably erythematous. A classic location contributes to the diagnosis and includes the popliteal, antecubital, and neck regions. (In children, eczema tends to be more generalized and commonly appears on the face.) Scratching may result in excoriations, scabbing, and areas of weeping secondary infection. When atopic

dermatitis has been present for years, the skin also becomes thickened and lichenified.

Pathogenesis involves an aberrant response to some sort of precipitant in an individual with compromised immune response systems. Abnormalities that have been detected include defective neutrophil and monocyte chemotaxis, abnormal cell-mediated immunity. elevated serum IgE, and increased susceptibility to secondary bacterial infection. Genetic factors are clearly involved as 70%–75% of these patients have a positive family history for atopy (atopic dermatitis, hay fever, asthma); this is not, however, a factor in contact or drug-induced dermatitis. Precipitants cannot always be identified, but those that have been implicated include cold weather, heat, or high humidity, physical exertion, contact sensitivity (wool clothing), infections (particularly those of the upper respiratory tract), emotional factors, and hyperhidrosis. A careful history and physical examination often reveal other factors. Particular attention should be given to discriminating between atopic and contact forms.

Atopic dermatitis during the teenage years usually is not characterized by progression to asthma as is common in infancy-onset disease. The prognosis varies; many cases clear with appropriate treatment. Some improve greatly but localized lesions persist or recur in many; less commonly, the disease may be disseminated over the entire body, posing major management problems both medically and psychologically.

Differential diagnosis includes seborrheic dermatitis, contact or drug-induced dermatitis, psoriasis, nummular eczema, dyshidrotic eczema, shoe dermatitis, tinea infections, lichen simplex chronicus, and scabies.

Atopic dermatitis usually can be controlled, but not cured, with a combination of lubricants (Lubriderm, Keri Lotion), mild soaps (Dove or Neutrogena) or cetyl alcohol preparations to avoid drying effects, topical steroids (hydrocortisone, Kenalog, Synalar, Cordran, Aristocort, others) and antihistamine sedation (diphenhydramine HCl, 5–25 mg at bedtime; hydroxyzine, 5–25 mg at bedtime). Wet compresses with Burow's solution (Domeboro packets) are soothing for acute weeping or crusted lesions. Erythromycin or other antibiotics are indicated for secondary infection, usually caused by staphylococcal organisms. A short course (7–10 days) of systemic steroids may be helpful for recalcitrant and disseminated lesions. Irritants such as hot baths, harsh soaps, and wool clothing or other irritating fabrics should be avoided. Nightly steroid occlusive dressings, avoidance of soap and water and greasy lubricants, and the use of photochemotherapy with oral psoralens and high-intensity long-wave ultraviolet light have all been employed with benefit in severe cases.

Scarring does not occur unless there has been serious secondary bacterial infection as well. Pigmentary changes (depigmentation in acute stages and hyperpigmentation in chronic disease) eventually resolve when the disease is controlled. Other complications sometimes encountered include pityriasis alba, dry skin, ichthyosis, keratosis pilaris, atopic cataracts, and/or keratoconus, alopecia areata, vitiligo, migraine headaches, and white dermatographism. Atopic dermatitis also may be seen as a component of such serious diseases as ataxia-telangiectasia, Wiskott-Aldrich syndrome, Job's syndrome, x-linked agammaglobulinemia, and others.

SEBORRHEIC DERMATITIS

Seborrheic dermatitis is due to sebaceous gland dysfunction that produces yellow, greasy scales or crusts and underlying erythema. Although patchy lesions can be noted in many places on the body, they are most common on the scalp, nasolabial folds, external ears, eyebrows, and eyelids. Severity varies, manifesting in anything from simple dandruff to extensive scaly plaques resembling psoriasis. Treatment includes avoiding associated irritants, brief soaks with mineral oil or petrolatum to remove scales, appropriate shampoos (tar, salicylic acid, sulfur, resorcinol, hexachlorophene, selenium sulfide, or zinc pyrithione), wet dressings followed by steroid ointments (avoiding fluoridated steroids on the face due to possible complications of atrophy, telangiectasia, or both), sunlight, and antibiotics if secondarily infected.

CONTACT DERMATITIS

Eczematoid lesions due to chemical contact usually are distinguishable by history and physical examination. They commonly begin with an area of erythema, itching, and blistering, which may progress to scaly, erythematous plaques resembling chronic stopic dermatitis (or any of the other differential considerations). Absence of disease in childhood or in other family members, distribution in a manner compatible with exposure (for example, on hands if offending agent is a dishwashing detergent, on face if an irritant cosmetic, or as demarcated by the dimensions of a new piece of clothing if due to dye) plus rapid clearing when the offending substance is identified and eliminated establish the diagnosis. Certain substances have a particularly high association with contact dermatitis. These include poison ivy, sumac, and oak (*Rhus* dermatitis), nickel (metal clasps, costume jewelry, earrings, watches), paraphenylenediamine dyes in furs and leathers, formaldehyde resins (used as mordant agents in new clothes), rubber, fiberglass, wool, Mycolog cream, Neomycin ointment, benzocaine products, hexachlorophene, perfumes, and detergents.

DRUG-INDUCED DERMATITIS

Drug-induced dermatitis may occur as a predictable or idiosyncratic skin eruption in response to the ingestion of almost any drug. Manifestations commonly are those of contact dermatitis but also may appear as erythema multiforme, erythema nodosum, any of the exanthems, exfoliative dermatitis, lichen planus, urticaria, discoid lupus, a photosensitivity rash, or virtually any other type of skin lesion. Treatment includes eliminating the offending agent plus saline or Burow's solution soaks, topical steroids, and other symptomatic measures.

DYSHIDROTIC ECZEMA

Dyshidrotic eczema (pompholyx) is an idiopathic recurrent dermatitis of the soles or palms; it probably is a variant of atopic dermatitis. Pruritus and small "tapioca" vesicles progress to a red, scaly, fissured dermatitis. The web spaces are clear in contrast to tinea pedis. Contact dermatitis due to shoes or socks also should be ruled out. Treatment includes topical emollients (Lubriderm, Keri Lotion) and topical steroids, and with wet soaks and antibiotics if secondarily infected.

LICHEN SIMPLEX CHRONICUS

Lichen simplex chronicus, or localized neurodermatitis, refers to localized, lechenified erythematous plaques anywhere on the body; the condition is often noted on the scrotum, vulva, or perianal region. In part it is due to repeated scratching of a normally itchy area. Emotional factors also are thought to play a role. Topical treatment as described for any of the eczemas plus cessation of scratching generally cures it.

Erythemas

The erythemas are characterized by inflammatory and vasodilatory reactions of small blood vessels within the skin or subcutaneous tissues. Usually they are secondary manifestations of some other primary and underlying process, which may be any one of a wide variety of diseases or drug reactions. Three forms of erythema have been identified: toxic erythema, erythema multiforme, and erythema nodosum.

TOXIC ERYTHEMA

Toxic erythema is characterized by flat or slightly raised erythematous skin lesions that vary in number, size, and location. They may be widely disseminated and merging (scarlatiniform) or relatively sparse and discrete; they may be fine or coarsely macular. Blanching on pressure is common. Mild pruritus is usually present. Drug reactions and infections such as scarlet fever or infectious mononucleosis are frequently associated. Treatment is directed at the underlying disorder. If pruritus is a problem, symptomatic measures include soothing baths (Aveeno, Domol bath oil, Lubath oil), calamine or Caladryl cream or lotion, and oral antihistamines.

ERYTHEMA MULTIFORME

Erythema multiforme is manifested in the rapid and often evanescent appearance of erythematous or violaceous macules or papules. Most commonly these are symmetrically located on the wrist, hands, elbows, face, knees, and/or ankles but may be found in other areas as well. Target or iris lesions are characteristic and consist of a central pale and edematous area with surrounding erythema. These lesions may extend in an annular pattern to eventually merge in a more serpiginous rash. Wheals, bullae, hemorrhagic necrosis, and ulceration also may occur.

Erythema multiforme is a nonspecific skin reaction sometimes seen with certain infections (*Mycoplasma pneumoniae*, herpes simplex, mumps, lymphogranuloma venereum, and others), drug reactions (antibiotics, anticonvulsants, thiouracil derivatives, analgesics, and others), vaccinations, topical irritants (*Rhus*), and collagen vascular disorders. Many other factors, singly or severally, also have been implicated. Treatment is directed at the underlying process. Symptomatic measures as outlined above for toxic erythemas may be employed if pruritus is a problem.

On occasion, erythema multiforme may present in a severe form comprising the Stevens-Johnson syndrome. Bullae, toxicity, fever, and widespread mucosal involvement is characteristic. A maculopapular or urticarial rash quickly progresses, first to target lesions, then to painful denuded mucosal and skin blisters, and finally to crusting and hemorrhagic necrosis. Almost any cutaneous or mucosal surface may be involved. Associated problems include corneal ulcerations, arthritis, convulsions, cutaneous bacterial infection, nephritis, lymphadenopathy, splenomegaly, and pulmonary lesions. Complications include dehydration, shock, and coma. Differential diagnosis includes pemphigus, bullous lupus erythematosus, bullous contact dermatitis, and dermatitis herpetiformis. Treatment includes attention to fluid balance, antiseptic compresses, prednisone, analgesics (viscous xylocaine for oral lesions), antibiotics for secondary cutaneous infection, and evaluation for and treatment of inciting factors (as for simple erythema multiforme). At least 20% of cases recur, and the mortality rate is 10%.

ERYTHEMA NODOSUM

Erythema nodosum consists of one, several, or many red and tender nodules of variable size, from one to several centimeters in diameter, involving the skin and subcutaneous tissue of the shins, anterior thighs, forearms, elbows, wrists, and/or face. It is a nonspecific sensitivity reaction sometimes seen in conjunction with bacterial (streptococcal) or fungal (histoplasmosis) infections, drug use (oral contraceptives), inflammatory bowel disease, collagen vascular disorders, sarcoidosis, Behçet's syndrome, tuberculin and other skin tests, as well as a wide variety of other conditions.

The lesions may enlarge, darken in color and becoming bruiselike, develop fine scales when healing, or go on to ulcerate with scarring (erythema induratum). Resolution usually occurs within 2–4 weeks, but the condition is recurrent in 10% of cases. The erythrocyte sedimentation rate is frequently elevated, reflecting underlying inflammation. Treatment of the skin lesions themselves is symptomatic but an underlying cause should be sought and managed appropriately.

MACULOPAPULAR RASHES

Maculopapular skin lesions are prominent features of many toxic states. Table 14-4 cites those conditions that should come to mind in establishing a differential diagnosis for an adolescent. Some of these conditions are discussed elsewhere (see index); others will require reference to an appropriate text. Table 14-4 should not be considered an exhaustive list and a number of rarer etiologies exist as well.

Henoch-Schönlein Purpura

Henoch-Schönlein purpura (anaphylactoid purpura) is a diffuse, generalized hypersensitivity angiitis characterized by a maculopapular-petechial (or ecchymotic) eruption in combination with other organ system involvement (nephritis, arthritis, and/or gastrointestinal bleeding). It occurs twice as often in males as females and is seen most commonly in those between 4 and 18 years of age. The etiology is not always clear. Implicated precipitants include upper respiratory tract infections, streptococcal disease, food or drug sensitivity, and insect bites.

The disease begins as an asymptomatic, erythe-

TABLE 14-4
DIFFERENTIAL DIAGNOSIS
OF MACULOPAPULAR RASH

1. Rubeola
2. Rubella
3. Enteroviral exanthems (ECHO virus and cox-sackievirus)
4. Scarlet fever
5. Erythema infectiosum (fifth disease)
6. Rocky Mountain spotted fever
7. Drug eruptions
8. Erythema multiforme (other erythemas)
9. Infectious mononucleosis
10. Adenovirus infections
11. Sunburn
12. Miliaria (heat rash)

matous, macular (or papular or urticarial) rash commonly spreading symmetrically over the buttocks, anterior legs, and posterior thighs, although the rash also can appear in such areas as the face, elbows, arms, hands, and/or feet. Characteristically, the lesions enlarge and become petechial; the petechiae then merge to form an ecchymotic patch. Differential considerations include meningococcemia, gonococcemia, septic emboli secondary to bacterial endocarditis or bacterial sepsis, toxic vasculitis due to such drugs as iodides or arsenicals, Rocky Mountain spotted fever, viral syndromes, hemorrhagic diathesis, and thrombotic thrombocytopenic purpura.

Forty to fifty percent of patients with Henoch-Schönlein purpura develop an acute nephritis; 25% of these progress to further renal disease. Anemia, hypertension, hematuria, pyuria, proteinuria, and urine casts may be noted. Soft tissue edema can develop in the hands, skin, feet, scalp, ears, or periorbital regions.

Transient nonhemorrhagic swelling and inflammation of large joints is another complication. This commonly involves the ankles and knees, but hands and feet may be involved as well. Although this arthritis usually is mild, it can be severe on occasion.

Rectal bleeding, melena, or hematemesis may occur with or without severe, colicky abdominal pain. Intramural intestinal hematomas can develop. Signs and symptoms often mimic an acute abdominal condition requiring surgery, and the purpuric rash is an important diagnostic point. Perforation and intussusception are rare complications. Other rare complications of Henoch-Schönlein purpura include encephalitis and convulsions or vasculitis of the spermatic cord simulating testicular torsion.

The clinical course of this syndrome varies but usually resolves over 3–4 weeks without sequellae. A few individuals may progress to chronic renal disease. Treatment is simply supportive unless symptoms are marked or there is evidence of progression in bleeding; in these circumstances, prednisone (1–2 mg/day up to 60 mg/day) may be given orally or intravenously. Aspirin should *not* be given due to its potential for causing gastritis and gastrointestinal bleeding as well as inhibiting platelet function.

Herpesvirus Infections
HERPES SIMPLEX
Herpes simplex virus causes primary gingivostomatitis, recurrent herpes labialis, keratoconjunctivitis, eczema herpeticum (all predominantly caused by type I), and herpes genitalis (90% due to type II; also see Chapter 17).

Primary type I infections usually are first noted in childhood with recurrent lesions occurring in adolescence. Type II lesions, however, are most likely to be transmitted through sexual contact and usually do not make their initial appearance until an adolescent becomes sexually active; thereafter, recurrences are possible throughout life.

Clinical signs of either type begin with an area of prutitus or hyperalgesia followed by the development of a small cluster of vesicles on an erythematous base. In about 24 hours these break down to form flat, shallow, painful ulcers. The history of vesiculation combined with local pain is an important point differentiating herpetic lesions from syphilitic chancres. Type I lesions tend to locate about the mouth and lips as fever blisters. Type II lesions may be found anywhere in the perineal, genital, or rectal region. Females with genital herpes also may have intravaginal lesions and/or an associated cervicitis with mucopurulent discharge; others may experience acute urinary retention when ulcers involve the urethral meatus. Perianal or rectal lesions in males may be an indication of homosexual relations.

Fever, headache, malaise, and tender regional lymphadenopathy may be associated systemic signs. On rare occasion, herpesvirus also can cause erythema multiforme, meningitis, encephalitis, or ascending myelitis. Herpetic keratitis may result in corneal scarring with blindness. Eczema herpeticum (Kaposi's varicelliform eruption) is a disseminated cutaneous infection due to herpesvirus hominis or vaccinia virus in an individual with atopic dermatitis or an immunodeficiency disease.

Diagnosis is largely made by clinical history and physical examination. Syphilis, however, should be kept in mind and ruled out by a dark-field examination of ulcer exudate for *Treponema pallidum* and serology in sexually active adolescents. Intranuclear inclusion bodies are diagnostic of herpesvirus and may be demonstrated by Giemsa or Wright stain of material obtained from a vesicle or ulcer (Tzanck test); multinuclear giant cells also may be evident on a Papanicolaou smear in genital forms. Other diagnostic tests include electron microscopy revealing viral particles, immunofluorescent studies, viral serology, and viral culture with typing.

No definitive treatment for herpes is available at this time, although current research efforts seem promising. Symptomatic measures to relieve pain include topical petroleum jelly, viscous xylocaine jelly or ointment (2%-5%), warm water sitz baths, or the application of povidone-iodine (Betadine) solution. Zinc sulfate solution, phosphoformic acid solution, or 2-deoxy-D-glucose solution are thought to possibly inhibit direct viral proliferation. A broad-spectrum antibiotic may be indicated in instances of secondary infection as suggested by bacterial cultures. Hospitalization may be necessary if lesions are excessively painful, cause urinary retention, or threaten a vital organ system. Pregnant females with active genital lesions during the third trimester may well be candidates for cesarean section to avoid exposing the infant to herpesvirus during birth; severe disseminated disease in the infant may result without such precautions.

HERPES ZOSTER
Herpes zoster is an acute viral infection of the sensory ganglion and corresponding cutaneous dermatome. It is caused by the varicella-zoster virus, the virus implicated in chickenpox. Indeed, herpes zoster only occurs in those who already had chickenpox some years previously; it represents a localized recrudescence of activity following an indeterminate period of viral dormancy in the related sensory ganglia. Increasing age and malignancy are two important activators.

After a prodromal period of fever and malaise combined with a burning or tingling sensation in the affected area, small erythematous macules appear and quickly become vesicular and painful. Cloudy vesicularization and crusting follow in sequence over a period of 5-10 days. Regional lymphadenopathy may be prominent. Although lesions usually are limited to one or two ipsilateral thoracic dermatomes, selected cranial nerves (trigeminal, IV or VI) also can be involved and may be complicated by meningeal irritation, encephalitis, paralysis, extra-ocular muscle weakness, ptosis, mydriasis, and/or keratoconjunctivitis. Zoster of the external ear with ipsilateral facial palsy is termed the Ramsay Hunt syndrome. Most patients recover from zoster without sequelae, although the pain may last from 2-4 weeks or more.

Diagnosis is based on clinical symptoms. Multinucleated giant cells and intranuclear inclusions may be demonstrated by the same techniques as for herpes simplex. There is no specific treatment. Burow's solution compresses followed by the application of zinc oxide lotion or calamine lotion may be soothing. Various topical anesthetic agents may offer temporary relief. If uveitis occurs, an ophthalmologist should be consulted immediately.

Hyperhidrosis
The complaint of excessive perspiration of palms, soles, and axillae is not uncommon among adolescents. Most frequently it is idiopathic or psychogenic. Hyperhidrosis also may be associated with systemic conditions such as hypoglycemia, Graves' disease, acromegaly, pheochromocytoma, certain infections (tuberculosis, brucellosis), and familial dysautonomia.

Treatment of idiopathic hyperhidrosis is symptomatic with topical agents the line of primary defense. These include the following:
1. Starch or talc to absorb excess moisture
2. 20% aluminum chloride (Drysol solution)
3. 2%-5% tannic acid in solution
4. 5%-20% formalin solution in water or alcohol
5. The stronger commercial antiperspirants (Mitchum)

When the above are unsuccessful and excessive perspiration is genuinely handicapping, systemic agents may be considered. These focus on inhibiting sympathetic nerve activity and include methenamine, diphemanil methylsulfate (Prantal), propantheline bromide (Propantheline), and sedation with barbiturates, antihistamines, or weak tranquilizers. In truly desperate cases surgical excision of the area of greatest sweat production and sympathectomy are potential options.

Nail Disorders
INGROWN TOENAIL
When the leading edge of a toenail (usually the lateral aspect of the large toenail) becomes imbedded in the skin, the result is an ingrown toenail. Usually this is due to improperly cut nails (too short) or tight shoes compressing the nail. The area becomes red, tender, and swollen; sometimes a purulent discharge may be present, sometimes granulation tissue. Acute treatment consists of warm soaks, topical or systemic antibiotics, and weekly cauterization of

granulation tissue with silver nitrate until the inflammation has quieted down. Calloused tissue should be pared at this time. Thereafter, the patient should be instructed to cut the nails straight across and to leave them long enough to extend beyond the soft tissue. A wisp of cotton can be placed under the nail to force growth outward and reduce chances of recurrence. In persistent cases, surgery may be necessary to remove part or all of the offending nail.

ACUTE PARONYCHIA

Acute paronychia is the superficial infection of a finger at the nail base and usually is due to *Staphylococcus aureus.* The involved area is painful, red, tender, and edematous; it may progress to an abscess with yellow-green purulent material collecting under the cuticle and nail. Black or greenish black purulent material suggests a *Proteus* or *Pseudomonas* infection. A paronychia should be distinguished from a deeper infection involving the digital pulp or a felon. This is a far more serious infection and may result in deep ischemic necrosis and osteomyelitis of underlying bone. Treatment of a paronychia involves warm soaks, nail puncturing, or incision of the lateral skin region to allow for drainage of any accumulated pus, and appropriate topical or systemic antibiotic administration. Treatment of a felon similarly involves soaks and drainage but with closer attention to systemic antibiotics and follow-up for possible complications.

CHRONIC PARONYCHIA

Candida albicans may cause a chronic infection in which all the nails are thick, grooved, and yellow-brown while the cuticle is red and edematous. The nail plate is not friable or cracked and there is no accumulation of subungual debris or purulent material, differentiating this condition from infection with tinea unguium or bacteria, respectively. Diabetes mellitus and frequent exposure to water are common precipitants. Treatment includes partial removal of the nail edge or nail plate with daily application of nystatin cream or amphotericin B ointment for several weeks.

Lichen Planus

Lichen planus is a chronic dermatitis characterized by scaly, polygonal, flat-topped papules variably but symmetrically distributed on the flexor surfaces of forearms or wrists, lateral aspects of the neck, or thighs and any aspect of the shins, lower back, or penis. The lesions are violescent or purplish and pruritic. Criss-crossed, faint gray lines (Wickham's striae) are usually evident on examination with a hand lens after application of mineral oil. With time, the papules may become umbilicated or may coalesce to form larger, extensive plaques. Additional lesions are apt to occur at sites of cutaneous injury or exposure to strong sunlight in predisposed individuals. Other manifestations of lichen planus include the formation of white linear lesions on the buccal mucosa, conjunctivae, pharynx or larynx, and follicular scalp papules that may atrophy and result in alopecia. Hypertrophic, atrophic, linear, annular, and bullous lichen planus are variations of the classic form.

Diagnosis is based on the clinical appearance and biopsy if the appearance is unclear. Differential considerations include leukoplakia, secondary syphilis, tinea infection, neurodermatitis, psoriasis, pityriasis rosea, and atopic dermatitis (eczema).

Treatment is symptomatic. Systemic or topical steroids, antihistamines (to counter pruritus), and/or griseofulvin (Table 14-5) are often used with variable benefit. In the majority of cases, the lesions resolve spontaneously within 12-18 months. In rare cases, however, the condition persists; squamous cell or epidermal cancer has been reported to occur in such chronic sites and periodic surveillance for this possibility is indicated.

Molluscum Contagiosum

Caused by a large pox virus with an incubation period of 2-8 weeks, molluscum contagiosum is spread by close physical contact of any sort, including sexual intercourse. Single or multiple lesions measuring 2-4 mm in diameter appear most commonly on the face, trunk, abdomen, groin, genitalia, and/or flexural areas. They appear as discrete, flesh-colored, or pearly gray papules with a central umbilication containing white curdy material. Several papules may coalesce to form a larger plaque. Some lesions may become inflamed and macerated due to secondary bacterial infection. Molluscum contagiosum poses special problems for patients with atopic dermatitis or on chronic steroid administration in their predisposition to develop thousands of widely disseminated lesions.

Clinical appearance alone often is sufficient for diagnosis. Supporting tests include the finding of intracytoplasmic inclusion bodies on microscopic examination of tissue from a lesion using potassium hydroxide or Wright, Giemsa, Gram, or Papanicolaou stain. A biopsy is definitive.

Many lesions resolve spontaneously over 4-9 months, but some remain for years. Treatment of unsightly or persistent papules may be by either of the following caustic agents:

1. Application of saturated (20%) trichloro-acetic acid at weekly intervals.

2. Application of 25% podophyllin tincture twice a week

In using either of these agents, considerable caution should be taken to avoid spillage onto normal tissue and instructing the patient to wash it off after 2-4 hours. Cantharidin, liquid nitrogen, curettage, and electrodesiccation may also be useful techniques. Puncturing the surface of a lesion with a scalpel and expressing the content with a comedo extractor before applying a topical agent may improve the potential for cure in resistant cases. Oral griseofulvin (Table 14-5) may help when lesions are large or extensive.

Pediculosis

Three types of lice may infest humans: *Phthirus capitis*, *P. corporis*, and *P. pubis*, involving the scalp, body, and genital regions, respectively. *P. pubis* (and sometimes *P. capitis*) also may locate on eyelashes and brows, causing phthiriasis palpebrarum. All produce a similar dermatitis, distinguishable only by location, consequent to the louse bite and the intradermal extrusion of an irritant salivary substance. Pediculosis consists of intensely pruritic, erythematous papules randomly distributed over the affected area. Both old and new lesions are evident at any one time. The picture may be complicated by extensive excoriations, hemorrhagic crustations, and/or secondary pyodermas due to scratching; these can mask the true state of affairs. Further diagnostic points are reviewed under appropriate subheadings.

Treatment varies somewhat, depending on the type of pediculosis, but a number of general measures should be taken in all cases:

1. Providing symptomatic relief of itching with any soothing lotion (calamine, Caladryl) or the use of systemic antipruritic agents (cyproheptadine).

2. Attention to any coexisting bacterial infection with topical or systemic antibiotics, depending on severity (*Staphylococcus aureus* is usually involved).

3. Laundering or dry cleaning all contact clothing, bedding, and so forth. DDT powder or equivalent may be dusted on objects that cannot be washed or cleaned.

4. Examining all family members and friends for nits (eggs) or lesions. A single application of a specific agent (see following discussion) if *P. capitis* or *P. pubis* is involved is a wise precaution for all contacts to take regardless of whether or not clinical evidence of infection exists.

PEDICULOSIS CAPITIS

The head louse inhabits the hair and scalp throughout its life cycle. Nits (eggs) are deposited near the base of hair shafts and are visible under a hand lens as single tiny white ovoid masses firmly adherent to the hair (this distinguishes nits from dandruff flakes, which are similar to the naked eye). Examination of nits under a microscope reveals either empty shells (if already hatched) or the larval form lying within. Treatment is with 1% gamma benzene hexachloride (Kwell), as shampoo or lotion. Two applications (4 minutes of the shampoo or overnight for the lotion) 1 week to 10 days apart (the second to kill unhatched eggs that survive the first application) are curative. Combing the wet hair after shampooing with a fine tooth comb is recommended to remove nits.

PEDICULOSIS CORPORIS

The body louse lives in seams of bedding and clothing, visiting humans only to feed. Neither lice nor nits will be found on physical examination, the only evidence being the rash. This may be located on any hairless part of the body but is commonly noted in the interscapular region of the back. Treatment consists only of the general measures previously described (gamma benzene hexachloride is not indicated). If dealing with an institutional situation and more than one or two residents are infected, special fumigation procedures with DDT or Lindane may be indicated.

PEDICULOSIS PUBIS (CRAB LICE)

Like *P. capitis*, *P. pubis* lives out its life cycle on the human body, predominantly in pubic hair. Usually sexually transmitted, it also may be disseminated in crowded schools and institutions simply through close contact. In addition to the presence of nits and louse-bite lesions, maculae caeruleae (sky-blue spots) may be noted; these are usually transient, nonblanching, bluish spots on the upper arms, trunk, or thighs and represent intradermal blood pigment or lice excretions. Treatment of pubic lice consists of two applications 1 week apart (as for *P. capitis*) of one of the following:

1. 1% gamma benzene hexachloride (Kwell, Lindane) as shampoo, cream, or lotion; 4 minutes for the shampoo and overnight for cream or lotion.

2. 25% benzyl benzoate lotion overnight.

3. DDT powder dusted on area.

The patient should also be examined for other sexually transmitted diseases, including gonorrhea and syphilis.

PEDICULOSIS PALPEBRARUM

Eyebrows and eyelashes are a less common, but noted location for *P. pubis* (or *P capitis*). Agents used to treat infestations of other sites cannot be used in this location. Simple petrolatum or yellow mercuric oxide should be applied to the brows and lashes twice a day for 7–9 days followed by removal of nits with a fine tooth comb. An alternative treatment is the application of a sterile 0.25% physostigmine ophthalmic ointment to the eyelid margin twice daily for 1–3 days; miosis, however, may be an undesirable side effect.

Pityriasis Rosea

Pityriasis rosea consists of a self-limited, symmetric papulosquamous rash of the trunk and proximal extremities. The onset is marked by a single large herald patch measuring several centimeters in diameter and appearing a few days or weeks before the onset of a generalized eruption; the herald patch may be missed easily by the patient, however, as it is asymptomatic and often located on body parts not readily seen such as the back. On the other hand, remnants of the herald patch may still be visible when the generalized rash emerges and should be looked for carefully as a specific diagnostic sign.

Generalized lesions measure several millimeters to a little over a centimeter in diameter but may be confluent and appear as larger irregularly shaped macules. The borders have loose rims of scales, which peel peripherally giving a "collarette" appearance. The long axis of ovoid macules tends to follow skin cleavage dermatome lines. Symptoms can include mild degrees of malaise, fever, and pruritus, or the patient may be asymptomatic. Nail pitting occurs in some cases.

Diagnosis is based on clinical findings. In the absence of historic or clinical evidence of a herald patch, differential considerations include tinea corporis, secondary syphilis, drug eruptions, viral exanthems, lichen planus, guttate parapsoriasis, pityriasis alba, and others.

Treatment is symptomatic. Distressing pruritus may be relieved by phenolated lotions or antihistamines. Steroids may be beneficial in rare instances of severe disease. Spontaneous clearing without sequellae usually occurs within 3–9 weeks.

Psoriasis

Psoriasis is a chronic papulosquamous dermatitis often first appearing during adolescence. It is characterized by a particularly rapid epidermal cell turnover rate with resultant epidermal hyperplasia. It affects 2% of the United States population and is inherited as an autosomal dominant trait with incomplete penetrance. Emotional and physical stress as well as a variety of other factors have been thought implicated in producing manifest disease in genetically vulnerable individuals, but in most instances there are no clear-cut precipitants.

The classic lesion consists of a discrete erythematous plaque or papule from several millimeters to several centimeters in diameter and covered with white or silvery scales. Even the gentlest removal of one or two scales will induce bleeding from capillary loops (Auspitz' sign). Psoriasis is most likely to appear on the scalp, elbows, knees, and lower back with the scalp a common site of initiation. Lesions also frequently develop on scratch marks or traumatized areas (Koebner phenomenon). The extent of the rash is unpredictable, varying from only one or several small, discrete, patches to extensive confluent disease covering a large portion of the body. The course tends to be equally unpredictable, marked by variable exacerbations and remissions, either of which may last from a few weeks or months to many years. The nails also are commonly involved with punctate pitting, subungual hyperkeratosis, oil spots, or onycholysis.

In most instances, the primary symptoms are pruritus and the emotional consequences of an unsightly chronic rash, a particularly serious issue in the adolescent. Severe forms of psoriasis, however, bear additional burdens in the potential complications of psoriatic arthritis and uveitis; either may be significantly handicapping.

Treatment of relatively limited disease can be carried out by the primary physician through the frequent application of steroid creams, coal tar ointments, or both. Sunlight also is beneficial, although appropriate precautions should be taken against sunburn through limited exposure or application of a PABA-containing tanning lotion. New treatment modalities include the use of psoralen with ultraviolet A light exposure (PUVA) and the use of etretinate (an experimental synthetic retinoid). Effective treatment of extensive disease, however, is a complex process and belongs in the hands of an experienced dermatologist. More severe forms also require continued monitoring for uveitis and psoriatic arthritis.

Scabies

Scabies, caused by the microscopic arthropod *Sarcoptes scabiei, var. hominis*, is transmitted by close contact with an infected individual or contaminated clothing and tends to have a predilection for the flexor surfaces of the wrists, finger web spaces, genitalia, axillae, intragluteal folds, umbilicus, and the periareolar region of the breast. It produces an intensely pruritic rash characterized by three different types of lesions. Fewest in number but most distinctive are the burrows of invading females, which appear as papular erythematous lines from 5-15 mm in length and 2-3 mm in width. Most numerous are erythematous circular papules accompanying the temporary intracutaneous invasion of larval forms. Some individuals also may demonstrate vesicles with an erythematous base due to host sensitization. In contrast to most nonarthropod papular rashes, both old and new lesions usually are present simultaneously. The dermatologic picture may further be complicated by excoriations, scabs, and pyodermas due to scratching. As scabies is commonly transmitted by sexual contact, other sexually transmitted diseases may be present as well.

Diagnosis can usually be made on the bases of the typical lesions and location. Scrapings of a burrow or papule (using a scalpel blade) placed on a slide with mineral oil or 10% KOH and examined under the microscope may reveal adult mites, eggs, or scybala (fecal pellets). A biopsy will reveal similar findings. The patient, the entire family, and intimate friends or sexual partners should be treated with an application of one of the following:

1. 1% gamma benzene hexachloride cream or lotion (Kwell, Lindane).

2. 10% crotamiton cream or lotion (Eurax).

3. 12.5%–25% benzyl benzoate emulsion.

4. 5%–10% precipitated sulfur in petrolatum.

The selected substance is applied to the entire body after a tepid shower and shampoo at bedtime and washed off the following morning. All family members, physically intimate friends, and sexual partners also should be treated once. The patient, however, should be treated again in 7 days to be sure of killing mites that have hatched since the first treatment. Clothing and bedding should be washed, dry cleaned, or thoroughly dusted with DDT or Lindane powder. The patient should be advised that pruritus due to the hypersensitivity state may persist for several days to weeks even though the mites have been killed and should not be mistaken for inadequate treatment (although the disease may recur if treatment of contacts, clothing, and so on have been incomplete).

Tinea (Dermatophytid) Infections

Superficial skin infections by the dermatophytid fungi are termed tineas. They are further subdivided according to the area involved: tinea capitis, corporis, cruris, manuum, and unguium of the head,

body, genital region, hands, or nails respectively. Two additional forms are identified by their production of characteristic pigmentary changes: tinea nigra and tinea versicolor. Tineas can pose difficult diagnostic and management problems; they can mimic a wide variety of other dermatoses, frequently resist standard treatment measures, and commonly recur after effective treatment. They also are associated with nonfungal hypersensitivity "id" reactions which appear as vesicular or squamous rashes, sometimes quite distant from the actual site of infection. An id reaction usually is coincident with the acute phase of the fungal lesion and fades with effective antifungal treatment.

Diagnosis is based on the clinical appearance as described in the following sections. Many of the causal fungi also fluoresce under a Wood's light. Scrapings of scales from the margin of a lesion placed in a drop of 10%–30% potassium hydroxide (KOH) on a slide, covered with a coverslip and examined under a microscope (after standing 10–20 minutes), will reveal hyphae and spores in positive specimens. (Note: Material from an id reaction will not be revealing.) Culture of scraped scales on Sabouraud's or Littman's media is another useful diagnostic tool.

Treatment of the tineas varies somewhat, depending on the site, and utilizes topical agents or systemic griseofulvin when the infection is extensive, severe, or recalcitrant. As a general principle, household contacts, including dogs and cats should be examined and treated if also infected. A new antifungal agent is now available, ketoconazole (Nizoral). It is proving to be very effective for many chronic and/or severe fungal infections.

TINEA CAPITIS

Tineas of the scalp produce localized scaly patches of variable appearance according to the causal agent. They are commonly associated with thinning or loss of hair, but this is differentiated from alopecia areata in that the hair breaks off at the base of the shaft rather than being lost in its entirety, giving a stubbled, rather than smooth, appearance. *Microsporum audouini* infection usually produces relatively circumscribed, noninflammatory lesions, whereas *M. canis* (from dogs and cats) or *M. gypseum* (from soil) causes more widespread inflammation. Diffuse scaling and thinning of the hair is characteristic of *Trichophyton vialaceum* or *T. tonsurans*.

Kerion is a deep suppurative boggy form of fungal infection occurring on the scalp, nape of the neck, and beard areas, sometimes resembling a carbuncle with follicular pustules, exudate, and crusting; most common organisms involved are *M. canis*, *M. gypseum*, *T. mentagrophytes*, and *T. verrucosum*.

Diagnosis is based on clinical appearance and the tests previously described; *T. mentagrophytes*, *T. verrucosum*, and *M. gypseum*, however, do not fluoresce.

To treat the condition, the hairs around the lesion should be clipped and the scalp washed daily with mild shampoo. If scaling, crusting, or matting is severe, 5%–10% ammoniated mercury ointment can be applied once or twice a day. Specific treatment consists of oral griseofulvin administered for 4–6 weeks or even longer (Table 14-5). Kerion, however, is not particularly responsive to griseofulvin; on the other hand, it usually is self-limited and clears with time, although scarring may result. Incision and drainage of kerion is *not* indicated.

TINEA CORPORIS

One or more mildly pruritic lesions tend to first appear on exposed areas of the skin, commonly on the arms or face. Initially measuring a centimeter or so, they expand slowly outward over weeks and months, ultimately covering quite large areas. Appearance is that of a faintly erythematous and slightly raised patch with finely vesicular and scaling borders. As a lesion progresses outward, central clearing occurs, giving an annular appearance.

Diagnosis is by clinical appearance, together with culture and KOH preparation (see previous discussion). *M. audouini* is most commonly involved. Differential considerations include pityriasis rosea, seborrheic dermatitis, psoriasis, tinea versicolor, pyoderma, neurodermatitis, nummular eczema, atopic dermatitis, contact dermatitis, and secondary syphilis.

Small lesions usually respond well to twice daily applications of one of the following topical antifungal agents. Treatment should be maintained for 2–4 weeks or even longer.

1. 1% clotrimazole (Lotrimin cream or solution).

2. 1% haloprogin (Halotex cream or solution).

3. 2% miconazole nitrate (MicaTin cream or lotion).

4. 1% tolnaftate (Tinactin cream or solution).

Systemic treatment usually is required for more extensive disease and employs griseofulvin for 2–8 weeks (Table 14-5).

TINEA CRURIS

Fungal infection of the groin can be due to *T. rubrum*, *T. mentagrophytes*, or *Epidermophyton floccosum*. The rash presents as a moderately pruritic

---

**TABLE 14-5
GRISEOFULVIN**

1. Characteristics: An antifungal antibiotic isolated from *Penicillium griseofulvin*, which accumulates in keratinizing cells and interferes with fungal nucleic acid synthesis.

2. Administration: It is best absorbed with lipids and should be taken after meals, particularly after drinking milk.

3. Usual dose:

a. microcrystalline form: 0.5–1.0 g/day (under 100 pounds: 5 mg/lb/day)

b. ultramicrosize form: 250–500 mg/day (under 100 pounds: 2.5 mg/lb/day)

4. Antagonistic drugs: Reduced blood levels are noted if taken with certain drugs such as phenobarbital.

5. Side effects: Headache, nausea, mild fatigue, dermatitis, photosensitivity, transient leukopenia; exacerbates or precipitates porphyria; reduces coumadin activity; and exacerbates liver failure.

---

eruption in the inguinal, perineal, and inner upper thigh regions. It may spread to the buttocks, gluteal cleft, or lower abdomen, but the labia and scrotum are usually spared. Most commonly, lesions are annular with raised, erythematous, scaly borders and clearing centers. But the pattern varies; some cases show no central clearing, some evidence a more inflammatory picture, while others have areas of vesiculation. *T. rubrum* characteristically presents with a nonspecific erythematous papular rash.

Particular conditions to be considered in the differential diagnosis are candidiasis, intertrigo, and erythrasma (infection with *Corynebacterium minutissimum*). Both candidiasis and tinea cruris will be positive for hyphae and spores on KOH preparations, but cultures using a dermatophyte test medium will only change color (orange to red) with tinea cruris. Other differential considerations are the same as those given for tinea corporis.

Treatment consists of a topical antifungal agent (see tinea corporis) or oral griseofulvin (Table 14-5). Preventive measures include attention to personal hygiene, the wearing of loose rather than tight-fitting clothing, and the application of powders that absorb perspiration, reduce maceration, and inhibit fungal growth (Cruex powder). If coexistent, tinea pedis should also be treated, as it may be a source of reinfection.

TINEA PEDIS

Usually due to *T. rubrum* (and sometimes *T. mentagrophytes* or *E. floccosum*), tinea pedis commonly starts in the web space between the fourth and fifth toes and then spreads to other toes. It is characterized by clusters of small vesicles with surrounding erythema and scaling, but this appearance may be masked by both tissue maceration and secondary infection. In the latter instance, typical pruritic symptoms may be accompanied by pain and discomfort. Differential considerations include moniliasis, vesicular dyshidrosis, atopic dermatitis, contact dermatitis, psoriasis of the palms and soles, soft corns, and plantar warts. A KOH preparation and fungal culture (including color change on special media; see tinea cruris) are positive.

Secondary bacterial infection should be eradicated with Burow's solution compresses and topical or systemic antibiotics. Topical antifungal agents or oral griseofulvin (see tinea corporis and Table 14-5) should then be used but often require administration from several weeks to 2-3 months to be effective. Undecylenic acid (Verdefam cream or solution) may be used as a peeling agent in areas of thickened skin where other topical agents will not penetrate. Preventive measures include frequent change of socks, reduction of hyperhidrosis (antiperspirant agents; dilute formaldehyde solutions), and frequent use of powdered starch, talcum powder, or antifungal powder (Desenex foot powder). Recurrence is common.

TINEA MANUUM

Dermatophytid infection of the palms with unilateral prominence of palmar creases and scaling is caused by the same agents as cause tinea pedis or cruris. Indeed, all three fungal forms of disease can coexist. The KOH preparation and cultures are positive. Treatment is as for other forms with topical antifungal agents, griseofulvin and undecylenic acid.

TINEA UNGUIUM

Tinea unguium (onychomycosis) is also caused by the agents that cause tinea pedis or cruris; one or two distal nail sections of either fingers or toes become thickened and cracked. Opaque, yellow material accumulates in the distal nail bed and the nails crumble easily. Differential considerations include chronic paronychia due to bacteria or *Candida albicans*, nail changes associated with vascular disease or psoriasis, and trauma. The culture is positive.

Treatment is with griseofulvin (Table 14-5). Since the drug is deposited in the nail plate matrix and only reaches the distal, infected region through growth, it must be given for 4-6 months for a fingernail and 6-12 months for a toenail. Surgical removal of the diseased nail is often necessary for recal-

citrant cases with oral griseofulvin continued for 2-3 months thereafter. Recurrences are common.

TINEA VERSICOLOR

Tinea versicolor is a superficial infection of the stratum corneum caused by *Pityrosporum ovale* (formerly *Malassezia furfur*), a dimorphic fungus normally present as a skin saprophyte in its yeast form. Factors precipitating the disease state include increased warmth and humidity, hyperhidrosis, poor hygiene, oral contraceptives, pregnancy, steroids, Cushing's disease, malnutrition, chronic infection, and genetic predisposition. Frequently no underlying cause can be found.

The disease interferes with pigment transfer and is manifested in noninflammatory, finely scaled hyperpigmented or hypopigmented lesions, which may demonstrate various color changes, including white, yellow-tan, light brown, and dark brown. Patches may be single and discretely round or ovoid or multiple and extensively confluent. They are most commonly noted on the upper chest, back, arms, and neck and are rare below the waist.

Differential diagnosis includes pityriasis rosea, drug eruptions, tinea corporis, seborrheic dermatitis, and vitiligo, among others. A KOH preparation is diagnostic in revealing spores surrounded by short plump mycelia or hyphae giving a "spaghetti and meatballs" appearance. Wood's light exposure produces a golden fluorescence.

Selenium sulfide suspension or shampoo (Selsun, Exsel) is effective for large areas. It is applied at bedtime and washed off in the morning for a total of three applications. The use of soap with sulfur and salicylic acid as well as selenium sulfide applications every 2-3 months is helpful to prevent recurrences. It should be kept in mind, however, that overzealous use of selenium may cause hair loss, brittle nails, skin irritation, nausea and vomiting, photosensitivity, eczema, hyperhidrosis, dizziness, and lethargy. Other treatment regimens include Tinver lotion (25% sodium thiosulfate, 1% salicylic acid, and other ingredients) or acrisorcin cream (Akrinol) applied twice a day for 7-14 days and other topical fungicides (see tinea corporis). The patient should be advised that it may take several months for the color change to resolve, even though the infection is well under control.

TINEA NIGRA

Tinea nigra, a superficial fungal infection, is caused by *Cladosporium wernecki* and manifests in flat dark-brown to blackish patches, which usually (but not invariably) appear on the hands. The major differential consideration is malignant melanoma; although tinea nigra is more often misdiagnosed as melanoma than vice versa. The KOH preparation demonstrates brown mycelia and culture is positive. Topical antifungal agents as for tinea corporis are effective.

Urticaria

The sudden onset of transient cutaneous wheals lasting from several to 48 hours is termed acute urticaria. Recurrent episodes over 2-6 weeks or more are called chronic urticaria. Giant hives extending below the dermis and involving subcutaneous tissue comprise angioedema.

Urticaria is a common phenomenon, with 20% or more of young adults having had at least one episode during their childhood or adolescence. The etiology is usually obscure, but there is an association in some cases with those factors cited in Table 14-6. Idiopathic and psychogenic factors account for the majority of instances of *chronic* urticaria.

Specific treatment is based on identifying and eliminating precipitating agents. Nonspecific, symptomatic measures primarily employ one or another of the antihistamines, for example, diphenhydramine hydrochloride (Benadryl), chlorpheniramine maleate (Chlor-Trimeton), cyproheptadine hydrochloride (Periactin), or hydroxyzine (Atarax, Vistaril). Daily dosage is adjusted to that which fully suppresses the hives and is then tapered slowly. If sedation is an unacceptable side effect with one agent, another can be tried. Cimetidine and terbutaline may help some patients with chronic urticaria.

Other potentially useful measures include a diet free of salicylates or penicillins or a 2-week trial of nystatin and tetracycline with a yeast-free diet; these measures should be followed by griseofulvin (Table 14-5). Special "elimination" diets are beneficial in some instances. Psychogenic causes should be looked for as well, although most adolescents evidence stress at some time or other and this etiology should not be oversubscribed.

In any event, chronic urticaria resolves by 6 months in half of all cases and by 5 years in 70%.

Verrucae

Verrucae, or warts, are benign epidermal tumors caused by the human wart virus (papilloma or polyoma virus; papovavirus). The virus enters the body through skin abrasions, with warts tending to occur nearby following an incubation period of 2-3 months. Other contributing factors to their development include hyperhidrosis, puberty, pregnancy, and diabetes mellitus. Autoinoculation can occur.

The peak incidence for the appearance of warts is between 12 and 16 years. Spontaneous cure is common with 20%-30% resolving in 6 months and 65% resolving in 2 years; only a few remain over 5 years. Table 14-7 gives specific clinical manifestations of various kinds of warts.

TREATMENT

Table 14-8 cites specific treatment modalities. No one method is effective in all cases, although treatment of single warts or warts of short duration usually is easiest. Other general measures include avoiding recognized precipitants (nail and hangnail biting, shaving, coitus, excessive heat, depending on the type and location of the wart) and the use of individual towels to reduce spread to others. Protective footwear may be needed for plantar warts. Common warts respond well to cryotherapy or topical agents such as salicylic acid with lactic acid, Cantharone, or 40% salicylic acid plasters. Flat warts often respond well to 30% trichloroacetic acid or one of the keratolytic agents. Plantar warts may do well if pared with a scalpel blade not quite to the point of bleeding; a 40% salicylic acid plaster should then be applied. The use of keratolytic agents requires some caution because excessive tissue lysis may progress to the point of ulceration. Daily application for 4–5 days should be followed by a rest period of similar duration to permit healing of any injured normal tissue. Treatment may be continued in this cyclical manner until all evidence of the wart is removed.

CONDYLOMATA ACUMINATA

Condylomata acuminata, or anogenital warts, are of particular significance for sexually active adolescents and comprise one of the sexually transmitted diseases (Chapter 17). This verrucous wart also is caused by a papilloma virus with an incubation period of several weeks to months. It often is associated with other sexually transmitted diseases as well, and the patient should be evaluated accordingly with gonococcal culture, syphilis serology, and other tests as symptoms indicate.

The lesions have a cauliflower or strawberry appearance and are white to pink-red in color. They can involve any part of the genitals (labia, vagina, urethra, penis, anus, anal canal) and also may appear in and around the oral cavity. Vaginal discharge, poor hygiene, hyperhidrosis, and pregnancy may contribute to furthering the lesion's growth. Resistance to treatment is noted in those with insulin-dependent diabetes mellitus and those with immunosuppressive disorders. It also is not uncommon for patients to delay presentation for treatment until

TABLE 14-6
ETIOLOGIC CLASSIFICATION OF URTICARIA

Type	Description	Treatment
Dermographism (factitious urticaria)	Exaggerated triple response of Lewis, elicited by stroking the skin. Very tight clothes may precipitate. Salicylates can be a major factor.	Salicylate-free diet if there is a measurable salicylate level in the blood. Antihistamines, especially hydroxyzine.
Cholinergic urticaria	Small (2–3 mm) evanescent wheals precipitated by sweat-producing stimuli (exercise, sauna, emotion). Intradermal injection of 0.02% Mecholyl or 1:100,000 nicotine produces a large wheal with flare and studding of smaller wheals.	Antihistamines: hydroxyzine.
Cold urticaria	Urticaria in response to cold (as ice on the skin, cold weather). Can be hereditary or acquired; can be associated with cryoglobulinemia, cryofibrinoginemia, systemic lupus erythematosus or paroxysmal cold hemoglobinuria.	Limited. Large penicillin doses. Cyproheptadine hydrochloride (Periactin).
Solar urticaria	Urticaria in response to sunlight. Face and hands usually spared.	Protective clothes, PABA sunscreens, antihistamines (high dose).
Infectious urticaria	Urticaria in response to various infections, including infectious mononucleosis, infectious hepatitis, *Candida albicans*, parasites (amoeba, helminths), tinea infections, and others. Look for occult bacterial infection of the teeth, sinuses, gallbladder, pelvis, prostate, urinary tract.	Treat underlying disease if possible. Antihistamines.
Inhalent urticaria	Urticaria in response to inhalent allergens: aerosols, animal danders, dust, mold, others.	Reduce exposure, desensitization program, antihistamines.
Food urticaria	Urticaria due to various foods: shellfish, strawberries, food additives (azo dyes, benzoates), alcohol, coffee, others.	Avoid offending food. Antihistamines.
Urticaria due to drug allergies	Many drugs may produce urticaria in sensitive individuals. Aspirin, indomethacin, tartrazine, penicillin, laxatives, analgesics, sedatives, others. Angioedema, respiratory obstruction, and urticaria occur with aspirin or indomethacin ingestion in some. Some patients have aspirin sensitivity syndrome: rhinitis, nasal polyposis, and asthma with aspirin allergy.	Avoid offending drug. Antihistamines. Treat the anaphylaxis.
Hereditary angioedema	Deficiency of inhibitor of complement C_1 esterase (either absolute deficiency or the presence of nonfunctional esterase). Development of edema in skin, mucous membrane (including bowel), airway, and others, either spontaneously or following trauma or infection. Positive serum Cylenol test.	*Prevention:* Danazol; epsilon aminocaproic acid; tranexamic acid. *Treatment:* 0.5 ml SQ 1:1,000 epinephrine; 15–30 mg ephedrine sulfate.
Miscellaneous	Collagen disease (SLE), vasculitis, malignancy (lymphoma), amyloidosis, thyrotoxicosis, psychogenic (25%), heat urticaria, aquagenic urticaria, urticaria pigmentosa, systemic mastocytosis, porphyria, others.	Identify the underlying etiology; treatment varies.

TABLE 14-7
TYPES OF VERRUCAE (WARTS)

Type	Description
Common wart (verrucae vulgaris)	Deep-seated, translucent, or flesh-colored or gray-brown shiny papules or nodules that appear on dorsum of fingers, hands, and distal forearms. They can become verrucous, hyperkeratotic lesions 0.5–1 cm in diameter. Multiple, small black dots (thrombosed capillary loops) are noted within the verrucous lesion. May become periungual or subungual. May be confused with keratosis or fibromas.
Flat or plane wart (verrucae planae)	Multiple, flat, tan to yellow-pink, 2–4 mm papules with a granular surface; common on the face, neck, forearms, and dorsa of the hand. Pruritus can occur, as well as plaques due to the warts coalescing. The differential diagnosis includes acne, seborrheic keratosis, epidermal nevi, and freckles.
Filiform wart	Slender, fingerlike, filiform warts on the face (especially around the eyes or the eyelids) and neck. Range is between 1–10 mm. Cornification can occur.
Condyloma acuminata	See text.
Plantar wart	Starts as a deep-seated, translucent papule on the plantar surface of the foot and does not become raised or verrucous due to constant weight bearing. Tends to be isolated, painful, smooth, sharply demarcated keratotic lesion with multiple capillary bleeding points if scraped with a surgical blade. Spreads to the surrounding area as several large, hyperkeratotic, less painful plaques (mosaic warts). Can occur on the fingers as well. Differential diagnosis includes corns, calluses, foreign body reactions, painful scars.

TABLE 14-8
TREATMENT MODALITIES FOR WARTS

1. Topical applications (o.d. or b.i.d.)*
   a. 16.7% salicylic acid with 16.7% lactic acid in a 5%–16% flexible collodion (Duofilm)*
   b. 0.7% cantharidin in flexible collodion (Cantharone)
   c. 40% salicylic acid plasters, with or without trichloroacetic acid or formalin
   d. 30% Trichloroacetic acid
   e. 5% ammoniated mercury ointment
   f. Benzoyl peroxide lotion (5%–10%)
   g. Retinoic acid (0.1% cream, 0.025% gel)
2. Cryotherapy (carbon dioxide snow or liquid nitrogen)
3. Surgery
   a. Curettage
   b. Cautery (electrocautery; silver nitrate)
   c. Diathermy
   d. Fulguration
4. Combinations (2 or 3 with 1 and others)
5. Immunotherapy
6. Time (leave alone; many resolve spontaneously)

*See text for precautions.

the lesions are very advanced due to the embarrassing location, the absence of associated symptomatology, and the predilection of some adolescents for denial.

The presence of lesions fitting the above description usually is sufficient for diagnosis. There may be only one or several warts less than a centimeter in diameter, but extensive confluent lesions measuring several centimeters or more are frequently seen. A biopsy can be done if in doubt, but there are few other conditions with a similar appearance. Condyloma latum, a manifestation of secondary syphilis, is the most serious contender and should be ruled out by syphilis serology and/or dark-field examinations. Bowen's disease can appear as multiple verrucous nodules and, if it seems a strong possibility, can be ruled out by biopsy.

Treatment is by the careful application of fresh 3%–25% tincture of podophyllin (podophyllin resin) to the lesion followed by the application of white petrolatum jelly to protect surrounding skin from exposure to this very caustic substance. Also when lesions are fairly extensive, treatment should be carried out in a segmental manner rather than all at once. Following the application of podophyllin and petrolatum, the patient is instructed to leave the material on for 2–4 hours and then to wash the area thoroughly with warm soap and water. Treatment should be at weekly intervals until all the warts are cleared. The patient also should be advised that the infection can be transmitted to a sexual partner and temporary restraint from sexual intimacy advised.

Topical chemotherapeutic agents (dinitrochlorobenzene, 5-fluorouracil) have been used to supplement podophyllin in resistant cases. Curettage, electrodesiccation, or surgical excision are required in some cases, particularly for singularly extensive lesions and those invading the urethra, vagina, or rectum, where podophyllin applications pose a formidable challenge. Immunotherapy with an autogenous vaccine prepared from excised warts also has been resorted to with variable success.

Vitiligo

Vitiligo is an idiopathic skin condition affecting 1%–2% of the population and manifesting in patchy areas of skin depigmentation. It often develops in a symmetric manner over such bony prominences as those of the wrists, knees, and ankles. The course is slow and unpredictable, but reversal of the process with repigmentation is unusual. Lesions appear as irregular patches of totally pigmentless skin. In dark-skinned individuals a partially depigmented or hyperpigmented border may be noted. An erythematous border is evident in an occasional case and can be mistaken for tinea corporis, tinea versicolor, pityriasis rosea, discoid lupus erythematosus, or lichen sclerosis et atrophicus. The etiology is unknown, and many cases are in otherwise normal, healthy individuals. Some instances of vitiligo, however, have been associated with Graves' disease (hyperthyroidism), chronic lymphocytic thyroiditis, pernicious anemia, diabetes mellitus, Addison's disease, hypoparathyroidism, and alopecia areata.

No treatment regularly results in normal repigmentation, although photochemotherapy (oral psoralens plus long-range ultraviolet light or PUVA) may be beneficial in some cases. Special custom cosmetics applied to mask the affected area offers the best approach. Vitiliginous patches are highly sensitive to sunburn and a 100% PABA sunscreen should be applied before sun exposure.

Bibliography

Ad Hoc Committee Report. 1975. Systemic antibiotics for treatment of acne vulgaris. *Arch. Dermatol.* 111:1630.

Callen, J. P., editor. 1982. Symposium on skin diseases. *Med. Clin. North Am.* 66(4):769–963.

Cohn, R. L. 1980. Current status of acne treatment. *Postgrad. Med.* 67:117.

Cram, D. 1980. Psoriasis. *West J. Med.* 133:226.

Flaxman, B. A. 1981. Pruritus: identifying and treating the causes. *Postgrad. Med.* 69:177.

Fragola, L. A., and Watson, P. E. 1981. Common groin eruptions: diagnosis and treatment. *Postgrad. Med.* 69:159.

Frank, S. B., editor. 1976. Symposium on acne. *Cutis* 17:421–608.

Gilchrest, B. A. 1982. Pruritus. Pathogenesis, therapy and significance in systemic disease states. *Arch. Intern. Med.* 142:101.

Hurwitz, S. 1982. Atopic dermatitis. *Pediatr. Ann.* 11:237.

Hurwitz, S. 1981. *Clinical pediatric dermatology. A textbook of skin disorders of children and adolescents.* Philadelphia: W. B. Saunders Co.

Jacobs, A. H., editor 1976. Symposium on pediatric dermatology. *Pediatr. Ann.* 5(12):6–108.

Jarratt, M. 1978. Viral infections of the skin: Herpes simplex, Herpes zoster, warts, and molluscum contagiosum. *Pediatr. Clin. North Am.* 25:339.

Knutson, D. D. 1974. Ultrastructural observations in acne vulgaris: the normal sebaceous follicle and acne lesions. *J. Invest. Dermatol.* 62:288.

Maguire, H. C. 1979. Drug-induced alopecia. *Am. Family Phys.* 19:178.

Mark, L. K. 1978. Chronic granulomatous disease in the adult. *J. Family Pract.* 7:445.

Mauro, J., and Lumpkin, L. R. 1977. Seborrheic dermatitis. *Am. Family Phys.* 15:116.

Melski, J. W., and Arndt, K. A. 1980. Current concepts: topical therapy for acne. *N. Engl. J. Med.* 302:503.

Millikan, L. E. 1976. Alopecia: a systemic approach to diagnosis and therapy. *J. Family Pract.* 3:313.

Monroe, E. W. 1980. Urticaria and urticarial vasculitis. *Med. Clin. North Am.* 64:867.

Norins, A. L., and Treadwell, P. A. 1982. The management of persistent pediatric skin problems. *Pediatr. Clin. North Am.* 29:37.

Olsen, T. G. 1982. Therapy of acne. *Med. Clin. North Am.* 66(4):851–872.

Orkin, M., and Maibach, H. I. 1978. Current concepts in parasitology: this scabies pandemic. *N. Engl. J. Med.* 298:496.

Pochi, P. E. 1982. Oral retinoids in dermatology. *Arch. Dermatol.* 118:57.

Price, V. H. 1978. Disorders of the hair in children. *Pediatr. Clin. North Am.* 25:305.

Quan, M. A.; Rodney, W. M.; and Strick, R. A. 1980. Treatment of acne vulgaris. *J. Family Pract.* 11:1041.

Roberts, S. O. B. 1980. The common fungal diseases of the skin. *Practitioner* 224:506.

Sauer, G. C. 1982. Dermatology: 1981 report. *Cutis* 29:167.

Schamberg, I. L. 1979. Dermatoses of the groin. *J. Family Pract.* 8:825.

Sibulkin, D. 1978. Drug eruptions. *Primary Care* 5:233.

Smith, S. Z. 1978. Contact dermatitis. *Primary Care* 5:653.

Solomon, L. M.; Esterly, N. B.; and Loeffel, E. D. 1978. *Adolescent dermatology*. Philadelphia: W. B. Saunders Co.

Stillman, M. A. 1978. Papulosquamous diseases. *Primary Care* 5:197.

Van Arsdel, P. P. 1979. An allergist looks at urticaria and angioedema. *Dermatology* 2(11):11.

Voorhees, J. J., and Orfanos, C. E. 1981. Oral retinoids. Broad-spectrum dermatologic therapy for the 1980's. *Arch. Dermatol.* 117:418.

–15–
Miscellaneous Infectious Diseases

Amebiasis
Enterobius Vermicularis
Exanthematous and Other Viral Illnesses of Childhood
Rubeola □ Rubella □ Mumps □ Varicella
Giardiasis
Hemophilus Influenzae Infections
Infectious Mononucleosis
Laboratory data □ Treatment
Influenza
Mycoplasma Infections
Rabies
Rocky Mountain Spotted Fever
Staphylococcal Infections
Impetigo □ Follicle infections □ Toxic shock syndrome
Streptococcal Infections
Erysipelas and cellulitis □ Scarlet fever

This chapter concerns selected bacterial, viral, and parasitic infections (in alphabetic order) that do not precisely fit into previous chapters. The reader also should refer to the index for specific organ system infections; for example, sinusitis and rhinitis are found in Chapter 4, endocarditis in Chapter 7, osteomyelitis and septic arthritis in Chapter 11, venereal disease in Chapter 17. Nor has any attempt been made to be comprehensive. Rather, discussion is limited to key aspects of those diseases occurring with some frequency in adolescence, or with specific implications for this age group, or which may pose diagnostic dilemmas. Even here, common minor infectious syndromes have been omitted on the assumption that a discussion of conditions such as the common cold or acute gastroenteritis is unnecessary. Additional diagnostic considerations and the management of complicated and particularly severe infections require further reference to the literature.

Amebiasis

Infection due to *Entamoeba histolytica* is found in 2%-5% of adolescents in the United States and is endemic in certain Indian reservations, mental institutions, and low socioeconomic areas in the south-central and southwestern states. It primarily involves the gastrointestinal mucosa but occasionally invades the liver, lungs, pericardium, central nervous system, or genital and perianal areas. Transmission is by ingestion of *E. histolytica* cysts, primarily through drinking contaminated water. As many as 95% of individuals with this infection are asymptomatic carriers.

Symptomatic individuals present with diarrhea ranging from a few loose stools to pronounced dysentery lasting days to weeks. Severe abdominal pain with tenesmus may be present. The most common extragastrointestinal manifestation of amebiasis (occurring in 5% of infected individuals) is liver abscess. Other complications include pericardial abscess, gastrointestinal perforations or stricture, anorectal fistula, and vaginal ulcer.

Diagnosis is by demonstrating cyst or trophozoite forms in stools; 80% of cases are confirmed in this manner after examination of three stool specimens and 90% after six specimens. *E. histolytica* should not be confused with leukocytes or the smaller and benign *E. hartmanni*. Other revealing tests include rectal biopsy, an indirect hemagglutination test ($\geq 1{:}128$), and an enzyme-linked immunosorbent assay. A liver scan or ultrasound is useful in instances of suspected hepatic abscess.

Both symptomatic and asymptomatic individuals should be treated with one of the following schedules: (a) metronidazole, 750 mg t.i.d. $\times$ 5–10 days together with diiodohydroxyquin, 650 mg t.i.d. $\times$ 20 days; (b) tetracycline, 500 mg t.i.d. or q.i.d. $\times$ 7–10 days; (c) diloxanide, 500 mg t.i.d. $\times$ 10 days. A hepatic abscess usually requires more vigorous treatment with intramuscular emetine or dihydroemetine. Needle aspiration or surgery also may be necessary in some cases.

Enterobius Vermicularis

Enterobius vermicularis, or pinworm, is the most common helminthic infestation in this country. It usually presents as a clinical problem in children with nocturnal perianal pruritus, vaginal discharge, cystitis, and/or enuresis. However, ova are ubiquitous in the household of the symptomatic member and one can be sure that other family members, including adolescent siblings, are infected as well. Diagnosis employs the cellophane tape technique: the sticky side of a piece of tape is pressed to the anus in early morning hours, placed sticky side down on an ordinary glass slide, and examined under a microscope for characteristic pinworm eggs. Treatment is with one of the following schedules: (a) pyrantel pamoate, 11 mg/kg in a single dose up to a maximum of 1 g (available as an oral suspension containing 50 mg/ml); (b) pyrvinium pamoate, 5 mg/kg in a single dose (available as 50 mg tablets or an oral suspension containing 10 mg/ml); (c) mebendazole (Vermox), a single 100 mg tablet. Nausea and vomiting sometimes may be encountered as side effects of these drugs. Treatment may be repeated in 2–3 weeks. All members of the household should be treated in addition to the diagnosed patient, and the house itself should be thoroughly cleaned with particular attention to dust-collecting corners.

Exanthematous and Other Viral Illnesses of Childhood

Although the following four diseases are classically noted in children, the lack of adequate immunization or loss of immunity may find them sometimes occurring in adolescents as well. They also may take an atypical form as in measles in an individual immunized with killed virus vaccine. In other instances there may be special considerations in adolescence not applicable to children, such as orchitis with mumps in pubertal males or the problems of possible fetal transmission of wild rubella virus or the attenuated virus of rubella vaccine in pregnant teenage girls.

RUBEOLA

Approximately one in three adolescents will not have been immunized against measles (rubeola) nor have acquired natural immunity. Such individuals are at risk of active disease. Following an incubation period of 10–16 days, initial signs include fever, headache, rhinitis, cough, photophobia, conjunctivitis, and Koplik spots (punctate red spots with a central white dot scattered over the pharyngeal and buccal mucosa). Shortly thereafter the rash appears as red maculopapules beginning on the face and spreading downward and outward to the trunk and extremities. Differential diagnosis primarily includes other viral exanthems, scarlet fever, erythema multiforme, and drug rashes. False-positive syphilis serology and false tuberculin tests may occur during acute measles infection. Treatment is symptomatic. Complications include otitis media, pneumonia, myocarditis, and encephalitis.

Exposure to the natural virus after immunization with killed vaccine (administered widely between 1962 and 1968) may result in atypical measles. Cough, myalgia, and abdominal pain are followed by a measleslike rash, often first appearing on the extremities, including palms and soles, and spreading proximally to the rest of the body. Pulmonary nodules are sometimes found on chest roentgenogram, can persist for months, and may be mistaken for neoplastic metastatic lesions, leading to an unnecessary thoracotomy. Diagnosis depends on the history of an atypical exanthematous illness, a high level of suspicion, and the finding of exceptionally high serologic measles antibody titers.

Infants, the elderly, and debilitated individuals who have not received measles vaccination and who have been exposed may receive passive, but temporary, protection through the use of human immune serum globulin (gamma globulin) at a dosage of 0.25 ml/kg given intramuscularly. Adolescents who have never been immunized should receive live measles vaccine; contraindications include compromised immunity from any cause and pregnancy.

RUBELLA

Although a substantial proportion of adolescents have not been immunized against rubella (German measles), the wild virus is still endemic, and a significant number will be immune from natural sources. Rubella has but minimal significance for the individual who gets it, having an exceptionally mild course. Following an incubation period of 16-22 days, rose-colored macules resembling rubeola or scarlet fever first appear on the face and then spread to the trunk and extremities. Posterior cervical chain and occipital lymphadenopathy are almost pathognomonic features. Fever and mild degrees of myalgia and malaise may also be present. Symptoms begin to clear within 3 days. Approximately 50% of females, however, go on to develop a mild, transient polyarthritis, most commonly involving the wrists and knees, some 5-10 days after the rash develops. Treatment of any aspect of this disease is symptomatic.

The major concern in rubella is the potential for serious fetal damage when a pregnant female contracts the virus during the first trimester. The fetal rubella syndrome includes mental retardation, cataracts, deafness, congenital heart disease, and other such serious defects. If a pregnant adolescent develops rubella during the first 24 weeks of gestation, the possibility of terminating the pregnancy should be carefully reviewed. The actual probability of fetal injury under these circumstances is difficult to ascertain, as the degree of risk appears to vary with the viral strain involved; the first epidemic in which an association with fetal defects was made occurred in Australia and demonstrated a 14% incidence of abnormalities. Subsequent epidemics have had a somewhat lower but still significant incidence.

Immunizing an adolescent girl against rubella also may be hazardous if she is pregnant at the time. Although no infant born to a female unwittingly receiving vaccine during the first trimester of pregnancy has yet demonstrated any defect (and some 250 such infants have been identified), studies of tissue obtained from abortions after such exposure have found that vaccine virus can be recovered from the fetus just as is wild virus, and one instance of cataracts has been identified. Current recommendations for immunizing adolescents for rubella are given in Chapter 3.

MUMPS

Following an incubation period of 15-25 days, mumps (epidemic parotitis) manifests in fever, malaise, headache, and pain on salivation, quickly followed by painful parotid swelling. This may be unilateral but most commonly (in 70%) is bilateral. Differentiation from cervical adenopathy may be made by observing for the obliteration of the angle of the jaw from swelling and edema. This occurs in mumps but not adenitis. Reddening and edema of Stensen's duct is another significant physical finding. Submaxillary and/or sublingual salivary glands also may be involved; on rare occasion they may be the only ones affected, with the parotid glands remaining normal. Differential diagnosis of parotid swelling includes salivary duct calculi, suppurative bacterial infection, uveoparotid fever, Mikulicz disease, or tumor, but all are considerably less common than simple mumps.

Forty percent of postpubescent adolescent males with mumps develop epididymoorchitis. The ultimate consequence may be an atrophic testis with impaired or absent spermatogenesis but normal Leydig cell function (testosterone production remains intact). Testicular involvement, however, is almost always unilateral with the uninvolved organ retaining full function; sterility or sexual performance usually is not compromised. Meningoencephalitis occurs in 10% of infected individuals of either sex, but full recovery without permanent central nervous system sequelae can be anticipated. Other complications of mumps include oophoritis, pancreatitis, myocarditis, facial nerve neuritis, and hearing loss; here too, however, full recovery can be expected. It should also be noted that at the other end of the clinical spectrum, 30%–35% of individuals with mumps have subclinical disease.

Treatment is symptomatic. Analgesics, ice bags, and steroids have been used, particularly in instances of orchitis. However, neither steroids nor surgical incision of the tunica alba (to release testicular compression) have been found to offer any appreciable benefit in minimizing permanent testicular damage.

Certainly, mumps prevention is a more rational approach than having to treat the disease. Even if morbidity is low, time lost from school or job may be significant. Some 20% of adolescents over 15 years of age are still susceptible to mumps. As there are few risks to the vaccine itself, any teenager—males in particular—who does not have a documented history of mumps or mumps immunization should receive the live attenuated vaccine.

VARICELLA

Varicella (chicken pox) is caused by the same virus that produces herpes zoster. Reinfection in an adolescent who previously had varicella may result in clinical herpes zoster. The incubation of chickenpox itself is 12–18 days. Prodromal symptoms are minimal, and the first sign usually is the appearance of small red macules scattered on the trunk. These quickly progress to clear vesicles with erythematous borders, then become pustular and eventually form scabs. Any area of the body may be involved with a succession of crops of lesions appearing at differing times (a sign that was used to differentiate from smallpox, in which the lesions all appeared at the same time and progressed in unison). Differential diagnosis includes Kaposi's varicelliform dermatitis (vesicular lesions on a chronic atopic dermatitis base) and Mucha-Habermann disease (crops of scattered scaling papules and papulovesicles due to a benign type of vasculitis).

Complications of chickenpox usually are minimal unless the patient has compromised immunity; in this circumstance the disease may be fatal. Human immune zoster serum is available for administration in such instances from designated centers. These may be identified by contacting the Center for Disease Control in Atlanta.

Giardiasis

Infection with *Giardia lamblia* may be asymptomatic, cause only mild epigastric cramps and diarrhea, or present as a severe malabsorption syndrome resembling sprue. Transmission is by drinking cyst-contaminated water or, less commonly, ingesting contaminated foods. Epidemics may occur in communities where the water supply has become a reservoir for *Giardia*, as has been reported in Leningrad. Even those adolescents and young adults who are wilderness enthusiasts may not escape. Recently, it has been determined that beavers may become carriers of *Giardia* and can contaminate isolated mountain streams on migrating from developed to undeveloped areas—an important note for backpacking youth, who should be advised to purify all drinking water from any source, no matter how remote. The use of iodine-containing tablets, available in most camping stores, is sufficient.

Diagnosis is by detecting the trophozoite or cyst form in a Giemsa-stained stool specimen. When the disease is suspected, serial specimens should be obtained and, if unrevealing, a purged specimen using a saline cathartic may be helpful.

Both symptomatic and asymptomatic individuals should be treated with quinacrine hydrochloride (100 mg t.i.d. × 5–10 days) or metronidazole (250 mg t.i.d. × 10 days).

Hemophilus Influenzae Infections

Hemophilus influenzae infections occur in adolescents and young adults as well as children. Type b organisms may produce otitis media, epiglottitis, bronchitis, pneumonia, pericarditis, endocarditis, septic arthritis, meningitis, etc. and should be considered a potential causal organism in any such apparent bacterial infection. Diagnosis is by bacterial culture and detection of the capsular antigen using countercurrent immunoelectrophoresis (CIE). Some strains are resistant to ampicillin due to beta-lactamase production; Cefaclor and trimethoprim-sulfamethoxazole are useful alternatives for treating otitis media; chloramphenicol is reserved for more serious forms of infection. Appropriate measures, however, for the early detection of chloramphenicol toxicity (aplastic anemia) should be taken. In any event, cultures for identification and antibiotic sensitivities are always indicated with therapy modified accordingly.

Infectious Mononucleosis

Infectious mononucleosis is a particularly common infectious disease among adolescents and young adults. Recently, considerable light has been thrown on the etiology and epidemiology of infectious mononucleosis through study of the Epstein-Barr (EB) virus. A cause and effect relationship between this agent and this disease is now all but confirmed. Previously, understanding had been clouded first by the fact that EB virus is not highly infectious and, second, infection in children rarely produces clinical signs but does produce protective antibody levels against future challenge. Further, even among susceptible adolescents and young adults, not all who demonstrate rising EB virus antibody titers manifest overt symptomatology. The predeliction of infectious mononucleosis for middle class young people in developed countries is now explained on the basis of their relative insulation from earlier exposure in contrast to those living in more crowded circumstances, where immunity is achieved early in life. The method of transmission appears to be due to airborne droplets or other close but not necessarily intimate contact, as evidenced by studies of families in whom a significant percent of siblings seronegative for EB virus antibodies became positive (with or without clinical disease) on exposure to a family member with documented infectious mononucleosis. We should now begin to think of this condition in broader terms than simply the "kissing disease."

Following an incubation period of 30–50 days the classic acute stage appears with fever, injected tonsils, pharyngitis, and rather pronounced cervical or generalized lymphadenopathy. Enlarged mediastinal nodes may also occur and are demonstrable on chest roentgenogram. Other more variable signs and symptoms include chills, headache, myalgia, nausea, diarrhea, weight loss, ocular muscle pain, photophobia, chest pain, and arthralgia. Hepatomegaly (with clinical and laboratory evidence of mild hepatitis) and splenomegaly are relatively common complications. The acute phase generally subsides spontaneously after 2–4 weeks but may be followed by a variable period of vague malaise and fatigability sometimes lasting for months. This latter phase may or may not be accompanied by periodic temperature elevations, an elevated sedimentation rate, splenomegaly, and/or signs of continued mild hepatitis.

Another common complication is observed in those patients who have been treated with ampicillin when the initial diagnosis was bacterial pharyngitis. More than half of these individuals develop an ampicillin-related rash after 7–10 days' treatment. Most commonly this is maculopapular, but in one out of three it is of the urticarial-angioedema type. The maculopapular form usually appears on the trunk, then spreads peripherally and clears within 3–5 days regardless of whether ampicillin is continued. The etiology of this rash is obscure, but the maculopapular form, at least, is not thought to be immunologic or allergic. It is also sometimes seen with ampicillin administration in other viral infections or in lymphocytic leukemia. Table 15-1 cites a wide variety of other far less common complications.

Differential diagnosis includes bacterial and other viral causes of pharyngitis, infectious lymphocytosis, infectious hepatitis, acute lymphocytic leukemia, and more obscure causes of infectious disease with similar symptoms such as brucellosis, leptospirosis, and tularemia. Indeed, infectious mononucleosis is a great mimicker of a variety of far more serious diseases. At the other end of the spectrum, however, misdiagnosis is just as likely to err on the side of the psychosomatic causation, and many an adolescent, suffering from the prolonged debility phase, has been advised that he or she is simply suffering from an adolescent adjustment reaction!

LABORATORY DATA

Classic laboratory findings include a leukocytosis with 50% lymphocytes, of which 10%–20% are atypical in form; atypical lymphocytes, however, may be seen in a number of other infectious diseases

TABLE 15-1
COMPLICATIONS OF INFECTIOUS MONONUCLEOSIS

HEMATOLOGIC	1. Hemolytic anemia 2. Thrombocytopenia 3. Agranulocytosis or granulocytopenia 4. Disseminated intravascular coagulation 5. Splenomegaly with splenic rupture
NEUROLOGIC	1. Guillain-Barré syndrome 2. Aseptic meningitis 3. Meningoencephalitis 4. Seizures 5. Peripheral neuritis 6. Cranial nerve palsies 7. Optic neuritis 8. Reye syndrome 9. Subacute sclerosing panencephalitis
MISCELLANEOUS	1. Pharyngeal obstruction 2. Pneumonia (interstitial) 3. Pericarditis 4. Myocarditis 5. Hepatitis (common) 6. Glomerulonephritis 7. Nephrotic syndrome 8. Monarticular arthritis 9. Psychotic behavior

(Table 15-2) and are not pathognomonic for infectious mononucleosis. The Paul-Bunnell-Davidsohn heterophil antibody test is positive in 85%–90% of individuals (as are titers for the Epstein-Barr virus). A positive heterophil test is characterized by an agglutination titer $\geq$ 1:56 against sheep erythrocytes with complete absorption by beef erythrocytes but not by guinea pig kidney erythrocytes. Titer elevation is first noted 7–9 days after onset of the disease, peaks in 3–4 weeks, and gradually disappears over 2–3 months. Modification of the heterophil test has resulted in a number of rapid slide agglutination "spot" tests (viz. Monospot), which sensitively and quickly screen for suspected cases. A positive spot test is significant, although false-positives also occur in other viral illnesses. A heterophil antibody test is indicated in suspected cases with a positive spot test but fewer than 10% atypical lymphocytes on the peripheral smears.

TREATMENT

Management of infectious mononucleosis is purely symptomatic. Bed rest and limited activity are pre-

TABLE 15-2
CAUSES OF ATYPICAL LYMPHOCYTES

TWENTY PERCENT OR
MORE ATYPICAL LYMPHOCYTES
1. Infectious mononucleosis
2. Viral hepatitis
3. Cytomegalovirus mononucleosis
4. Drug sensitivity (PAS or phenytoin)

FEWER THAN 20% ATYPICAL LYMPHOCYTES
1. Common viral infections (childhood exanthems, herpes, influenza)
2. *Mycoplasma* infections
3. Tuberculosis
4. Rickettsial infections
5. Lead intoxication
6. Radiation effects
7. Stress reactions
8. Other infections

scribed as indicated by the patient's symptoms and degree of fatigability. Strenuous physical activity and sports likely to result in abdominal trauma should be avoided as long as the spleen is enlarged; splenic rupture is a possibility during this time. No specific measures relative to associated liver involvement are required. Improvement usually is noted within several weeks, although, as previously indicated, fatigue and general malaise may persist for several months. Prognosis is favorable, with complete recovery expected in all but those with the most serious (and, fortunately, exceptionally rare) complications. Steroids may be helpful in these circumstances. Death due to fulminant meningoencephalitis has been reported.

Influenza

Adolescents are particularly prone to influenza in that it occurs in 10–11 year pandemic cycles. Adolescents therefore have no preexisting immunity from prior infection, as each pandemic is caused by a strain with slightly different antigenicity than the previous one and immunity is only partial. Influenza is caused by variants of influenza virus A, and the incubation period of 1–4 days is followed by variable degrees of fever, headache, malaise, prostration, myalgia, rhinitis, conjunctivitis, and pharyngitis. Ocular symptoms include tearing, burning, and photophobia. Cough may be severe. Toxic symptoms last 7–10 days, whereas cough and/or easy fatigability may last for a number of weeks. Diagnosis is usually based on clinical and epidemiologic grounds, but various specific laboratory tests are available and include viral isolation, immunofluo-

rescent studies, enzyme-linked immunosorbent assays, and serologic tests employing acute and convalescent serum.

Treatment is symptomatic. Amantadine hydrochloride (Symmetrel), 100 mg b.i.d. × 5-7 days, may be helpful in severe cases and, when given daily throughout an epidemic, as prophylaxis in unvaccinated individuals at high risk for severe influenza and its major complication, pneumonia. But amantadine hydrochloride is not without potential serious side effects; depression, psychotic behavior, congestive heart failure, orthostatic hypotension, urinary retention, convulsions, neutropenia, headaches, and blurred vision have been encountered.

Healthy adolescents may be quite uncomfortable with influenza but are not at serious risk; therefore neither amantadine nor influenza vaccine are recommended for this age group in general. On the other hand, young people with serious chronic illness, particularly chronic pulmonary or cardiovascular disorders, are candidates and should be vaccinated each fall.

Mycoplasma Infections

Mycoplasma pneumoniae is the most frequent bacterial cause of pneumonia in adolescents. It often appears in late fall or early winter epidemics occurring every 1-6 years and is disseminated by close contact with contaminated airborne droplets, as with coughing. The disease is communicable during the symptomatic acute phase and, in some instances, for several months thereafter, when the infected individual may be in an asymptomatic carrier state.

Following an incubation period of 14-21 days, *Mycoplasma* pneumonia sometimes begins with fever, chills, headache, malaise, sore throat, and anorexia, although a hacking dry cough is the dominant feature and often the presenting symptom. Substernal pain, pharyngeal edema, cervical lymphadenopathy and, sometimes a nonspecific dermatitis also are seen. Patchy or reticular pulmonic infiltrates are demonstrable by roentgenogram in 10% of these patients, and pleural effusion is present in 25%. Rales may or may not be heard on auscultation. The presence or absence of auscultory signs and the appearance of the chest roentgenogram, however, do not always correlate with the degree of clinical toxicity. The course is quite variable, but it is not uncommon for signs and symptoms to persist for weeks, with easy fatigability continuing even longer. Although serious complications are relatively rare, a wide variety of conditions have been implicated on occasion, including severe pneumonia with massive effusion (particularly in patients with chronic lung disease or sickle cell anemia), lung abscess, hemolytic anemia, thrombocytopenic purpura, paroxysmal cold hemoglobinuria, disseminated intravascular coagulation, myocarditis, acrocyanosis, meningoencephalitis, Guillain-Barré syndrome, cranial nerve palsies, transverse myelitis, Henoch-Schönlein purpura, Stevens-Johnson syndrome, erythema nodosa, erythema multiforme, hepatitis, pancreatitis, arthritis, renal failure and tuboovarian abscess.

M. pneumoniae also may cause otitis externa, bullous myringitis, and bronchitis. *M. hominis* and T-strain mycoplasma (*Ureaplasma urealyticum*) have been implicated in sexually transmitted diseases, particularly nonspecific urethritis in males and some instances of salpingitis in females (see Chapter 17).

Significant laboratory findings in *Mycoplasma* pneumonia vary and may include an elevated white blood count (but only in about one-third of the patients) and a leukemoid reaction on occasion. Streptococcal MG agglutinins ($\geq$ 1:40), cold isohemagglutinins for human type O erythrocytes ($\geq$ 1:40), complement fixation titers ($\geq$ 1:64, or a fourfold titer rise), indirect immunofluorescent antibodies, positive counterimmunoelectrophoresis, and a positive metabolic inhibition test have all been noted. The combination of elevated cold agglutinins and complement fixation titers, both at levels of 1:64 or more, is suggestive for *M. pneumoniae* infection; elevated cold agglutinins alone, however, are nonspecific and also may be encountered in infectious mononucleosis, influenza, rubella, adenovirus, and a variety of other disorders.

Treatment with tetracycline or erythromycin at a dosage of 1–2 g per day in divided doses for 7–14 days is recommended and may hasten resolution. Although these agents have clear in vitro antibiotic activity against *M. pneumoniae*, their in vivo specificity is less clear, and clinical results are not dramatic. Symptoms do seem to improve, although the organism is not eradicated. Otherwise, management is supportive and symptomatic.

Rabies

Rabies itself is a rare disease among humans in the United States, but managing those with a bite from a potentially rabid animal is a common clinical problem. It is most often encountered among adolescents who have interests in biology, nature, camping, and a propensity for collecting wild pets, as the pool of infected animals includes bats, skunks, raccoons, and foxes, as well as domesticated and stray dogs and cats.

When an individual is bitten by a potentially rabid animal, every attempt to recover the animal should be made. Wild animals should be sacrificed and a brain biopsy carried out immediately. Domestic pets that have not been vaccinated against rabies, have no evidence of sickness or abnormal behavior, and that bit the victim consequent to reasonable provocation should be confined and observed for 10 days; sacrifice and brain biopsy should take place when signs of aggressive changes or other suggestive symptoms are present. As the rabies virus migrates to the brain along neuronal pathways at a constant speed, the distance of the bite from the central nervous system determines the urgency of the treatment decision; bites on the face or proximal upper extremity bear more urgency than those on the legs.

Antirabies treatment is clearly indicated with documented infection in the offending animal and probably indicated in the instance of an unprovoked bite by a wild animal or stray cat or dog that is not caught. Current treatment is given in Chapter 3 and employs the new human diploid cell vaccine with fewer side effects and more immunogenicity than the older duck embryo vaccine. It generally can be obtained through departments of health or the Center for Disease Control in Atlanta, Georgia.

Local therapy of the bite itself also is important and involves copious flushing, cleansing with benzalkonium or other antiseptic soap, tetanus prophylaxis, and possible antibiotic therapy.

Rocky Mountain Spotted Fever

Rocky Mountain spotted fever is an acute exanthematous disease caused by *Rickettsia rickettsii* that is transmitted by the bite of a tick. It is widespread in this country and occurs in all locales during the warm months when ticks are active. Since it has a predilection for the southeastern United States, the geographic appellation is misleading. Although tick is the vector, mice and dogs are thought to play a role as the host reservoir. The tick does not survive its own infection for more than a few days.

Clinical signs begin with fever, lethargy, and toxicity quickly followed by the appearance of a macular rash on the extremities, wrists, palms, ankles, and soles; the rash shortly becomes petechial or purpuric and spreads centripetally. The original tick bite may have gone wholly unnoticed and the disease is often mistaken for meningococcemia, measles, coxsackievirus infection, or drug eruption. Various complications include thrombocytopenia, hyponatremia, meningismus, hepatitis, and pneumonia. Diagnosis is confirmed by a rise in the Weil-Felix agglutination titer 10–14 days after onset. A complement fixation test is also available.

Treatment is with chloramphenicol (100 mg/kg/

day) or tetracycline (25 mg/kg/day) together with supportive measures. The mortality rate can be high, particularly when appropriate antibiotic treatment is delayed.

Staphylococcal Infections

Staphylococcus aureus is implicated in a wide variety of infections, ranging from mild to severe. Some of this variability is due to host resistance factors and some to the presence of penicillinase-producing strains. Skin infections such as folliculitis, furunculosis, impetigo, and carbuncles are the most common manifestations. More serious staphylococcal diseases include pneumonia, endocarditis, osteomyelitis, toxic epidermal necrolysis, etc. Recurrent staph infections, particularly if occurring in more than one family member, suggest someone in the household is a chronic carrier of a pathogenic strain.

Treatment of staphylococcal infections usually is with one of the semisynthetic antibiotics such as oxacillin sodium, dicloxacillin sodium, nafcillin sodium, and methicillin sodium or with broad-spectrum antibiotics such as erythromycin. It is always wise to obtain an initial culture before instituting treatment to confirm the etiologic agent and to be able to test for antibiotic sensitivities if treatment failure suggests a resistant organism. Vancomycin is often used for these resistant staphylococcal infections.

IMPETIGO

Impetigo (pyoderma) is an indolent and slowly expanding pustular eruption of the skin further characterized by discrete, large, tender crustations and regional lymphadenopathy. Bullous impetigo, generalized dermatitis, or toxic epidermal reactions may develop. Although usually caused by *S. aureus* alone, beta-hemolytic streptococcus may be involved as the sole agent or in combination. Transmission is by close contact with contaminated material or fomites. In addition to systemic antibiotics, treatment involves soaks to remove crusts and topical antibiotic ointments.

FOLLICLE INFECTIONS

Infection of plugged hair follicles or sebaceous or sweat glands with small, localized, and superficial cutaneous abscesses comprises folliculitis. Lesions may be single, multiple, or recurrent. A furuncle involves more extensive and deeper abscess formation, most frequently occurring on the face, neck, back, groin, or extremities. Complications of furunculosis include septicemia, septic arthritis, and cavernous sinus thrombosis. A very large and painful furuncle occurring in the region of the posterior neck or upper back is termed a carbuncle and also may be associated with fever and positive blood cultures. Infection of plugged apocrine glands in the axilla, groin, or perineum may result in multiple chronic abscesses with draining sinuses and is termed hidradenitis suppurativa. This is more commonly seen in tropical than temperate climates.

Treatment of any of these manifestations involves systemic or topical antibiotics or both, local heat, and incision and drainage when indicated. Prevention of recurrences includes good hygiene as well as eliminating apparent precipitants such as oils, dust, cosmetics, abrasive soaps, shaving, and the like. Such measures may not always be effective in an individual who is a chronic carrier or is repeatedly exposed to a family member with this condition. Treatment in such instances may be particularly difficult.

TOXIC SHOCK SYNDROME

This newly recognized symptom complex, linked to *Staphylococcus aureus* infection, has been described in menstruating women, usually in the second and third decades of life. There is an abrupt onset of fever, often with a variety of symptoms including emesis, diarrhea, headache, irritability, conjunctivitis, and/or muscular aches. A sunburnlike macular erythema develops on the body, especially the trunk and the thighs. Hyperemia of the conjunctivae, mouth, pharynx, and vagina can also occur. An adolescent girl can present to the clinician with severe prostration and hypotension (or overt shock). As the course progresses, variable laboratory tests may become noteworthy: leukocytosis, thrombocytopenia, elevated blood urea nitrogen (and creatinine), elevated creatine phosphokinase, and/or increased liver enzymes. In 7–10 days, desquamation occurs, especially about the distal extremities, and spontaneous recovery ensues in the majority. Serious complications, however, can occur, including renal failure, diffuse intravascular coagulation and the respiratory distress syndrome, with a 10%–15% mortality rate. Differential diagnosis should also consider various viral syndromes, Stevens-Johnson syndrome, scarlet fever, meningococcemia, Rocky Mountain spotted fever, mucocutaneous lymph node syndrome (Kawasaki's disease) among others.

The etiology of toxic shock syndrome is believed due to a toxin produced by *S. aureus*. It usually occurs within 5 days of the onset of menses and is not noted in women who use tampons continuously, although it has also been noted in other individuals of either sex unassociated with tampon use. Treatment is supportive, including hydration and vasopressor medications for the shock state. Pure cultures of *S. aureus* are often obtained from the cervix or other sites but not the blood. Semisynthetic penicillins (as nafcillin or oxacillin) are used, but their real value in this disease is unclear. Vaginal lavage has also been used in very ill patients in an attempt to remove *S. aureus;* the value of this procedure is not known. Toxic shock syndrome can be reduced in incidence if menstruating women use tampons intermittently and change them three to four times a day; continuous tampon use should be avoided. One recommended pattern is to employ tampons during the day and pads at night. A brand of tampon that was associated with a high percentage of cases has now been removed from the commercial market, and the actual incidence with currently available brands is quite low, regardless of how they are used.

Streptococcal Infections

A wide range of infections is caused by streptococci, particularly the group A, beta-hemolytic strain. This includes impetigo (see previous discussion), erysipelas, cellulitis, pharyngitis, otitis media, pneumonia, and others. The complications of rheumatic fever or acute glomerulonephritis following streptococcal pharyngitis (Chapter 4) are well known.

ERYSIPELAS AND CELLULITIS

Superficial infection of the skin alone is termed erysipelas, or St. Anthony's fire, whereas the additional involvement of deeper tissue is termed cellu-litis. The affected area usually is red or violacious, edematous, and tender. Fever, toxicity, and septicemia are common accompaniments. Although group A streptococcal organisms are most commonly implicated, group C *Streptococcus, S. aureus,* and *H. influenzae* may be causal on occasion. Positive cultures usually may be obtained from the blood or from aspirates of saline injected into the advancing border. Antibiotic therapy is indicated and should be given until the infection is entirely clear and, under any circumstance, for at least 10 days. Septicemia, septic arthritis, osteomyelitis, pneumonia, and other such severe infections may be complications of inadequate treatment. Penicillin is the drug of choice. Alternatives include ampicillin, amoxicillin, semisynthetic penicillin, or erythromycin.

SCARLET FEVER

Streptococcal infection occasionally manifests in pharyngitis together with a fine sandpapery, scaling, or erythematous rash on the face, trunk, inner arms, legs, axillae, and groin; the rash is caused by an erythrogenic toxin. Circumoral pallor, a strawberry tongue, and marked toxicity may be present as well. Resolution is associated with extensive desquamation. Scarlet fever is less commonly seen today than in the preantibiotic era, but when it does occur, it bears the same risk of postdisease rheumatic fever or glomerulonephritis, as does streptococcal pharyngitis alone. Treatment is with penicillin for a minimum of 10 days or one of the other antibiotics mentioned previously.

Bibliography

Alcoff, J. M. 1981. Group B Streptococcus. *Am. Family Phys.* 23(2):117.

Allhiser, J. N.; McKnight, T. A.; and Shank, J. C. 1981. Lymphadenopathy in a family practice. *J. Family Pract.* 12:27.

Causey, W. A. 1979. Staphylococcal and streptococcal infections of the skin. *Primary Care* 6:127.

Dan, B. B., and Shands, K. N. 1981. Toxic-shock syndrome. *Pediatr. Ann.* 10(12):29.

Demert, M. L. 1981. Giardiasis. *Am. Family Phys.* 23(2):137.

Dirckx, J. 1976. Childhood diseases: what to do when they strike adults. *Consultant* 16:31.

Ellenbogen, C. 1981. The common cold. *Am. Family Phys.* 24:181.

Fedson, D. S. 1977. Influenza: the continuing need and justification for immunization. *Primary Care* 4:761.

Fekety, R. 1981. Prevention and treatment of viral problems and current recommendations. *Postgrad. Med.* 69(1):133.

Fozard, G. 1978. Major helminthic diseases of North America: a review. *J. Family Pract.* 6:1195.

Geyman, J. P., and Erickson, S. 1978. The ampicillin rash as a diagnostic and management problem. *J. Family Pract.* 7:493.

Gysler, M. 1981. Toxic shock syndrome—a synopsis. *Pediatr. Clin. North Am.* 28:433.

Hinman, A. R. 1982. Measles and rubella in adolescents and young adults. *Hosp. Pract.* 17:137.

Katz, M. 1975. Parasitic infections. *J. Pediatr.* 87:165.

Kelsey, D. S. 1979. Rocky Mountain spotted fever. *Pediatr. Clin. North Am.* 26:367.

Knight, P. J.; Mulne, A. F.; and Vassy, L. E. 1982. When is lymph node biopsy indicated in children with enlarged peripheral nodes? *Pediatrics* 69:391.

Koblenzer, P. J. 1978. Common bacterial infections of the skin in children. *Pediatr. Clin. North Am.* 25:321.

Krogstad, D. J.; Spencer, H. C.; and Healy, G. R. 1978. Amebiasis. *N. Engl. J. Med.* 290:262.

Leipzig, B., and Obert, B. 1979. Parotid gland swelling. *J. Family Pract.* 9:1085.

Levine, D. P., and Lerner, A. M. 1978. The clinical spectrum of *Mycoplasma pneumoniae* infections. *Med. Clin. North Am.* 62:961.

Mccubbin, J. H., and Smith, J. S. 1981. How to diagnose rubella during pregnancy. *Am. Family Phys.* 23:205.

Markell, E. K. 1978. Diagnosis of the more common parasitic diseases. *Primary Care* 5:57.

Melish, M. E.; Hicks, R. V.; and Reddy, V. 1982. Kawasaki syndrome: an update. *Hosp. Pract.* 17:99.

Norden, C. W. 1978. Hemophilus influenza infections in adults. *Med. Clin. North Am.* 62:1037.

Pegram, P. S. 1981. *Staphylococcus aureus* antibiotic resistance. *Am. Family Phys.* 24:165.

Peter, G., and Smith A. L. 1977. Group A streptococcal infections of the skin and pharynx. *N. Engl. J. Med.* 297:311; 365.

Rapp, C. E., and Hewetson, J. F. 1978. Infectious mononucleosis and the Epstein-Barr virus. *Am. J. Dis. Child.* 132:78.

Riley, H. D. 1981. Rickettsial diseases and Rocky Mountain spotted fever. *Curr. Probl. Pediatr.* 11(5):3–46; 11(6):3–38.

Stollerman, G. H. 1982. Global changes in Group A streptococcal disease and strategies for their prevention. *Adv. Intern. Med.* 27:373.

Ziring, P. R. 1977. Congenital rubella: the teenage years. *Pediatr. Ann.* 6:11.

–16–
Collagen Vascular and Other Miscellaneous Disorders

Collagen Vascular Disorders
Juvenile rheumatoid arthritis □ Systemic lupus erythematosus □ Scleroderma
Dermatomyositis □ Polyarteritis nodosa □ Miscellaneous collagen vascular diseases
Sarcoidosis
Amyloidosis
Marfan's Syndrome

Collagen Vascular Disorders
JUVENILE RHEUMATOID ARTHRITIS
See Chapter 11.

SYSTEMIC LUPUS ERYTHEMATOSUS
Systemic lupus erythematosus (SLE) is the second most commonly encountered collagen vascular disease in adolescence, being exceeded only by juvenile rheumatoid arthritis. It predominantly affects females between the ages of 10 and 60 years and is characterized by an autoimmune disorder of connective tissue with multiple system involvement and a highly variable course. The etiology is unknown, but various factors have been implicated, including sunlight, virus infections, and certain drugs (hydralazine, procainamide, antibiotics, oral contraceptives), among others.

Diagnosis is made on the basis of clinical findings and supportive laboratory data (Table 16-1). A characteristic rash, fever, polyarthralgia, polyserositis, nephritis, idiopathic thrombocytopenia, and/or an autoimmune hemolytic anemia constitute the classic presenting signs. Suspicion should be raised, however, in any adolescent female (or male on occasion) with signs of an unexplained systemic disease, only one or two of the major criteria (Table 16-1), or persistent fever of unknown origin. One out of every five cases presents with fever as the only sign.

Laboratory tests supporting the diagnosis of SLE include low hemoglobin or hematocrit levels, low white blood cell count, elevated erythrocyte sedimentation rate, abnormal urinalysis, low complement levels (C3, C4, or total complement), positive antinuclear antibodies (ANA), positive anti-DNA antibodies, and the presence of LE cells. The last two tests are relatively specific for SLE, although they need not be positive for a diagnosis. Other contributory findings include a persistent biologically false-positive syphilis serologic test (syphilis itself being ruled out by a negative fluorescent treponema antibody test), positive rheumatoid factor, cryoglobulinemia, elevated serum muscle enzymes (CPK, LDH, SGOT, aldolase), and immunofluorescence of complement and/or immunoglobulin at the dermal-epidermal junction of a normal or abnormal skin biopsy (the lupus band test). A kidney biopsy also may demonstrate abnormalities although of a nonspecific nature.

The differential diagnosis includes many of the other collagen vascular disorders; acute rheumatic fever, juvenile rheumatoid arthritis, polyarteritis nodosa, polymyositis, and scleroderma have some features in common. SLE also may be confused with *mixed connective tissue disease* manifesting in variable symptomatology of all the foregoing conditions, for example polyarthritis, Raynaud's phenomenon, sclerodermalike skin changes, fever, esophageal motility abnormality, myocarditis, peri-

TABLE 16-1
DIAGNOSTIC CRITERIA FOR SYSTEMIC LUPUS ERYTHEMATOSUS (SLE)*

Criteria	Comment
Facial butterfly rash	Flat or raised malar erythema with or without edema. May develop vesicles, crusting, or ulcerations. Present in half of all cases.
Discoid lupus	Scaly erythematous plaques predominating on face and scalp with or without scarring, atrophy, pigment changes, and telangiectasia. May be an isolated cutaneous disorder or part of systemic disease. Other skin lesions that may be seen with SLE include urticaria, tender nodules on palms, fingertips, and soles, digit gangrene, and periungual erythema.
Raynaud's phenomenon	See Chapter 7.
Alopecia	With normal underlying skin.
Photosensitivity	
Oral or nasopharyngeal ulceration	May result in epistaxis and/or perforation of the septum.
Joint swelling	Polyarthritis similar to juvenile rheumatoid arthritis but without joint destruction. Present in 9 out of 10 cases.
Nephritis or nephrotic syndrome	Renal involvement occurs in half of all cases.
Pleuritis, pericarditis, and/or peritonitis	Also may develop myocarditis, endocarditis, or parenchymal lung disease.
Psychosis, convulsions, and/or mononeuritis	Other CNS manifestations that may be seen include cranial nerve neuropathy, chorea, myelopathy, aseptic meningitis, and cerebrovascular accidents.
Hemolytic anemia, leukopenia, and/or thrombocytopenia	Coombs test will be positive if hemolytic anemia present. Splenomegaly also seen.
LE cells	See text for other, less specific tests.
Persistent false-positive serologic test for syphilis	Verify that patient indeed does not have syphilis with FTA test.

*Established by the American Rheumatism Association in 1971. The presence of four or more of the criteria is associated with a positive pathologic diagnosis in 9 out of 10 cases.

carditis, dermatitis, proximal muscle inflammation, renal disease, thrombocytopenic purpura, and hepatospenomegaly among others. High titers of ANA and hemagglutination antibody to ribonucleoprotein antigen usually are noted.

Treatment depends on the organ systems involved. Polyarthritis may respond to such medications as aspirin, nonsteroidal antiinflammatory agents, antimalarials (hydroxychloroquine), or gold therapy. Topical or oral steroids are effective in SLE dermatitis; exposure to sunlight or the use of a 100% paraaminobenzoic acid sunscreen is important as well. Steroids and/or immunosuppressive agents (azathioprine, cyclophosphamide) may be necessary for renal complications. Steroids alone or in combination with other drugs as indicated by symptomatology (for example, digitalis for heart failure, antiepileptic agents for seizures) usually are employed in managing other major manifestations. Patients receiving steroids also should be monitored for secondary infections such as tuberculosis, fungal disorders, and septic arthritis.

The prognosis, although often guarded, remains highly variable and unpredictable. Some patients experience only a mild, chronic disease, others an episodic illness with periodic acute exacerbations, and yet others a severe protracted or rapidly fulminating course.

SCLERODERMA
Scleroderma is a rare disorder of unknown etiology. It predominates in females and is characterized by

varying degrees of cutaneous and multisystem inflammatory changes with subsequent fibrosis and tissue atrophy. Several forms have been identified. Progressive systemic sclerosis is reviewed in Table 16-2. About 5% of these patients have a specific symptom complex called the CREST syndrome (calcinosis, Raynaud's phenomenon, esophageal motility abnormality, sclerodactyly, and telangiectasia); this bears a better prognosis than when other organ systems are involved, although biliary cirrhosis or Sjögren's syndrome (keratoconjunctivitis with recurrent salivary gland swelling, often in association with rheumatic diseases) may develop. Diffuse scleroderma is characterized by truncal cutaneous changes and fulminating visceral involvement but without Raynaud's phenomenon.

Sclerodermalike skin changes may occur in a variety of other disorders as well. Differential considerations include systemic lupus erythematosus, dermatomyositis, mixed connective tissue disease, Werner's syndrome, carcinoid tumor, porphyria, and amyloidosis among other conditions. Contact with silica or polyvinyl chloride or certain infectious processes (Buschke's scleroderma) may result in similar lesions.

Treatment of scleroderma is difficult, involving symptomatic measures as indicated. Steroids, immunosuppressive drugs, and various supportive and rehabilitative techniques have been employed with variable results. The best outcome is with the use of steroids for the sclerodermalike skin changes seen in mixed connective tissue disease.

DERMATOMYOSITIS

Dermatomyositis is a rare autoimmune disorder that predominates in females and largely affects skin and skeletal muscle. The characteristic rash consists of an erythematous or violaceous dermatitis most often located on the face in a butterfly distribution. The neck and shoulders may be involved as well, with or without progression to other body parts, particularly the extensor surfaces. Alternatively, there may be a heliotrope rash or a dark, purplish discoloration about the eyelids, and periorbital edema. A scaly erythema with dermal atrophy and linear streaks over the knuckles, knees, and elbows (Gottron's sign) also may be seen, as may dilated capillaries in the nail beds. Later dermatologic changes vary and may include a scaly dermatitis, thin or atrophic skin, sclerodermalike thickening, telangiectasia, pigmentary changes, and ulcerations. The polymyositis usually is manifested in tender, "indurated," and weak muscles with decreased deep tendon reflexes; muscles of the proximal extremities, trunk, and pharynx are most likely to be involved.

TABLE 16-2
SIGNS AND SYMPTOMS OF
PROGRESSIVE SYSTEMIC SCLEROSIS

1. Raynaud's phenomenon (see Chapter 7)
2. Cutaneous manifestations; cycles of edema followed by thickening and then atrophy, particularly of hands, forearms, face, and neck
3. Abnormal distal esophageal motility with esophageal reflux and esophagitis
4. Reduced intestinal motility
5. Cardiac disorders (fibrinous pericarditis among others)
6. Pulmonary disorders (manifested in reduced pulmonary function tests and pulmonary hypertension)
7. Renal disorders with failure due to widespread fibrosis
8. Polyarthralgia with stiffness or polyarthritis
9. Proximal muscle weakness and atrophy
10. Hypergammaglobulinemia
11. Positive antinuclear antigen test with nucleolar or "speckled" pattern
12. Cutaneous calcinosis, distal digit pad atrophy, thickened mucous membranes
13. Skin biopsy demonstrating sclerodermalike changes
14. Pigment changes in skin, telangiectasia

Other organ systems may or may not be affected. Recurrent abdominal pain, gastrointestinal bleeding, ulcers, infarction and perforation may occur due to alimentary tract vasculitis. Myocarditis, arrhythmias, congestive heart failure, subcutaneous calcium deposits, pneumonitis, Raynaud's phenomenon, arthritis, joint contractures, muscle atrophy, lymphadenopathy, and hepatosplenomegaly, have been reported as well.

Findings of characteristic skin manifestations, polymyositis, elevated serum muscle enzymes (CPK, LDH, SGOT, aldolase), and decreased muscle conduction with normal nerve conduction on electromyography are diagnostic. The erythrocyte sedimentation rate is usually elevated during active disease. Nonspecific tests for collagen vascular disorders (ANA, LE cells, rheumatoid factor, others) may or may not be positive. A muscle biopsy is helpful in ruling out other causes of myopathy.

Treatment employs steroids and other supportive and rehabilitational measures as indicated. Immunosuppressive agents (methotrexate, azathioprine) have been used in steroid "resistant" cases with inconsistent results. Prognosis varies and is difficult to predict. Some patients fully recover even without treatment; others continue with a chronic downhill course. Adults with dermatomyositis bear an increased risk of developing a neoplastic disease; it is unknown whether this is true for adolescents as well.

POLYARTERITIS NODOSA

Polyarteritis nodosa (PAN, periarteritis nodosa) is an uncommon idiopathic vascular disorder manifested in widespread inflammation of small and medium blood vessels. Signs and symptoms are diverse, depending on which organ systems are involved (Table 16-3), but fever, hypertension, abdominal pain, calf pain, nodules, and renal disease are among the more frequent findings.

Diagnosis can be difficult on clinical grounds alone because syndrome specificity is lacking. In addition to all the collagen vascular disorders, other differential considerations include primary arterial disorders (giant cell, temporal, cranial, and Takayasu's arteritis), disorders of small vessels (Henoch-Schönlein purpura, serum sickness, hypersensitivity angiitis), and subacute bacterial endocarditis. A PAN-like illness has been described with rheumatoid arthritis, Crohn's disease, and hepatitis B infection. Periarteritis has been reported several times among methamphetamine abusers in other countries, but this has not been confirmed among North American youth and other factors are thought to be operative.

Supportive laboratory data depend on which organ system is involved, although anemia and an elevated erythrocyte sedimentation rate are common findings. Evidence of renal disease (hematuria, proteinuria, creatinemia, azotemia, etc.) eventually occurs in most patients. Confirmation of a provisional diagnosis requires a biopsy from involved tissue, whether skin, muscle, gastrointestinal tract, or kidney. Angiography may be helpful in demonstrating the extent of gross vascular abnormalities.

Treatment primarily is with high-dose steroids and often produces a good response. Immunosuppressive drugs may be necessary on occasion. The prognosis varies with possibilities ranging from full recovery to a fulminant downhill course.

MISCELLANEOUS COLLAGEN VASCULAR DISEASES

Takayasu's arteritis. Takayasu's arteritis (pulseless disease) is a rare disorder marked by an inflammatory reaction of the aorta and its major branches; it predominates in females. Signs and symptoms vary but may include fever, dermatitis, arthritis, myalgias, pericarditis, and pleurisy. Major complications result from the dilation, obstruction, or both of the involved vessels. Aortic aneurysm, reduced or absent pulses, general hypertension or reduced blood pressure in the lower extremities, renal artery involve-

TABLE 16-3
SIGNS AND SYMPTOMS
OF POLYARTERITIS NODOSA

1. Fever
2. Weight loss
3. Malaise
4. Calf pain and other musculoskeletal complaints
5. Abdominal pain, gastrointestinal bleeding, gastrointestinal infarction
6. Painful nodules
7. Dermatitis (petechial rash among others)
8. Renal disease (glomerulitis among others)
9. Peripheral neuropathy
10. Papilledema
11. Raynaud's phenomenon (see Chapter 7)
12. Hypertension
13. Thromboses and aneurysm formation particularly at vascular bifurcation points

ment (contributing, in part to an elevated blood pressure), and cerebral ischemia may be seen. Diagnosis is by angiography demonstrating the vessel abnormalities; a dilated, tortuous aorta is characteristic. Treatment varies, with steroids, vascular surgery and other measures employed as indicated by manifestations.

Wegener's granulomatosis. Wegener's granulomatosis is an unusual autoimmune collagen vascular disorder in which destructive granulomatous lesions develop in the upper and lower respiratory tract in association with vasculitis of the lungs, kidneys, and other organ systems. Signs and symptoms can include refractory sinusitis, nasal discharge, otitis media, nasal or pharyngeal ulcers, epistaxis, arthritis, ocular diseases (exophthalmos), glomerulonephritis, and parenchymal lung infiltrates with cavitation among others. Sinus and lung roentgenograms may reveal a granulomatous process; biopsy of a lesion is diagnostic. The prognosis is poor despite treatment with steroids, nitrogen mustard, cyclophosphamide, or other agents.

Granulomatosis of Churg and Strauss. The allergic granulomatosis of Churg and Strauss is a rare systemic vasculitis most often involving the skin, peripheral nerves, and lungs. Eosinophilia and bronchial asthma are common accompaniments. Extravascular granulomas may develop in any organ system. Differentiation must be made between this syndrome and polyarteritis nodosa, Henoch-Schönlein purpura, Löffler's syndrome, allergic bronchopulmonary aspergillosis, and Wegener's granulomatosis, among other conditions. Diagnosis is by biopsy. The presence of eosinophils in perivascular infiltrates is characteristic and distinguishes between this and Wegener's granulomatosis in which neutrophil infiltrates predominate.

Weber-Christian disease. Weber-Christian disease (relapsing nodular nonsuppurative panniculitis) is an uncommon idiopathic disorder (or collection of disorders) characterized by systemic vasculitis of any organ system and successive crops of tender, erythematous nodules in the subcutaneous fat of thighs, trunk, or breasts. The nodules appear over months or years and may undergo fat liquification with rupture and discharge of oily material. Infections, trauma, diabetes mellitus, glomerulonephritis, systemic lupus erythematosus, bromides, iodides, and steroid withdrawal are among those factors that have been implicated as possible precipitants. The nodules must be differentiated from those seen with erythema nodosum, erythema induratum, erythema multiforme, subcutaneous fat necrosis, and pancreatic fat necrosis. Treatment usually is with steroids, again with variable results.

Sarcoidosis

Sarcoidosis is an uncommon granulomatous multisystem disorder of unknown etiology predominantly affecting persons of Swedish extraction, other Northern Europeans, and American blacks. Although the age of onset usually is between 20 and 50 years, adolescents may be affected on occasion. Intrathoracic granulomas occur in 90% of all patients; thus cough, chest pain, dyspnea, and/or hemoptysis may be presenting signs. Other common complaints are weight loss, anorexia, lethargy, abdominal pain and, sometimes, fever. Erythema nodosum occurs in 33%; ocular and skin changes in 25%. General lymphadenopathy as well as findings referable to the musculoskeletal and central nervous systems may develop in some patients (Table 16-4). The differential diagnosis is manifold and includes tuberculosis, the pulmonary mycoses, Hodgkin's disease, other lymphomas, allergic alveolitis, Crohn's disease, phlyctenular conjunctivitis, and many other conditions.

Laboratory data vary, but significant findings include leukopenia with decreased T lymphocytes, eosinophilia, thrombocytopenia, elevated erythrocyte sedimentation rate, hypercalcemia with hypercalcuria, negative delayed hypersensitivity skin tests (mumps, *Candida*, tuberculosis, others), hyperglobulinemia, and hyperproteinemia. Intradermal injection of material derived from a sarcoid lesion may produce a granuloma, indicating the presence

TABLE 16-4
MANIFESTATIONS OF SARCOIDOSIS

1. Pulmonary
   a. Parenchymal infiltrates
   b. Miliary nodules
   c. Hilar and paratracheal lymphadenopathy
   d. Pleural effusion

2. Enlarged lymph nodes (generalized or local: cervical, epitrochlear, inguinal, others)

3. Ocular
   a. Uveitis or iridocyclitis
   b. Keratoconjunctivitis sicca
   c. Cataracts
   d. Glaucoma
   e. Choroidoretinitis

4. Dermatologic
   a. Erythema nodosum
   b. Maculopapular lesions
   c. Lupus pernio
   d. Scars

5. Musculoskeletal
   a. Polymyositis
   b. Arthritis
   c. Bone cysts (hands, feet, others)
   d. Myopathies
   e. Polyarthralgia

6. Neurologic
   a. Cranial nerve involvement
   b. Peripheral neuritis
   c. Papilledema
   d. Meningitis
   e. Space-occupying lesions

7. Gastrointestinal
   a. Splenomegaly
   b. Hepatic granulomas
   c. Crohn-like presentation

8. Miscellaneous
   a. Uveoparotid fever (uveitis, painless swelling of parotid or salivary glands, fever, and/or peripheral facial paralysis)
   b. Cardiomyopathy
   c. Cardiac arrhythmias
   d. Renal calculi
   e. Uremia
   f. Disseminated sarcoidosis

of active disease (the Kveim or Kveim-Siltzbach-Nickerson test). A chest roentgenogram commonly demonstrates parenchymal infiltrates with hilar and paratracheal lymphadenopathy; miliary nodules and pleural effusion also may be seen. Slit lamp examination of the eyes may reveal keratoconjunctivitis, iridocyclitis, uveitis, choroidoretinitis, cataracts, or glaucoma.

Treatment is nonspecific. Topical or systemic steroids often are effective with ocular lesions, and systemic use may benefit other lesions as well. Reduction of calcium and vitamin D intake are indicated to minimize the consequences of hypercalcemia and hypercalcuria. Antibiotics may be required for intercurrent infections. The prognosis varies. Although spontaneous recovery after a prolonged and chronic course is more common, obstructive lung disease, blindness, and other irreversible complications may occur.

Amyloidosis

Infiltration with amyloid, a complex protein secreted by reticuloendothelial cells, may involve the tissues of the heart, liver, spleen, kidneys, and gastrointestinal tract among other organs. Additional clinical findings variably include urticaria, deafness, peripheral neuropathy, thyroid carcinoma, and trophic skin lesions. Primary and secondary forms of amyloidosis have been identified. Primary disease may be idiopathic or, rarely, the autosomal recessive Familial Mediterranean fever. The latter is characterized by episodes of fever, abdominal or chest pain, and severe renal disease; pleurisy, peritonitis, arthritis, splenomegaly, and lower extremity erythema are other variable findings. Secondary amyloidosis is more common and may be associated with any of a number of chronic illnesses, including osteomyelitis, bronchiectasis, tuberculosis, rheumatoid arthritis, Crohn's disease, and Hodgkin's disease. Diagnosis is by suspicion, rapid uptake of intramuscular Congo red, and a rectal biopsy (or biopsy of other involved tissue) demonstrating amyloid deposits with Congo red staining.

Marfan's Syndrome

Marfan's syndrome (arachnodactyly), an autosomal dominant defect in connective tissue formation, most commonly manifests in musculoskeletal abnormalities. Affected individuals are tall and thin with a long narrow head, high-arched palate, and unusually long extremities. The last characteristic is particularly noticeable in the fingers and toes, hence the term arachnodactyly, or spider fingers. From 40%–75% of these patients develop scoliosis. Ligament laxity, pectus carinatum, pectus excavatum, and pes planus may be encountered as well. Manifestations involving other organ systems are highly variable in occurrence and age of onset; these include luxation of the lens and other eye abnormalities (myopia, strabismus, nystagmus, cataracts, coloboma, megalocornea), cardiac valvular disorders, aortic dilation, and aneurysmal formation (which may dissect), and renal ectopia. Nearly all those with Marfan's syndrome have the prolapsed mitral valve syndrome.

Differential diagnosis includes idiopathic scoliosis, homocystnueinuria, Ehlers-Danlos syndrome (cutis hyperelastica), and arthrogryposis. Occasionally, healthy adolescents who are constitutionally tall and slender may be misdiagnosed as potential Marfan's cases during the growth spurt in that arm and leg growth predominate in the accelerational phase giving a disproportionate appearance until trunk growth catches up.

Prognosis depends on the nature of the abnormalities present. Skeletal manifestations alone generally permit normal function. Scoliosis usually requires spinal fusion if more than of a mild degree. Pectus deformities may require cosmetic correction (see Chapter 5). Cardiovascular features pose the most serious set of complications, with aneurysmal complications a potential life-time threat. Eye problems and cardiac valvular disease are treated accordingly. Management also must take into consideration the genetic aspects of this disease with appropriate counseling on future child-bearing.

Bibliography

Athreya, B. H.; Norman, M. E.; Myers, A. R.; et al. 1977. Sjögren's syndrome in children. *Pediatrics* 59:931.

Blau, E. B.; Morris, R. F.; and Yunis, E. J. 1977. Polyarteritis nodosa in older children. *Pediatrics* 60:227.

Callen, J. P. 1981. Cutaneous vasculitis and its relationship to systemic disease. *D.M.* 28:3–48.

Callen, J. P. 1979. Dermatomyositis. *Intern. J. Dermatol.* 18:423.

Canoso, J. J. 1979. A review of the use, evaluations and criticisms of the preliminary criteria for the classifications of systemic lupus erythematosus. *Arthrit. Rheum.* 22:917.

Chumbley, L. C.; Harrison, E. G.; and DeRemee, R. A. 1977. Allergic granulomatosis and angiitis (Churg-Strauss syndrome): report and analysis of 30 cases. *Mayo Clin. Proc.* 52:477.

Cupps, T. R. 1982. The vasculitic syndromes. *Adv. Intern. Med.* 27:315.

Decker, J. L. 1979. NIH conference. Systemic lupus erythematosus; evolving concepts. *Ann. Intern. Med.* 91:587.

Hochberg, M. C. 1981. The spectrum of systemic sclerosis—current concepts. *Hosp. Pract.* 16:61.

Kaplan, D., and Sadovsky, R. 1978. Diagnosis and management of systemic lupus erythematosus. *Am. Family Phys.* 17:133.

Kassan, S. S. 1978. Sjögren's syndrome: an update and review. *Am. J. Med.* 64:1037.

Lell, M. E., and Swerdlow, M. L. 1977. Dermatomyositis of childhood. *Pediatr. Ann.* 6:115.

Orlowski, J. P.; Clough, J. D.; and Dyment, P. G. 1978. Wegener's granulomatosis in the pediatric age group. *Pediatrics* 61:83.

Patrick, G. B. 1982. An approach to vasculitic syndrome. *Hosp. Pract.* 17:47.

Pyeritz, R. E., and MuKusick, V. A. 1979. The Marfan syndrome: diagnosis and management. *N. Engl. J. Med.* 300:772.

Siegel, R. C. 1977. Scleroderma. *Med. Clin. North Am.* 61:283.

Sills, E. M. 1975. Juvenile rheumatoid arthritis and systemic lupus erythematosus in the adolescent. *Med. Clin. North Am.* 59:1497.

Singsen, B. H.; Bernstein, G. H.; Kornreich, H. K.; et al. 1977. Mixed connective tissue disease in childhood. A clinical and serologic survey. *J. Pediatr.* 90:893.

Synkowski, D. R.; Mogavero, H.; and Provost, T. T. 1980. Lupus erythematosus: laboratory testing and clinical subsets in the evaluation of patients. *Med. Clin. North Am.* 64:921.

Vickery, D. M., and Quinnell, R. K. 1977. Fever of unknown origin. An algorithmic approach. *J.A.M.A.* 238:2183.

Waldo, R. T. 1981. Dermatomyositis: cutaneous clues to subclinical myositis. *Am. Family Phys.* 24:151.

Wiggelinkhuizen, J. 1978. Takayasu's arteritis and renovascular hypertension in childhood. *Pediatrics* 62:209.

PART THREE

SPECIAL ADOLESCENT HEALTH ISSUES

–17–
Adolescent Sexuality and Related Health Problems

Richard R. Brookman

Evaluation of Sexuality-Related Health Problems
The sexual history □ Physical examination and screening procedures

Sex Education
Overview □ Educational content

Sexuality Counseling
Masturbation □ Dating behavior □ Sexual performance □ Premarital counseling
Genital abnormalities □ Homosexuality □ Transsexualism □ Cross-dressing
Sexual asphyxia syndrome □ Acting-out sexual behavior

Sexual Assault
Rape □ Sexual abuse □ Incest

Menstrual and Pelvic Disorders
Menstrual physiology □ Amenorrhea
Dysfunctional uterine bleeding □ Dysmenorrhea and pelvic pain
Pelvic masses □ In utero estrogen exposure □ Cervical neoplasia

Genital Infections
Sexually transmitted diseases □ Other sexually transmitted infections
Other genital infections and problems

Contraception
Contraceptive counseling □ Oral contraceptives □ Intrauterine devices
Medroxyprogesterone acetate injection (depoprovera) □ Diaphragm
Vaginal spermicides (foams, jellies, suppositories) □ Condom
Postcoital contraception □ Abstinence □ Sterilization

Pregnancy
Diagnosis □ Counseling the pregnant adolescent □ Continuation to term □ Termination

Sexual thoughts, feelings, and behaviors, although present throughout the life cycle, become accentuated during adolescence. The visible changes of puberty proclaim physical maturity, sex specificity, and reproductive capacity. Genital changes and associated functions have major psychologic implications. They often are unpredictable as well; spontaneous erections and ejaculations, menarche and menstrual periods are all outside the adolescent's conscious control.

Each year, an increasing number of teenagers are experimenting with a greater variety of sexual experiences at ever younger ages. The marked discrepancy between the traditional moral teaching of premarital chastity on the one hand and the excessive sexual stimuli that pervade the adolescents' milieu on the other only adds to their sense of confusion and frustration. All too often this leads to impulsive, poorly thought out sexual behavior and serious health consequences: unwanted pregnancy, sexually transmitted infections, adverse psychologic sequellae. Considerate attention, complete evaluation, and comprehensive treatment—including preventive education and services—are essential for any adolescent having sex-related concerns.

Evaluation of
Sexuality-Related Health Problems

THE SEXUAL HISTORY

The sexual history expands on the general medical history (Chapter 2) to assess the adolescent's understanding about puberty, reproduction, sexual behaviors and their implication, as well as to explore the young person's feelings, attitudes, and personal value system. The identification of inadequate or incorrect information, past or present health risk behaviors, or psychologic conflict will define the nature and extent of needed sex education, counseling, preventive or remedial therapies, and clarification of sexual values.

Admittedly, these functions are time consuming and may take more than the span of a single visit to accomplish. The busy practitioner may wish to delegate selected aspects to some other appropriately trained health professional, for example, nurse, nurse practitioner, or nurse midwife. Female practitioners, whether physician or nurse, often are more effective in counseling female adolescents than are male practitioners and often are preferred by the patients.

Table 17-1 provides detailed outlines of points comprising a complete sexual history. Obtaining this information will be facilitated if the adolescent is first assured of privacy and advised that what is said is confidential, not to be shared with others without permission. Second, both patient and interviewer need to be sure they understand each other. Although this may require resorting to the vernacular in facilitating communication, correct terms and definitions should be provided as well. The clinician also will find it advantageous to the trust relationship if overreaction to explicit language or candid details of sexual behavior can be avoided.

Questioning is best initiated with the least sensitive topics, progressing to more sensitive ones as mutual comfort and trust develop; for example starting with age of pubertal onset, moving on to seminal emissions or menarche, and then to masturbation or sexual intercourse. Within this sequence, questioning should be direct and nonjudgmental rather than circuitous or by inuendo. "Do you and your partner have sex together?" will be more productive than "Do you two do anything you shouldn't be doing?" Anxiety about discussing sex-related matters often is considerably greater for the professional than the adolescent.

PHYSICAL EXAMINATION
AND SCREENING PROCEDURES

Tables 17-2, 17-3, and 17-4 outline the physical examination and screening procedures appropriate to sexuality issues and the reproductive tract. A number of specific techniques can be employed that will facilitate this examination and reduce patient anxiety. The following apply to both sexes unless otherwise specified.

The nature and reasons for the examination should be explained while the adolescent is still dressed. The use of appropriate models, cross-sectional drawings, and diagrams is particularly helpful and enhances the likelihood of profitable education about bodily and reproductive functions.

During the examination itself, modesty, privacy, and comfort should be preserved with proper draping and strategic coverage to the degree possible. Parents should be absent unless their presence is specifically requested by the patient. Requests for a same-sex examiner should be honored if staffing permits. The presence of female chaperons when male physicians examine females often is preferred by the patient and is a customary, although not mandatory, procedure. Reciprocally, some males may wish a male chaperon when the examiner is female; this, however, is not customary procedure.

In examining young females, an unhurried, gentle approach, with advance description of each step, showing the instrument to be used, is essential. Draping should not prevent eye contact between the adolescent and examiner. Allowing the patient to watch the procedure through an extension mirror can be both educational and reassuring, particularly when anatomical parts are pointed out. If a third person is not to be present, instruments, swabs, culture media, glass slides, and other required equipment should be placed conveniently in advance. When inserting the speculum, discomfort primarily comes when the urethra is compressed against the pubic bone. Introducing the speculum into the vagina with the blades slightly angled and then rotating them into proper position with a forward and downward motion can minimize this distress. Although comfort might be further enhanced by a surgical lubricant, this should not be used due to its bactericidal activity; the speculum should be moistened with warm tap water. (Lubricants can be used for the bimanual examination, as cultures already will have been taken.) Once in place, gentle opening of the speculum blades usually finds the cervix readily coming into view.

Young males may experience penile erections as a reflex response to the rectal or genital examination. Recognition of this embarrassing phenomenon is indicated; simply reassure the youth that this is a common, normal, and perfectly healthy event, well beyond his control and nothing to be concerned

TABLE 17-1
CONTENTS OF A COMPLETE SEXUAL HISTORY

1. Puberty: age of onset, current stage, knowledge about, questions about.
2. Sex education: sources, amount; extent of communication with parents, parental awareness of adolescent's sexual behavior (from adolescent's perspective).
3. Dating patterns: past and present status; extent of sexual experience, including intercourse, actual or contemplated (also see item 7).
4. Consequences of sexual activity:
   a. History of sexually transmitted disease(s); which one(s), when, how treated, followup tests, complications, treatment of partner, emotional reactions.
   b. History of contraception: knowledge and/or use, which one(s), when, complications, partner's participation in decision/use.
   c. History of pregnancy/paternity: when, outcome, how decision was made, partner's involvement in decision, parental reaction, patient's reaction and current feelings.
   d. History of genital trauma: when, how caused, treatment, outcome, feelings about.
   e. Plans for parenthood: child care experience; acceptance of responsibility for sexual behavior and family planning.
5. Female-specific topics:
   a. Menarche: age (month and year), preparation, reaction, family's reaction.
   b. Menses: frequency, duration, amount (number of pads/tampons per day; amount of blood on each); menstrual patterns in female relatives; questions and concerns about menstruation.
   c. Menstrual and perineal hygiene: type of sanitary protection used; use of douches, deodorants, vaginal suppositories, bubble bath, tight underwear; frequency of bathing; wiping habits after defecation.
   d. Menstrual symptoms: cramps (duration, severity, treatment), midcycle bleeding, midcycle pain (mittleschmertz), premenstrual discomfort (symptoms, duration).
   e. Vaginal discharge: amount, color, odor, itching, pain; frequency, duration; perineal rash, lesions.
   f. Urinary tract: dysuria, frequency, urgency, hematuria; relation of symptoms to sexual intercourse.

g. Abdominal/flank/back pain: frequency, duration, nature, location, relation to menses, relation to intercourse.
6. Male-specific topics:
   a. Ejaculation: age at onset (nocturnal emission—"wet dreams"), preparation for; questions and concerns about erection, ejaculation.
   b. Urinary tract: dysuria, hematuria, penile discharge.
   c. Genital/scrotal: pain, rash, lesions, inguinal pain, swellings, perineal or rectal discomfort.
   d. Sexual responsibility: attitudes toward role in protecting self and partner against pregnancy, sexually transmitted disease; decision-making about degree of intimacy.
7. Sexual behaviors: both males and females.
   a. Masturbation: method, frequency, satisfaction, concerns.
   b. Sexual intimacy: type (light petting, heavy petting, mutual masturbation, oral-genital, anal), satisfaction, concerns; decision-making skills in determining values and degree of intimacy desired.
   c. Sexual intercourse: frequency, problems (impotence, premature ejaculation, anorgasmia, guilt, ambivalence), satisfaction, concerns; responsibility for adverse consequences.
   d. Homosexual experience: motivation, when, frequency, type (mutual masturbation, oral-genital, anal), feelings, concerns.
8. Information from parents. The foregoing will have been obtained from the patient privately. It also is helpful if additional history is obtained from the parental perspective.
   a. Concerns about adolescent's dating, nondating.
   b. Knowledge or suspicion about adolescent's sexual behavior and complications (sexual intercourse, pregnancy, paternity, sexually transmitted disease, contraceptive use, masturbation).
   c. Feelings about their adolescent's sexuality.
   d. Comfort in discussing sex-related topics with their adolescent; amount of sex education in home; attitude about sex education outside the home.
   e. Concerns about menstruation, menstrual problems, other health problems.

TABLE 17-2 PHYSICAL EXAMINATION AND SCREENING: FEMALES

1. Signs and stage of puberty (see Chapter 2).
2. Axillary hair, acne.
3. Breasts: size, shape, symmetry, masses, tenderness, nipple discharge (see Chapter 5).
4. Pubic hair: skin lesions, excoriations, nits/lice.
5. External genitalia: skin lesions, hymenal patency, labial size, clitoral size, Bartholin's and periurethral glands, discharge.
6. Inguinal region: adenopathy, hernia.
7. Anus: discharge, lesions.
8. Pelvic examination*:

   a. Speculum examination[†] (warm tap water lubrication only; surgical lubricants are bactericidal): vaginal canal discharge, mucosal lesions, foreign body, cervix color, cervical erosions/other lesions/bleeding/discharge.

   b. Bimanual examination: cervical tenderness, pain on motion; uterus size, consistency, position, mobility; adnexal tenderness, masses; ovarian size.

   c. Rectovaginal examination: cul-de-sac or rectal tenderness, hemorrhoids, rectal masses, stool blood.

   d. Test procedures (performed if symptomatic and as recommended in health maintenance schedule given in Chapter 3).

   (1) Endocervical culture for *N. gonorrheae* (Table 17-4).

   (2) Endocervical culture for *Chlamydia trachomatis* (if available in laboratory).

   (3) Papanicolaou smear.

   (4) Wet mount of vaginal pool swab (suspended in saline) for trichomonads, yeast, and "clue cells" (Figure 17-1).

---

*Indications for a complete pelvic examination are: (a) history of sexual intercourse; (b) suspicion of sexually transmitted disease (may be present even if no penile penetration); (c) request for contraceptive method; (d) evaluation for possible pregnancy; (e) lower abdominal or pelvic pain (to assess gynecologic vs. other cause); (f) evaluation of menstrual disorder; (g) request for education and/or assistance with tampon use; (h) history of in utero exposure to diethylstilbestrol or related estrogen; (i) introduction as a component of the complete preventive health evaluation in mid to late adolescence in the virginal female.

[†]Use Huffman speculum in virginal females; its narrow blades slip easily through a narrow hymenal opening yet provide good visualization.

TABLE 17-3 PHYSICAL EXAMINATION AND SCREENING: MALES

1. Signs and stage of puberty (see Chapter 2).
2. Axillary hair, acne, gynecomastia.
3. Penis: meatal location, circumcision, phimosis, discharge, skin lesions.
4. Pubic hair: skin lesions, excoriations, nits/lice.
5. Scrotum and testes: skin lesions, testicular size,* consistency, tenderness, cord, abnormal masses.
6. Inguinal region: adenopathy, hernia.
7. Anus: discharge, lesions.
8. Rectal[†]: prostate size, tenderness, hemorrhoids, stool blood.
9. If history of sexual activity or clinical evidence of infection present:

   a. Culture and Gram stain of anterior urethra with calcium alginate swab for *N. gonorrheae* (Table 17-4). (Spun sediment of first 5 ml of freshly voided urine is a satisfactory alternative culture specimen for the above.)

   b. Culture for *Chlamydia trachomatis* (if available in laboratory).

   c. Microscopic examination of sediment of spun fresh urine specimen for trichomonads.

   d. Serologic test for syphilis; dark-field examination if chancre present.

   e. Cultures of anal canal and/or pharynx for *N. gonorrheae* when indicated by symptoms or nature of sexual practices.

---

*When precision is desired in assessing testicular size, the best method is by volumetric comparison with the orchidometer, a string of ovoid beads of differing calibrated size. This is available from Professor Andreas Prader, Dept. of Pediatrics, Kinderspital, Steinweisstrasse 75, Zurich 8012, Switzerland.

[†]Indications for a rectal examination in males are (a) signs and/or symptoms of genitourinary, prostatic, or gastrointestinal disease, (b) sign and/or symptoms of inadequately treated gonorrhea (may have asymptomatic prostatic enlargement), (c) annually in sexually active males, (d) introduction as a component of the complete adult preventive health evaluation in mid to late adolescence in the virginal male.

about. Joking, studied silence, or other indicators of the examiner's discomfort should be avoided.

Some adolescents deal with the genital or pelvic examination well. For others, it can be a distressing prospect they are not yet ready to accept. The young person's right to refuse examination should be respected whenever possible. In any circumstance, examination should never be coerced.

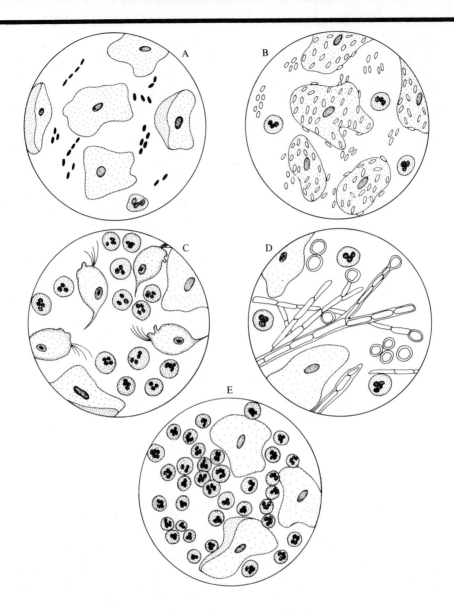

FIGURE 17-1
DIFFERENTIAL DIAGNOSIS OF VAGINAL DISCHARGE BY EXAMINATION OF WET MOUNT (FOOD COLORING MIXED IN 1:10 DILUTION WITH SALINE IMPROVES CONTRAST).
A, Normal epithelial cells, lactobacilli. No infection—physiologic leukorrhea.
B, Bacilli-studded epithelial cells (clue cells); *Hemophilus*.
C, Motile flagellated cells, WBCs; trichomonas.
D, Hyphae, spores, WBCs; *Candida*.
E, Numerous WBCs, no other organisms; suspect gonorrhea, *Chlamydia*.

TABLE 17-4
TECHNIQUES FOR OBTAINING SPECIMENS

CULTURES FOR *N. GONORRHEAE*

1. Obtain specimen
   a. Endocervix: insert sterile cotton-tipped swab into canal, rotate and move side to side, allow 10–30 seconds to absorb secretions.
   b. Urethra: insert sterile calcium alginate swab ¼ to ½ inch beyond meatus, rotate gently, allow 10–30 seconds to absorb secretions.
   c. Anal canal: insert sterile cotton-tipped swab 1 inch into canal, move side to side, allow 10–30 seconds to absorb secretions; try to avoid fecal contamination.
   d. Oropharynx: swab posterior pharynx and tonsillar crypts with sterile cotton-tipped swab.
2. Streak out on Thayer-Martin or other appropriate media.
3. Place in candle jar, light candle (will provide appropriately reduced oxygen tension environment).
4. Place in incubator with all cultures clearly labeled with patient ID and source.

CULTURES FOR *CHLAMYDIA TRACHOMATIS*

1. Obtain specimen from endocervix or urethra as above; must use calcium alginate swab and firm pressure on endothelium.
2. Place swab in transport media properly identified.
3. Transport to laboratory for tissue culture on McCoy cells.

CYTOLOGIC SMEARS

1. Papanicolaou smear
   a. Gently scrape endocervical canal and endocervix by 360-degree rotation of a "cervical scraper" or with a sterile moist cotton-tipped swab (endocervix) and a flat "Pap stick" (ectocervix).
   b. Smear swab or stick on a clean, dry glass slide and dry.
   c. Spray with Papanicolaou spray fixative or any plain hair spray and send to laboratory.
2. Maturation index (estrogenization)
   a. Gently scrape lateral wall of middle third of vagina with moist cotton-tipped swab.
   b. Prepare slide as for Papanicolaou smear.

WET MOUNT

1. Absorb secretions from the cul-de-sac on a cotton-tipped swab.
2. Mix with 1–2 drops of saline on a clean slide; apply cover slip. (Adding food coloring to saline improves contrast.)
3. Examine under low- and high-power magnification with microscope for trichomonads, "clue" cells, and yeast spores or hyphae (see section on vaginitis for details).
4. A second slide prepared with 10% KOH will dissolve cellular material but not hyphae, rendering the latter more visible.

Sex Education

OVERVIEW

Sex education of the young is the shared responsibility of parents, health professionals, educators, clergy, and other appropriate youth-serving adults. All contribute in important ways, directly and indirectly, to the adolescent's understanding of and attitude toward his or her own sexuality and its expression. But the anxiety, ambivalence, and taboo surrounding human sexuality on all fronts, both personal and societal, often results in more confusion than clarification. The normal distancing process of adolescence adds to the problem in making it sometimes difficult for parents to continue as effective sex educators, even if they had been such during their offspring's younger years. The primary care physician occupies a unique position and can be an important source of information for the adolescent, the supporter of intrafamily communication, and an ally of responsible sex education programs in the community and schools.

Teenagers obtain most of their sex *information* from peers, books, magazines, and the media. Much of this information is mythical, distorted, or false. Their sexual *attitudes*, however, are derived from those of their parents, at least in the long run. Although transient rejection often accompanies the emancipation process, family values usually form the core of the young person's own postadolescent morality. Particular confusion in the adolescent's mind can result when two parents openly express conflicting values, when parents' attitudes and societal norms diverge widely, or when parents' stated views are inconsistent with their behavior.

Many parents are anxious about sex education outside the home. This may activate the parents' own sexual ambivalences, stir feelings of inadequacy in meeting their adolescent's needs, or challenge perceived rights of control and indoctrination with parental values. Sex education programs may be seen as threatening to family unity or as activating adolescent sexual drives that otherwise would be contained.

These perceptions are incorrect. There is no evidence that sex education undermines a young person's moral base but rather strengthens it. Nor is there indication that sexual intercourse is more prevalent among young people exposed to good sex education programs that teach mutual respect, responsibility, and effective decision making. To the contrary, evidence indicates that such programs tend to inhibit premature sexual intimacy rather than promote it. Hopefully, parents can be reassured and will come to the perspective that sex education programs are far more often supportive of their primary role in moral development than antagonistic.

Who provides sex information outside the family is a critical matter. Sex educators must be properly trained and aware of the ways their own value systems and beliefs may enter into and prejudice teaching. On one hand is the tendency to dictate a traditional morality or avoid controversy, fearful of parental alienation. On the other, is the propensity for overidentifying with adolescents, espousing total freedom for young people to make up their own minds or expressing hostility toward parents, who are perceived as jeopardizing teenagers' healthful development. Obviously educators face no fewer pitfalls than do parents.

Professional and parent collaboration in adolescent sex education is essential. Parents can be helped to clarify their views about adolescent sexuality and to be more open with their teenager through conferences with the physician or through discussion groups sponsored by church, PTA, or other community organizations. Useful references on human sexuality are listed at the end of this chapter.

Sex education for adolescents needs to be geared to their developmental stage. Preadolescents and early teens, rapidly approaching or progressing through puberty, are primarily concerned about their changing bodies and the associated changes in feelings and function. They are insatiably curious about the "what, why, how, when, and where" of every conceivable aspect of their physical growth. Their curiosity may be accompanied by exhibitionistic or provocative language or behavior. Although social appropriateness should be reinforced and the family's value system supported, such testing is best handled by tolerance or even ignoring. Another problem commonly encountered at this time is the reactivation of sexual conflicts in parents (and professionals as well!) triggered off by the advent of puberty and all it implies. This only adds to the anxiety experienced by many adults in dealing with adolescent sexuality.

Midadolescents, virtually complete in their physical development, turn to explore the nature of their maleness or femaleness and the complexities of heterosexual relationships. Experimentation is the usual means of defining these issues, but it is not always carried out with forethought or consideration of consequences. Education should provide facts about all aspects of human sexuality. Guided forums must be available for adolescents of both sexes to exchange views together, clarify their own value systems, and develop strategies to resist opposing pressures.

Older adolescents are concerned with putting their sexuality into adult, autonomous terms and with exploring mutuality and reciprocity in relationships. They may want a sounding board to test the validity of their own ideas and a source of factual information on various issues. They welcome suggestions and carefully considered responses to their inquiries but rarely appreciate gratuitous advice.

Sex education techniques include one-to-one discussion, group "rap" sessions, role playing and rehearsal, literature, audiovisual materials, and assigned topics for group, individual, or family research. Whatever methods are employed, discussions with teenagers should be by open-ended, two-way exchange. Inquisitions or preaching lectures only create distance and polarization between educator and youth. Methods for establishing the therapeutic relationship and interviewing in general, as presented in Chapters 2 and 23, are as applicable to this issue as to any other. Opportunities should be provided to discuss feelings and how to handle difficult situations. An important goal is to help the adolescent clarify his or her own values and to develop skills enabling him or her to live by them.

Regardless of the adolescent's personal decisions about his or her sexual behavior, three cardinal rules governing sexual intimacy must be reinforced:

1. No individual has the right to harm or exploit another or allow himself or herself to be harmed or exploited.

2. No one has the right to create an unwanted life.

3. No one has the right to spread disease through sexual behavior.

EDUCATIONAL CONTENT

If young people are to develop responsible sexual attitudes and behavior based on established values, understanding, and fact, then by the advent of puberty children should be introduced to the following information in a manner consistent with their cognitive capacity.

1. The events of puberty, including ejaculation and menstruation.

2. The physiology of reproduction, conception, pregnancy, and delivery.

3. The recognition, treatment, and prevention of sex-related infections.

4. Normal adolescent sexual activity: masturbation, experimentation, exploration; facts and myths about their effect on physical and emotional health.

5. Appropriate responses to sexual advances by peers or adults.

By midadolescence, young people should be introduced to concepts relating to the following:

1. The range of sexual intimacy, including sexual intercourse.

2. Appropriate feelings and attitudes surrounding sexual intimacy.

3. Methods of pregnancy prevention: advantages/disadvantages; how and where to obtain; male responsibility in family planning; how to remain abstinent.

4. Legal issues surrounding minors' rights to consent to fertility-related care.

5. Signs and symptoms of pregnancy; what to do if pregnancy suspected.

6. Options should pregnancy occur: delivery versus abortion; parenthood versus adoption; marriage versus remaining single.

7. Marriage and parenthood preparation, parenting skills.

8. Varieties of sexual behavior: homosexuality; socially unacceptable patterns; sexual abuse, rape, incest.

9. Common concerns about sexual performance, common sexual dysfunctions.

10. Community resources for sexuality-related counseling or health services.

Sexuality Counseling

Counseling a young person about specific sexual issues requires (a) thorough knowledge of sexual anatomy, physiology, and behavior; (b) awareness of local peer influences; and (c) understanding of the family's ethnocultural background. The approach to any problem depends on the adolescent's stage of intellectual and psychosexual maturation, using the same guidelines cited for sex education and techniques as described in Chapter 23. If discussions are initiated in a comfortable and nonjudgmental manner, the adolescent usually is willing to express his or her concerns.

MASTURBATION

Masturbation is a normal, widely practiced sexual activity but all too often engenders much guilt and concern due to historical proscriptions and antiquated, but still persistent, beliefs in disastrous mental and physical consequences. Young adolescents, heavily focused on body changes, are likely to feel that any perceived deviation from normal, particularly in the genital region, is caused by masturbation. But associated embarrassment and guilt often inhibits questioning. If there is suspicion that the adolescent has such fears but is unable to express them the subject should be gently introduced by the

physician at an appropriate time; usually this is when pubertal development is discussed. Parents or adolescents who believe that masturbation is abnormal or harmful should be assured that it is a normal, universal behavior causing neither physical nor mental harm, that it is a natural part of learning about human sexuality and is a useful means of relieving sexual tension.

DATING BEHAVIOR

Most midadolescents are interested in dating for companionship and for physical and emotional closeness. Degrees of intimacy run the gamut from hand-holding to kissing, embracing, or petting, to outright sexual intercourse. Currently, two-thirds of all teenage males and one-half of all teenage females have had intercourse at least once. The interpersonal commitment that develops between two young people may be intense and a serious part of their lives. Few adolescents are promiscuous (multiple partners with little or no commitment), although many have a series of close, committed single-partner relationships, each lasting weeks, months, or longer. Some relationships persist and lead to marriage.

Intimate sexual behavior usually is multidetermined, serving two or more functions at the same time. For a relatively mature and committed teenage couple, the reasons are similar to those of healthy adults: it is an expression of warm, tender feelings, a method of interpersonal communication, and a means of gratifying sexual drives and providing physical pleasure. Although these factors may be operative in younger, less mature adolescents, other reasons may be as an announcement of independence, conformity with peer group behavior or pressure, developmental experimentation in the formation of sexual identity, challenge to parents or society, escape from loneliness, or in response to stress. Counseling approaches may need to be varied, depending on which of these factors are operative (as determined by the sexual history and psychosocial assessment).

Most professionals working with adolescent sexuality agree that intercourse between young teenagers is a complex issue with many emotional and physical ramifications that complicate rather than simplify many developmental tasks. Young people who are still in a stage of emerging sexual identity and emancipation, primarily preoccupied with self-discovery and learning to stand on their own two feet, all too often encounter more anxiety and confusion than emotional reward by such intimacy. If counsel will be heeded, most early and midadolescents would be well advised to remain abstinent until a somewhat later time when their ultimate identity is more consolidated. But this is not always the case and it is virtually impossible for anyone, parents included, to prevent adolescents who wish to have intercourse from doing so unless someone is willing to act as chaperon 24 hours a day. If intercourse is likely, it is important to discuss it in a nonjudgmental manner (otherwise most adolescents will not discuss it at all), ensuring that appropriate steps are taken to prevent pregnancy or the transmission of infectious diseases.

Many adolescents do not wish to have intercourse but feel they must due to peer or partner pressure. Reviewing sexual feelings, behavior, and motives with a nonjudgmental professional may enable the young person to remain or return to being abstinent until he or she feels mature enough to handle a more intimate sexual relationship. Greater tolerance by parents and professionals of masturbation and noncoital heterosexual behavior might allow many adolescents to postpone intercourse to a more appropriate age and circumstance. When discussing the consequences of premature sexual intimacy, the young person should be helped to clarify his or her own feelings and offered various alternatives for meeting sexual and developmental needs.

Much parental and societal attention is given to the adolescent seeming to be overpreoccupied with sex. Little attention is given to the one reluctant to engage in dating behavior at all. As heterosexual interest and involvement (with appropriate limits as to degree) is a normal, natural, and necessary part of adolescent development, the young person who fails to express or evidence any such interest may well have serious psychosocial problems and warrants careful evaluation.

One of the more difficult issues to deal with is the adolescent involved in sexual intercourse because of emotional disturbance or less than mature reasons. Although abstinence may seem the best alternative, it is highly unlikely that the admonitions of adults will be heeded. Once virginity has been dispensed with, moral persuasion has little appeal. Although the potential for harm and the inappropriateness of the relationship can and should be reviewed, the probability of continued sexual intimacy will need to be accepted and attendant health risks responded to while instituting longer-range treatment plans for the underlying disturbance.

SEXUAL PERFORMANCE
Adolescents seldom complain directly of sexual dysfunction. They may be embarrassed to reveal a personal "flaw," fearful of discovery of their specific sexual practices, or naive about what is supposed to be normal sexual functioning. Because of biologic immaturity and situational anxieties (fear of failure, fear of discovery, guilt), many young people experience impotence, premature ejaculation, insufficient lubrication, painful intercourse, or lack of orgasm. A single such episode may be devastating if the adolescent fears this to be indicative of permanent dysfunction or disability. When such concerns are discovered, reproductive function and dysfunction should be explained; the use of illustrations from a reference text can be a helpful adjunct. The frequency of dysfunction in youth, the relationship to existent extrinsic or intrinsic stress factors (including performance expectancies), and the usually favorable prognosis need to be emphasized. The current place of sexual intercourse in the young person's life and the possibility of alternative satisfactions can then be reviewed.

PREMARITAL COUNSELING
Even if a premarital visit is solely for the mandatory serologic test and health statement, it also is important to take time to meet with both partners and explore their sexual knowledge and attitudes in order to avert possible marital difficulties related to sexual dysfunction or dissatisfaction and to discuss other important issues. Marriages between adolescents often are associated with premarital pregnancy, lower socioeconomic level, low general motivation, and an unhappy family life. They bear an increased risk for divorce, financial difficulties, large family size, and child-rearing problems. There are, of course, exceptions, particularly when the partners come from very happy homes where early marriages have been the rule and when they have known each other for some time. In any event, all these young couples are almost invariably in need of family planning services and sexuality counseling. Many need psychosocial support services as well. The same parameters should apply to those who choose to live together without marriage.

GENITAL ABNORMALITIES
Body image concerns related to congenital or acquired genital defects are greatly enhanced in adolescence and may prompt extreme denial, marked anxiety, overcompensation by sexual heroics, or dysfunctional withdrawal, and social isolation. Even when full correction has been accomplished by childhood surgery and normal pubertal maturation has occurred, the adolescent may continue to perceive that he or she is abnormal in genital develop-

ment or sexual functioning. When abnormalities persist (for example, neurogenic lesions, micropenis, epispadias, ambiguous genitalia), patient concerns can be overwhelming. Intercurrent genital problems, even with favorable outcomes, also may threaten body image and sexual identity. Such problems range from simple phimosis to minor genital surgery (herniorrhaphy, hydrocoelectomy, and cautery of genital warts or cervical erosion) to major, possibly mutilating situations (serious perineal trauma, testicular torsion with infarction, salpingo-oophorectomy for infection or ectopic pregnancy, and genital malignancies).

Complicating psychologic factors include guilt over the role of past or present "forbidden" sexual practices, fears and fantasies about future fertility and sexual performance, and marked anxiety over the possible compromise of sex-role definition and attractiveness. Whether such concerns are matters of fantasy alone or have a basis in fact, they require a considered response. Guidelines for counseling are as follows:

1. The physician should initiate discussion about the abnormality and typical adolescent concerns, for example, effect on masculinity or femininity, ability to function sexually (even if not sexually active), effect on fertility, urinary tract function, etc. The patient often finds it difficult to raise these issues. It should not be assumed that they do not exist simply because nothing is said.

2. Ample time is needed for a comfortable un-hurried approach in encouraging the young person to express concerns and ask questions once the topic has been introduced. Appropriate direction of the discussion can be encouraged by enquiring whether the adolescent has experienced masturbation or sexual intercourse since the problem's onset, how these events transpired, and how he or she felt about them. Reported normal functioning can be used to reassure while dysfunctionality, when brought out into the open, can be dealt with appropriately.

3. Discussion of the patient's own concerns is followed by specific education about the disorder or about the procedure to be performed, together with the expected outcome and implications for future health and sexual function.

4. Referral to an appropriate specialist is indicated for disorders requiring evaluation and treatment skills beyond those of the primary care physician or when prior surgery has had unsatisfactory cosmetic or functional results. It should not be assumed, however, that the specialist will provide sexual functioning counseling to an *adolescent*. This is seldom the case and the primary care physician must continue to take an active supporting role.

5. Patients with untoward emotional reactions unresponsive to the counseling approach should be referred for psychotherapy. It should not be assumed that the young person will "grow out" of his emotional problems; more often they become consolidated, causing even more difficulty at a later date.

6. See Chapter 21 on chronic illness for additional points.

HOMOSEXUALITY

Some degree of homosexual experience is part of the psychosexual developmental history of many individuals and is the sole expression of sexuality for a small minority of the adult population. Because of society's unresolved position about the meaning of homosexuality and the stigma often attached to it, the adolescent who is especially affectionate with a same-sex peer or adult may engender considerable parental concern. The adolescent who has engaged in, fantasized, or even been curious about homosexual behavior may feel extremely guilty and anxious, yet too embarrassed to have ever discussed this with a parent or other trusted adult. Reassurance may be offered by sharing these points:

1. Strong attraction to same-sex adults is a normal event for most adolescents, representing displacement of such feelings for parents onto others in the separation-individuation process.

2. Strong attraction to same-sex peers is the first step in the shifting of one's love-object relationship from the parents to age-mates and an intermediate early adolescent stage in the development of the capacity to form intimate interpersonal relationship. A further shift to heterosexual interests typically occurs in midadolescence.

3. Exhibitionism, voyeurism, and mutual masturbation are common experimental experiences, especially among boys aged 8–13 years. Group masturbation and ejaculation, often as a contest, are frequent methods of declaring maturity and superiority in the peer group.

4. In many cultures, the expression of affection between same-sex friends and relatives through embracing and kissing is a normal and accepted practice for males as well as females.

5. Few persons who have had a homosexual episode in adolescence retain a homosexual preference as adults. There is nothing predictive in such an act alone.

6. Adult sexual identity is not solidified until late adolescence, but as this is most influenced by early childhood factors, ultimate sexual gender

preference is well established, albeit nascent, by the advent of adolescence. Homosexual experiences during the early years will not alter a basic heterosexual orientation.

A small percentage of adolescents, however, become homosexual or bisexual adults. These young people usually begin to be aware of their different feelings by the medteens, although retrospectively most state they have been "different" for many years. It may be difficult for homosexual adolescents to secure appropriate medical and counseling services. The health professional who is accepting and reasonably comfortable in communicating with homosexual youths can play a major role in providing essential emotional support and medical care at a time of great difficulty for them. Practitioners who are not comfortable with these patients should refer them to professionals or agencies who can meet their needs. Appendix II lists several national resource organizations.

Sexually related medical conditions encountered in homosexuals include the same ones seen in heterosexuals plus those due to intestinal microorganisms transmitted during oroanal or genitorectal activity. The high incidence of sexually transmitted infections reported in this population may be attributed to the greater likelihood of having multiple sexual partners, the greater likelihood of having absent or minimal symptoms with pharyngeal or anorectal infections, and the psychosocial barriers to seeking medical care, all resulting in a significant pool of untreated individuals. Anorectal trauma resulting from such sexual practices as fist insertion or the masturbatory use of rectal foreign objects also may be seen.

The emergent homosexual adolescent faces additional stresses in psychosocial development. He or she initially tends to be greatly confused as to his or her true orientation and then must come to accept and define a sexual identity that is unacceptable to most of society. He or she feels exceptionally isolated in his or her dilemma, often having no opportunity to share thoughts with others in a similar plight and few available counseling services. Very much alone, the homosexual youth must adapt to the social consequences of belonging to a minority group with particularly limited rights and opportunities and often the target of community vilification. He or she faces great conflict and difficulty in resolving decisions about "coming out," telling parents, siblings, and friends, and the extent of involvement in political activism. Counseling support from within the gay community can be a valuable adjunct to whatever the health professional can provide.

TRANSSEXUALISM

The primary care physician will encounter an occasional adolescent requesting a sex change operation. The history most often reveals much sex role confusion and intense homosexual concerns. A deep-rooted, confirmed feeling of being the wrong sex is relatively rare. In the first instance, psychotherapy and sexuality counseling by an appropriately trained professional is indicated. A few adolescents, however, have always felt that their gender was wrong and express the strong conviction that sex change is the only resolution. They should be referred to a medical center that provides comprehensive evaluation of transsexuals and all components of sex reassignment. This by no means commits the adolescent to inevitable surgery; indeed such would not even be entertained during the patient's minority. But it does ensure that he or she is provided with the most experienced source of evaluation and counseling.

CROSS-DRESSING

Adolescent boys who repetitively dress in female clothing may fall into any one of the following categories.

1. Transvestites: accepting masculine identity but wishing to *appear* as a girl. Psychodynamically thought to represent the desire to win the mother's affection in families where femaleness is particularly valued.

2. Fetishists: using aberrant objects, thoughts, or practices, including the wearing of female clothing during sexual stimulation, particularly masturbation. Thought to represent the adoption of a hostile defense against maternal seductiveness.

3. Transsexuals: rejecting masculine identity, perceiving self to be a female mistakenly placed in a male body, and wishing to reconcile biological with psychological gender.

4. Sexually immature: lacking internal and/or external controls against immature and inappropriate behaviors; experimentation with female dressing is as a far younger child might normally do.

5. Homosexuals: accepting masculine identity, but desired love object is also male. May dress in an effeminate manner to attract males (uncommon in teenagers).

Evaluation should assess the frequency, intensity (casual or committed), duration, significance (isolated or part of a symptom pattern), and family response. All but mild, sporadic cases should be referred for psychological evaluation, sexuality counseling, and individual and family psychotherapy.

SEXUAL ASPHYXIA SYNDROME

The practice of self-strangulation during autoerotic activity recently has reached medical awareness due to occasional asphyxiation deaths. The most frequent victims are adolescent males, possibly due to their propensity for risk-taking behavior and ignorance of the potential lethal consequences. The syndrome, usually a private and well-kept secret, variably includes arranging a rope or belt in a manner that will compress the neck, binding the extremities, wearing female clothing, viewing sexually explicit pictures, and masturbating with neck compression at orgasm to heighten the effect. Initially, adolescents engaging in this behavior appear to be heterosexual in orientation and do not manifest depression or suicidal ideation. Those who avoid death tend to engage in repeated acts, in time involving a partner and developing a homosexual orientation. Any evidence of preoccupation with ropes and bondage or attempts at self-hanging deserves investigation for this practice and evaluation for abnormal psychosexual development. Treatment requires both protective and psychiatric intervention.

ACTING-OUT SEXUAL BEHAVIOR

Provocative sexual behavior includes the open use of sexually explicit language or gestures, the wearing of highly revealing clothing, seductive flirting with peers, adults, or both, and public display of sexual intimacy (kissing, hugging, petting). Adults frequently overreact and interpret this behavior as evidence of sexual promiscuity, a symptom of sexual disorder, or an act of delinquency and defiance. These behaviors commonly have a far less threatening meaning and represent a means of nonverbal communication, a method of testing the response of others, or a reactive symptom of anxiety or depression. The sexually provocative adolescent often is sexually inexperienced, struggling with psychosexual developmental issues, or simply attempting to win peer approval and notice. In other instances, clothing and behavior termed "seductive" by adults may only reflect the normal showing off of physical development and assertion of sexual identity characteristic of midadolescence. Flirting most often is a form of experimentation with interpersonal relationships and testing one's attractiveness to others. Thus, adolescent "sex offenses" often represent relatively innocuous developmental sex play or peer-urged experimentation brought to public or police attention. Retarded adolescents especially are vulnerable to being viewed as sex offenders when they behave appropriately for their delayed intellectual and psychosocial development despite physical maturity consistent with their chronological age.

Prostitution often begins in mid to late adolescence and frequently comprises part of a constellation of delinquent behaviors, including running away, truancy, shoplifting, and substance abuse. Many young female prostitutes have borderline character disorders. Their behavior provides escape from an intolerable home situation without having to become autonomous, since dependence shifts from parent to pimp. Prostitution also can be a survival adaptation for male and female adolescent runaways and drug users, practiced to obtain shelter, money, protection, and companionship.

Flagrant promiscuity (multiple partners without discrimination or commitment), repeated exhibitionism, repeated voyeurism, and the commission of rape or child sexual molestation go well beyond the range of adolescent experimentation and almost always indicate serious underlying psychosocial problems. Past history often reveals that the offenders were themselves victims of incest, rape, and child abuse, and had, as well, limited educational and vocational skills, an unstable home life, and a high degree of geographic mobility. Their problems frequently are compounded by being in trouble with the law consequent to their sexual behaviors.

Evaluation and management of any problematic sexual behavior first requires further definition in terms of frequency, duration, circumstances, and meaning. The psychosocial history (Chapters 2 and 23) will reveal whether symptoms fall within the realm of provocative normalcy or minor acting-out or reflect significant deviancy. Counseling by the primary care physician usually is sufficient for lesser issues. The goal of treatment is to help the young person modify the more provocative aspects of his or her behavior and to enable parents or other adults to feel less threatened and more tolerant. Chapters 23 and 24 provide specific techniques.

Prostitution and other serious deviant behaviors usually require psychiatric and social work assistance in resolving emotional and environmental difficulties. Legal services may also be required, as commission of prostitution and many sexually deviant acts are criminal offenses with clear judicial consequences if the individual is caught by police. Regardless of the nature of the problem, these adolescents also require attention for the possible medical consequences of pregnancy and infection.

Sexual Assault

RAPE

Up to 50% of female rape victims are adolescents. Each is potentially subject to serious physical or psychologic harm or both. Immediate emotional reactions, varying from stoicism to panic and hysteria, are not predictive of long-range effects. Regardless of initial manifestations, these young women commonly develop various phobias, depression, denial of the rape, and multiple psychosomatic symptoms. Adolescent males also may be assaulted (usually homosexually) and experience the same range of symptoms.

Effective management of the raped adolescent is based on a calm, reassuring, and supportive approach and the perception that he or she is indeed the victim of a particularly traumatic assault. Every effort should be made to minimize the emotional and physical discomfort of necessary legal and medical procedures as outlined in the following rape management protocol:

1. Identify and manage serious acute trauma: This includes physical (lacerations, hematomas, fractures) and emotional needs (panic state, extreme withdrawal, suicidal ideation).

2. Institute emotional support and advocacy: A trained peer counselor, rape counselor, psychiatric social worker, or nurse counselor can initiate the process and then accompany the victim throughout all steps.

3. Determine whether forensic evidence is to be obtained: The patient or parent has the right to request medical attention only and refuse legal examination.* If there is any stated or implied reason to believe the case will be pursued, special requirements govern the conduct and recording of the history and physical examination, as well as the collection of clothing and other specimens in evidence. Failure to follow these requirements precisely will seriously impair the strength of the patient's case and her ability to obtain legal redress. Legal procedures differ from one jurisdiction to another and should be ascertained before proceeding. Some states require a law officer in attendance at all times, others that the examination be performed only by designated persons such as a coroner or hospital-based gynecologist. Optimally, rape evidencial procedure should be posted in every hospital emergency room. Alternatively, most urban police departments have a rape crisis division that can provide appropriate information.

4. Obtain the history: Record all data in the patient's words ("The patient stated . . . ."). Note the alleged time, date, and place of the rape; the use of threats, force, weapons, or restraints; the occurrence and location of ejaculation; the insertion of any foreign object; loss of consciousness; prior consumption of drugs or alcohol; injuries inflicted on the rapist by the victim. Also obtain a complete gynecologic and sexual history; note time and date of last voluntary coitus; note any postrape bathing, douching, or clothing change.

5. Perform the physical examination: Note mental status. Carefully measure, describe, and diagram all cutaneous, perineal, pelvic, rectal, and other internal or external injuries. Take photographs when possible. Do a complete pelvic examination.

6. Collect specimens as needed for medical and/or legal purposes (see item j):

a. Scrape and preserve any material suggestive of semen from abdomen, thighs, or other reported ejaculation site. Comb or clip suspect areas in the pubic hair. Collect any apparent foreign head or pubic hairs. Take nail scrapings if patient reports scratching assailant.

b. Use a Wood's lamp to detect bright fluorescence of semen (urine, saliva, and feces only fluoresce dimly); scrape area or clip hairs and preserve.

c. Aspirate pooled secretions from vaginal vault or swab with cotton applicator. Air dry material on two slides (for sperm, acid phosphatase); place aspirate in sterile tube and/or swab in 1–2 ml sterile saline; irrigate vault with 10-20 ml sterile saline and preserve washings.

d. Culture endocervix for *N. gonorrhoeae*; *Chlamydia trachomatis* (if available).

e. Take Papanicolaou smear. (Motile sperm may be found in cervical mucus for several days, morphologically intact sperm for up to 2 weeks after coitus.)

f. Obtain similar specimens from oral cavity and/or anus for sperm, acid phosphatase, and cultures if patient reports assault at these sites.

g. Examine small amount of suspect secretions for motile sperm, trichomonads.

h. Obtain blood for syphilis serology, drug/alcohol screen, typing. Obtain urine for pregnancy test (or serum beta subunits for very early pregnancy).

---

*An increasing number of states have enacted laws providing for minors who have been raped to obtain medical care on their own as if adult. Consult hospital counsel about appropriate consent procedures in the jurisdiction. Emergency provisions pertain to urgently required medical and psychiatric care.

i. Save all clothing in sealed bag (have patient obtain other clothing from home).

j. Seal all specimens, marking with source, date and time obtained, patient's and examiner's names. Deliver all evidence to police or handle as directed by police protocol.

7. Prevent gonorrhea and syphilis: See standard treatment for uncomplicated gonorrhea and incubating syphilis.

8. Prevent pregnancy (if postmenarchal, not pregnant, and raped within past 72 hours: See postcoital contraception.

9. Arrange counseling for victim, family: Local rape crisis centers often are able to assist with immediate and ongoing counseling.

10. Observe patient closely for possible infection, pregnancy, emotional sequellae.

SEXUAL ABUSE

Sexual abuse has been reported with increasing frequency due to both public and professional awareness. Sexual abuse comprises up to 50% of all cases of child abuse and must be reported, when suspected, according to local child abuse laws (usually covering minors up to 18 years of age). Single nonviolent episodes by strangers usually have few long-term adverse emotional effects, but violent or chronic sexual abuse has a serious psychologic prognosis. The spectrum of sexual abuse by an adult on a minor ranges from exhibition of genitals without physical contact to manual manipulation of the minor's genitals, genital apposition, or outright penetration. A variety of differing terms for sexual abuse is employed in legal definitions, varying somewhat among jurisdictions (for example, "molestation" or "sexual misuse"). All imply the use of force, deceit, coercion, or persuasion to induce a minor to participate in sexual activity to which he or she cannot give legal consent. Evaluation and management follow the steps outlined for rape with the additional assessment of the minor's continuing vulnerability to sexual imposition. Sexual abuse committed by a relative comprises incest and introduces additional issues.

INCEST

Incest is increasingly recognized as a much more common problem than previously thought. Sexual activity between siblings is the most frequent form but also the least consequential, often falling within the realm of experimental sex play, and seldom reported. The most common relationship of serious significance is between father or stepfather and

TABLE 17-5
"RAPE KIT" CONTENTS

1. Rape manual
   a. Medical protocol.
   b. Psychologic support protocol.
   c. Legal protocol, including reporting requirements: who may take evidence (hospital personnel or coroner only); who must be present (hospital personnel only or police observer); statutory status of minor's consent; points to be covered in history and how to record; points to be covered in physical examination and how to document, including photographs; specimens required for evidence and how to obtain, preserve, label; what should be done with record, specimens.
   d. Telephone numbers of hospital/clinic rape counselors, local rape crisis centers, local police rape division.
2. Plastic bags, envelopes, seals, labels to contain evidence.

The following should be available in the emergency room, clinic, or office and should be assembled and prepared prior to assessment of the victim:
3. Speculum, gloves, and other equipment needed for pelvic examination.
4. Polaroid camera, color film (not outdated).
5. Wood's lamp (to detect semen).
6. Sterile swabs, glass slides, cover slips, test tubes with removable screw tops.
7. Scissors, tweezers, comb (for pubic hair, foreign material).
8. Sterile saline, irrigation catheters and syringes.
9. Pregnancy test kit (2-minute slide type).
10. Culture media for *N. gonorrhoeae* (candle jar unless using transport media); transport media for *C. trachomatis* (if testing available).
11. Syringes, needles, test tubes (for syphilis serology, drug screen, blood type).
12. Appropriate antibiotics for prophylaxis of gonorrhea, syphilis.
13. Appropriate estrogen preparations for postcoital contraception; antiemetics.
14. Sanitary napkins.

daughter or uncle and niece, with "step" relations more frequently involved than blood relations. Father-son incest is not uncommon. Other relative combinations are encountered less frequently. Incest usually begins when the girl is between 10 and 12 years of age. Initial paternal voyeurism may progress to fondling the genitals to outright sexual intercourse. Obviously, the interpersonal dynamics of incest families are greatly disturbed. The father, often with an alcoholic problem, is defective in psychosocial maturation with poor control of sexual impulses. The mother also has difficulty in heterosexual relationships and frequently has abdicated from her role as mother and wife, leaving the daughter to be her surrogate. The girl herself, although usually a reluctant partner, commonly sees herself as responsible for the father's attentions. She rarely reveals the situation willingly out of fear of parental retribution or rejection or out of concern that she precipitate a breakup of the family unit. Outwardly many of these families appear pillars of society. The father, often rigid and controlling over his daughter, is seemingly concerned about her welfare; the mother tends to be heavily committed to employment or community work. Another pattern is the totally disorganized family in which incest is simply one of many manifestations of acting-out behaviors by all its members.

The consequences to the victim of incest include a wide variety of emotional disturbances, which can make effective heterosexual relationships as an adult singularly difficult. These include mistrust of men, sexual dysfunction, sexual promiscuity, conversion reactions, phobias, chronic depression, and suicidal behavior. From the medical perspective there also is the more immediate risk of pregnancy or sexually transmitted disease.

Incest should be considered as a possible operative factor in any of the following situations, with two or more usually present in varying combinations.

1. Reversal of roles within a family, with the adolescent acting as mother in caring for the household and the father, combined with parental estrangement and cessation of marital sexual activity.

2. Running away.

3. *Serious* adolescent rebellion against the parent of the same sex.

4. Very low self-esteem in an adolescent.

5. Frequent psychosomatic complaints in an adolescent without obvious environmental stress, often severe enough to precipitate hospitalization (and thus secret sanctuary).

6. Paternal alcoholism and/or other parental dysfunctional behaviors.

7. Evidence of physical abuse of the adolescent.

8. Sexually transmitted infection in a young or retarded adolescent.

9. Pregnancy in a young or retarded adolescent. Any report or suspicion of possible incest should be taken seriously and investigated. At the same time, however, tact and sensitivity are needed to avoid unjust accusations. This can be a narrow tightrope to negotiate, made particularly difficult by the conspiracy of silence that usually obtains. Facts may be difficult to elicit, both parents and victim being most reluctant to reveal the situation. Truth often remains hidden until a solid trust relationship has been established between the helping professional (physician, social worker, psychiatrist) and adolescent.

Alternatively, the situation may present as a crisis, the father and daughter having been caught by some other family member or visitor to the home. Sometimes this is the mother herself, no longer able to escape dealing with reality through avoidance and denial.

The following guidelines are recommended in management:

1. Any report or suspicion of incest should be taken seriously.

2. Suspicion should prompt family evaluation for various risk factors and taking steps toward establishing a trust relationship with the adolescent and, if possible, her parents as well (Chapter 23).

3. If presenting as a crisis, the first requirement is to bring calm and order to the situation, preventing precipitate, poorly thought out actions that could lead to irreversible fragmentation of the family. Hasty actions are now regarded as ill advised for the adolescent's ultimate emotional health, although temporary removal of the father (or, less desirably, the daughter) from the home often is necessary for the adolescent's protection until the father can control his impulsiveness.

4. When facts begin to emerge, the duration, frequency, nature, and circumstances of the sexual activity should be defined, together with the degree of involvement and response of each family member, other family problems and, of equal importance, family strengths.

5. Accusations, assigning blame, or precipitating disruption of the family (except as necessary to protect the adolescent from further harm) should be avoided, as they tend to polarize family members and create an intrafamilial adversarial situation that only makes later therapy more difficult.

6. Any recent sexual contact should be evaluated for medical and legal purposes (when requested) as outlined under the previous sections on rape and sexual molestation. Incest is a criminal offense and, in a minor, also constitutes child abuse.

7. Referral for family therapy and individual therapy of both victim and offender is always indicated. The best outcome for the adolescent is the reconstitution of the family unit along healthier, more appropriate lines.

8. Report in compliance with local legal requirements pertaining to child abuse.

9. Provide ongoing support and closely observe for any physical or emotional consequences; ensure continued psychotherapy.

Menstrual and Pelvic Disorders

MENSTRUAL PHYSIOLOGY

Menstrual periods often are irregular in timing, duration and amount for 1-2 years after menarche. They may range from 2-4 days of flow every 10-14 days to no flow for many months. Cycles may be anovulatory or ovulatory with short luteal phases in which little progesterone is available to convert the endometrium from a proliferative to secretory stage. These cycles tend to be associated with milder cramps and fewer premenstrual symptoms than mature ovulatory cycles. Many adolescents are relatively infertile during this time, although there is no guarantee that ovulation and conception will not occur. All sexually active females are candidates for contraception regardless of the interval since menarche or irregularity of periods.

Once established, mature menstrual periods last from 2-7 days (average 5), with the heaviest flow occurring near the onset. Cycles can be as short as 21 days or as long as 45 days and still be normal, although the interval is consistent for the individual. A common pattern in adolescents is a 30-35 day cycle with prolonged proliferative and shortened secretory phases due to more gradual estrogen production and limited progesterone production. Ovulation is later in the cycle than would be expected for adults. Blood loss averages 30-40 ml. Four well-soaked pads or tampons per 24 hours are usual. More than six suggests an unusually heavy flow. Less than four is common, especially toward the end of the period.

AMENORRHEA

The absence of menstrual flow may be due to an anatomic defect or physiologic dysfunction at any point in the hypothalamic-pituitary-ovarian-endometrial-vaginal axis. Delayed menarche is a preferred term when a menstrual flow has never occurred (primary amenorrhea) and postmenarchal amenorrhea when menses cease after at least three menstrual flows in a 3-6 month time span (secondary amenorrhea).

Delayed menarche. The mean age of menarche in the United States is 12½ years, occurring 1-5 years after the onset of puberty (average 2½ years). Menarche usually follows the growth spurt, precedes full sexual maturity, and occurs between sexual maturity (Tanner) stages III and IV (Chap-

ter 2). Fifteen percent of females achieve menarche only after reaching stage V.

Evaluation of delayed menarche (Table 17-6) is highly dependent on the timing of puberty. The direction of investigation is determined by the following relationships.

1. Puberty absent at or after age 13½: Evaluate for delayed puberty (Chapter 12).

2. Puberty present, onset late, progression normal: Constitutionally delayed puberty and menarche likely; seek family history of delayed puberty (frequent) and rule out anatomic defect.

3. Puberty present, onset normal, progression delayed: Investigate for physical or emotional illness, significant weight gain or loss.

4. Puberty present, onset normal, progression normal, no menses after 4 or more years since onset: Anatomic obstruction to flow likely.

Genital anatomic defects generally are detected by a combination of genital inspection, pelvic and/or rectal examination, and chromosomal studies as indicated. Sonography and laparoscopy are definitive procedures. The patient also should be screened for associated cardiac, renal, and musculoskeletal abnormalities in cases of sex chromosomal abnormalities. Evaluation frequently is facilitated by endocrinologic and/or gynecologic consultation. Referral for surgical correction, when indicated, should be as early as possible. Counseling also is essential to lessen the potential for serious psychologic effects of an abnormal genital tract or infertility on developing self-image, formation of sexual identity, and sexual activities. The inability to procreate and alternatives to child-bearing should be discussed in later adolescence or any time the patient specifically asks.

Postmenarchal amenorrhea. The most frequent cause of cessation of menses in an adolescent is inhibition of the secretion and/or function of follicle-stimulating hormone (FSH) and luteinizing hormone (LH) with anovulation. This may be due to many factors, including immaturity, pregnancy, extreme physical stress such as competitive athletics, severe emotional stress, sudden environmental change, hyperthyroidism or hypothyroidism, chronic systemic illness, extreme weight loss or gain, anorexia nervosa (even before marked weight loss), polycystic ovaries, or extrinsic pharmacologic agents (prescribed medications, abused substances, hormones). The history of prior menstrual periods establishes the presence and patency of a uterus and vagina.

The following approach is suggested:

1. Pregnancy always should be ruled out, even with a history of only one late or absent menstrual period and despite denial of sexual activity.

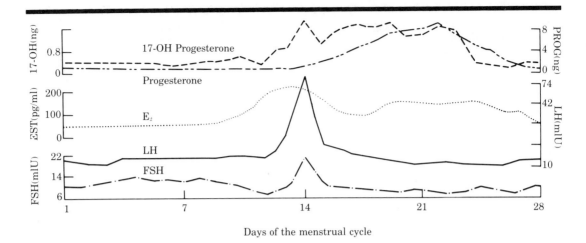

Days of the menstrual cycle

FIGURE 17-2
SCHEMATIC REPRESENTATION OF THE INTERRELATIONSHIP OF ENDOMETRIAL CHANGES, OVARIAN FUNCTION, AND PATTERNS OF HORMONE SECRETION THROUGHOUT A MATURE MENSTRUAL CYCLE.

(From Brookman, R. R. 1981. *Pediatric and adolescent gynecology case studies,* New Hyde Park, N.Y.: Medical Examination Publishing Co., Inc.)

2. Investigate for medical conditions or emotional stress by complete health assessment (Chapters 2 and 3). If detected, treat as indicated.

3. If no medical condition is present administer a single dose of progesterone in oil, 100 mg IM, or medroxyprogesterone acetate, 10 mg/day p.o. for 5 days, provided there is *no chance of pregnancy.* Withdrawal bleeding within 4–7 days demonstrates an intact endocrine axis and an estrogen-primed endometrium. Diagnosis is functional anovulation.

4. If withdrawal bleeding occurs, reassure the patient (and parents) that her reproductive system is

TABLE 17-6
DIFFERENTIAL DIAGNOSTIC APPROACH TO DELAYED MENARCHE

External inspection	Uterus (rectal exam)	Likely diagnosis	Confirmatory investigations
Common			
Normal immature female	Present	Delayed puberty	Evaluation as in Chapter 12
Normal mature female			
Patent introitus	Present	Normal with late onset Vaginal septum	Speculum exam normal Speculum exam difficult
Nonpatent introitus	Present	Imperforate hymen	Bulging membrane, midline mass
Nonpatent introitus	Present/Absent	Congenital absence of vagina	Flat membrane, ± mass Surgical exploration
Rare			
Normal mature female			
Patent introitus	Absent	Congenital absence of uterus	Karyotype: 46 XX
Normal female, no hair	Absent	Testicular feminization syndromes	Karyotype: 46 XY
Virilized female	Absent	Partial testicular feminization	Karyotype: 46 XY
Ambiguous genitalia	Absent	Hermaphroditism	Karyotype: variable

normal. Try to eliminate or alleviate any causal factor or factors through health education, nutritional intervention, and/or psychosocial counseling. Await resumption of menses.

5. Progesterone administration can be repeated every 6–12 weeks to reinforce normalcy and prevent excessive endometrial proliferation consequent to unopposed estrogens and the possibility of menometrorrhagia. This will not inhibit gonadotropin cycling or the return of ovulation.

6. Estrogen-progestin combinations (oral contraceptives) also can be used for regulating chronic menstrual irregularity (see section on contraception for prescription). They should not be used, however, during the first 6–12 months after menarche, as some investigators believe this will suppress maturation of the hypothalamic-gonadal axis.

7. When hypoestrogenization is suspected (decreased breast size, vaginal dryness), obtain a lateral vaginal wall cytologic smear for maturation index (Table 17-4). Due to high sensitivity of vaginal cells to low levels of estrogen, a report of absent or low estrogen effect suggests extreme hypothalamic suppression or primary ovarian failure.

8. Evidence of other than simple functional amenorrhea requires further investigation, often with endocrinologic, gynecologic, and/or neurologic consultation (Table 17-7).

Anorexia nervosa. Amenorrhea often precedes weight loss and may not resolve until long after the weight returns to normal. Even then, a predisposition to anovulation and amenorrhea remains, with even minimal stress. Starvation results in hypothalamic suppression with low serum FSH, LH, and estrogens, lack of the midcycle LH surge, a hypoestrogenic vaginal smear, and no response to the progesterone withdrawal test. Ovulation can be induced with clomiphene or LH-releasing hormone and will restore menses. However, a precipitous return of signs of female maturity can be emotionally counterproductive and only should be considered in light of the total medical and psychiatric management plan (Chapter 19).

Primary ovarian failure. Amenorrhea and loss of estrogenization following at least a few menstrual cycles can occur in some variants of gonadal dysgenesis, instances of ovarian damage from irradiation or chemotherapy for malignancy, and as the rare syndrome of premature menopause. The last condition may be part of an autoimmune, multiple endocrine disorder with circulating antiovarian antibodies. Biopsy is diagnostic, revealing a lack of functioning follicles. Regardless of cause, treatment of primary ovarian failure requires replacement of estrogen and progesterone until the desired time of menopause,

TABLE 17-7
DIFFERENTIAL DIAGNOSTIC APPROACH TO POSTMENARCHAL AMENORRHEA

Associated physical findings	Likely diagnoses	Confirmatory investigations
Abnormal stature		
Tall	Partial gonadal dysgenesis	Karyotype: 45 XO, 46 XY, mosaicism, variants
Short	Gonadal dysgenesis (premature menopause)	Gonadotropins: markedly elevated
Abnormal weight		
Excess	Obesity	Diet history
	Polycystic ovary syndrome	Serum androgens, gonadotropins
Insufficient	Starvation	Diet history
	Anorexia nervosa	Vaginal smear; psychosocial evaluation
Hirsutism	Polycystic ovary syndrome	Serum gonadotropins, androgens
	Cushing's syndrome	Serum cortisol
Virilization	Late adrenogenital syndrome	Serum androgens, 17-hydroxypro-gesterone
	Polycystic ovary syndrome	Serum gonadotropins, androgens
	Virilizing tumor (adrenal/ovarian)	Serum androgens; radiography
Systemic symptoms/signs	Chronic illness	
	Endocrinopathy	Specific tests as indicated
	Pregnancy	
Galactorrhea and/or neurologic symptoms	Pituitary tumor	Serum prolactin; neurologic exam; skull films
	Drug-induced hyperprolactinemia	Serum prolactin; history; toxic screen
	Severe hypothyroidism	Serum T_4, TSH
No other findings	Early pregnancy	Pregnancy test: urine, serum
	Emotional stress	History; psychosocial evaluation
	Premature menopause	Vaginal smear; serum gonadotropins; biopsy

together with counseling about self-image, sexual function, and infertility.

Polycystic ovary syndrome (formerly, Stein-Leventhal syndrome). Beginning any time after the onset of puberty, variable manifestations include hirsutism, obesity, and chronic anovulation with amenorrhea or irregular bleeding. There is erratic or inappropriately elevated LH secretion, low constant FSH secretion, androgen excess, and normal estrogenic activity. Pelvic examination, pelvic ultrasound, and/or laparoscopy reveal bilateral polycystic and, often, enlarged ovaries. Definitive treatment to restore fertility consists of ovulation induction by the administration of clomiphene or LH-releasing hormone or by ovarian wedge resection. Oral contraceptive steroids provide temporary "normal" menstrual cycles, suppress hyperandrogenism, and prevent further hirsutism. Electrolysis is the only method to remove existing hair. Reduction of excess

weight is recommended. The differential diagnosis of postmenarchal amenorrhea with hirsutism includes the late presentation of variants of the adrenogenital syndrome (Chapter 12).

Amenorrhea-galactorrhea syndrome. The association of milky nipple discharge with amenorrhea raises suspicion of a pituitary microadenoma or other pathologic condition, especially in an adolescent who has never been pregnant. The symptoms are caused by hyperprolactinemia, which stimulates lactation and suppresses midcycle gonadotropin elevations, producing anovulatory cycles. Points to be considered in evaluation include the following:

1. History of recent pregnancy carried to term or aborted; can result in amenorrhea and galactorrhea, which ultimately is self-limited.

2. History of oral contraceptive use; this may produce oligomenorrhea or amenorrhea with sensitization of the mammary tissue and lactation even

in the face of normal prolactin levels. This is most likely to occur in parous females.

3. History of drug use that may cause hyperprolactinemia (phenothiazines, tricyclic antidepressants, reserpine, haloperidol, amphetamines, opiates, marijuana, among others).

4. Evaluate for CNS-hypothalamic-pituitary lesion, especially pituitary microadenoma.

a. Complete neurologic exam, visual fields, fundoscopy.

b. Serum prolactin level.

c. Lateral skull film, CT scan.

5. Evaluate for thyroid dysfunction by examination and serum T_4, T_3, TSH levels.

6. Treat specific etiologies as indicated (stop medication, correct thyroid status, remove tumor). When no explanation for the prolactinemia can be demonstrated and pituitary microadenoma is suspected, bromocriptine therapy often is effective; referral to an experienced endocrinologist or gynecologist is indicated.

7. Due to the high prevalence of adenomas in nulliparous females who develop galactorrhea while taking oral contraceptives, these individuals should be observed closely for signs or symptoms of this lesion.

DYSFUNCTIONAL UTERINE BLEEDING

Dysfunctional uterine bleeding in adolescents is almost always due to acute or chronic anovulation. Menstrual cycles may be immature, with irregular bleeding patterns occurring for months to several years after menarche. Normal menstrual function also may be altered by any of the same factors causing postmenarchal amenorrhea. Occasionally, following ovulation, the corpus luteum degenerates prematurely, causing excess flow, or functions excessively with the next flow delayed in onset but then heavy and/or prolonged. The various patterns of dysfunctional bleeding are defined as follows:

□ Amenorrhea: no flow for 3 or more months after a normal flow

□ Oligomenorrhea: low to normal amount, increased intervals

□ Hypomenorrhea: decreased amount, regular intervals

□ Polymenorrhea: low to normal amount, decreased intervals

□ Hypermenorrhea: increased amount, regular intervals

□ Menometrorrhagia: increased amount, irregular intervals

□ Breakthrough bleeding: small amounts between normal menstrual flows

The pattern itself is not diagnostic or even suggestive as to cause. Evaluation includes the following:

1. Investigate for a nonuterine source of bleeding, for example, urinary tract, vagina, rectum: trauma, infection, tumor, granulomatous disease.

2. Investigate for pregnancy, even with denial of sexual activity. If early spontaneous abortion or ectopic pregnancy suspected, may need serum pregnancy test.

3. Confirm that cycles are anovulatory.

a. Look for estrogenization of vaginal cytology, stretchability (spinnbarkeit) and ferning of cervical mucus (pattern when dried on slide).

b. Record daily basal body temperature for 2–3 months. The adolescent can take her temperature each morning before arising and record it on plain paper for the clinician to transcribe to the temperature chart.

4. Establish the pattern of bleeding by having the patient keep a menstrual calendar. What some adolescents term irregular (for example, "two periods last month") may turn out to be simple misunderstanding of normal physiology (menses began on the first and twenty-ninth).

5. Exclude other etiologies or contributory factors. Although considerably less common than simple dysfunctional bleeding, other causes (and diagnostic procedures) that should be considered include:

a. Oral contraceptive problems (breakthrough bleeding, missed pills); history

b. Intrauterine device (IUD) side effects; history, pelvic examination, abdominal roentgenogram/ultrasound

c. Endometritis; history, pelvic examination, cultures (suspect when irregular bleeding is associated with pelvic pain, fever, vaginal discharge, and/or IUD in place)

d. Chronic anemia, thrombocytopenia, blood dyscrasias; history, physical examination, CBC, blood smear, platelet count (suspect when bleeding is very heavy, especially at or soon after menarche)

e. Ovarian cyst/tumor; abdominal and pelvic examination, ultrasound, laparoscopy

f. Endocrinopathy; history, physical examination, thyroid and other hormone levels as indicated

g. Clotting disorders; history, clotting studies (some coagulopathies may first present or only manifest in excessive menstrual flow—see Chapter 13)

Treatment is determined by the etiology, pattern of bleeding, severity of blood loss and degree of expressed concern. Dysfunctional bleeding due to

TABLE 17-8
TREATMENT OF DYSFUNCTIONAL UTERINE BLEEDING*

Regimen	Acute bleeding	Cyclic therapy[†]
Enovid (norethynodrel-mestranol), 5 mg Norlutin (norethindrone), 5 mg Norlestrin (norethindrone acetate-ethinyl estradiol), 2.5 mg	4–6 tabs/day until flow stops; then 2 tabs/day for 3 weeks	1–2 tabs/day for 20 days; cycle every 28 days
Norlutate (norethindrone acetate), 5 mg	2–3 tabs/day until flow stops; then 1 tab/day for 3 weeks	1 tab/day for 20 days; cycle every 28 days
Estinyl (ethinyl estradiol), 0.05 mg	10–20 tabs/day until flow stops; then 1–3 tabs/day for 2 weeks	1–3 tabs/day for 14 days; cycle every 28 days
Provera (medroxyprogesterone acetate), 10 mg	2–3 tabs/day for 5–10 days; await withdrawal flow	1 tab/day on days 15–19 of cycle beginning with withdrawal flow; repeat every 28 days
Conjugated estrogen, 20–25 mg (for example, Premarin)	IV or IM dose, repeat in 2–4 hours, then every 4 until flow stops (usually 2–4 doses needed)	

*Note: a. None of the above should be given if there is evidence or strong suspicion of pregnancy.
b. Volume expansion, blood replacement may be needed with shock, acute anemia.
c. Iron replacement may be indicated with secondary chronic anemia.
d. Parenteral estrogen recommended if oral medication not tolerated due to nausea or vomiting; administration in hospital setting preferred.
e. Dilatation and curettage rarely indicated except for cases refractory to hormonal therapy.

[†]Begin cyclic therapy on fifth day after withdrawal flow begins.

physiologic immaturity need not be treated unless the frequency or amount of blood loss risks anemia or interferes with school attendance and social activities. Simple reassurance and having the patient record her bleeding pattern on a menstrual calendar usually is all that is required; a normal pattern typically emerges within 6–24 months. Treatment of chronic dysfunctional bleeding beyond the period of immaturity similarly depends on the degree of blood loss and interference with daily life. The psychologic impact also needs to be taken into account. Stress-related irregularity often reverts to a normal pattern when the stress itself is reduced or removed. Treatment, when indicated, largely depends on the use of cyclic hormonal therapy (Table 17-8). Such treatment, however, will not alter the underlying problem, and irregularity (with potential fertility problems) may return once treatment is stopped; the patient should be so advised. There is no evidence, however, that the use of cyclical therapy will either aggravate or cause a fertility problem.

An unusually heavy or prolonged flow, even from a single menstrual period, can be sufficient to produce acute anemia and/or shock requiring emergency treatment. Patients not on cyclical treatment

should be advised to seek medical attention promptly if they experience excessive blood loss. Patients with frequent or prolonged episodes of bleeding, even if not pronounced, should have periodic monitoring of their hematocrit and reticulocyte count and may be candidates for iron supplementation.

Regulation by the induction of ovulation with clomiphene or similar agents is not recommended for most adolescents. Since sexual activity may be unpredictable and concealed, treatment could lead to a multiple as well as unintended pregnancy. Those with chronic anovulation who seriously wish to become pregnant should be referred to a gynecologist specializing in infertility problems.

DYSMENORRHEA AND PELVIC PAIN

Functional dysmenorrhea. Menstrual cramps characterize cycles in which the postovulatory rise and fall of progesterone prompts the release of prostaglandins. These substances, in turn, increase uterine contractions and irritate endometrial nerve endings. Half of all ovulating females experience discomfort for 1–3 days of most menstrual periods. Twenty-five percent have severe cramps, the most common single cause of school and job absence among females.

Such individuals tend to have particularly high levels of circulating prostaglandins during menses when compared to those with lesser discomfort. Although the pain clearly is mediated by physiologic mechanisms, cultural and familial attitudes about menses and individual psychosocial adjustment factors often strongly influence the nature and extent of an adolescent's response. Regardless of the degree of pain, some adolescents continue normal daily routines and others become quite incapacitated, perceiving cramps as an illness. Menstrual discomfort also may be accompanied by nausea, vomiting, diarrhea, backache, headache, and/or general malaise.

Although most dysmenorrhea in adolescents is functional in origin, differential considerations include anatomic genital defects, ovarian cysts, endometriosis, and postinfectious adhesions. Increased menstrual discomfort in a sexually active adolescent may be due to endometritis. "Retroverted uterus" and "cervical stenosis," however, are normal variants having no significance.

Functional dysmenorrhea is a definite physiologic phenomenon, not simply the exaggerated response of a hysterical female. Any adolescent experiencing significant discomfort is entitled to reduce her symptoms by any effective method, including strong analgesics, antiprostaglandins, and, in some instances, the lesser narcotics such as codeine. Use of these agents for 1-3 days a month is far different than chronic daily administration and bears low abuse potential. However, limited prescriptions for narcotics should be given to adolescents suspected of drug abuse or drug dealing.

Numerous compounds relieve menstrual cramps by analgesia and/or suppression of prostaglandin release. Prostaglandin synthetase is inhibited by aspirin, acetaminophen, phenacetin, indomethacin, ibuprofen, and naproxen. Fenamates not only inhibit prostaglandin synthesis but also block myometrial receptors. Each agent's potential for gastrointestinal, cutaneous, neurologic, and/or hematologic complications should be weighed against the degree of dysmenorrhea and resulting incapacitation.

The following management protocol for functional dysmenorrhea is suggested:

1. Investigate patient, familial, and cultural attitudes about menstruation.

2. Rule out anatomic abnormalities and endometritis by complete pelvic examination; rule out endometriosis in *severe* dysmenorrhea (see below).

3. Dispell myths and reassure the patient and her parents about the normalcy of menstrual symptoms.

4. Try aspirin in adequate doses (650-1000 mg)

every 4 hours for 2-3 days, beginning with onset of bleeding or cramping (not simply on an as needed basis).

5. If no response in two or three cycles, select a more potent agent. Because many such products are available today, it is desirable to become familiar with the use and potential toxicity of a limited number such as the following.

    a. Ibuprofen, 400 mg t.i.d.

    b. Sodium naproxen, 275 mg q.i.d.

    c. Mefenamic acid, 250 mg t.i.d.

    d. Indomethacin, 25-50 mg t.i.d. (high rate of GI side effects, headaches)

Although more expensive than aspirin or acetaminophen, these compounds are effective and often abort cramps after only one or two doses. They are best reserved for moderate to severe cramps and taken only as long as needed. In unresponsive cases, aspirin or acetaminophen compound with codeine may be tried.

6. In severe dysmenorrhea, relief may be provided by the induction of anovulatory cycles for 3-6 months through the use of cyclic hormones (if there are no contraindications). The greater comfort experienced with anovulatory cycles for a limited time may break a hyperresponsive pattern. This also comprises specific therapy for endometriosis, which often resolves with such treatment (see section on contraception for prescription).

7. Significant benefit also can be obtained from the use of self-hypnosis, meditational techniques, relaxation techniques, or biofeedback.

8. Avoid the use of intrauterine devices as these tend to increase menstrual cramps. If an IUD is the only acceptable contraceptive, select a progesterone-releasing device. Prescribe aspirin or other antiprostaglandins with some caution because they inhibit platelet adhesiveness and tend to exacerbate IUD-induced menorrhagia.

9. Encourage normal activity and exercise. There are no contraindications to any athletics except as aesthetics and the adolescent's own preferences dictate. Exercise often has an ameliorating effect on cramps.

Mittelschmerz. Midcycle lower quadrant pain sometimes occurs in association with ovulation and is believed due to pelvic irritation from discharged ovarian follicular contents. The discomfort tends to be unilateral, alternating sides each month, and often is accompanied by mild bleeding or changes in vaginal secretions. The pain may last from several hours to 3-4 days. Treatment consists of education, reassurance, analgesia as needed, and ovulation inhibition when the symptoms are severe and incapacitating.

Endometriosis. Endometriosis is much more common in adolescents than previously thought. Recent laparoscopic studies have found this condition present in up to 65% of adolescents with severe chronic pelvic pain. Endometrial tissue refluxed from the oviducts during menstruation or developing from embryonic cell rests may be seeded anywhere in the pelvis and form multiple small cysts on the ovaries, uterine surface, pelvic ligaments, or peritoneum. Pain occurs when these cysts swell during the menstrual cycle, create adhesions between pelvic structures, or are located so as to irritate nerve endings. The pain may be cyclic or acyclic, can be aggravated by coitus, and is relieved by rest. Pain may be localized to the lower abdomen, back, groin, thigh, and/or deep pelvis. The pelvic examination may be entirely within normal limits or may detect tenderness and/or nodularity of any structure, thickened broad ligaments, and/or a fixed, immobile uterus. Ultrasonography may demonstrate multiple scattered cysts in the pelvis. Laparoscopy is confirmatory. Treatment with cyclic hormones for 3–6 months often produces shrinkage and disappearance of the aberrant tissue. Endometriosis tends to be a chronic, recurring condition. Referral to a gynecologist for continuing management is indicated. Various surgical procedures may be necessary but are postponed whenever possible until completion of childbearing.

Premenstrual tension. Numerous symptoms may precede the onset of menstrual bleeding, including headache, tiredness, irritability, bloating, and edema. The etiology is unclear, although water retention resulting from hormone-induced sodium retention appears to be a significant factor in this physiologic variant. There is no evidence that this is simply a figment of female imagination or a psychogenic response. In some cases, however, psychological factors may exacerbate the physiologic state consequent to the negative attitudes of the adolescent and her family toward menses ("the curse").

Therapy is controversial and produces inconsistent results, but relief often is obtained by decreasing the fluid load. Water retention may be relieved by salt restriction or use of a mild diuretic during the week preceding menstrual flow; hydrochlorothiazide, 25 mg once a day or once every other day, can be tried.

Differential diagnosis of pelvic pain. Common causes of acute and chronic pelvic pain in adolescents are individually discussed in detail elsewhere. Table 17-9 summarizes a more extensive listing of differential considerations. Many of the rarer conditions require additional gynecologic, urologic, and/or surgical evaluation for definitive diagnosis and management.

PELVIC MASSES

A pelvic mass may be discovered in an adolescent under any of the following circumstances:

1. During evaluation of acute, chronic, or intermittent abdominal or pelvic pain
2. During evaluation of menstrual dysfunction
3. With a history of progressive abdominal enlargement
4. During evaluation of suspected pelvic inflammatory disease
5. As an unexpected finding in the routine health assessment of an asymptomatic female
6. As an unexpected finding of pelvic calcification on roentgenograms taken for other reasons

The most common pelvic mass is an enlarged uterus due to pregnancy, even in patients denying sexual activity. Other masses include cysts, tumors, abscesses, and complications of anatomic defects or physiologic function (Table 17-10).

The most frequent ovarian mass* is a cyst, which may be asymptomatic or present as chronic pelvic pain, dysfunctional bleeding, or both. An acute abdominal emergency also is possible, either through spontaneous rupture or torsion and infarction. Ovarian cysts may become quite large, producing abdominal distension, or remain small and disappear after one to three menstrual cycles. Small cysts may be simply observed over several months for spontaneous resolution, with appropriate reassurance of the adolescent. Symptomatic, enlarging, or very large cysts at the time of discovery require surgical removal. The differential diagnosis of ovarian masses includes tuboovarian abscess (especially in the presence of an IUD and/or evidence of pelvic infection), ectopic pregnancy, and tumors. Most ovarian tumors are benign, but even those which are malignant have a good prognosis when diagnosis and treatment occur early. In any instance, referral to a cancer specialist is advisable.

Ultrasonography followed by laparoscopy, if needed, are particularly useful in the detection and differentiation of pelvic masses. Standard roentgeno-

*Note: For comparison, the ovaries are palpable as bilaterally equal, ovoid masses slightly larger than almonds; in tense or obese adolescents it may be difficult to feel them at all.

TABLE 17-9
DIFFERENTIAL DIAGNOSTIC APPROACH TO PELVIC PAIN

Characteristics of pain	Likely diagnoses	Confirmatory investigations
Midline location		
Cyclic, normal bleeding	Physiologic dysmenorrhea	History, pelvic examination (normal)
	Endometriosis	Pelvic exam; sonography; laparoscopy
Acute, irregular bleeding	Endometritis	Pelvic exam, cultures; CBC; sed rate
	Threatened/septic abortion	History; pelvic exam; pregnancy test
Unrelated to menses, urinary symptoms*	Cystitis	History; urinalysis, urine culture
	Normal uterine pregnancy	History; pregnancy test
Lateral location		
Cyclic, normal bleeding	Mittelschmerz	History (timing, nature); pelvic exam (normal)
	Endometriosis	Pelvic exam; sonography; laparoscopy
Acute, postmenstrual	Salpingitis/pelvic inflammatory disease	History; pelvic exam, cultures; CBC, sed rate; laparoscopy
Acute, abnormal bleeding	Ectopic pregnancy	History; pelvic exam; pregnancy test
Unrelated to menses, acute	Appendicitis	History; physical exam; CBC; radiography
	Ureteral colic	History; urinalysis; radiography
Unrelated to menses, chronic	Constipation	History; rectal exam
	Pelvic osteomyelitis	Physical exam; radiography; gallium scan
	Psychogenic	History; exclusion of others; psychosocial evaluation

*Dysuria, urinary frequency, may be associated with infection, pregnancy, psychogenic factors.

grams are helpful only in detecting calcifications. Computerized axial tomography is expensive and indicated mainly for complete evaluation of the tissues surrounding a suspected malignant mass. The ease and safety of laparoscopy warrant its frequent use for direct observation of pelvic structures and obtaining cultures or biopsy material. Gynecologic or surgical consultation is almost always indicated and will direct further evaluation and management.

IN UTERO ESTROGEN EXPOSURE

Daughters of women who took diethylstilbestrol (DES) or a related estrogen during pregnancy have a high incidence of benign anatomic changes, including ectopic glandular tissue (vaginal adenosis, cervical ectropion), and surface epithelial changes (transverse vaginal ridges, pseudopolyps, cervical hood). Clear

cell adenocarcinoma is a far less common complication, occurring in 0.25-1.4/1000 young women with benign changes. Current opinion is that benign changes rarely progress to malignancy and frequently resolve spontaneously over several years. Of greater concern in these young women are uterine structural abnormalities, which increase their chances for infertility, premature delivery, and fetal wastage. When there is a history of in utero exposure to estrogens or suspicious anatomic findings observed during pelvic examination, the young woman should be referred to an experienced gynecologist for further evaluation, including colposcopy and possible biopsy. Exposed females should have their first evaluation soon after menarche or by age 14 if asymptomatic, but at younger ages if there is irregular vaginal bleeding. Psychologic reactions to the

TABLE 17-10
DIFFERENTIAL DIAGNOSIS OF PELVIC MASSES

Characteristic of mass	Differential diagnosis	Confirmatory history/findings/procedure
Midline location		
With amenorrhea/abnormal menses	Pregnancy	History of sexual activity; positive pregnancy test; positive pelvic exam
	Hematocolpos, hematometra	History of no menses, cyclic pelvic pain; perineal exam reveals imperforate hymen, vaginal stenosis
	Uterine sarcoma (rare)	Negative pregnancy test; uterine enlargement; sonography, computerized tomography; tissue diagnosis
With normal menses	Bladder	History of acute retention; findings of herpetic or other lesions precipitating retention; catheterization
Lateral location		
With amenorrhéa/abnormal menses	Functioning ovarian cyst Ovarian tumor	History of menstrual irregularity; negative pregnancy test; unilateral mass; physical/laboratory evidence of hormonal abnormalities; sonography, laparoscopy, tissue diagnosis
	Polycystic ovary syndrome	As above with bilateral ovarian enlargement
	Ectopic pregnancy	History of sexual activity; pregnancy test may or may not be positive; sonography; may or may not have pain/tenderness; may present as acute emergency
With normal menses	Tuboovarian abscess	History and findings compatible with pelvic inflammatory disease; sonography, laparoscopy
	Nonfunctioning ovarian cyst	History of pain or asymptomatic; unilateral mass; may be very large; sonography, laparoscopy, tissue diagnosis
	Appendiceal abscess	History of appendicitis (or acute abdominal condition); positive rectal/abdominal exam; may be difficult to distinguish from pelvic inflammatory disease; sonography, laparotomy
	Fecal impaction	History of constipation; positive rectal/abdominal exam; abdominal roentgenograms

discovery of the problem should be evaluated and responded to with counseling. Guilt feelings in the adolescent's mother are particularly prevalent.

CERVICAL NEOPLASIA
Between 1% and 4% of sexually active adolescents have early neoplastic changes on cervical cytologic smear (severe dysplasia, carcinoma in situ). Up to 40% have mild atypia or inflammatory changes, usually secondary to cervicitis. High-risk factors for early neoplasia include history of pregnancy, early onset of sexual activity, multiple partners, low socioeconomic status, repeated genital infections, and nonuse of barrier contraception. Mildly abnormal Papanicolaou smears should be repeated in 3 months after treatment of any existing infection. Severely or persistently abnormal cytology warrants referral to a gynecologist for further evaluation.

Adolescents with early onset of sexual activity, multiple sexually transmitted infections, or both should have frequent Papanicolaou smears. Controversy exists over the precise periodicity. Some recommend annual tests for life; others suggest that the frequency in high-risk adolescents should be every 6 months. In any event, a history of previous cervical dysplasia clearly warrants annual or semiannual monitoring indefinitely.

Genital Infections
SEXUALLY TRANSMITTED DISEASES
Infections are the most frequent cause of genital-related complaints in adolescents. A significant proportion of these are classifiable as a sexually transmitted disease (STD). This term now supplants the term venereal disease (VD) because it encompasses all conditions that may be spread by intimate sexual

contact, and because VD has a more limited (and pejorative) connotation.

Many factors contribute to the current prevalence and epidemiology of STDs in adolescents, including increasing rates of sexual intercourse, the likelihood of multiple partners, the high incidence of asymptomatic carrier states, the relatively low use of protective barrier contraceptive methods, the relatively low rate of use of medical sources (and associated screening for carriers) for contraception, the low rate of screening adolescents for STDs as a component of routine health care and health maintenance, the propensity of even symptomatic adolescents to deny the possibility of STD and delay treatment, barriers to obtaining care by the young because of limited availability of services and associated social stigmata, and a tendency to stop medication when symptoms abate, leading to incompletely treated disease and persistence of infectivity. In combination, these reasons have led to a widespread incidence of STDs among the adolescent population, second only to the 20–25 year old age group. Examination and testing for STDs must be part of the routine health assessment of all sexually active adolescents.

Any genital infection must be potentially considered an STD and investigated accordingly. This includes not only the diagnosis and treatment of the infected individual, but also the identification, location, and treatment of contacts. Syphilis and gonorrhea are reportable conditions in virtually every state. The physician must report these diseases together with the patient's name and address to the local department of public health. This does not necessarily compromise the patient's confidence, as such reporting is governed by strict privacy regulations; parents will not be advised and the information can only be used for epidemiologic control and statistical purposes. Any direct followup of contact cases usually is limited to persons with syphilis. Gonorrhea is ubiquitous and the number of investigators too few to adequately pursue eradication of this disease through case-finding methods.

STD in an adolescent may come to the attention of the physician in a number of ways. The patient, either aware or unaware of the significance of his or her symptoms, may present with clear clinical signs. Alternatively the patient may think he or she has an STD but in fact the condition turns out to be something else. An example is the female with candidal vaginitis who believes herself to have gonorrhea. Then there is the asymptomatic adolescent who has been exposed to a known contact and presents for evaluation or the patient without a known contact but discovered to be a carrier on routine screening tests (VDRL, gonococcal cultures). But it is also possible that an STD may be entirely missed by both patient and physician when symptoms are atypical, as in gonococcal pharyngitis.

In managing adolescents with STDs, the potential adverse effects of this diagnosis on self-image, reputation, family interactions, and/or sexual relations need to be assessed with appropriate counseling, empathy, and support. Conversely, a patient who believes himself or herself to have VD but who does not needs to be thoroughly reassured on this count and educated about STD prevention.

GONORRHEA
Uncomplicated gonorrhea
Agent: Neisseria gonorrhoeae
Popular names: Clap, drip, dose, strain
Transmission: Sexual only in physically mature individuals.
Incidence: Frequent.
Presentations:
- *Male:* Urethritis—marked dysuria; frequency of urination; thick, creamy penile discharge
  Prostatitis—rectal pain; perineal discomfort; enlarged, tender prostate
  Epididymitis—unilateral scrotal pain; groin pain; fever, chills; tender swelling above a nontender testis
  Orchitis—tender, enlarged testis (uncommon)
  Asymptomatic in 10%–40%
- *Female:* Cervicitis—thick, creamy endocervical discharge; tender cervix
  Urethritis, cystitis—dysuria; frequency of urination
  Bartholinitis—tender, swollen Bartholin's gland
  Asymptomatic in 50%–80%
- *Both:* Proctitis—rectal pain, itching, discharge; history of anogenital sexual contact common in males, less common in females, in whom contamination by infected vaginal secretions may be causal
  Pharyngitis—sore throat; erythema, exudate on tonsils and/or pharynx; history of orogenital contact, but pharyngeal colonization commonly asymptomatic
Diagnosis:
- *Gram stain:* Gram-negative, intracellular diplococci in urethral or endocervical discharge. This finding is diagnostic in males but only suggestive in females, in whom nongonococcal *Neisseria* saprophytes may be found (these, however, are usually extracellular; intracellular diplococci constitute presumptive evidence). In either sex, a negative Gram stain does not exclude the diagnosis.

□ *Culture:* Essential for confirmation of diagnosis, followup of treatment, and identification of resistant strains. Use special media (Thayer-Martin or equivalent) incubated under reduced oxygen and increased CO_2 (candle jar), humidity, pH of 7.2–7.6, and at temperature of 35–37°C. Growth is inhibited by delay in placing in proper environment, overgrowth by other organisms, the presence of inappropriate antibiotics in the media, poor technique, or contamination of the specimen with bactericidal or surgical lubricants used during examination.

Culture all suspected sites, including endocervix, urethra, anal canal, and pharynx (as described in Table 17-4). Colonization may be symptomatic or asymptomatic in any of these locations. Indications are based as much on the nature of sexual practices as on clinical findings or complaints.

Differential diagnosis: Chlamydia trachomatis, genital mycoplasmas (*Ureaplasma urealyticum*); *Trichomonas* (often concurrent)

Treatment (Center for Disease Control recommended schedules, 1982):

□ Aqueous procaine penicillin G, 4.8 million units IM with probenecid 1.0 g p.o.

or

□ Amoxicillin 3.0 g; ampicillin, 3.5 g p.o. with probenecid 1.0 g p.o.

or

□ Tetracycline hydrochloride, 500 mg p.o. 4 times daily for 7 days

or

□ Spectinomycin, 2.0 g IM; best reserved for (a) penicillin allergy plus pregnancy or tetracycline allergy or intolerance, or poor compliance with oral therapy and (b) treatment failures with other agents or in the presence of penicillinase-producing strains. Note: Spectinomycin has a high failure rate for pharyngeal gonorrhea, no effect on incubating syphilis, and a high rate of producing bacterial resistance.

General:

1. Identify, examine, obtain culture from, and treat all sexual contacts.
2. Obtain posttreatment cultures from all infected sites in 3–10 days.
3. Obtain syphilis serologic test at time of treatment. Repeat in 4–6 weeks if therapy is not adequate for incubating syphilis (for example, treatment with spectinomycin or failure to complete course of tetracycline).
4. Report to local health department for epidemiologic purpose.

Complications: Disseminated gonorrhea, pelvic inflammatory disease, perihepatitis.

Pregnancy complications: Increased risk for septic abortion, premature delivery, amionitis, ophthalmia neonatorum, neonatal disseminated infection. Gonorrhea cultures schould be performed for pregnant women at first prenatal visit, in last month, and during labor. The infant should receive prophylactic antibiotic ointment or silver nitrate drops in each eye before leaving the delivery room.

Disseminated gonorrhea

Incidence: 1%–3% of untreated cases of gonorrhea; onset usually 15–30 days following exposure; increased incidence during pregnancy, with pharyngeal or anorectal gonococcal infection (see comment), and in homosexual males (due to high incidence of pharyngeal and anorectal primary infection sites).

Presentation: Migratory polyarthralgia followed by multiple tender swollen small joints or one to several septic large joints (knee, ankle); tenosynovitis common; dermatitis (papules, pustules, vesicles, purpuric spots; usually few in number and tend to be located on extremities, often over involved joints); fever, malaise.

Diagnosis: Gram stain and culture. Take smears and cultures from all possible primary sites, aspirate of septic joints, blood, incised skin lesions, and, if indicated, spinal fluid (see *Complications*). Usually positive from point of entry (urethra, cervix, anus, pharynx) and from large septic joints; only 25%–50% positive from blood, skin lesions, small joints (small joint involvement may be either septic or hypersensitivity reaction).

Differential diagnosis: Rheumatic fever, rheumatoid arthritis, postviral arthritis, acute Reiter syndrome, bacterial endocarditis, meningococcemia, serum sickness.

Treatment (Center for Disease Control recommended schedules, 1979):

□ Amoxicillin, 3.0 g, or ampicillin, 3.5 g, p.o. plus probenecid, 1.0 g p.o. stat, followed by either antibiotic, 500 mg four times daily for 7 days

or

□ Tetracycline hydrochloride, 500 mg p.o. four times daily for 7 days

or

□ Erythromycin, 500 mg p.o. four times daily for 7 days

or

□ Aqueous crystalline penicillin G, 10 million units/day IV until improved; then ampicillin or amoxicillin, 500 mg p.o. four times daily to complete 7–10 day treatment course.

or

□ Cefoxitin 1.0 g or cefotaxime 500 mg IV four times daily for 7 days (choice for disseminated infections caused by penicillinase-producing strains).

General:

1. Hospitalization strongly recommended, even for oral regimens.
2. Bed rest, elevation of septic joints, orthopedic consultation.
3. Posttreatment cultures of all positive sites 3–7 days after treatment completed.

Complications: Gonococcal endocarditis, meningitis (both rare); mild hepatitis (common); osteomeylitis, joint destruction (if arthritis untreated). Treatment is with high-dose intravenous antibiotics (penicillin, ampicillin, tetracycline) for 10–14 days or longer for bone involvement.

Comment: Strains of gonorrhea that disseminate are relatively resistant to host responses yet very sensitive to antibiotics. Hence they often remain asymptomatic at entry site (with a predeliction for the pharynx and rectum), become blood-borne easily, and respond well to oral therapy alone. Gonococcal arthritis is the most common septic arthritis in sexually active young people and should be thought of even if sexual intimacy is denied. The coexistence of characteristic skin lesions, if present, gives an additional clue.

Pelvic Inflammatory Disease (PID); salpingitis, salpingo-oophoritis, endometritis.

Incidence: 15%–20% of females with gonorrhea develop PID, but numerous other microorganisms also have been isolated from the cervix, endometrium, cul-de-sac, and/or salpinx in these patients, suggesting multiple or mixed etiologies; 90%–95% of first cases but only 50% of repeat cases of PID are associated with gonorrhea; *Chlamydia trachomatis* appears to be a primary cause when this association exists.

Presentation and findings: Onset commonly occurs during or just after menses with intense cramps, pelvic pain, and, sometimes, abnormal bleeding. Other complaints include lower quadrant abdominal pain (95%), vaginal discharge (50%), fever (35%), and dysuria (20%). Malaise, weakness, fainting, dizziness, nausea, and vomiting also may be seen. Adnexal tenderness and pain on cervical motion are classic findings present in 90%–95%. Perihepatitis (Fitz-Hugh–Curtis syndrome) occurs in 15%–30% and is marked by right upper quandrant pain and/or mildly elevated transaminases; shoulder pain, pleuritic pain, hepatic friction rub also occur. An adnexal mass is palpable in 10%–15% and indicates pyohydrosalpinx or tuboovarian abscess.

Diagnosis: Usually a clinical diagnosis with supportive evidence.

□ *Cultures:* Cervix; also consider taking from pelvic interior by culdocentesis or laparoscopy.
□ *ESR:* elevated in 50%–75%.
□ *WBC:* elevated in 35%–50%.
□ *Pelvic ultrasound:* Thickened pelvic structures, often unilateral.
□ *Laparoscopy:* Provides definitive visual diagnosis; peritoneal cultures aid in treatment (some recommend laparoscopy for all cases, others only for chronic, recurrent, or resistant disease).

Comment: Most cases of PID in adolescents are due to gonococcal and/or chlamydial infection. A gonococcal etiology is more likely with a first episode, young age, nulliparity, no history of IUD, presence of dysuria, evidence of perihepatitis, onset in summer, and/or onset close to menses. Other organisms should be suspected with repeated episodes of PID, multiparity, evidence of abscess, and/or presence or history of IUD. Other organisms that have been implicated besides gonococcus and *Chlamydia* include aerobic and anaerobic streptococci, coliforms, and *Bacteroides* sp.

Differential diagnosis: Appendicitis, ectopic pregnancy, ovarian cyst, urinary tract infection, septic abortion.

Treatment (Expanded Center for Disease Control Recommendations, 1982):

□ *Outpatient* (for mild to moderate acute salpingitis in compliant adolescent). Treat as for uncomplicated gonorrhea followed by doxycycline 100 mg twice daily, or tetracycline, 500 mg 4 times daily for 10–14 days. Reevaluate clinical condition in 2–3 days and after completion of therapy.
□ *Inpatient:* Hospitalization and parenteral treatment is recommended for the following situations.
  1. Uncertain diagnosis, possible surgical condition
  2. Abscess suspected or diagnosed
  3. Salpingitis in the presence of pregnancy
  4. Severe systemic symptoms: fever, chills, vomiting
  5. Peritonitis diagnosed
  6. Probable or previously demonstrated inability to tolerate or comply with an oral regimen
  7. Failure to respond to outpatient therapy
  8. IUD in place (controversial)

Parenteral regimens (with broad activity against major pathogens associated with PID) *include:*

1. Doxycycline 100 mg IV twice daily plus cefoxitin 2.0 g IV four times daily for at least 4 days followed by doxycycline 100 mg p.o. twice daily to complete 10–14 days. (Optimal coverage for N. gonorrhoeae, including penicillin-resistant strains, and C. trachomatis.)
2. Clindamycin 600 mg IV 4 times daily plus genta-

micin 1.5 mg/kg IV 3 times daily for at least 4 days, followed by clindamycin 450 mg p.o. 4 times daily to complete 10–14 days. (Optimal against organisms other than N. gonorrhoeae and C. trachomatis.)

3. Doxycycline 100 mg IV twice daily plus metronidazole 1.0 g IV twice daily for at least 4 days followed by both drugs at same dosage p.o. to complete 10–14 days. (Excellent coverage only for anaerobes and C. trachomatis.)

(The treatment of choice has not yet been established. Currently, combined therapy should be selected based on the suspected or isolated pathogens and the clinical response of the patient.)

General:

1. Bed rest, analgesics.
2. Consultation with surgeon and/or gynecologist as indicated.
3. Consider removal of an IUD, especially if patient responds poorly to therapy.
4. Consider laparoscopy or surgery for diagnostic purposes, drainage of large abscess, or with poor patient response to triple antibiotic therapy after 48 hours.
5. After patient discharge follow up all initially positive cultures, and reculture those patients at high risk for repeat PID at frequent intervals. Avoid use of IUD.

Complications: Peritonitis, tuboovarian abscess, perihepatitis with adhesions; increased risk of ectopic pregnancy; sterility due to tubal damage (risk increases with repeated episodes of PID).

Comment: Pelvic inflammatory disease is a significant cause of sterility, days lost from school or work, major hospitalization costs, chronic menstrual dysfunction, and chronic pelvic pain. A high index of suspicion and aggressive management, especially in young, nulliparous women, may reduce these consequences.

CHLAMYDIA

Agent: Chlamydia trachomatis.
Transmission: Sexual contact.
Incidence: Frequent.
Presentations:

☐ *Males:* Urethritis—mild dysuria; watery penile discharge (most common cause of nongonococcal (NGU) or postgonococcal urethritis).
Prostatitis—as with uncomplicated gonorrhea.
Epididymitis—as with uncomplicated gonorrhea.
Asymptomatic in 25%–50%.

☐ *Females:* Cervicitis—mild erythema, variable endocervical discharge.
Asymptomatic in at least 50% (common in partners of males with NGU).

☐ *Both:* Proctitis and pharyngitis—mild symptoms (increasing rates being reported).

Diagnosis: Tissue culture (McCoy cells)—excellent diagnosis within 3 days when available. Rapid immunoassay of serum, genital secretions; but a high percentage of individuals have positive titers from past chlamydial infections of all types and serologic tests are only useful in diagnosis if rising titers are demonstrated in acute and convalescent phase sera.

Differential diagnosis: Gonorrhea; genital mycoplasmas (*U. urealyticum*); *Trichomonas.*

Treatment:

☐ Tetracycline hydrochloride, 500 mg p.o. four times daily for 7–10 days.

or

☐ Doxycycline, 100 mg p.o. twice daily for 7–10 days.

or

☐ Erythromycin, 500 mg p.o. four times daily for 7–10 days (especially if pregnant).

Complications: Acute Reiter syndrome; salpingitis; perihepatitis; possible contributor to premalignant changes in cervix.

Pregnancy complications: Neonatal conjunctivitis, infant interstitial pneumonitis.

Comment: Genital chlamydial infection is common and a significant cause of infant morbidity and, possibly, of PID and sterility. When possible, specimens should be cultured as carefully as for gonorrhea; when the organism has been isolated, the patient should be treated. Followup cultures will indicate adequacy of therapy. All pregnant women should be routinely screened.

NONGONOCOCCAL URETHRITIS

Nongonococcal, or nonspecific, urethritis in males appears to be dominantly caused by *Chlamydia* (50%–60%). Another 20%–30% of cases are caused by genital mycoplasmas, primarily *U. urealyticum.* In other cases, no organism is isolated. Because *Chlamydia* and *Ureaplasma* are often transmitted along with gonorrhea and also respond to tetracycline, males treated for gonococcal urethritis with this antibiotic seldom develop persistent symptoms; however, 25% or more treated with penicillin or ampicillin continue to be symptomatic (postgonococcal urethritis). Because tetracycline is effective against all organisms implicated in urethritis, clinical differentiation is unnecessary. In adolescents with symptoms of urethritis resistant to treatment and no identified organism, urethral irritation from masturbatory practices should be considered.

ACUTE REITER SYNDROME

Incidence: Uncommon; may be associated with

chlamydial infection and/or *Salmonella, Shigella,* and other enteritides.

Presentation: Constellation of urethritis, conjunctivitis, mucocutaneous lesions, and arthritis.

Diagnosis: Cause unknown; cultures should be taken for *Chlamydia,* gonorrhea; stool cultures when indicated.

Differential diagnosis: Gonococcal arthritis, rheumatoid arthritis, inflammatory bowel disease with arthritis, psoriatic arthritis.

Treatment:

1. Tetracycline as for uncomplicated chlamydial infections.
2. Bed rest, analgesia, elevated joints, physical therapy.
3. Orthopedic consultation.

Note: Also see Chapter 9 for additional information.

TRICHOMONIAS

Agent: Trichomonas vaginalis.

Popular name: Trich.

Incidence: Frequent; often associated with gonorrhea in females.

Transmission: Sexual primarily; fomites rarely.

Presentation:

☐ *Male:* Urethritis—mild dysuria, itching (uncommon); most often asymptomatic.

☐ *Female:* Vaginitis—variable discharge (often frothy, watery, white-yellow-green); itching, vaginal odor.

Cervicitis—erythema, edema, erosion, red punctate "strawberry cervix" (the latter, although often cited as a diagnostic hallmark, is an uncommon finding).

Urethritis/cystitis—dysuria, frequency of urination (15%–20%).

Asymptomatic in 25%–50%.

Diagnosis: Wet mount of vaginal secretions (Table 17-4) and/or spun sediment of urine (male and female) reveals motile organisms, numerous WBCs (Figure 17-1). Culture is usually unnecessary, expensive, and limited in availability.

Differential diagnosis: Candidiasis, chemical vaginitis; urethritis, cystitis; *Hemophilis vaginalis* (*Gardnerella vaginalis*) vaginitis.

Treatment: Metronidazole (Flagyl); 2 g single dose p.o. usually effective; resistant cases, 250 mg three times daily for 7 days or 500 mg twice daily for 5 days. May cause nausea, vomiting and should be taken with food; alcohol should be avoided for 24 hours.

General:

1. Treat partner(s) whenever possible.
2. Repeat examination in 7–10 days for test of cure.

3. Use condom during intercourse until repeat examination reveals infection cleared.
4. Topical therapy is not effective.

Complications: May contribute to premalignant changes in cervix.

Pregnancy complications: Postpartum endometritis; neonatal vaginitis. Metronidazole should be avoided. Clotrimazole intravaginally for 7 days may relieve symptoms with occasional cures.

GENITAL HERPES

Agent: Herpes simplex type 2, type 1.

Incidence: Frequent.

Transmission: Sexual primarily, including orogenital contact; autoinoculation.

Presentation: Painful vesicles progressing to flat ulcers on an erythematous base located on penis, vulva, introitus, vagina, cervix, perineum, perianal region, mouth, lips, or pharynx; severe dysuria even to the point of urinary retention if urethral; local lymphadenopathy; fever, malaise (especially with primary infections). Recurrent lesions are uncommon but may occur at variable intervals (weeks or months) for months or years after the primary infection in a small percent of patients. These episodes tend to be less severe but pose significant hazards to child-bearing.

Diagnosis: Smear of lesion—giant cells may be seen with Wright's stain or on Papanicolaou smear. Tissue culture—results available in 48–72 hours. Paired serologic testing for type rarely necessary.

Comment: Formerly, genital herpes was mainly due to type 2 virus, whereas herpes above the waist was predominantly type 1. This segregation is gradually disappearing, presumably due to increasing frequency of orogenital contact. Currently, either type may be responsible for any sexually transmitted herpes, including orolabial and anal lesions. Clinical manifestations and treatment are identical for both types.

Differential diagnosis: Primary syphilis, molluscum contagiosum, allergic reaction, chancroid.

Treatment (only symptomatic at present):

1. Cold compresses, topical solutions (Burow's), possibly topical anesthetics; dry heat from home hair dryer.
2. Analgesics, bed rest as needed, catheterization if urinary retention from pain.
3. Avoid sexual intercourse or use condom; no orogenital activity; vaginal spermicides may be virucidal; careful handwashing.
4. Avoid sitz baths and occlusive ointments, as these may lead to spread.

Comment: Of many treatments proposed, few show

significant results, although a strong placebo effect has been observed. Photoinactivation is currently considered questionable in efficacy and safety. Recent work with arabinocides (Ara A) in herpes meningitis may make virucidal agents available for herpes genitalis. Acyclovir, a specific inhibitor of herpes virus replication, has been used to treat complicated infections and now is available in topical form. While it shortens the course and lessens the severity of initial infections, it does not appear to affect significantly or to prevent recurrent infections. Judicious use for severe cutaneous or systemic infections has been advised due to the possibility of inducing mutant strains that will be resistant to acyclovir. Vaccines are also under investigation. Nervous system infections (recurrent neuralgia, meningitis) are rare complications. Disseminated infection may occur in those with eczema or immunosuppression.

Pregnancy complications: Neonatal infection, especially if membranes rupture. (Should deliver by cesarian section before or within 4 hours of rupture if herpes still cultured from cervix in last prenatal week.)

GENITAL WARTS (CONDYLOMATA ACCUMINATA)

Agent: Human papillomavirus.

Incidence: Frequent.

Transmission: Sexual; autoinoculation.

Presentation: Warty lesion(s); firm, gray to pink, fimbriated, single or multiple, variable in size from several millimeters to extensive lesions measuring several centimeters; located on penis, vulva, introitus, vagina, cervix, perineum or perianal region; painless.

Diagnosis: Clinical appearance.

Differential diagnosis: Condyloma latum (secondary syphilis), molluscum contagiosum.

Treatment:

1. 10%-25% podophyllum in tincture of benzoin (Podophyllin) carefully applied to warts only and washed off after 4-6 hours and repeated weekly as needed; should not be used on mucous membranes, and normal tissue surrounding the wart may be protected by applying petroleum jelly before using podophyllum; do not use during pregnancy.
2. Excision, electrodesiccation, cryosurgery for extensive or resistant lesions.
3. Avoid moisture; improve hygiene to prevent recurrence.

Complications: Warts may be premalignant; perianal or urethral obstruction can occur from very large lesions.

Pregnancy complications: Obstructed delivery if lesions are very large; laryngeal papillomas in infants.

Comment: Genital warts may resolve spontaneously but can recur, even after treatment. Perianal location in males may signify homosexual activity.

SYPHILIS

Agent: Treponema pallidum.

Popular names: Siff, lues, bad blood.

Incidence: Infrequent in United States except in endemic areas or among homosexual males.

Transmission: Sexual primarily; careless hygiene. Infected persons are contagious during all early stages of the disease and through approximately the first 2 years of the latent stage.

Presentations:

☐ *Primary:* Painless ulcer or chancre on penis, vulva, introitus, vagina, cervix, perineum, perianal region, lip, tongue, or extremities with local adenopathy occurring 10-90 days after contact. The ulcer lasts 2-6 weeks if untreated, then clears spontaneously. Intravaginal and rectal lesions may be missed.

☐ *Secondary:* Fever, sore throat, headache, rhinitis, arthralgias, malaise; diffuse adenopathy; hepatosplenomegaly; anogenital condylomata lata; rash (variably papular, macular, pustular, and/or annular) anywhere on body, including palms, soles; mucous patches; alopecia. Symptoms last 10 days to 2 weeks, then spontaneously clear.

☐ *Asymptomatic* (majority of cases):

1. Incubating syphilis: average 3 weeks from contact, with a range of 10-90 days.
2. Asymptomatic period between primary and secondary stage; ranges from 6 weeks to 6 months.
3. Latent syphilis follows the secondary stage and lasts until signs of late syphilis appear, with a range of 2-20 years or even for life (not all cases develop late clinical disease).

Diagnosis:

☐ *Dark-field microscopy*—spirochetes seen on scrapings or washings from the primary lesion (chancre); repeat two or three times if no organisms seen initially (requires special techniques and microscope modification).

☐ *Serologic tests:* Detect asymptomatic disease; confirm symptomatic disease.

1. Nontreponemal tests (VDRL, RPR) are low cost, easily performed.
   a. Detect nonspecific antigens; quantifiable.
   b. Become positive within 2-4 weeks after appearance of chancre, remain positive throughout secondary and early latent stages, may become negative in late stage.

c. Gradually return to normal in most cases within 6–12 months after treatment, particularly if disease is of less than 2 years' duration.

d. Use to screen, diagnose (repeat weekly two or three times if negative in face of suggestive symptoms or signs), detect reinfection (rising titers), and to test cure (falling titers or disappearance).

e. May yield false-positive reactions due to
  (1) Laboratory error (frequent); repeat test is usually negative.
  (2) Following an acute infectious illness or after immunization; positive response is transient.
  (3) Parenteral narcotic abuse (common).
  (4) Chronic "benign" reactor; often a precursor of collagen vascular disease.

2. Treponemal tests (FTA-ABS) are more expensive, time consuming.

a. Detect treponemal antigens; greater specificity than nontreponemal tests.

b. Become positive within 2–4 weeks after onset of primary stage; remain positive throughout life if untreated.

c. Return to normal in 50%–70% if treated early; in very few if treated late.

d. Used to confirm positive and check false-positive nontreponemal tests.

e. False-positive reactions considerably less common than with nontreponemal tests but may be seen in same situations on occasion, including laboratory error.

f. False-negative reactions (nonreactivity) occur in up to 18% of individuals with primary syphilis and up to 5% with late syphilis.

Comment: Although syphilis is not common in adolescents in the United States, all who are sexually active should be screened annually, with those at particularly high risk (multiple partners, homosexual contacts) being checked every 6 months. Serologic tests must be interpreted in context with the clinical history, epidemiology, and physical findings; as noted above, these tests are by no means absolute in their reactivity or specificity.

Differential diagnosis:

□ Primary: Genital herpes, chancroid, lymphogranuloma venereum, granuloma inguinale.

□ Secondary: Mononucleosis, infectious hepatitis (systemic); the tineas, "id" eruptions, drug sensitivity reactions, the exanthems, pityriasis rosea, psoriasis, erythema multiforme (rash); condylomata acuminata (condylomata pata); alopecia from any other cause.

Treatment (Center for Disease Control recommended schedules, 1982: For primary, secondary, or early latent (incubating syphilis will be eradicated by penicillin or ampicillin at dosages recommended for uncomplicated gonorrhea).

□ Bicillin, 2.4 million units IM at one visit (New York State schedules recommend a repeat dose 1 week later)

or

□ Tetracycline, 500 mg p.o. four times daily for 15 days (do not use in pregnancy)

or

□ Erythromycin, 500 mg p.o. four times daily for 15 days.

General:

1. Serologic tests should be repeated at 1, 3, 6, and 12 months.

2. Examination of cerebrospinal fluid 1 year after treatment is recommended by some, particularly if treatment not instituted until latent stage.

3. Because primary and secondary stages are highly contagious, health professionals should wear gloves and take other precautions against accidental contamination or innoculation during examination, venipuncture, treatment. Particular care is required in disposing of needles, syringes, or other equipment.

4. Sexual partners should have physical examination and serologic testing.

Complications: Thirty to forty percent of individuals with untreated disease develop late syphilis within 2–20 years; 60%–70% remain in the latent stage. Among those who do develop late disease, 50% have benign (gummatous) syphilis, 30% cardiovascular syphilis, and 20% neurosyphilis; some individuals may have more than one form.

Pregnancy complications: Congenital syphilis (the spirochete does not cross the placenta until the last trimester; detection and treatment in early pregnancy will fully protect the fetus from harm).

OTHER SEXUALLY TRANSMITTED INFECTIONS

Chancroid (*Hemophilus ducreyi*). Rare in the United States; primarily occurs in males. Signs and symptoms include painful penile ulcers with local adenopathy that may progress to suppuration. The organism is difficult to isolate; culture results only confirm an essentially clinical diagnosis. Treatment is erythromycin 500 mg p.o. four times daily for 10 days, local soaks, and cleansing.

Granuloma inguinale (*Calymmatobacterium granulomatis*). Rare in the United States and low infectivity. Signs and symptoms include painless genital and/or inguinal ulcers, nodules, and granulation tissue that slowly increase in size and extent. Organisms may be demonstrated in tissue smears and biopsy specimens. Treatment is tetracycline or ampicillin, 500 mg every 6 hours for 3 weeks.

Lymphogranuloma venereum (*Chlamydia trachomatis strains*). Rare in the United States. Signs and symptoms include transient painless, shallow genital ulcers (in up to 40%); significant inguinal adenopathy with suppuration (cervical nodes can be involved when transmission is through orogenital contact, fever, chills, malaise, arthralgias, and myalgia. Diagnosis is confirmed by complement fixation titer; cultures are positive in 50%; the Frei test is no longer used. Treatment is tetracycline, 500 mg p.o. four times daily for 2-3 weeks.

Enteric organisms. Shigellosis, salmonellosis, amebiasis, and giardiasis may be transmitted by oral-anal or oral-genital contact and mainly occur among male homosexuals. Abdominal cramps, nausea, and watery diarrhea, often with blood, should raise suspicion, but some infected individuals remain asymptomatic. Diagnosis is confirmed by stool culture and examination for parasites. Shigella infections often resolve spontaneously, becoming asymptomatic in 1–3 weeks and noncontagious in 2–3 months; treat with ampicillin or tetracycline, 500 mg every 6 hours for 5–7 days. Amebiasis responds to metronidazole, 750 mg 3 times daily for 10 days. Metronidazole, 250 mg 3 times daily for 7 days, is used for giardiasis. Partners of individuals with sexually transmitted enteric disease should be evaluated and treated if infected and the couple instructed about improved hygiene and increased care in sexual practices.

OTHER GENITAL INFECTIONS AND PROBLEMS

The following may or may not be sexually transmitted.

CANDIDIASIS (MONILIASIS)

Agent: Candida albicans.
Popular name: Yeast.
Incidence: Frequent in females, occasionally in males; especially common with use of oral contraceptive, antibiotics, metronidazole, during pregnancy, in debilitating illness, in diabetes, and in other endocrinopathies.
Transmission: Overgrowth of normal flora present in 30%–50% of all females; by direct contact, including sexual.

Presentation:
□ *Male:* Erythematous, itching rash on genitalia and/or in groin.
□ *Female:* Vulvitis—erythema, itching, excoriations. Vaginitis—thick white curdlike patches on cervix, vaginal walls, and as curdy discharge; itching.
Diagnosis:
□ *Wet mount*—hyphae with budding, branching (more evident on 10% KOH preparation per Table 17-4). (See Figure 17-1.)
□ *Culture*—Nickerson's media incubated at room temperature for 24–48 hours (seldom necessary).
Differential diagnosis: Chemical balanitis, vulvitis, or vaginitis; vaginitis due to other infections; tinea cruris.
Treatment:
□ *Females:* Fungicidal vaginal cream (Monistat, Gyne-Lotrimin, Vanobid, Sporostacin), one applicator full inserted into vagina one or two times daily for 1–2 weeks; careful genital hygiene; attention to any predisposing cause; if condition is secondary to oral antibiotics for acne, try topical antibiotics.
□ *Males:* Apply cream to affected area plus previously indicated measures.

HEMOPHILUS VAGINITIS

Agent: Hemophilus vaginalis (or *Gardnerella vaginalis,* according to recent efforts at reclassification).
Incidence: Frequent.
Transmission: Normal flora in 35% of females; sexual.
Presentations: Vaginitis—mild nonspecific discharge, often foul odor. Asymptomatic in 10%–40%.
Diagnosis:
□ *Wet mount*—few WBCs, many epithelial cells covered with bacilli ("clue cells"; see Figure 17-1).
□ *Culture*—Blood agar; provides specific identification.
Differential diagnosis: Trichomonas, chemical vaginitis, candidiasis.
Treatment: (necessity for treatment controversial).
□ Metronidazole 500 mg p.o. twice daily for 7 days (recently approved by FDA).
□ Ampicillin 500 mg p.o. four times daily for 7 days (choice in pregnancy).
□ *Comment:* Response to topical therapy with antibiotic vaginal creams limited at best. When infection is resistant or recurrent, treating partner with systemic antibiotics also recommended.
Complications: none reported, including during pregnancy.

BETA-HEMOLYTIC STREPTOCOCCUS

Group A strains may be transmitted by autoinoculation or sexual contact from a pharyngeal site and cause vaginitis on rare occasion. When organisms are cultured from the vagina, treatment with penicillin, 250 mg four times daily for 10 days, is indicated whether patient is symptomatic or not. Group B and other types usually comprise normal vaginal flora but may be involved in PID and postpartum infections; when present during pregnancy, treatment with penicillin plus continuous monitoring of mother and newborn is indicated.

PINWORMS

Pinworms may invade the vagina and cause itching, particularly at night. Diagnosis is by stool examination or an early morning anal cellophane tape test. Treatment is with pyrvinium pamoate (Povan) or mebendazole (Vermox) (see Chapter 15).

CUTANEOUS INFECTIONS AND INFESTATIONS

These commonly are distributed more widely than the genital region alone. See Chapter 14 for details of manifestations, diagnosis, and management.

Pediculosis pubis. Infestation with pubic lice. Eggs ("nits") or active adult forms are evident on examination of pubic hair with a hand lens. Also may be found on perineal and axillary hair or eyelashes. Intense pruritis invites scratching and excoriation.

Scabies. Intensely pruritic, papular rash with excoriations caused by burrowing and egg laying of the mite, Sarcoptes scabiei. Common sites of involvement include intertriginous areas, external genitalia, buttocks, beltline, breasts, and between digits.

Tinea cruris. Common superficial fungal infection most often seen in male athletes with less than optimal hygiene. Also colloquially known as "jock itch." Manifested by a flat, erythematous, pruritic rash involving the scrotum and adjacent thighs and groin.

Molluscum contagiosum. Asymptomatic umbilicated papules, singly or in crops, variably scattered over the body. May be located on external genitalia, but this site is less common than other regions.

Contact dermatitis. Dermatitis of the external genitals, urethritis, vaginitis, and/or proctitis may develop from sensitization or exposure to genital hygiene products or other agents such as soaps, vaginal deodorants (sprays, suppositories), douches, perfumes, chemicals in spermicides, rubber in condoms or diaphragms, dyes in underclothing, patterned toilet tissue or saliva. Treatment is by identifying and eliminating the source or recommending a less allergenic alternative. Topical compresses (Burow's solution), sitz baths, and/or mild topical steroids may be used for symptomatic relief.

Foreign body. Retained tampons or toilet tissue in the vagina may produce a significant discharge, which often is brown or bloody and usually has a foul odor. Treatment is by removing the foreign material and mild douching for hygiene (1 tablespoon vinegar in a quart of warm tap water or a commercial preparation administered by a gravity-feed type douche bag).

Physiologic leukorrhea. Many adolescents normally have an intermittent or persistent physiologic vaginal discharge. This is a characteristic response to estrogen stimulation, commonly beginning several months before menarche and persisting for several years. It also is apt to increase with the use of estrogen-dominant oral contraceptives. The discharge varies from clear to white in color, mucoid to watery in consistency, and scant to moderate in amount. Of particular significance is that it is nonirritating and without odor. Variation in character may parallel the menstrual cycle.

Physical examination reveals entirely normal perineal and pelvic structures and normal vaginal secretions, as previously described. Microscopic examination of a wet mount demonstrates only mucus and sloughed-off epithelial cells (Figure 17-1).

It is common for a young adolescent with physiologic leukorrhea to present with complaints of an "excessive" discharge, believing this to be a pathological state. In virginal females not yet ready for a pelvic examination, the clinical history, external genital inspection, and a wet mount obtained by an introital swab are sufficient for the diagnosis. Treatment consists of reassurance, instruction in perineal hygiene, and avoiding excessive washing, douching, or the use of vaginal perfumes and deodorants.

Perineal hygiene is accomplished by regular bathing, daily changing of underpants (cotton preferable to synthetic types), avoiding tight panty hose or other constricting garments worn for prolonged periods of time, and preventing fecal contamination of the introital region by wiping in a posterior direction after defecation.

Contraception

Most adolescents do not expect or want pregnancy to follow sexual intercourse, yet few use any contraceptive method for the first 6–12 months of coital experience. Initial contraceptive efforts often follow peer advice and are relatively ineffective (Saran wrap condoms, cola douches, and withdrawal). Some adolescents use effective methods improperly such as sporadically taking a friend's oral contraceptive, intermittent use of barrier methods, or attempts at periodic abstinence ("rhythm method") without having accurate knowledge about the timing of ovulation. Consulting a reliable medical source for an effective method and proper education tends to be a late event, often following a first conception or "pregnancy scare" (late menstrual period).

The primary health care provider plays a critical role in identifying contraceptive needs and introducing sexuality counseling as routine components of adolescent health care. Approximately 50% of all unintended pregnancies to teenagers occur within the first 6 months following the initiation of coital activity, the time when they are least likely to use contraception of any kind. Every opportunity should be taken to identify those adolescents at actual or potential risk rather than waiting for the consequences.

Lack of contraceptive use by adolescents may be due to one or a combination of factors. These include a sense of invulnerability; denial of the potential consequences of or responsibility for one's actions; ignorance of contraceptive methods, their proper use, or how to get them; barriers to obtaining methods (legal, financial, geographic, societal); and ignorance of reproductive physiology. Many adolescents, male and female, believe they are too young to be fertile. At least 50% believe that pregnancy is most likely to occur during menses and least likely when coitus is at midcycle! Intercourse tends to be sporadic and unpredicted, decreasing the motivation for planning ahead. High value often is placed on romantic "spontaneity." Due to the lack of regular ovulation and/or luteal insufficiency during the first year or two after menarche, unprotected intercourse without resulting in conception during this relatively brief period is often misinterpreted as "proof" of indefinite immunity (or feared as evidence of infertility). Immature cognitive development and an existential orientation tend to preclude awareness by these adolescents that regular ovulation will sooner or later occur, bringing an end to their invulnerability.

CONTRACEPTIVE COUNSELING

Adolescents in need of contraception may either present for this particular reason or be identified as in need during the course of any health contact. Counseling teenagers about contraception is more involved than counseling adults. It not only requires education about and counseling on method selection and use, providing a method, and continuing support, but also attention to a variety of developmental and psychosocial issues. Education and knowledge have considerably less impact on contraceptive use in adolescents than do cognitive and developmental stage, personal beliefs, internal conflict, life-style, cultural background, and external support systems. A number of "hidden agenda" factors also may be at work and, if present, require close attention (see Part IV) in the overall management plan. Consider the impact on contraceptive compliance of the following, all commonly encountered in many teenagers:

1. Fatalistic attitudes, alienation, apathy, a sense of helplessness.

2. Low self-esteem, feelings of incompetence, chronic depression.

3. Dependency, passivity.

4. Risk-taking life-style, hedonistic orientation, impulsivity.

5. High anxiety levels.

6. Problems in establishing sexual identity, handling sexual feelings.

7. Fear of contraceptive side effects (personal, familial, religious, medical).

8. Valuation of fertility (impregnation, pregnancy, childbirth) by self, partner, peers, family, culture.

9. Ambivalent desire for pregnancy in confirmation of insecure femininity, as a remedy for loneliness, to escape from an indifferent adolescence into instant adulthood, to escape from an intolerable home or school situation.

In establishing any contraceptive management plan, the following general points should be kept in mind by the physician and adolescent:

1. Any contraceptive is better than none.

2. There is no ideal contraceptive; none combines 100% efficacy and safety, complete acceptability, unrelatedness to coitus in timing of use, and low cost. In addition, combined methods may be needed to prevent both pregnancy and sexually transmitted infections.

3. The best contraceptive is the one the adolescent will use correctly and consistently (Table 17-11).

4. The adolescent may need to try several methods before selecting one for long-term use. However, method-free intervals without abstinence risk pregnancy.

5. The morbidity and mortality of adolescents using *any* contraceptive method is considerably less than that resulting from teenage pregnancy.

TABLE 17-11
CONTRACEPTIVE METHODS WITH REGARD TO ADOLESCENTS

Method	Theoretical effectiveness (%)	Actual (use) effectiveness (%)	Advantages	Disadvantages
Abstinence	100	?	Nonprescription; available; no cost; safe; little infection	High motivation needed; emotionally difficult
Depo-Provera	100	99–100	Very effective; little motivation needed; no estrogen risks	Not FDA approved; delayed resumption of menses, ovulation
Foam and condom	99	95	Nonprescription; available; antiinfective; no side effects	High motivation needed; high cost if intercourse frequent
IUD	97–99	95	No motivation needed; no interference with intercourse	Side effects; expulsion, replacement needed; possible risk of PID, ectopic pregnancy
Pill	99.5	80–95	Noncoital method; relief of acne, cramps, excess menses	Daily motivation needed; estrogen side effects; possible estrogen risk
Condom	97	90	Nonprescription; male responsible; antiinfective; easy to use	Coital-related; motivation needed; coital interference?
Minipill	97	90	No estrogen risks	Very irregular menses; ovulation frequent; discontinuation high
Diaphragm	97	85	No side effects; little infection; little interference with intercourse	Needs medical visit; motivation needed; messy, cumbersome
Foam/cream/ suppository	97	80	Nonprescription; no side effects; antiinfective	Motivation needed; messy, care needed; interference with coitus, orogenital sex

6. Contraception in the adolescent is a dymanic issue requiring periodic reevaluation and change as warranted by changes in sexual behavior, nature of the partnership, or increasing psychosocial maturity. Different methods will have their proper time and place in a single patient over a number of years.

Specific steps in implementing contraception are outlined below:

1. Determine contraceptive need. Define the parameters of current and anticipated sexual activity (coital frequency, practices, circumstances, satisfaction or dissatisfaction, feelings about, concerns (see Table 17-1). Explore the possibility of abstinence and the feasibility of achieving satisfaction through noncoital means. Many adolescents choose to abstain from coitus for indefinite periods, even if previously experienced. Additionally, some parents request contraception for their daughters even though they are virginal or no longer sexually active. Ensure that contraception actually is needed. In the latter instance, promoting intrafamily communication and understanding of emerging adolescent sexuality is indicated.

When parents are unaware of the young person's contraceptive need, the possibility of their involvement should be reviewed. If adolescents, particularly those who are very young, can receive the benefit of parental support, the parents' participation should be encouraged. Mandatory parental notification, however, will only risk alienating the patient and increase the probability of pregnancy. The confidential physician-adolescent relationship should be breached only with the young person's permission.

2. Obtain a medical and sexual history (see Chapter 2; Table 17-1). Details of pubertal development, menstrual patterns, and any medical contraindications to or side effects from specific methods (see discussions of specific methods) are particularly important.

3. Obtain a psychosocial history (Chapter 2). Particularly evaluate factors influencing selection of method and compliance; inquire about contraceptive experience and attitudes of patient, partner, parents, siblings, and friends.

4. Conduct health assessment (Chapter 3; Table 17-2).

5. Discuss methods (with both partners together, if possible). Points to be covered include the following:

    a. All effective methods, proper use, efficacy, common side effects, possible risks, and comparative benefits; illustrate with diagrams, models, and contraceptive samples.

    b. Which methods work best for adolescents under various circumstances; what problems may be encountered in use.

    c. Which ones are medically contraindicated for the particular patient, if any.

    d. Benefits of barrier methods in preventing spread of disease.

    e. Ineffective methods (withdrawal, rhythm, "home remedies," popular myths).

Reinforcement with appropriate reading material the adolescent can take home is particularly helpful. No patient of any age can be expected to remember everything that is discussed in this first counseling session.

6. Institute method. Help the adolescent select a method that she (and her partner, if possible) feels comfortable with, is best able to comply with, and suits her coital patterns. Instruct about specific steps for use of the chosen method. If the adolescent is not yet ready to select a method or wishes to discuss her options with others, encourage interim abstinence or the combined use of condom and foam; arrange a return appointment as soon as possible.

7. Educate about method. Elaborate on the correct use, advantages, minor side effects, major side effects, and potential serious risks plus what symptoms to look for and what to do. Provide the patient with the printed package insert (as required by FDA regulation) or, more suitably, a set of directions and symptom check list geared to her or his level of comprehension.

    Review techniques by which the patient can check that she is using her method properly. Provide information about backup methods either as required during the first contracepting month or months or if use is interrupted for any reason.

8. Obtain consent and document visit. In most instances, it is legally permissible for adolescents to consent on their own to fertility-related medical services (Chapter 22). It is a good practice to obtain this consent in writing both at the time of the initial examination and when a particular method is prescribed. The record should also document in writing (with the date and physician's signature) that the correct use, benefits, and risks have all been explained and appear to be fully understood.

9. Provide for followup. Before leaving, the patient should have a definite appointment at the appropriate interval for the specific method to be used or as indicated by the adolescent's own particular needs, whichever is sooner. She also should be given appropriate telephone numbers and counseled to contact the physician promptly at any time symptoms of major side effects occur, if she has questions or concerns about either method use or minor side effects, even if expected, or if she becomes dissatisfied with the method for any reason and thinks she might stop. Unprotected coitus at any time must be avoided.

ORAL CONTRACEPTIVES
Pills with estrogen and progestin
Action: Prevents ovulation (suppresses midcycle surge of FSH, LH); alters cervical mucus, tubal motility, endometrium.

Indications: Contraceptive of choice for many adolescents.

Contraindications:

Absolute:
- ☐ Past or present history of thromboembolic disorder; prolonged bed rest, leg cast.
- ☐ Impaired liver function (acute hepatitis, drug abuse).
- ☐ Undiagnosed abnormal vaginal bleeding.
- ☐ Pregnancy known or suspected.

Relative:
- ☐ Vascular or migraine headaches; collagen vascular diseases.
- ☐ Severe hypertension; chronic heart disease; sickle cell disease.
- ☐ Diabetes; chronic renal failure.
- ☐ Gynecologic immaturity (first 6–12 months after menarche—controversial).
- ☐ Unreliability; strong ambivalence about use of contraception or desire for pregnancy; problems in remembering to take pill every day.
- ☐ (Note: Smoking increases the risk of cardiovascular disease in persons using the pill if over 30 years of age. This association is not present in younger individuals.)

Complications:
- ☐ Thromboembolic disease (rare in adolescents).
- ☐ Blood pressure elevation (reversible upon stopping).
- ☐ Cholestatic jaundice (uncommon).
- ☐ Post-pill menstrual irregularities (uncommon if none previously present).
- ☐ Hepatomas (rare, particularly in first 5 years of use).
- ☐ Contact lens problem (decreased tearing, corneal edema).
- ☐ Increased water retention, mild weight gain.

TABLE 17-12
ORAL CONTRACEPTIVES COMMONLY USED FOR ADOLESCENTS*

Contraceptive	Estrogen	Progestin
Estrogen-dominant		
Enovid-E	Mestranol, 100 μg	Norethynodrel, 2.5 mg
Ovulen	Mestranol, 100 μg	Ethynodiol diacetate, 1 mg
Norinyl/Ortho-Novum 2	Mestranol, 100 μg	Norethindrone, 2 mg
Norinyl/Ortho-Novum 1+80	Mestranol, 80 μg	Norethindrone, 1 mg
Balanced		
Demulen	Ethinyl estradiol, 50 μg	Ethynodiol diacetate, 1 mg
Norinyl/Ortho-Novum 1+50	Mestranol, 50 μg	Norethindrone, 1 mg
Norinyl/Ortho-Novum 1+35	Ethinyl estradiol, 35 μg	Norethindrone, 1 mg
Progestin-dominant		
Ovral	Ethinyl estradiol 50 μg	Norgestrel, 0.5 mg
Norlestrin 2.5	Ethinyl estradiol, 50 μg	Norethindrone acetate, 2.5 mg
Low-dose		
Brevicon	Ethinyl estradiol, 35 μg	Norethindrone, 0.5 mg
Lo-ovral	Ethinyl estradiol, 30 μg	Norgestrel, 0.3 mg

*Notes:

a. Norinyl and Ortho-Novum are identical formulations by different companies.

b. Mestranol is two-thirds as potent as ethinyl estradiol at equivalent doses.

c. Pills lower than 35 μg ethinyl estradiol are likely to cause break-through bleeding, patient discontinuation, and risk of pregnancy if a single pill is missed. Their use is discouraged except for older adolescents with strong motivation to prevent pregnancy and low tolerance for estrogen side effects.

Recommendations:

1. A "balanced" pill containing 50 μg mestranol or 35 μg ethinyl estradiol is best tolerated by most adolescents (Table 17-12).

2. Side effects are most frequent with the first cycle and generally improve within three cycles; the patient should not switch to another type prematurely. Indications for changing to an estrogen-dominant or progestin-dominant type plus other recommendations for managing side effects are given in Tables 17-13 and 17-14.

3. Memory is aided by use of a 28-day package with four rows of seven pills each, paralleling the days of the week.

4. Begin the first pack on the first Sunday after the onset of a menstrual period. (If menses begin on a Sunday, start pills the next week.) Start each new pack every fourth Sunday. (Relating the pill cycle to the fifth day of a menstrual period tends to lead to confusion in subsequent months.)

5. Discuss where the adolescent will keep her pills and how she will remember to take them, for example, as part of the wakeup or bedtime routine.

6. A backup method such as foam and/or condom always should be used with each coital episode for the first month of pill taking (ovulation may occur) and at any time errors are made or disruption occurs during the balance of the cycle.

7. If one pill is missed, it should be taken as soon as remembered (but within the same 24 hours) and the schedule continued. If two or more are missed, they can be made up by taking two pills a day (b.i.d.) until caught up to the schedule, *but* a backup method must be used for the rest of the cycle. Missing two or more pills early in the package may cause break-through ovulation, bleeding, or both.

8. Approach side effects rationally (Table 17-14); be realistic but do not alarm the patient excessively.

9. Advise the adolescent not to discontinue the pills without calling, but to call at once if there are any possible adverse effects.

10. Discontinue pills and consider another method if any of the following occur:

a. Blurred vision or loss of vision, numbness, paralysis, severe headaches, exacerbation of migraine

b. Thrombophlebitis, emboli (documented or suspected)

c. Hypertension, hyperlipidemia

d. Pregnancy (documented or suspected)

TABLE 17-13
SELECTION OF ORAL CONTRACEPTIVES FOR ADOLESCENTS

First choice	Indications
Balanced pill	Most adolescents, including first-time users and those with previous satisfactory experience with balanced pills
Estrogen-dominant	Androgenic females: moderate-marked acne, hirsutism, small breasts, menses usually short and scant
Progestin-dominant	Estrogenic females: large breasts, leukorrhea, premenstrual edema/weight gain, menses long and heavy

TABLE 17-14
MANAGEMENT OF COMMON ORAL CONTRACEPTIVE SIDE EFFECTS

- ☐ Nausea, vomiting, abdominal pain: Take pill with food; use lower estrogen pill.
- ☐ Headache, fatique: Evaluate for psychosocial concerns; use lower estrogen pill.
- ☐ Weight gain: Limit caloric intake, increase activity; use lower progestin pill.
- ☐ Leukorrhea: Investigate for infection; use lower estrogen pill.
- ☐ Amenorrhea/oligomenorrhea: Investigate for pregnancy; use higher estrogen pill.
- ☐ Hypermenorrhea: Investigate for infection; use lower estrogen pill.
- ☐ Irregular bleeding: Investigate for infection, incorrect pill-taking.
- ☐ Galactorrhea: Investigate for pregnancy, CNS-pituitary lesion, drug use.
- ☐ Early cycle break-through bleeding: Use higher estrogen pill.
- ☐ Late cycle break-through bleeding: Use higher progestin pill.
- ☐ Breast discomfort: Use lower estrogen pill.

e. Documented pill-related depression, dysphoria

f. Hepatitis (viral, drug-induced)

11. Schedule the first followup visit in 4–6 weeks with a phone contact after 2–3 weeks to discuss correct use and initial side effects.

12. Follow up every 3 months (or more often if patient needs additional support) for first year of use, then every 3–6 months according to the maturity, reliability, and medical status of user. Monitor weight, blood pressure each time, with a breast exam annually and Papanicolaou smear according to the schedule suggested in Chapter 3.

Progestin-only pills

Action: Prevents implantation, alters cervical mucus; *may* inhibit ovulation.

Indications: When oral contraception is desired but estrogen use is contraindicated or rejected.

Contraindications:

- ☐ Undiagnosed abnormal uterine bleeding (will mask)
- ☐ Intolerance of irregular menstrual bleeding (common side effect)

Complications: Irregular menses, ranging from daily to no flow.

Recommendations:

1. Progestin-only pills are only rarely indicated for adolescents due to their lower efficacy, particularly if a pill is delayed or missed, and the anxiety and confusion resulting from the fairly high incidence of menstrual irregularities.

2. When use is indicated (adolescents with severe headaches, hypertension, or media-induced fear of estrogen and no other method is acceptable, strongly urge use of a backup method (foam and/or con-

dom) during the first 6 months of use (highest failure rates), at every midcycle, and whenever a pill is delayed or missed.

3. Follow schedule as described for combined oral contraceptives with frequent reassurance about the irregular bleeding.

INTRAUTERINE DEVICES

Action: Prevents implantation (alters endometrium, alters tubal motility).

Indications: May be best method for adolescent who is at high-risk for poor compliance or who cannot take pills and will not use a barrier method or who needs a method not likely to be discovered by parents.

Contraindications:

- ☐ Acute pelvic infection or infection within past 6 months; pregnancy suspected; for 6–8 weeks postpartum.
- ☐ History of ectopic pregnancy.
- ☐ Uterine abnormalities: severe dysmenorrhea; severe dysfunctional bleeding.
- ☐ Valvular heart disease; blood dyscrasias.

Complications:

- ☐ Perforation during insertion (rare in experienced hands).
- ☐ Pregnancy more likely to be ectopic when it occurs (1%–3% pregnancy rate).
- ☐ Expulsion frequent in young women, particularly if nulliparous.

□ Increased menstrual flow, cramps.

□ Increased risk of pelvic inflammatory disease complicating cervicitis.

Comment: IUD users who acquire gonococcal or chlamydial infection have a significantly higher risk of complicating pelvic inflammatory disease (PID) than nonusers. PID, particularly if chronic or repeated, carries a risk of permanent sterility. For this reason many clinicians feel that IUDs should not be used in those who have not completed their families, especially adolescents and other nulliparous females. Nonetheless, considering the serious consequences of pregnancy in adolescence, we believe the IUD does have a definite place for teenagers unable to use other methods for medical or psychological reasons. It is best, however, to avoid use, if at all possible, for young women at significant risk for infection (multiple partners, poor judgment, poor compliance with followup and treatment, history of previous infection). If unavoidable, an IUD may be tried with careful and frequent monitoring for infection, prompt and aggressive treatment if infection occurs (including removal of the device), and persistent encouragement and education in the use of alternate methods.

Recommendations:

1. Consider the IUD for the adolescent needing effective contraception but who is not a pill candidate (medical contraindication, immature menstrual function, and/or poor compliance) and is at low risk for infection (monogamous, reliable partner, aware of risk of infection).

2. IUDs should be inserted by a person with experience (for example, gynecologist or trained primary care practitioner), especially in nulliparous females.

3. IUDs are inserted most easily within 1 week of menstrual onset (the cervix is dilated, pregnancy unlikely, cramps and bleeding already present).

4. Copper-containing IUDs appear best for nulliparous females (lower expulsion rate and lower blood loss than others but replacement needed in 3–4 years).

5. Hormone-releasing devices may help control menstrual cramps and/or heavy bleeding when these side effects are troublesome, but yearly replacement is required.

6. After insertion, followup visits are indicated at 2, 6, and 12 weeks, then every 3 months. At each visit, check position of string and a wet prep for possible infection. Culture for gonorrhea and chlamydia whenever suspected and at each visit in patients felt to be at risk. Check hematocrit yearly, more often in those with anemia history. Obtain Papanicolaou smears as described under "cervical neoplasia."

7. Instruct the adolescent to check for the IUD string after each menses. Urge her to phone at once if the string cannot be located and to use a backup method (foam and condom).

8. A missing IUD string is most often retracted into the cervical canal and can be retrieved by gentle probing with a cotton swab or small hook. When the string is not retrievable, pelvic roentgenogram or ultrasound will indicate whether the device is still within the uterus or has been expelled (all IUDs are radioopaque). If still present, a gynecologist's help usually is needed to remove it and replace it with a new one, with the string correctly positioned.

9. A partially expelled device may cause cramps and bleeding or no symptoms at all. The plastic stem will be seen in the cervical os or felt with the tip of a cotton swab. Such location is less effective in preventing pregnancy (contact with the uterine fundus is needed to prevent implantation); it should be removed and replaced with a new, properly positioned device.

10. All side effects should be reported and investigated thoroughly. Cramps, painful coitus, discharge, abnormal bleeding, and abdominal pain may be secondary to placement of the device but also may indicate infection. Amenorrhea usually indicates pregnancy.

11. Pregnancy with an IUD in place bears a risk of septic abortion. The device should be removed as soon as possible after pregnancy is diagnosed. Removal may stimulate spontaneous abortion but the chance of abortion is even greater if the device remains.

12. To minimize the risk of infection, insert the IUD only after recent negative gonorrheal and chlamydial cultures have been obtained.

MEDROXYPROGESTERONE ACETATE INJECTION (DEPO-PROVERA)

Action: Inhibits ovulation; alters cervical mucus; atrophies endometrium.

Indications: When a high degree of protection is desired and no other method is acceptable or medically safe; when cessation of menses is desired; when future fertility is of minimal concern.

Contraindications: Not approved for use as a contraceptive in the United States by the FDA.

Complications:

□ Irregular menses for 3–6 months, amenorrhea frequent thereafter.

□ Headache, nausea, weight gain.

□ Delayed return of ovulation/menses after discontinuation.

Recommendations:

1. Consider for adolescents with moderate to severe mental retardation (both as contraceptive and in eliminating problems related to menstrual hygiene), severe physical disability, severe coagulopathy, or severe sickle cell disease; that is, in situations where there is need for highly effective contraception with minimal compliance requirements, a desire for elimination of menstrual flow, and strong recommendation against natural child-bearing.

2. Give 150 mg IM initial dose, repeat in 1 month, then every 3 months. Narrow the interval if there is break-through bleeding.

3. Monitor blood pressure at each visit. Check breasts, Papanicolaou smear periodically (Chapter 3).

DIAPHRAGM

Action: Prevents fertilization.

Indications: Good method for the older adolescent in a committed relationship or any adolescent who is comfortable with insertion and cannot or will not use hormonal or IUD methods.

Contraindications:

□ Lack of privacy for insertion/removal.

□ Hesitation in handling genitals, using tampons, inserting creams.

□ Immediate postpartum period (problems with proper fitting).

Complications:

□ Pregnancy due to improper usage, incorrect fit; higher failure rate than oral contraception.

□ Topical allergic reaction to rubber, spermicidal jelly.

Recommendations (Table 17-15):

1. Fitting for correct diaphragm size should be done by an experienced practitioner.

2. Reassessment for a new size is indicated if weight changes by 15 or more pounds and following pregnancy.

3. A new diaphragm is recommended after 2 years of use.

4. The diaphragm should always be used with a spermicidal cream or jelly liberally applied to the center and around the edge. Additional spermicide should be applied vaginally before each repeated coitus.

5. Petroleum products should not be used for additional lubrication as they will cause rubber deterioration.

6. The diaphragm can be inserted up to 6 hours before coitus. It should remain in place for at least 6–8 hours after the last coitus. After use, it should be cleaned, dried, dusted with plain powder or cornstarch, and stored.

7. New diaphragm users should have insertion and removal explained and demonstrated carefully. They should not leave until they have tried insertion themselves and the practitioner has checked for proper positioning.

8. Followup visits in 1, 3, and 6 months and at least annually thereafter with a Papanicolaou smear and breast examination as indicated in Chapter 3.

VAGINAL SPERMICIDES
(FOAMS, JELLIES, SUPPOSITORIES)

Action: Prevents fertilization.

Indications: Best for the adolescent having infrequent intercourse or as an interim or backup method for oral contraception and the IUD; very effective if consistently used with a condom.

Contraindications:

□ Low motivation for use with each coitus.

□ Concern about handling genitals, messiness.

□ Uncooperative partner.

Complications:

□ Topical allergic reaction (infrequent).

□ Interference with orogenital sexual activity.

Recommendations (Table 17-15):

1. Foams are more effective than creams or suppositories; they are best distributed over the cervix and have the longest efficacy.

2. Suppositories are easiest to insert but the least consistent in distribution and, consequently, lowest in protection rate; they frequently remain in the solid state for many hours. If used, it is important that the adolescent recognize the difference between those which are spermicidal and those only intended for use as vaginal deodorants (for example, Norforms).

3. Spermicides should be inserted no longer than 10–20 minutes before coitus, not be douched out for 6–8 hours after coitus, and reapplied in the full amount 10–20 minutes before each repeat coitus.

4. Vaginal spermicides may offer some protection against infectious agents.

CONDOM

Action: Prevents insemination.

Indications: Best for the adolescent having infrequent intercourse or as interim or backup method; very effective if used consistently with vaginal spermicide; recommended as additional method whenever there is high risk of sexually transmitted infection and/or desire to stress male responsibility.

Contraindications: Should not be relied on as only method when motivation is low for consistent and/or correct use. Deemed to interfere with pleasure by many males.

TABLE 17-15
EXAMPLES OF BARRIER CONTRACEPTION

Method	Brands	Comments
Diaphragm	Koromex,** Ortho,[†] Ramses[‡]	Kit with variable size rings used for fitting and establishing proper size.
Spermicides		
Jellies	Koromex-A,* Preceptin,[†] Orthogynol,[†] Ramses[‡]	To be used with diaphragm only.
Creams	OrthoCreme,[†] Delfen,[†] Conceptrol[†]	Used alone or with condom (latter preferred); OrthoCreme and Delfen available in multiple dose tubes with or without applicator; Conceptrol available as prefilled, single-dose applicators.
Foams	Delfen,[†] Emko,[§] Because	Most effective in dispersion over cervix; used alone or with condom (latter preferred); Delfen and Emko available in multiple dose form with or without applicator; Because available as pre-filled, single dose applicators.
Suppositories	Encare-Oval[‖]	Effervesces on insertion, uncertain distribution; tendency to remain partly in solid state for excessively long time.
	Semicid[¶]	Melts on insertion; uncertain distribution; tendency to partly remain in solid state.
Condoms	Nuform,[‡] Ramses,[‡] Sheik,[‡] Trojan-Enz,[#] Horizon Nuda,** Horizon Prime**	Used alone or with spermicide (latter preferred); prelubricated types with terminal reservoir preferred.

*Holland-Rantos Co., Inc.
[†]Ortho Pharmaceutical Corp.
[‡]Schmid Products Co.
[§]The Emko Company.
[‖]Norwich-Eaton Pharmaceuticals.
[¶]Whitehall Laboratories.
[#]Youngs Drug Products Corp.
**Akwell Industries, Inc.

Recommendations Table 17-15):

1. Condom should be applied before any penile contact with the perineal area, as sperm are present in preejaculation secretions. It should be held in place during penile withdrawal and removed from the penis only after complete separation from the introital region.

2. A 1 cm reservoir should be left at the end to avoid rupture or spillage during use. Some types are manufactured with a terminal nipple for this purpose.

3. Condoms should not be reused or subjected to heat (automobile glove compartments in the summer, back trouser pockets for prolonged periods) and should be purchased from a reliable source.

4. Lubrication with petroleum products will damage rubber, but water-soluble surgical lubricants may be used. Prelubricated condoms often are preferred.

5. Decreased sensation with a condom can be an asset by delaying male orgasm and increasing pleasure for both partners. Modern brands have minimal interference with sensation.

6. The condom is the most effective means of preventing the spread of infection; however, infections can be transmitted during foreplay.

7. All sexually active males and females should be instructed in proper use. Bulk quantities are available at low cost to health care facilities and should always be on hand for "starter supplies."

POSTCOITAL CONTRACEPTION

Action: Prevents implantation.

Indications: Unprotected coitus at midcycle (3-4 days before to 3-4 days after the presumed day of ovulation) *and* no more than 72 hours following coitus.

Contraindications: Possible existent pregnancy.

Complications:

□ Effect on fetus if pregnancy exists (DES daughters).

□ Nausea, vomiting.

□ Medical contraindications against estrogen use (see oral contraceptives).

Recommendations:

1. Used properly postcoital methods have a very low failure rate of 0.03%-0.3%.

2. Treatment is with diethylstilbestrol 25 mg, *or* conjugated estrogens 25 mg, *or* ethinyl estradiol 2.5 mg p.o. twice a day for 5 days.

3. Nausea and vomiting are common side effects and may be controlled by giving an antiemetic (for example, prochlorperazine 5-10 mg) 1-2 hours before each dose.

4. The use of diethylstilbestrol for postcoital contraception has become controversial due to the complications of DES exposure in utero. When DES is used postcoitally, the practitioner should be certain that the patient is not already pregnant and that no more than 72 hours have elapsed since coitus. The patient should be informed of the possible risk to the fetus should the method fail. Some feel that postcoital DES should be given only to those who agree to abortion if the method fails; others feel it should be abandoned in favor of other estrogens.

5. If oral therapy is rejected or estrogens are contraindicated and the patient wants to initiate regular contraception with an IUD, a copper-containing IUD can be inserted provided there is no evidence of infection and cultures are taken.

6. Menstrual extraction is an alternative to postcoital estrogen or IUD insertion. (See No. 7).

7. Because the risk of pregnancy from a single act of coitus is low and because first trimester abortion is generally safe and readily available, many advocate withholding postcoital methods and offering abortion to those few who become pregnant. The emotional effects of waiting, the difficulty of deciding to abort, or personal opposition to this procedure should be considered in each case and the decision must be individualized.

ABSTINENCE

Action: Prevents insemination.

Indication: Any adolescent uncertain about his or her readiness for sexual intercourse.

□ Any adolescent unprepared to prevent and/or cope with the consequences.

Contraindications:

□ Strong ambivalence about capacity for self-restraint or wish to avoid pregnancy.

□ Any other psychological risk factor cited at the beginning of this section.

Complications: Interference with noncoital sexual intimacy and/or interpersonal relationships.

Recommendations:

1. Abstinence always should be discussed during contraceptive counseling and supported as the safest, least expensive, most effective and, often, most psychosocially appropriate method.

2. The adolescent choosing abstinence needs emotional support and assistance through rehearsal and role playing techniques to deal with partner and peer pressures to have intercourse.

3. When abstinence is chosen, education should include alternate means of sexual gratification, the need to avoid genital closeness during ejaculation if other forms of physical intimacy are used, the risks of transmitting infection by noncoital sexual activity, and complete information about *all* contraceptive methods for reference in case abstinence is not sustained.

STERILIZATION

An adolescent or parent may request vasectomy, tubal ligation, or hysterectomy. Unless there are compelling medical reasons, this is strongly discouraged (and of questionable legality) for anyone under 21 years old due to the low chance of reversibility and the improbability of an adolescent being able to make an irrevocable decision to forego childbearing for the rest of his or her life without regret. Effective contraception is a far better alternative.

Sterilization of severely retarded or multiple handicapped adolescents, for whom childbearing or parenthood are clearly impossible options, may be indicated in carefully selected cases. A complete diagnostic evaluation and multidisciplinary review of all circumstances are essential. The sole consideration is enabling the patient to live a healthier, fuller, and less restricted life. Continued counseling of the family and sex education of the handicapped adolescent before and after sterilization are mandatory to deal with parental guilt feelings and continued vulnerability to sexual exploitation. However, sterilization in any minor (or in any adult unable to give an informed consent), regardless of other factors no matter how compelling, is highly controversial. The current status of the law is reviewed in Chapter 22.

Pregnancy

Pregnancy in teenagers can have significant obstetric risks and major psychosocial impact (Table 17-16). Complications primarily correlate with delayed and inadequate prenatal care, less so (if at all) with young chronologic age, young gynecologic age, or low socioeconomic status. Complications increase in frequency with subsequent pregnancies below age 19 years.

Psychologic responses to the discovery of being pregnant correlate with the adolescent's developmental stage. Early adolescents evidence disbelief, disassociation, and denial, an attitude which may persist well into the last trimester. Late diagnosis, late onset of prenatal care, and poor compliance with recommendations are characteristic. There is a tendency to let parents and other adults decide whether the pregnancy is to be continued or terminated, once it is revealed.

Midadolescents also may deny pregnancy and often fear the consequences of discovery; both factors combine to delay medical attention. Ambivalence is most characteristic—ambivalence about themselves, their sexual identities, and their pregnancies—and has a significant impact on pregnancy prevention and resolution. Self-recrimination and adverse psychological reactions are common, whatever the chosen course. Compliance with prenatal care generally is good if the young mother's independence and maturity are acknowledged. A highly individualized approach is necessary, however, due to great variation in cognitive development, emotional maturity, and sociocultural backgrounds.

Late adolescents usually are more rational about their situation and make firm decisions about pregnancy outcome early in the course with little outside help. Their dominant concerns are practical and include selection of an appropriate treatment facility, information about the anticipated medical course, relative costs, and most importantly, effects on all parameters of their future.

DIAGNOSIS

Pregnancy should be suspected in any adolescent, whether she admits to being sexually active or not, if menses are delayed, scanty or irregular; if one or more periods have been missed; or if there are symptoms of nausea, vomiting, headaches, backache, breast tenderness, urinary frequency, and/or lower abdominal pain. It is critical to interview any female having any of these complaints (even if amenorrhea is initially denied) in private without parents present and to inquire specifically about the date of the last menstrual period. Many adolescents fearing pregnancy are so worried about the prospect of discovery by others that they may present with a cover com-

TABLE 17-16
INCREASED RISKS WITH PREGNANCY IN TEENAGERS*

Maternal	Infant
Medical	
First/third trimester bleeding	Prematurity
Significant anemia	Low birth weight
Prolonged, difficult labor	Neonatal mortality
Need for cesarian section	Neurologic defects
Toxemia of pregnancy	Sexually transmitted infections
Psychosocial	
Interrupted adolescence	Retarded development
Interrupted/incomplete education	Poor school performance
Limited career options/income	Physical abuse, neglect
Unstable marriage/divorce	Delinquency
Large family	Stigma of illegitimacy
Child-raising difficulties	
Depression, suicide risk	

*Comment: Increased risk of medical complications is greatest at the youngest maternal ages, primarily under age 15. Intensive prenatal care begun early will lessen the risks, even for young teenagers. Increased risk for psychosocial complications applies throughout the teenage years but varies with emotional maturity, motivation for and acceptance of pregnancy, and availability of external support systems.

plaint and not reveal their true concern unless these specific steps are taken.

The diagnosis is confirmed by immunoassay for chorionic gonadotropin on a random urine specimen using either the 2-minute slide test or 2-hour tube test; both are readily available in commercial kits. Testing can be quickly carried out in the office setting and results known before the end of the visit; test kit insert directions are clear and easily followed. If a random specimen is negative, repeat testing should be carried out on a first morning concentrated specimen after withholding fluids overnight. Urine pregnancy tests usually become positive 10–14 days after the first missed menstrual period but may be negative up to 21 days. False-positive results may be encountered with 3-4+ proteinuria, use of narcotics, phenothiazines, or marijuana, or at the time of the midcycle LH surge when normal ovulation follows an anovulatory, amenorrheic cycle.

Serum immunoassay for the beta-subunit of human chorionic gonadotropin (HCG) may be employed if the urine test is ambiguous or in situations in which earlier detection is desired. It has a high degree of sensitivity and specificity, becoming positive within 7–10 days after conception, and is increasingly available in commercial and hospital laboratories.

If the pregnancy test is positive, the adolescent should be so advised and the diagnosis confirmed by pelvic examination, which reveals the characteristic bluish tinge and softer consistency of the cervix and early uterine enlargement. These signs, however, also take several weeks after conception to appear, and pregnancy cannot be immediately ruled out by their absence. If the primary care physician is uncertain of his or her skills in detection, referral to a gynecologist is indicated.

If the urine pregnancy test is negative, a serum assay can be performed. Alternatively, the urine test may be repeated in 7–10 days. In instances of persistent negativity, testing should be repeated at similar intervals until a normal period arrives or until 4–5 weeks have elapsed. (Note that scanty bleeding or spotting can occur at the time of an expected period for the first month or two of pregnancy and this should not mislead.) The continuing lack of pregnancy signs or elevated gonadotropins for 1 month beyond a missed period suggests some other cause of amenorrhea (Table 17-7). The single exception is an ectopic pregnancy, in which placental insufficiency may produce insufficient gonadotropins for detection. Ectopic pregnancy is most likely to occur in individuals with a prior history of pelvic infection or in those using an IUD. Examination commonly reveals a tubal mass.

When the diagnosis is uncertain, effective barrier contraception (foam and condom, diaphragm) or abstinence is indicated until the situation is resolved. Oral contraception should be discontinued; moreover, if the patient is indeed pregnant, a history of a missed pill or improper use should be present. An IUD may be left in place until pregnancy is confirmed, at which time it should be removed; in this instance, however, additional observation for an ectopic pregnancy or spontaneous abortion is indicated.

Diagnosing pregnancy by the progesterone withdrawal test (no bleeding following a single test dose) is not recommended due to the association of congenital defects with in utero exposure to this substance and the current availability of equally sensitive serum pregnancy tests.

Home pregnancy test kits are *not* recommended for adolescents. They are expensive, subject to error in performance or interpretation, still require a visit to the physician for confirmation, and, most importantly, may delay seeking appropriate care with the consequences of specific health detriment and limitation of options.

COUNSELING THE PREGNANT ADOLESCENT

The first step is to discuss the reality of the pregnancy and its estimated duration. The adolescent needs help in accepting the situation and its medical, emotional, and social implications. The practitioner should encourage the teenager to involve the parents and partner and should offer to inform the parents independently or to be present when the adolescent does so herself. Many parents are highly supportive, once over the initial shock, and adolescents who enjoy this support adjust much more effectively regardless of their chosen outcomes. In addition, decisions made without actual knowledge as to how the family or partner will respond often are based on mistaken presumptions and can cause the adolescent to take an inappropriate course. These individuals commonly react very differently than the adolescent expects.

All concerned should review advantages and disadvantages of all alternatives (although there is never an "advantageous" solution to an unintended teenage pregnancy, only a "least disadvantageous") and discuss the specific implications of each option for the particular adolescent. Optimally, a final decision should only be made after the girl herself has had time to thoughtfully reflect on her choices as well as obtain counsel from her parents, her partner, and others in clarifying her position. It should not be put off any longer than absolutely necessary. If continuation is selected, optimal prenatal care and planning for parenthood or adoption are best instituted in the first trimester. If abortion is selected, it is safest and easiest to arrange during the first 10–12 weeks of pregnancy and has minimal consequences for future childbearing at that time.

Counseling a newly diagnosed pregnant adolescent about her options can be a difficult task. It is not a moment of singular rationality. It is essential, however, to present all her alternatives in a balanced, nonjudgmental manner, with careful review and rereview in terms she fully understands. No attempt should be made to influence her decision, regardless of the physician's personal views toward teenage pregnancy and its solution; all questions should be answered honestly. Decisions based on the pressure or bias of another do not reflect the adolescent's true feelings and are much more commonly associated with long-term adverse psychologic consequences, regardless of what that decision might be. If it appears to be particularly difficult for the adolescent to make a choice or if the situation is complicated by environmental, intrafamilial, or psychological factors beyond those normally encountered, referral to an agency specializing in pregnancy, adoption, or abortion counseling is indicated.

Although family involvement should be supported as a general rule, this is not always possible due, first, to the resistance of the adolescent to such revelation (and the likelihood of serious inpairment to the therapeutic relationship if confidentiality is violated) and second, when there is a reasonable probability that parental knowledge will result in physical or emotional harm to the adolescent or even to parents themselves if they are unwell. Laws in many states permit diagnosis and prenatal care with only the minor's consent. Abortion also may be performed with the minor's sole consent, but parental notification is increasingly required for dependent minors and, with some probable exceptions, now has constitutional standing (see Chapter 22).

CONTINUATION TO TERM

The adolescent who elects to continue with her pregnancy is best cared for by an experienced hospital, clinic, or obstetrician known to have a caring, comprehensive approach to pregnant teenagers. Special adolescent maternity programs that include strong psychosocial and developmental supports have the most success in reducing physical and emotional complications and preventing recidivism. When available, special school programs for pregnant teenagers can be helpful in furthering education and preparing for parenthood; some adolescents, however, may prefer to stay in their regular classroom and often are supported in this decision by state law. Young adolescents particularly are predisposed to medical complications with even modestly compromised prenatal care and should be referred to a medical center with a high-risk obstetric service. This also is true for those teenagers having closely spaced second, third, or more pregnancies, whatever their outcomes.

Prenatal care. In many instances, the experienced primary practitioner will be the one to provide pregnant teenagers with their initial prenatal care, at least while arranging for referral to a special program. Management should include the following:

1. Screen by examination and appropriate tests for gonorrhea, *Chlamydia*, cervical cytology, herpes, syphilis, rubella immunity, blood type, anemia, proteinuria, and diabetes. Treat underlying disorders; plan for RhoGAM administration if Rh negative; do *not* give rubella vaccine.

2. Prescribe a multiple vitamin with iron (numerous prenatal formulations available).

3. Provide reassurance and diet advice for nausea and vomiting (small frequent meals, simple nonfatty foods, adequate fluids). Use an antinauseant such as Bendectin sparingly, if at all, due to recent concern about potential teratogenic effects.

4. Urge the patient to avoid any drugs not prescribed or cleared by a physician who is aware of the pregnancy. Alcohol, cigarettes, aspirin, coffee, tea, cola drinks, and all over-the-counter preparations should be avoided. If substance abuse is known or suspected, begin planning for any necessary special management issues related to the last trimester, delivery, and possible neonatal addiction.

5. Provide instruction and educational materials about diet (see Table 19-1), exercise, rest, signs and symptoms of a normal prenatal course, and signs and symptoms of possible complications.

6. Evaluate the adolescent's preparation for parenthood (previous training, experience in child care), subsistence needs, continued education, and emotional support systems (family, partner, community) and institute planning as indicated. A social worker is particularly helpful here.

7. Make plans to resume general health care, including contraception, after delivery.

Ectopic pregnancy. Almost always tubal, ectopic gestation is a significant cause of maternal death if rupture occurs before diagnosis. Suspect an ectopic pregnancy if there is a positive pregnancy test together with lower quadrant pain and tenderness, an adnexal mass with tenderness, abnormal bleeding, and/or less than expected uterine growth. However, the pregnancy test is not always positive due to a compromised placenta; even if negative, physical signs and symptoms alone should be sufficient to raise suspicion. The risk of an ectopic pregnancy increases when the patient has a history of pelvic inflammatory disease or second trimester abortion and/or the presence of an IUD at the time of conception. The presence of any of these factors gives additional weight to the diagnosis.

Ruptured ectopic pregnancy should be considered when the sudden onset of severe pain and shock follow the diagnosis of pregnancy or a period of amenorrhea. When suspected, refer the patient to an emergency room or gynecologist for immediate evaluation and management.

Adoption. Although this alternative might seem an optimal solution, it is now rare for adolescents who elect to continue a pregnancy to term to surrender their infant for adoption. Ninety-five percent keep the infant at home or in the care of a relative; this decision is the young mother's exclusive legal right, even if a minor. Those who do wish to consider adoption should be referred to an adoption agency early in pregnancy for ongoing counseling and planning. Adolescents who are pressured into giving up their babies against their will are likely to have deep regrets, depression, suicidal ideation, and early repeat pregnancy.

Parenthood. Few teenage mothers or fathers are able to make the smooth, rapid transition to parenthood that they fantasize or that others may expect. The developmental needs and as yet to be completed tasks of normal adolescence do not disappear simply because of parenthood and often complicate adjustment. Adolescent tendencies toward risk-taking, denial, experimentation, and low frustration tolerance may cause their children to be poorly protected from accidents and poisonings, to be exposed to a variety of infections and environmental hazards, and sometimes to be victims of abuse and neglect. On the other hand, given ample support, guidance, and encouragement, particularly from their own families, young parents and their infants can do surprisingly well. Attention should focus particularly on child-rearing skills, economic needs, continued education or vocational training, and opportunities for socialization, with provision for child care in the young mother's absence. The role of the teenage father must be defined. If the young couple marry, ongoing marital counseling is recommended in light of the high incidence of divorce among adolescent couples. Family planning is essential. An adolescent, once pregnant, is particularly vulnerable to repeat pregnancy, yet the chance of a favorable outcome for young families, either couples or single parents, diminishes with the arrival of each additional child during these early years.

TERMINATION

It is a pregnant adolescent's legal right to elect and secure an abortion on her own consent. If termination is contemplated, she should be referred to a facility known to provide comprehensive services to young women. Local Planned Parenthood agencies often provide or can recommend abortion services. The physician or other health professional personally opposed to abortion certainly should make his or her position known, but he or she is not entitled to provoke inordinate guilt, coerce, or otherwise obstruct the young woman from securing an abortion to which *she* is not opposed. This is her constitutional prerogative. In such cases, the clinician should refer the adolescent to a neutral source of information, such as a hospital adolescent medical clinic, a local physician specializing in adolescent health care,

the county medical society, or a clergymen's consultation service.

If abortion is to occur, most adolescents require and should have a great deal of advance preparation, ongoing psychosocial support, and postabortion counseling to help them work through this difficult time. (Few teenagers make this decision lightly; for most it is a painful, stressful choice.) Some abortion clinics may not offer counseling to this extent. The primary practitioner who is comfortable with the patient's choice is in an optimal position to supplement their services. Alternatively, adolescent medical clinic social workers or those in community service and mental health programs can be an excellent referral source. The involvement of supportive parents is particularly helpful and should be encouraged.

Therapeutic abortion. Forty to sixty percent of adolescents elect to terminate their pregnancies, with the larger proportion occurring in those under age 15. For gestations of less than 12 weeks, outpatient abortion by dilatation and suction-curettage usually is possible and bears minimal risks—far fewer than those associated with pregnancy going to term. Past 12 weeks, hospitalization for dilatation and extraction (12-15 weeks) or saline or prostaglandin induction (16-20 or 24 weeks) is required. The later option has a complication risk rate tenfold higher than early procedures but is still far safer than bearing a child. Referral should be instituted as soon as the decision is made, the earlier the better. But continuing support and followup by the primary care provider is important as well.

When parents are not involved, payment may be a problem. Medicaid today is not a viable resource except in those few states willing to apply their own funds to this purpose. However, many abortion clinics are quite low cost, particularly for early procedures, and offer installment payment plans.

The adolescent who is or feels coerced or pressured into choosing abortion against her personal feelings is at high risk for emotional repercussions as well as rapid repeat pregnancy. On the other hand, those who choose abortion freely, while commonly experiencing a normal mourning period of several months, usually have few long-term psychological sequelae, particularly if provided continuing emotional support and a chance to discuss feelings and reactions as they arise.

Menstrual extraction. Gentle suctioning of the uterine contents may be done easily up to 14-16 days after a missed menstrual period, even without a pregnancy test. Indications include the adolescent's desire to eliminate any possibility of pregnancy as early as possible or her preference not to know whether she is pregnant or not (although the pathology report on suctioned tissue will reveal trophoblastic and/or placental tissue if conception has occurred). Menstrual extraction also may have a place in postcoital contraception.

The procedure is highly effective, low cost, simple, and low risk, particularly when performed by an experienced physician. Unfortunately, its use in adolescents often is hindered by their frequent delay in seeking attention for a missed menstrual period until it is too late for extraction to be performed.

Although charges that the term "menstrual extraction" is simply a euphemism for an early suction abortion have some basis, these charges are not always accurate. Tissue studies reveal that from 40%–60% of young women undergoing this procedure are not pregnant at all, the delayed menses being due to some other reason. Nonetheless, both of these issues (misdirection and the possibility of performing an unnecessary procedure) have made menstrual extraction controversial.

Spontaneous abortion. Ten percent of all adolescent pregnancies end in miscarriage. A spontaneous or threatened abortion should be suspected when lower abdominal cramps, abnormal bleeding, or both follow a diagnosis of pregnancy, especially if pelvic examination reveals cervical dilatation and blood in the os. Refer the patient to an emergency room or gynecologist for management.

References for Adolescents and Their Parents*

Balis, A. 1981. *What are you using? A birth control guide for teenagers.* New York: Dial. (MA, LA)

Barlow, D. 1979. *Sexually transmitted diseases: The facts.* New York. Oxford University Press. (MA, LA, P)

Bell, R., Women's health collective. 1980. *Changing bodies, changing lives: A book for teens on sex and relationships.* New York: Random House. (MA, LA)

Block, W. A. 1974. *What your child really wants to know about sex and why.* Greenwich, Conn.: Fawcett-Crest. (P)

Bode, J. 1980. *Kids having kids: The unwed teenage parent.* New York: Franklin Watts. (EA, MA)

Burkhart, K. W. 1981. *Growing into love: Teenagers talk candidly about sex in the 1980s.* New York: G. Putnam's & Sons. (LA, P)

Carrera, M. 1981. *Sex: The facts, the acts, and your feelings.* New York: Mitchell Beazley. (LA, P)

Calderone, M. S., and Johnson, E. W. 1981. *The family book about sexuality.* New York: Harper & Row. (P)

Comfort, A., and Comfort, J. 1979. *The facts of love: Living, loving, and growing up.* New York: Thomas Crown. (MA, P)

Corsaro, M., and Korzeniowsky, C. 1980. *S.T.D.: A common sense guide.* New York: St. Martin's Press. (MA, LA, P)

Eagan, A. B. 1979. *Why am I so miserable if these are the best years of my life?* New York: Avon. (MA, LA)

Fairchild, B., and Hayward, N. 1979. *Now that you know: What every parent should know about homosexuality.* New York: Harcourt Brace Jovanovich. (P)

Gardner-Loulan, J.; Lopez, B.; Quackenbush, M. 1979. *Period.* San Francisco: New Glide Publishers. (EA, P)

Gordon, S. 1978. *Facts about sex for today's youth.* Fayetteville, N.Y.: Ed-U-Press. (EA)

Gordon, S. 1978. *Facts about VD for today's youth.* Fayetteville, N.Y.: Ed-U-Press. (EA)

Gordon, S. 1979. *Let's make sex a household word: A guide for parents and children.* Fayetteville, N.Y.: Ed-U-Press. (EA, P)

Gordon, S. 1978. *You would if you loved me.* New York: Bantam. (EA, MA)

Gordon, S., and Wollin, M. M. 1975. *Parenting: A guide for young people.* New York: Oxford University Press. (MA, LA, P)

Hanckel, F., and Cunningham, J. 1979. *A way of love, a way of life.* New York: Lothrop, Lee & Shepard. (MA, LA, P)

Hunt, M 1979. *What is a man? What is a woman?* New York: Farrar, Straus, & Giroux. (MA)

Johnson, E. W. 1977. *Love and sex in plain language.* Philadelphia: Lippincott. (EA)

Johnson, E. W. 1978. *V.D. Venereal disease and what you should do about it.* Philadelphia: Lippincott. (EA)

*These books are keyed according to the author's recommendations for the most appropriate readers. EA = early adolescents; MA = mid-adolescents; LA = late adolescents; P = parents (also teachers, non-health professionals). The practitioner is advised to review these books in the local library or book store before recommending to specific patients or families and to base the recommendations on cognitive, psychosocial, and ethnocultural appropriateness. Parents may wish to review specific books before they are recommended to their children.

Justice, B., and Justice, R. 1979. *The broken taboo: Sex in the family.* New York: Human Sciences Press. (P)

Kaplan, H. S. 1979. *Making sense out of sex.* New York: Simon & Schuster. (MA, LA)

Kelly, G. F. 1977. *Learning about sex: A contemporary guide for young adults.* Woodbury, N.Y.: Barron's. (MA)

Langone, J. 1980. *Like, love, lust: A view of sex and sexuality.* Boston: Little-Brown & Co. (MA)

Lewis, H. R., and Lewis, M. E. 1980. *The parent's guide to teenage sex and pregnancy.* New York: St. Martin's Press. (P)

Lieberman, E. J., and Peck, E. 1981. *Sex and birth control: A guide for the young,* 2nd ed. New York: Harper & Row. (MA, LA, P)

McCoy, K., and Wibbelsman, C. 1978. *The teenage body book.* New York: Pocket Books. (MA, LA)

Nourse, A. E. 1980. *Menstruation: Just plain talk.* New York: Franklin Watts. (EA, P)

Oettinger, K. B. 1979. *Not my daughter: Facing up to adolescent pregnancy.* Englewood Cliffs, N.J.: Prentice-Hall. (P)

Pomeroy, W. B. 1981. *Boys and sex.* New York: Dell. (EA, MA)

Pomeroy, W. B. 1981. *Girls and sex.* New York: Dell. (EA, MA)

Silverstein, C. A. 1977. *A family matter: A parent's guide to homosexuality.* New York: McGraw-Hill. (P)

Wear, J., and Holmes, K. K. 1976. *How to have intercourse without getting screwed.* Seattle: Madrona. (MA, LA, P)

Bibliography

COMPREHENSIVE

Brookman, R. R. 1981. *Pediatric and adolescent gynecology case studies.* Garden City, N.Y.: Medical Examination Publishing Co., Inc.

Capraro, V. J., editor. 1977. Symposium: Pediatric and adolescent gynecology. *Clin. Obstet. Gynecol.* 20(3):531–663.

Cowell, C. A., editor. 1981. Symposium: Pediatric and adolescent gynecology. *Pediatr. Clin. North Am.* 28(2):245–530.

Emans, S. J. H., and Goldstein, D. P. 1982. *Pediatric and adolescent gynecology.* 2nd ed. Boston: Little-Brown & Co.

Huffman, J. W.; Dewhurst, C. J.; and Capraro, V. J. 1981. *The gynecology of childhood and adolescence,* 2nd ed. Philadelphia: W. B. Saunders Co.

Kreutner, A. K. K., and Hollingsworth, D. R. 1978. *Adolescent obstetrics and gynecology.* Chicago: Year Book Publishers.

SEX EDUCATION-SEXUALITY

Chilman, C. S. 1978. Adolescent sexuality in a changing American society: Social and psychological perspectives. Rockville, Md.: U.S. Dept. of Health, Education and Welfare (NIH 79-1426).

Craft, A., and Craft, M. 1981. Sexuality and mental handicap: A review. *Br. J. Psychiatr.* 139(5):494–505.

Gordon, S.; Scales, P.; and Everly, K. 1979. *The sexual adolescent: Communicating with teenagers about sex,* 2nd ed. N. Scituate, Mass.: Duxbury Press.

Katchadourian, H. 1980. Adolescent sexuality. *Pediatr. Clin. North Am.* 27(1):17-28.

Litt, I. F., and Cohen, M. I. 1979. Adolescent sexuality. *Adv. Pediatr.* 26:119-136.

Lloyd, R. 1976. *For money or love: Boy prostitution in America.* New York: Ballantine.

Lothstein, L. M. 1980. The adolescent gender dysphoric patient: An approach to treatment and management. *J. Pediatr. Psychol.* 5(1):93–109.

Robinault, I. P. 1978. *Sex, society, and the disabled: A developmental inquiry into roles, reactions, and responsibilities.* New York: Harper & Row.

Rosenblum, S., and Faber, M . M. 1979. The adolescent sexual asphyxia syndrome. *J. Am. Acad. Child Psychiatr.* 18:546-558.

Sarrel, L. J., and Sarrel, P. M. 1979. *Sexual unfolding: Sexual development and sex therapies in late adolescence.* Boston: Little-Brown & Co.

Zelnik, M., and Kantner, J. F. 1976 and 1971. Sexual and contraceptive experience of young unmarried women in the United States. *Fam. Plan. Perspect.* 9(2):55-71.

SEXUAL ASSAULT

Burgess, A. W.; Groth, A. N.; Holmstrom, L. L.; and Sgroi, S. M. 1978. *Sexual assault of children and adolescents.* Lexington, Mass.: D. C. Heath & Co.

Halpern, S. 1978 *Rape. Helping the victim.* Oradell, N.J.: Medical Economics Publishers.

Schultz, L. G., editor. 1980. *The sexual victimology of youth.* Springfield, Ill.: Charles C Thomas, Publisher.

MENSTRUAL-PELVIC DISORDERS

Goldstein, D. P.; De Cholnoky, C.; and Emans, S. J. 1980. Adolescent endometriosis. *J. Adol. Health Care* 1(1):37-41.

Hein, K.; Schreiber, K.; Cohen, M. I.; et al. 1977. Cervical cytology: The need for routine screening in the sexually active adolescent. *J. Pediatr.* 91(1):123-126.

Henzl, M. R., editor. 1980. A new perspective on dysmenorrhea: The role of prostaglandins and prostaglandin inhibitors. *J. Reprod. Med.* 25(4):191-242.

Klein, J. R. 1980. Update: Adolescent gynecology. *Pediatr. Clin. North Am.* 27(1):141-152.

Mishell, D. R., Jr., and Davajan, V., editors. 1979. *Reproductive endocrinology, infertility, and contraception.* Philadelphia: F. A. Davis.

Yen, S. S. C., and Jaffe, R. B., editors. 1978. *Reproductive endocrinology: Physiology, pathophysiology, and clinical management.* Philadelphia: W. B. Saunders Co.

GENITAL INFECTIONS-SEXUALLY TRANSMITTED DISEASES

Catterall, R. D. 1981. Biological effects of sexual freedom. *Lancet* 1(8215):315-319.

Govan, D. E., and Kessler, R. 1980. Urologic problems in the adolescent male. *Pediatr. Clin. North Am.* 27(1):109-124.

Noble, R. C. 1979. *Sexually transmitted diseases: Guide to diagnosis and therapy.* New Hyde Park, N.Y.: Medical Examination Publishing Co., Inc.

Schacter, J., and Dawson, C. R. 1978. *Human chlamydial infections.* Littleton, Mass.: PSG Publishing Co.

Shafer, M. B.; Irwin, C. E.; and Sweet, R. L. 1982. Acute salpingitis in the adolescent female. *J. Pediatr.* 100(3):339-350.

Solomon, L. M.; Esterly, N. B.; and Loeffel, E. D. 1978. *Adolescent dermatology.* Philadelphia: W. B. Saunders Co.

St. John, R. K., and Brown, S. T., editors. 1980. International Symposium on Pelvic Inflammatory Disease. *Am. J. Obstet. Gynecol.* 138(7):845-1112.

St. John, R. K.; Neu, H. C.; and Thompson, S. E., editors. 1979. Gonorrhea therapy 1979. *Sex. Transm. Dis.* 6(2):87-194.

U.S. D.H.H.S. Public Health Service. Centers for Disease Control. 1982. Sexually transmitted diseases treatment guidelines 1982. Morbidity and Mortality Weekly Report 31(25):355-605.

CONTRACEPTION

Bergman, A. B. 1980. Condoms for sexually active adolescents. *Am. J. Dis. Child.* 134(3):247-249.

Edelman, D. A.; Berger, G. S.; and Keith, L. 1979. Intrauterine devices and their complications. Boston: G. K. Hall Publishers.

Greydanus, D. E. 1981. Alternatives to adolescent pregnancy: A discussion of the contraceptive literature from 1960 to 1980. *Seminars Perinatol.* 5(1):53-90.

Greydanus, D. E., and McAnarney, E. R. 1980. Contraception for the adolescent: Current concepts for the pediatrician. *Pediatrics* 65(1):1-12.

Hatcher, R. A.; Stewart, G. K.; Stewart, F.; et al. 1980. *Contraceptive technology 1980-1981.* 10th ed. New York: Irvington Publishers. (11th edition available).

Klaus, H. 1982. Natural family planning: A review. *Obstet. Gynecol. Surv.* 37(2):128-150.

Lyle, K. C., and Segal, S. J. 1979. Contraceptive use-effectiveness and the American adolescent. *J. Reprod. Med.* 22(5):225-232.

Ory, H. W.; Rosenfield, A.; and Landman, L. C. 1980. The pill at 20: An assessment. *Fam. Plan. Perspect.* 12(6):278-283.

Tatum, H. J., and Connell-Tatum E. B. 1981. Barrier contraception: A comprehensive review. *Fertil. Steril.* 36(1):1-12.

Torres, A.; Forrest, J. D.; and Eisman, S. 1980. Telling parents: Clinic policies and adolescents' use of family planning and abortion services. *Fam. Plan. Perspect.* 12(6):284-292.

Zelnik, M., and Kantner, J. F. 1979. Reasons for nonuse of contraception by sexually active women aged 15-19. *Fam. Plan. Perspect.* 11(5):289-296.

PREGNANCY-ABORTION

American College of Obstetricians and Gynecologists, Task Force on Adolescent Pregnancy. 1979. *Adolescent Perinatal Health: A Guidebook for Services.* Chicago: A.C.O.G.

Cates, W., Jr. 1980. Adolescent abortions in the United States. *J. Adol. Health Care* 1(1):18-25.

Chilman, C. S., editor. 1980. *Adolescent pregnancy and childbearing: Findings from research.* Rockville, Md.: U.S. Dept. of Health and Human Services (NIH 81-2077).

Alan Guttmacher Institute. 1981. *Teenage pregnancy: The problem that hasn't gone away.* New York.

McAnarney, E. R., and Stickle, G., editors. 1981. *Pregnancy and childbearing during adolescence: Research priorities for the 1980s.* Birth Defects Foundation Original Article Series, XVII(3). New York: Alan R. Liss.

Ooms, T., editor. 1981. *Teenage pregnancy in a family context: Implications for policy.* Philadelphia: Temple University Press.

Scott, K. G.; Field, T.; and Robertson, E., editors. 1981. *Teenage parents and their offspring.* New York: Grune & Stratton.

Smith, P. B., and Mumford, D. M., editors. 1979. *Adolescent pregnancy: Perspectives for the health professional.* New York: G. K. Hall.

Tryer, L. B., editor. 1978. Symposium: Complications of teenage pregnancy. *Clin. Obstet. Gynecol.* 21(4):1135-1232.

Zabin, L. S.; Kantner, J. F.; and Zelnik, M. 1979. The risk of adolescent pregnancy in the first months of intercourse. *Fam. Plan. Perspect.* 11(4):215-222.

–18–
The Adolescent Athlete

Ira M. Sacker, M.D.
Shepard H. Splain, D.O.

Conditioning
Sleep □ Nutrition □ Strength □ Endurance □ Flexibility □ Skills
Developmental Matching
Disqualification
The Female Athlete
Equipment
Common Sports Injuries
Fractures □ Strains and sprains
Principles of management applicable to all acute injuries
Chronic Musculoskeletal Problems Related to Sports
Osgood-Schlatter's disease □ Chondromalacia patellae
Slipped femoral epiphysis □ Shin splints □ Tendinitis
Heat Disorders

Sports medicine involves male and female athletes at all levels of play: Little League, secondary school, college, semiprofessional, and professional—although the latter two categories are uncommon foci of attention for the primary care physician. General health concerns include preseason evaluation, physiologic and psychologic development, conditioning, nutrition, injuries, and rehabilitation (Table 18-1). The extent of the physician's involvement depends on whether he or she is functioning as the young athlete's personal doctor, as the team physician, or both. In the first instance, responsibilities variably include preparticipation evaluation, management of intercurrent or chronic health conditions that affect the young person's capacity for play, and the management of various injuries after emergency care has been rendered on the field. In the second two instances, added responsibilities include establishing health standards for the team as a whole; educating athletes, parents, school and sports personnel about

adolescent health and safety requirements; promoting an integrated and comprehensive approach toward adolescent sports participation by all concerned; the emergency management of accidents or other medical problems as they occur on the field; and being the final arbiter in clearing a young person for play.

This chapter responds to both sets of concerns but emphasizes the team physician's role. In this regard the following basic principles should prevail:

1. The primacy of medical concerns: It is essential that all involved agree about the primacy of health protection and the inviolateness of the team physician's decisions about player participation, conditioning requirements, equipment safety, and health standards.

2. The importance of conditioning: Improperly conditioned players and injured players who are improperly reconditioned are most vulnerable to injury. Preparticipation health evaluations should

TABLE 18-1
AN ATHLETE'S CHECKLIST

1. Preparticipation history and physical examination
2. Preseason conditioning
3. Proper, correctly fitting equipment
4. Proper psychologic orientation
5. Proper matching on a developmental basis
6. Coordinated team approach of all involved
7. Proper playing conditions
8. Immediate medical attention to any injury
9. Appropriate medical assessment before return to game
10. Appropriate emergency care by specialist trained in care of serious injuries
11. Reconditioning and medical clearance before resuming participation after injury
12. Recognition of alternative sports when disqualification from one activity necessary

occur early enough (ideally 2 weeks in advance) to allow indicated remediation and conditioning to take place.

3. An appropriate health evaluation: Assessment of an adolescent before his or her participation in sports must be more than simply a heart and lung check on the first day of practice. A relatively detailed evaluation should be carried out. The history may be obtained in advance by a self-administered questionnaire (Figure 18-1), then reviewed before the examination (by paramedical personnel if available), ensuring that particular attention will be given to potential problem areas. The physical examination itself should include assessment of musculoskeletal integrity (Figure 18-2), as well as those elements appropriate to adolescents in general (Chapter 2).

4. The team physician during the game: All injured players should be promptly examined no matter how minor the injury appears to be. When the adolescent returns to the game it should be the team physician's exclusive decision. The physician also is responsible for instituting appropriate emergency measures on the field, calling in indicated consultants, and supervising movement and transport of those who are seriously injured to the hospital. At this point it becomes the responsibility of the parent (or patient if over age 18) to determine who should continue with care. In many instances, the team physician is also the adolescent's general physician.

5. Return to sports after injury or illness: Return to play should only be with proper medical clearance and after completion of appropriate reconditioning steps.

6. Alternatives for limited adolescents: Some young people are limited as to what sports they may participate in because of permanent injury or chronic health problems. Disqualification from one type of sport does not mean disqualification from *all* sports (Table 18-2). Many alternative sports can be physically and psychologically rewarding.

Conditioning

Only in romantic novels or late night movies does the untrained, unconditioned, but naturally gifted performer step up from the role of spectator to that of Olympic champion without the benefit of years of training. At the other extreme, no amount of training will transform one who is not endowed with natural ability into a world record holder. Conditioning, however, will enable each participant to reach the highest point attainable with a particular genetic endowment and degree of motivation. Simplistically, conditioning can be divided into general conditioning and athletic conditioning. The latter can be further subdivided into overall conditioning and specific measures as determined by the demands of a particular sport. Here the discussion concerns only general conditioning and overall athletic conditioning, leaving specific sport concerns to more specialized texts.

SLEEP

An obvious point is that it is difficult to be in top form or protect against injury if chronically fatigued. An adequate number of hours of sleep is a basic condition for effective play.

NUTRITION*

Dietary fads come and go. Unfortunately these often depend on the endorsement contracts of professional athletes or other unscientific word-of-mouth "gospel." No scientific evidence indicates that any diet, other than one that is well balanced and meets minimal daily requirements, advantageously affects performance in the long run. Potentially harmful trends such as excessively high protein diets, quick weight loss diets or dehydration to make a weight class, and other deviations from sound health practices are to be condemned. Caloric intake should be sufficient to meet basal growth and activity requirements apportioned as follows: protein 10%–20%, carbohydrate 50%–55%, and fat 30%–35%. The higher figure for protein is appropriate for rapidly growing youths. Vitamin supplementation is unnecessary, provided intake of appropriate food substances is adequate. Although vitamin megadoses

*Also see Chapter 19.

Athlete's Medical History Questionnaire for Sports Participation

Name _____

Home Address _____

Telephone _____ Sex _____ Age _____ Birth Date _____

Parents' Names _____

Parents' Business Telephones   Father _____ Mother _____

Person to Notify in Emergency _____

    Address _____ Telephone _____

Personal Physician _____

    Address _____ Telephone _____

Health Insurance Company _____

    Name of Insured _____ Policy Number _____

Sport(s) Will be Playing _____

Supervisor/Sponsor (school, community recreation program, etc.)

    Name _____

    Address _____ Telephone _____

Check All That Apply and Describe as Indicated:

During sports participation do you wear any of the following?

_____ Contact lenses

_____ Glasses

_____ Dental appliance

_____ Mouth protector

_____ Brace, splint, ace bandage, or any other orthopedic appliance

If so, describe _____

_____

Have you ever had any injury or other problems with any of the following?

_____ Head	_____ Shoulder/clavicle	_____ Ribs	_____ Knee, knee cap
_____ Neck	_____ Arm, elbow, wrist	_____ Hips, pelvis	_____ Leg
_____ Back	_____ Hand	_____ Thigh	_____ Ankle
			_____ Foot

Give date or age of occurrence of any checked items and describe problem.

Do you have any bone grafts, spinal fusions, plates, screws, etc.? _____

Describe _____

Do you have any health conditions that might give you problems in sports? _____

Describe _____

Have you ever been in the hospital or had any operations?

Problem   Date   Hospital   Doctor's name and address

Continued

General Health History

Have you ever had any of the following?   Give date and describe

_____ Birth defect
_____ Absent organ (eye, kidney, etc.)
_____ Anemia, other blood problem
_____ Infectious mononucleosis
_____ Pneumonia
_____ Hepatitis, jaundice
_____ Other serious infection
_____ Diabetes
_____ Cough up or vomit blood
_____ Sugar, protein, pus, blood in urine
_____ High blood pressure
_____ Concussion, knocked out
_____ Headaches, blackouts
_____ Blurred vision
_____ Dizzy spells
_____ Styes, eye infections
_____ Frequent nose bleeds
_____ Other bleeding problems
_____ Skin infections, boils
_____ Heart disease, rheumatic fever, murmurs
_____ Appendicitis
_____ Hernia
_____ Chest pain during exercise
_____ Tuberculosis
_____ Chronic cough
_____ Frequent indigestion, heartburn
_____ Stomach ulcer
_____ Kidney or bladder problems
_____ Heat exhaustion, heat stroke
_____ Hearing problems
_____ Ear infections
_____ Allergies to drugs, foods, insect stings, etc.
_____ Mental health problems
_____ Any other health problem or illness not listed

Are you taking any medications regularly? What kind? _____

How much? _____

Female Health History Supplement

Menstrual history. Age started menstruating (having periods) _____

  Are your periods regular; how frequent? _____

  Do you have cramps? _____   Any other problems? _____

  Date of last period? _____   Have you ever been pregnant? _____

  Do you use birth control? _____   What type? _____

_____   _____
Signature of Athlete   Date

FIGURE 18-1
SELF-ADMINISTERED ATHLETE'S HISTORY QUESTIONNAIRE FOR PREPARTICIPATION SPORTS HEALTH EVALUATION

Modified and adapted from Marshall, J., and Tischer, L. 1978. Screening for Sports. *N.Y. State J. Med.* 78:243.

Musculoskeletal Examination Checklist for Sports Participation

Neck
_____ Normal

_____ Pain on motion
_____ Limited rotation
_____ Limited flexion
_____ Limited extension

Spine
_____ Normal

_____ Pain on motion
_____ Excess lordosis
_____ Excess kyphosis
_____ Scoliosis
_____ Limited motion
_____ Weakness

Shoulders
_____ Normal

_____ Pain on motion
_____ Limited range of motion
_____ Atrophy
_____ Weakness

Elbows
_____ Normal

_____ Hyperextension (extends >180 degrees)
_____ Flexion contracture (extends < 180 degrees)
_____ Pain on motion
_____ Weakness

Wrists
_____ Normal (extension and
flexion = 90 degrees)

_____ Limited flexion
_____ Limited extension
_____ Limited rotation
_____ Pain on motion
_____ Weakness

Hands
_____ Normal

_____ Pain on grasp
_____ Limited digit extension
_____ Limited digit flexion
_____ Weakness of grasp

Hips
_____ Normal

_____ Limited in flexion
_____ Limited in extension
_____ Limited in rotation
_____ Pain on motion
_____ Weakness

Knees
Alignment
_____ Normal

_____ Varus (bowlegged)
_____ Valgus, 0–14 degrees (normal range)
_____ Valgus, > 15 degrees (knocked knee)
_____ Flexion contracture (extends < 180 degrees)
_____ Hyperextension (extends > 180 degrees)

Range of motion
_____ Normal

_____ Limited in flexion (< 90 degrees)
_____ Limited in extension (< 180 degrees)
_____ Pain on motion
_____ Weakness

Thigh size
_____ Equal

_____ 1–2 cm smaller than opposite side
_____ > 2 cm smaller than opposite side

Stability
Lateral collateral ligament
(Varus stress test)
_____ Normal (= opposite knee)
_____ Mild instability in flexion
_____ Moderate instability in flexion
_____ Instability in extension
_____ Gross laxity

Medial collateral ligament
(Valgus stress test)
_____ Normal (= opposite knee)
_____ Mild instability in flexion
_____ Moderate instability in flexion
_____ Instability in extension
_____ Gross laxity

Continued

Anterior cruciate ligament
(Anterior drawer sign)
_____ Normal (= opposite knee)
_____ Slight jog
_____ Moderate jog
_____ Gross movement

Palpation and observation
_____ Normal

Posterior cruciate ligament
(Posterior drawer sign)
_____ Normal (= opposite knee)
_____ Slight jog
_____ Moderate jog
_____ Gross movement

_____ Scar
_____ Pain (location _____)
_____ Swelling (location _____)
_____ Crepitation

Patellae
_____ Normal

_____ Pain on motion
_____ Positive apprehension test (patient tenses, flinches when
     examiner starts to palpate or move patella)
_____ Deviates from midline on isometric hamstring contraction
     with knee in extension
_____ Crepitation

Range of excursion: _____ 1/2 "   _____ 1 "   _____ 1 1/2 "   _____ 2 "   _____ > 2 "

Ankles
_____ Normal

_____ Pain on motion
_____ Limited range of motion
_____ Weakness
_____ Instability
_____ Positive anterior drawer sign
_____ Positive medial/lateral talar shift

Feet
_____ Normal

_____ Pes cavus (high arches)
_____ Pes planus (flat feet)
_____ Pronated
_____ Splayed

Functional Tests
(Score: 0 = cannot perform; 1 = can perform with discomfort; 2 = can perform well)

Walk up and down stairs _____
Running in place _____
Half squat _____
Full squat _____
Hop on left leg only _____   Hop on right leg only _____
Rise up onto toes, left leg only _____   right leg only _____
Palms to floor: _____ 10 " from floor
                _____ Fingertips touch floor
                _____ Fingers touch floor in entirety
                _____ Palms touch floor

FIGURE 18-2
MUSCULOSKELETAL EXAMINATION CHECKLIST FOR THE PREPARTICIPATION SPORTS HEALTH EVALUATION
Normal or abnormal findings may be indicated by placing an "L" or "R" in the appropriate spaces. The presence of abnormal findings in any joint requires further orthopedic evaluation and appropriate conditioning prior to sports participation.

Modified and adapted from Marshall, J., and Tischer, L. 1978. Screening for sports. *N.Y. State J. Med.* 78:243.

TABLE 18-2
DISQUALIFYING CONDITIONS FOR SPORTS PARTICIPATION*

Condition	Contact[†]	Noncontact[‡]	Others[§]
General			
Acute infections: respiratory, genitourinary, infectious mononucleosis, hepatitis, active rheumatic fever, active tuberculosis	X	X	X
Obvious physical immaturity in comparison with other competitors	X	X	
Obvious growth retardation	X		
Hemorrhagic disease: hemophilia, purpura, other bleeding tendencies	X		
Diabetes, inadequately controlled	X	X	X
Jaundice, whatever cause	X	X	X
Eyes			
Absence or loss of function of one eye	X		
Severe myopia	X		
Ears			
Significant hearing impairment	X		
Respiratory			
Tuberculosis (active or under treatment)	X	X	X
Severe pulmonary insufficiency	X	X	X
Cardiovascular			
Mitral stenosis, aortic stenosis, aortic insufficiency, coarctation of the aorta, cyanotic heart disease, recent carditis of any etiology	X	X	X
Hypertension on organic basis	X	X	X
Previous heart surgery for congenital or acquired heart disease	X	X	
Liver			
Enlarged liver	X		
Spleen			
Enlarged spleen	X		
Skin			
Boils, impetigo, herpes simplex gladiatorum	X		
Hernia			
Inguinal or femoral hernia	X	X	
Musculoskeletal			
Symptomatic abnormalities or inflammations	X	X	X
Functional inadequacy of the musculoskeletal system, congenital or acquired, incompatible with the contact or skill requirement of the sport	X	X	
Neurologic			
History or symptoms of previous serious head trauma, repeated concussions, or controlled convulsive disorder	X		
Incompletely controlled convulsive disorder	X	X	
Previous surgery on head or spine	X	X	
Renal			
Absence of one kidney	X		
Renal disease	X	X	X
Genitalia[‖]			
Absence of one testicle	X		
Undescended testicle	X		

Continued

TABLE 18-2
DISQUALIFYING CONDITIONS FOR SPORTS PARTICIPATION* (CONTINUED)

AMA Committee on Medical Aspects of Sports. 1972. *Guide for medical evaluation of candidates for school sports*, rev. ed. Chicago: American Medical Association. Copyright 1980 American Medical Association.

*Some of the disqualifying conditions listed above are subject to evaluation and consideration by the responsible physician with respect to anticipated risks, the otherwise athletic fitness of the candidate, special protective preventive measures that might be utilized, and the nature of the supervisory control. Disqualification, moreover, does not necessarily imply restriction from all sports at that time or from the sport in question in the future. If the decision is disqualification, however, the physician vested by the school with the authority to disqualify should not be overruled by any other person. This is a direct and unavoidable responsibility and needs the full support of the institution and all personnel involved.

†Lacrosse, baseball, soccer, basketball, football, wrestling, hockey, rugby, etc.

‡Cross country, track, tennis, crew, swimming, etc.

§Bowling, golf, archery, field events, etc.

‖The absence of one testicle or an undescended testicle should be evaluated by the physician with the school authorities, the parent, and the athlete who should be fully informed and involved. Should such an athlete be permitted to play in contact sports, he should be properly fitted with a protective device or athletic supporter.

enjoy popularity in some circles, there is no evidence that these are beneficial and vitamin A or D toxicity is possible.

Nutritional status can be grossly estimated by comparing the adolescent's height and weight to standard norms (Appendix I, Tables 1 and 2). More precise estimates of body fat can be achieved through triceps fold measurements (Appendix I, Table 3). Weight and height should be monitored throughout the conditioning period and the sport season. Rapid weight loss usually indicates inadequate caloric intake unless it occurs in an overweight youngster who is slimming down. Weight gain variably depends on normal growth factors, increasing muscle mass consequent to training, and/or accumulation of excess body fat. Optimally, the triceps skin fold measurement should be at or less than the fiftieth percentile for age and sex. The leaner values are more desirable in runners than in, say, weight lifters. It is now recognized that females can achieve a lean body mass close to that of males with proper conditioning.

STRENGTH

Strength is developed by progressively overloading muscles through isometric, isotonic, or isokinetic means. Isometric contracture occurs when a muscle contracts against a resistance, but it does not shorten, for example, straight leg raising efforts while restrained by weight. Isotonic contracture occurs when a muscle contracts and moves the skeleton, as in knee extension with weights. Isokinetic contracture allows the muscle to work at a maximum effort through the entire range of motion by matching resistance to effort.

ENDURANCE

Muscular endurance refers to the ability of a single muscle to sustain rapid repetitive contractures at or close to peak efficiency. This is closely correlated with strength and is promoted by increasing the work done during each exercise period.

Similarly, cardiovascular endurance is promoted and maintained by the overload principle, according to the following observations by Scheuer and Tipton:

1. Little cardiovascular effect is achieved if a heart rate does not reach 130–150 beats per minute.

2. Three to four sessions per week lasting 30–45 minutes per session at a level of 60% maximum oxygen consumption will improve cardiovascular fitness.

3. Vigorous exercise once a week has been reported to cause beneficial effect on some cardiovascular parameters.

How much endurance training is enough? Unfortunately, we have no answer as to what the upper biologic limits of human achievement might be. From a practical viewpoint, however, the degree of endurance possible in a given case largely depends on the individual's own level of aspiration and the degree to which he or she is willing to engage in conditioning.

FLEXIBILITY

Flexibility, or mobility, is the range of motion through which a joint can move without injury. Much has been written by Nicholas and others regarding tightness and looseness, but the data concerning this concept and its relation to injury are contradictory. It is universally accepted, however, that every person should spend some time going through flexibility and stretching exercises before participating in any sport.

SKILLS

Skill derives from the continuing practice of the sport in question coupled with innate talent, coaching, training, study, and sacrifice in enhancing knowledge, judgment, and the effective performance of required motor responses.

Developmental Matching

When is a 14-year-old not a 14-year-old? This apparent riddle raises a real issue for adolescents in light of the wide variation in parameters of normal pubertal growth. All 14-year-olds do not reach the same level of physical maturity at the same time. In any group of young and midadolescents there are major differences among individuals, not only in height and weight but also in total muscle mass, upper-lower body segment ratio, the degree to which epiphyses are open or closed, musculoskeletal strength, cardiovascular capacity, and so on. A 14-year-old at Tanner stage II is a far different individual physiologically than one who is Tanner stage IV or V (Chapters 1 and 2), even if both are identical in height and weight.

Developmental matching is particularly desirable in contact sports, in which fulcrum forces, open epiphyses, and muscle mass are important factors, or in which a pubertally slow adolescent would be disadvantaged by his or her physical immaturity, as in long-distance running. Assessment is by Tanner staging in males and premenarcheal females. The time elapsed since menarche is a sufficient indicator in those who have reached this landmark; although all females will be fully physically developed by 2 years after this time.

Of course, developmental matching is not an invariable requirement or the only requirement in determining the makeup of a team. In many instances, the developmental stage has less relevance than other factors, such as actual size, inherent skill, conditioning, and motivation. It is important, however, to bring attention to this issue, because developmental status is a significant element in the overall assessment of an adolescent's placement in sports.

Disqualification

The question of disqualification from sports is a serious one. Over the past several years there have been changes in what were once considered absolute indications for disqualification, for example, the absence of a paired organ. Table 18-2 cites the current recommendations of the American Medical Association regarding disqualifying conditions for sports participation. The list is rather extensive, and it must be emphasized that each case needs to be assessed individually. Exercise tolerance tests can be particularly helpful in evaluating pulmonary and cardiac reserves. Considerable challenge also has been offered to such exclusions as epileptics, those having had head or spinal surgery, or those with asymptomatic renal disease. The American Medical Association emphasizes flexibility in applying these recommendations (see table footnote).

The Female Athlete

For many years women in sports were rarely taken seriously or given much attention. Only a few fields, such as tennis and track, recognized the female athlete. A girl with keen competitive interest in baseball, basketball, soccer, and other fields considered exclusively male was labeled unfeminine—a "tomboy." School budgets for female athletics were miniscule compared to those for males. Female varsity sports were virtually nonexistent. In 1971, the National Federation of State High School Associations estimated that there were only 14 interscholastic sports for girls, with but 287,000 participants nationwide, despite the 1970 census finding of 20 million young women between 10 and 20 years. This picture has changed dramatically in the past decade. Federal funding regulations now mandate equal expenditures for men's and women's athletics. In 1974, the number of recognized interscholastic sports for women in high school had increased to 25, with 1.3 million participants.

Many misconceptions exist about the female athlete. These are often given as reasons for not allowing full female athletic participation. The following are some of the myths and rebuttals to them:

1. "Physiologic differences in body build, strength, and cardiovascular endurance due to endocrine differences make it unwise for females to compete vigorously." FALSE. Although it is true that endocrine differences modify the potential of each athlete, the above statement has no basis in fact. Moreover, until the age of 13 or 14, there is *no* physiologic difference between male or female competitors. The earlier onset of maturity in females may even place them at a physiologic advantage for a short period of time. At maturity however, the average female is 5 inches shorter, 40–50 pounds lighter, and has 10% more body fat (25%:15%) than males. But conditioning can alter the latter figure significantly and, as studies of long-distance female runners have shown, the proportion of body fat can

be drastically reduced. Weight-lifting training programs for female athletes have shown them also to be capable of significant gains in strength. Interestingly, females do not develop the large muscles seen in weight-lifting males. This phenomenon is probably due to the effects of higher circulating levels of testosterone on the male musculature. We can conclude that if muscle bulk is a determinant of strength, the female athlete, although capable of increasing her strength greatly, will probably lag behind her male counterpart.

The average female does have a smaller cardiac stroke volume and lower hemoglobin concentration than her male counterpart. In the past this was felt to be extremely important in limiting her potential for endurance, but recent evidence indicates that, with proper training, females indeed can approximate the maximal oxygen uptake of males but not quite catch up. There is no physiologic reason that females cannot compete in strenuous, competitive athletics.

2. "Females should not compete due to potential injury to primary or secondary sex organs." FALSE. No evidence exists to support this notion. Few reports in the literature indicate injury to ovaries or breasts from athletic competition. In fact, the intrapelvic position of the female ovary makes it less vulnerable to injury than the exposed male testes.

No evidence exists linking athletic competition or trauma to the breasts to lesions, either malignant or benign. The comfort of the participant should be the only consideration. For larger-breasted girls this means a good support brassiere. A word of caution: an overly constrictive support may diminish oxygen consumption to a significant degree. Girls electing to compete without bras will occasionally develop irritation over the nipple from friction against their jerseys. Simple measures such as a Band-Aid or Vaseline over the nipple often solve the problem.

3. "Competition during menses is not healthy and will lead to diminished performance." FALSE. Certainly no girl should be forced to compete during menstruation, or at any time, if she does not wish to. The literature, however, fails to reveal any evidence that harm can occur. Physical activity often diminishes dysmennorrhea. World records and Olympic gold medals have been won during all phases of the menstrual cycle. It is important for the physician counseling the young female athlete to understand how the girl psychologically views her menstruation and counsel her accordingly. Continuing all usual physical activity, however, is preferred.

4. "The pregnant female should not compete."

FALSE. No ill effects from exercise during pregnancy, including strenuous competition, have been observed in the female or fetus. Often delivery is easier and more rapid than in the non-physically fit woman. The amount of exercise permitted during pregnancy is an individual consideration for the patient and her physician; the sedentary female may well benefit by an increase in activity, and the marathon runner appropriately might be advised to diminish her training program to some degree.

Equipment

Every sports participant is entitled to effective protection against injury. This applies as much to novices as to the varsity player and to females as well as males. Although hand-me-down equipment may ensure a balanced budget, it also ensures that no player will be truly well fitted and thus bears a higher injury potential. The team physician can play an important role in seeing that schools properly respond to their student's protective equipment requirements. This means purchasing such items as helmets and dental guards specifically fitted for each player and ensuring that these are of the latest design. In general, equipment should be bought from a reputable dealer who is established in the community and has a good record for abiding by the service agreement. Special bargains at very low prices should be avoided as they usually indicate that obsolete equipment is being unloaded. There is no escape from the observation that the best equipment generally costs the most.

Many sports have few protective equipment requirements beyond appropriate proper fitting footwear and suitable, comfortable clothing. Participants in sports with collision potential (surfing, cycling, motorcycling) also need protective helmets. Some sports have additional mandatory protective requirements such as the following:

☐ Football
  Individually fitted helmet
  Face mask appropriate to position
  Custom-made dental guard
  Shoulder, hip, and knee pads
☐ Ice hockey
  Face guard
  Custom-made dental guard
  Shoulder, hip, elbow, and knee pads
  Padded gloves
  Face mask and special pads for goaly
☐ Baseball
  Batting helmet
  Rubber cleat shoes only; no steel spikes
  Catcher's mask and helmet

□ Boxing and wrestling
Athletic supporter
Headgear to prevent cauliflower ears

In addition, the coaching staff should be instructed to insist on the proper use of equipment and to place stringent penalties on those athletes who misuse equipment in dangerous ways or fail to use it at all. Examples include use of the football helmet for spearing, grabbing the face mask for tackling, or forgetting to wear a dental guard in hockey. It also is important to guard against athletes taking foolish risks consequent to feelings of invincibility conveyed by well-fitting protective gear.

Common Sports Injuries
FRACTURES
Fractures in growing adolescents commonly involve the epiphyseal plate. By general consensus these injuries are described according to the Salter and Harris classification scheme (Figure 18-3). Type I and II fractures generally heal uneventfully and have few serious sequelae. Anatomic reduction usually is not necessary, as continued growth will remodel the bone. Types III and IV, however, are more serious, as they involve the articular surface as well as the epiphyseal plate and have implications for long-term joint mobility, as well as ultimate bone growth. Expert primary and followup care is essential; operative intervention often is required. Type V fractures carry a poor prognosis, with permanent deformity a common late result due to crushing and destruction of growing cells. This potential often goes unrecognized at the time of the injury itself.

STRAINS AND SPRAINS
The terms strain and sprain often are used interchangeably, but they each describe a separate entity. Strain refers to injury of a muscle-tendon unit and sprain to ligamentous injuries. The distinction is important to management. Strains are graded according to degree. Mild (first degree) strain implies no anatomic disruption of the injured part. Recovery can be expected with rest, avoidance of activity, and proper rehabilitation. Moderate (second degree) strain implies actual damage to the muscle or tendon, but some degree of anatomic continuity remains. The extent of disruption is often a diagnostic problem. Ice and protection will give immediate relief. Protection until complete healing has occurred and proper reconditioning therapy are the hallmarks of treatment. Too early a return to activity may cause rerupture and form the basis for a chronic, incapacitating condition. Severe (third degree) strain implies

complete rupture of some part of the musculotendinous apparatus, with resultant loss of function. Surgical intervention to restore anatomic continuity usually is required.

Sprains are similarly classified. A mild (first degree) sprain involves tearing some ligamentous fibers, producing hemorrhage but no functional loss. Immediate treatment is by ice and compression with subsequent therapy being symptomatic. Moderate (second degree) sprain involves a more severe tearing of ligamentous fibers with some functional loss. Immediate treatment is ice and compression. In general, moderate sprains heal without surgical intervention but must be protected for varying periods; the patient subsequently returns to activity at a graduated pace while undergoing vigorous physical therapy. Severe (third degree) sprain implies complete ligamentous disruption with complete loss of function. Surgical treatment is invariably indicated.

PRINCIPLES OF MANAGEMENT APPLICABLE TO ALL ACUTE INJURIES
Certain principles of management prevail in most instances of acute injury on the playing field. Because they apply to each of the specific injuries in the following section, they will not be repeated.

1. Examine the player where he or she lies; ascertain the location and approximate nature of injury and approximate degree of seriousness.
a. Ensure that further injury will not occur if patient moves or is moved. Particularly check neurovascular status distal to injury.
b. Carefully note the position of the affected part and inquire about how the injury occurred. Much useful diagnostic information can be obtained before further tissue swelling occurs and while the events are clear in the player's mind and other participants are available for questioning.
2. Remove taping, padding, and other gear for more definitive examination (see specific injury section). In extremity injuries, compare with opposite normal joint.
3. Promptly apply moderate compression and ice to all fresh sprains and strains. Be sure not to restrict blood flow; frequently check to see that distal color and pulses are good.
4. Reduction may be tried with dislocations and certain other injuries, but should *not*, however, be attempted unless the physician is familiar and experienced with these maneuvers (see specific injury section). It is safer to splint the patient and later transport him or her to an orthopedist or hospital if doubtful of one's capability.

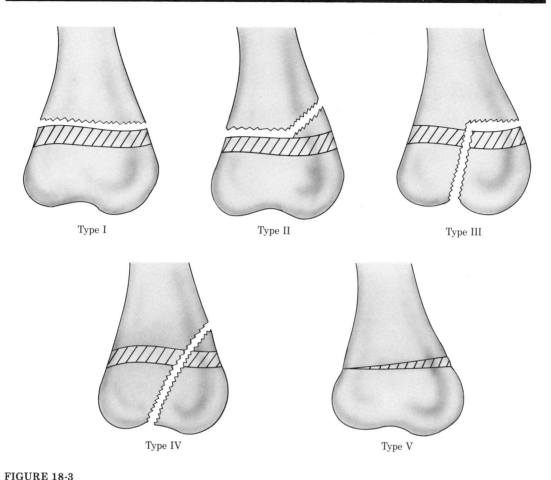

FIGURE 18-3
SALTER-HARRIS CLASSIFICATION OF FRACTURES
Type I, separation through the epiphyseal plate without a bony fracture. Type II, fracture through the epiphyseal plate and through a portion of the metaphysis. Type III, fracture extends from the articular surface to the epiphyseal plate and then parallel with the plate to its periphery. Type IV, fracture extends from the articular surface through the epiphysis, the epiphyseal plate, and a segment of the metaphysis. Type V, crush injury of some or all of the epiphyseal plate.

Salter, R., and Harris, R. 1963. Injuries including the epiphyseal plate. *J. Bone Joint Surg.* 45A(3):587.

5. Splint all possible fractures and second- and third-degree sprains and strains well above and below the affected joint to achieve full immobilization prior to removal from the field. Follow the same injunction about overtight splints as noted for compression bandages. Note that further swelling aggravates a tight splint. The top and bottom edges should easily admit several fingers; distal pulses and color should be good.

6. Any patient requiring splinting should be transported to an appropriate facility (a hospital emergency room or an orthopedist's office) for further evaluation and management. If the team physician is not qualified in this area, he or she should establish an appropriate linkage with a physician who is qualified.

7. First-degree strains and sprains may be managed by avoiding weight-bearing or applying a sling;

TABLE 18-3
EQUIPMENT LIST FOR FIELD EMERGENCIES

1. Stethoscope
2. Blood pressure cuff and manometer
3. Flashlight
4. Scissors
5. Airways (assorted sizes)
6. Portable suction apparatus
7. Portable ventilation apparatus
8. Portable oxygen and mask
9. Assorted dressings, gauze pads, adhesive tape
10. Triangle slings
11. Elastic bandages
12. Safety pins
13. Assorted splints (inflation and traction types and simple padded boards of appropriate length for arms and legs)
14. Short and long spine board
15. Ice, instant cold packs
16. Adjustable crutches
17. Stretcher

the patient should be referred to the orthopedist or skilled generalist's office for further evaluation and management.

8. The patient with transient loss of consciousness, head or neck injury, spinal injury, possible intraabdominal injury, shock, heat disorder, or any other potentially serious condition must be transported immediately by ambulance with the necessary life support systems to a hospital.

9. No player, even if only sustaining a minor injury, is to return to the game unless there is a full range of painless motion of the affected joint or joints and no swelling or joint tenderness. In addition, he or she must be able to perform all maneuvers relative to the sport in question without discomfort or feelings of instability.

Table 18-3 lists supplies that should be available to the physician for on-field management of injuries.

DIAGNOSIS AND MANAGEMENT OF SPECIFIC ACUTE INJURIES

All general principles cited in the last section also apply to the following injuries as clinical judgment indicates.

Head injuries. In actual or suspected head injury:

1. Remove the adolescent from play and do not allow reentry that day, even if he or she is seemingly unaffected.

2. Test mental status for time, space, recent and past memory.

3. Question about headache, nausea, and dizziness.

4. Check pupil size, pulse, respirations. Look for possible motor and/or sensory changes.

5. If the patient is unconscious, establish an airway; transport in a semiprone position to hospital by ambulance.

Persons with mild concussion, no neurologic signs, and no amnesia usually can return to sports when all headache is gone. More serious concussions need to be individually evaluated. Two or more concussions of any type may be cause for exclusion from contact sports; each case should be individually evaluated (with neurologic consultation) if the sport is very important to the youth.

Neck and spine injuries. Handle the patient with utmost care, avoiding motion until properly assessed to avoid further cord injury in the case of spinal fracture or compression.

1. Initial management on field where player lies.

2. Remove helmet with extreme caution (if football or other sport requiring same). Be sure neck is neither flexed, extended, or subject to excessive traction. Use cutters.

3. Stabilize neck or back immediately; do *not* put patient through range of motion or force beyond the pain level.

4. Palpate areas of tenderness.

5. Note existence and extent of pain, paresthesias, hyperesthesias, motor loss, sensory loss.

6. Immobilize neck with spine board or sandbags and transport the patient from the field on a rigid support (stretcher, door, boards).

7. The adolescent may reenter play only if he or she has no neurologic signs and has full, painless range of motion.

Clavicle fractures. Major complications are rare but include injury to regional vessels and nerves.

1. Look for classic diagnostic signs of pain, crepitation, and deformity at the fracture site.

2. Check neurovascular status of ipsilateral arm.

3. Apply ice and sling and refer patient for further evaluation.

Acromioclavicular injuries. Anything from mild sprain to complete disruption may occur. Usually, the injury results from a fall directly on the acromion process with the arm in adduction.

1. Check for extent of injury.

First degree: only mild tenderness and swelling over joint.

Second degree: Swelling, tenderness, pain, and abnormal laxity of distal clavicle on motion.

Third degree: Severe pain and free floating distal clavicle.

2. Apply ice and sling and send patient for further evaluation.

Shoulder injuries. Salter I and Salter II type fractures readily occur during rapid growth due to the open epiphysis of the proximal humerus. This is a common injury in early and midadolescents.

1. Examine for characteristic signs: severe pain and an inability to move the affected joint.

2. Check neurovascular status of ipsilateral arm.

3. Apply ice and sling and send patient for further evaluation.

This epiphysis has a great capacity for molding in the growing adolescent, and even displaced fractures usually can be expected to heal without sequellae.

A dislocated shoulder is a common injury of late adolescence and adulthood. More than 90% are anterior and usually result from a combined abduction-external rotation force. Posterior dislocations result from the opposite force and are only rarely encountered.

1. Determine the type of injury.

a. Anterior dislocation: Severe pain, arm held slightly abducted and externally rotated; a hollow can be palpated in the glenoid.

b. Posterior dislocation: May be missed on first examination; severe pain; arm held abducted and internally rotated.

2. Check neurovascular status, particularly distribution of the axillary nerve.

3. If anterior, the physician may be able to reduce by applying immediate gentle traction in line with the deformity.

4. Whether reduced or not, place arm in sling and send patient for further evaluation to ensure there are not additional injuries.

Unfortunately a first dislocation in an adolescent often sets the stage for recurrent dislocation, regardless of the treatment rendered.

Elbow injuries. Strains, sprains, and contusions of the elbow are relatively common. Dislocations and all types of Salter fractures also may occur. X-ray evaluation of a fracture may be difficult due to the confusion provided by the many epiphyseal centers at this joint. Comparison roentgenograms of the opposite arm are helpful.

1. Assess the extent of injury; major injuries usually are evident with severe pain, rapid swelling,

limitation of movement and, in some instances, deformity and/or crepitus.

2. If circulation is impaired following dislocation or fracture with displacement, immediately reduce by straight downward and forward traction of the arm with the shoulder fixed.

3. Apply ice, splint, and refer patient for further evaluation if serious injury exists or if doubt exists about diagnosis.

4. If the injury is assessed as less serious, try gentle range of motion and check for ligament injuries. These may be detected by applying gentle valgus (outward) and varus (inward) stress, or pressure, at the elbow while it is in extension and slight flexion; variable degrees of laxity will be encountered in second- and third-degree sprains.

5. With lesser injuries, use clinical judgment about returning individual to play.

Radius and ulnar fractures. These usually are evident.

1. Look for characteristic signs.

a. Shaft fractures; pain, deformity, crepitus.

b. Colles fracture; typical silver spoon deformity. Usually is Salter type I or II.

2. Apply ice and send for further evaluation.

Wrist and hand. Sprains, strains, and fractures of the wrist and hand are all possible. Fractures of the carpals, metacarpals, and phalanges should be carefully evaluated and treated even if seemingly minor. Long-term complications and permanent disability are possible, particularly if initial management is inadequate.

1. Assess type of injury.

a. Fracture of the carpal navicular may be difficult to detect. It often only manifests in vague wrist tenderness after a fall on outstretched hand. Pain on palpation of the anatomic snuffbox (on the dorsum of the hand at the base of the first and second metacarpal) should arouse suspicion.

b. Fracture of metacarpals: pain and tenderness over the involved bone, sometimes with deformity.

c. Phalangeal fractures: usually present with point tenderness and swelling. Mallet finger (drooping of the distal phalanx with an inability to extend) occurs on avulsion of the insertion of the extensor digitorum longus.

d. Phalangeal dislocations: a common injury marked by pain, immobility, and deformity at the affected joint. (Usually reduced easily by

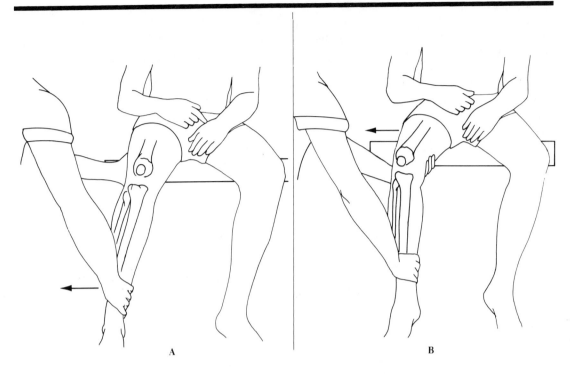

A   B

FIGURE 18-4
EXAMINATION OF THE KNEE: VALGUS AND VARUS STRESS TESTS.
A, VALGUS TESTING. B, VARUS TESTING.
These maneuvers detect disruption of the collateral ligaments. Grasp the ankle with one hand and stabilize. Apply inward pressure (valgus stress) to the lateral aspect of the knee with the other hand to test integrity of the medial collateral ligament; apply outward pressure (varus stress) to the medial aspect to test the lateral collateral ligament. Perform with knee in both extension and 30-degree flexion. The degree of "give," or laxity, parallels the degree of disruption. No movement should be encountered in the normal knee.

longitudinal traction before the onset of swelling.)

2. Apply ice, splint or sling, and send patient for further evaluation if fracture or significant other injury thought to be present.

Hip. The hip joint itself is rarely injured in sports. Strains, sprains, and epiphyseal avulsions may be seen, including the sartorius muscle from the anteriosuperior iliac spine, the iliopsoas from the lesser trochanter, and hamstring tendons from the ischium.

1. Assess seriousness of the injury according to pain and limitation of movement.

2. If more than a minor strain, stop weight-bearing, apply ice, and send patient for further evaluation.

Most hip injuries respond well to symptomatic treatment alone, but if faced with a painful hip in a rapid-ly growing adolescent of either sex or one who is chubby and is early pubertal or prepubertal, a slipped femoral epiphysis should not be overlooked. Slippage can be provoked by an athletic injury, thus the history of an antecedent traumatic event does not rule it out. Lateral as well as anterior hip roentgenograms are necessary to the diagnosis of milder forms. Chapter 11 provides further details.

Knee. The knee is the most exposed and vulnerable joint in the body. Injuries therefore are common. A prompt examination of the knee can be critical to the diagnosis. Techniques for evaluation is as follows:

1. Try to reconstruct the mechanism of injury.

2. Examine the patient immediately; there usually is a short lag time before edema, muscle spasm, and pain intervene.

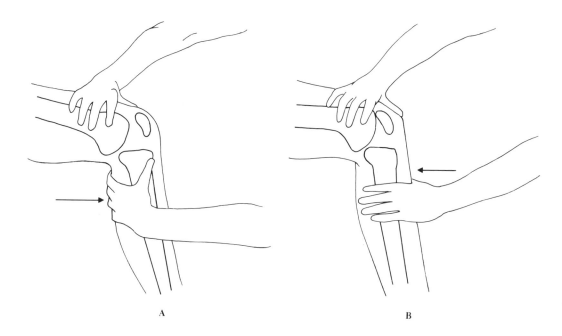

A   B

FIGURE 18-5
EXAMINATION OF THE KNEE: ANTERIOR AND POSTERIOR DRAWER SIGNS.
A, ANTERIOR DRAWER SIGN. B, POSTERIOR DRAWER SIGN.
These maneuvers detect disruption of the cruciate ligaments. With the thigh fixed and knee at 90-degree flexion, grasp the calf just below the knee joint and exert firm pressure in the direction indicated by the arrow. Anterior movement indicates disruption of the anterior cruciate ligament; posterior movement the posterior cruciate ligament. A slight jog with firm end point is encountered in partial tears; moderate to marked laxity with a soft end point suggests a total disruption. No movement should be encountered in the normal knee.

3. Observe the knee. Notice the position of the tibia in relation to the femur and the patella relative to its normal position.

4. Test the knee in full extension and at 30 degrees of flexion with valgus and varus stress (Figure 18-4) to define the status of medial and lateral collateral ligaments.

5. Attempt to elicit anterior and posterior drawer signs (Figure 18-5) to define the status of the anterior and posterior cruciate ligaments.

6. Gently test range of knee flexion and extension motion. Meniscal injuries may result in a locked knee.

7. Check for tenderness to pressure along the medial or lateral joint line. This finding may also indicate possible meniscal tears.

Characteristic findings in various knee injuries are as follows:

1. Medial collateral ligament: a common injury.
a. Injury produced by forceful stress applied to the lateral aspect of the knee, often with a component of external rotation.
b. Findings variably include tenderness over the course of the ligament, instability on valgus stress testing, and joint effusion, depending on the degree of sprain.

2. Lateral collateral ligament: less common than the above.
a. Produced by forceful stress applied to the medial side of the knee, often with an internal rotation component.
b. Findings are similar to the above, only on the opposite side; instability is elicited by the varus stress test.

3. Anterior cruciate ligament injury: often seen as the second component in the triad of O'Donoghue,

which consists of this injury plus injury to the medial collateral ligament and medial meniscus.

a. Produced by external rotation of the knee while the foot is firmly planted on the ground; clipping in football is a frequent cause.

b. The player frequently hears a "pop" at the time of injury.

c. Findings include rapid onset of effusion and a positive anterior drawer sign if the patient is relaxed.

4. Posterior cruciate ligament: less commonly injured.

a. Usually the result of a direct blow to the anterior knee.

b. Demonstrates pain, effusion, and a positive posterior drawer sign.

5. Meniscal injuries: the medial meniscus is injured two to ten times more frequently than the lateral meniscus.

a. Medial injury often occurs from forceful internal rotation of the femur in combination with external tibial rotation. Lateral injury most often results from internal rotation of the tibia with external rotation of the femur.

b. Mobility may or may not be limited; the knee may even be locked.

c. Tenderness along the joint line on the affected side is common.

d. Internal and external rotation of the tibia while holding the femur stable may produce pain with lateral or medial tears respectively.

After evaluation and the finding of a significant knee injury, ice, splinting, non-weight bearing, and immediate referral for further treatment are indicated.

Ankle and foot. Ankle sprains are extremely common injuries. Salter fractures also are common in adolescents; type I may go undetected.

1. Evaluate before swelling intervenes. Look for gross deformity; define areas of tenderness; establish range of motion.

2. Test for laxity and pain on inverting the foot (inversion test) and by an anterior drawer sign, using the heel as the point of forward pressure to establish ligament status.

3. Check for fractures of metatarsals; indicated by ecchymosis and pain over the fracture site.

4. Ice, splint, and send all patients with significant injuries for further evaluation.

Chronic Musculoskeletal Problems Related to Sports

OSGOOD-SCHLATTER'S DISEASE

Osgood-Schlatter's disease consists of epiphysitis of the tibial tubercle; it is presumably related to repeated tendinous stress. See Chapter 11 for a detailed description.

CHONDROMALACIA PATELLAE

Irritation, inflammation, and erosion of the undersurface of the patella consequent to maltracking within the femoral groove secondary to congenital malformation or acquired laxity in supporting structures constitutes chondromalacia patellae. See Chapter 11 for a detailed description.

SLIPPED FEMORAL EPIPHYSIS

See Chapter 11 and discussion of the hip in this chapter. Also note that pain referred to the knee is common and may mislead during diagnosis.

SHIN SPLINTS

Shin splints is most commonly seen in poorly conditioned individuals in the acute form; the chronic form is seen in anyone who runs frequently on very hard surfaces, as in jogging. It also is seen in divers and is caused by diving board action. Shin splints appears to be due to excessive, repetitive stretching and jarring of leg muscles, particularly the anterior and posterior tibial groups. Manifestations are swelling and pain. Stretching of the muscles before and after exercise to achieve flexibility in the first instance and relaxation in the second instance is helpful, as is wearing a shoe with a well-cushioned sole to absorb shock.

TENDINITIS

Tendinitis can occur at any joint and usually results from repeated stress to key muscle-tendon units employed in a particular sport. "Tennis elbow" is an example seen in any racquet sport. Tendinitis of the shoulder or elbow also may be seen in archery, gymnastics, and swimming. Swimming also can produce tendinitis about the knee, as may bicycling. The pain usually resolves with rest and oral anti-inflammatory medication. Particular attention should be given to reconditioning before play is resumed.

Heat Disorders

Heat disorders are particularly prevalent when a nonacclimated individual engages in strenuous athletics during hot weather, as is most apt to happen when initiating spring, summer, or early fall training for a seasonal sport requiring a sustained heavy work load. Football is most commonly implicated, but other sports also can be involved. Past heat acclimation is lost after 2 months' exposure to temperate climates, and it takes approximately 1 week to become heat-acclimated again. Prevention is through adequate water and salt intake, frequent

TABLE 18-4
GUIDELINES FOR ATHLETIC ACTIVITY
ACCORDING TO WET BULB TEMPERATURE*

Wet bulb temperature	Action
Under 60 F	No precaution necessary
61–65 F	Alert observation of all squad members, particularly those who lose considerable weight
66–70 F	Insist that salt and water be given on the field
71–75 F	Alter practice schedule to provide rest periods every 30 minutes in addition to above precautions
76 F and higher	Practice postponed or conducted in shorts

From Murphy, R., and Ashe, W. 1965. Prevention of heat illness in football players. *J.A.M.A.* 194(6):180. With permission. Copyright 1965, American Medical Association.

*Whenever relative humidity is 95% or higher, great precaution should be taken.

rests, and a gradual buildup of the daily work load during this period.

Even conditioned and heat-acclimated athletes are vulnerable to heat disorders if the temperature is excessive for the work demanded. Table 18-4 provides guidelines for the conduct of football practice according to wet bulb temperature; these can be applied to other sports requiring comparable work loads as well. As a general rule, a 3% loss of body weight through sweating is safe, 5% is borderline, and anything over 7% is dangerous; needless deaths can and do occur with failure to recognize the effect of heat and following traditional spartan practices of full work in full uniform and the withholding of fluid during a practice or game. Adherence to the following principles will go a long way toward preventing serious heat disorders:

1. Provide unlimited water during practice and games. Players will not overhydrate themselves. The use of salt supplements is controversial. Some advocate their use; others feel the ordinary use of table salt and the salt content of regular meals are sufficient. Potential problems with salt tablet supplementation rest in the possibility that the athlete will take an excessive amount without adequate fluid to effect renal clearance of the extra solute load. Dilute electrolyte solutions are recommended by some.

2. Clothing and timing of practice should be geared to weather conditions. On hot, humid days sessions should be held in early mornings or late afternoons with light clothing, leaving as much of the body exposed as possible.

3. The use of rubber or plastic suits to sweat off weight should not be allowed. This prevents the dissipation of body heat and cooling by evaporation, leading to a potentially fatal rise in body temperature.

Despite even these precautions, heat disorders still occur. Table 18-5 reviews the most common disorders.

TABLE 18-5
HEAT DISORDERS: TREATMENT AND PREVENTION

Disorder	Cause	Clinical features and diagnosis	Treatment	Prevention
Heat cramps	Hard work in heat Heavy and prolonged sweating Inadequate salt intake	Low serum/sodium/chloride Muscle twitching, cramps and spasms in arms, legs, and abdomen—usually after mid-day	Severe case: intravenous administration of 500 ml of normal saline Light case: oral administration of saline Rest in cool environment Salt foods used Delay 24–48 hours before reentering hot area	Ensure acclimatization Provide extra salt at meals Drink saline when working
Heat syncope	Peripheral vasodilation and pooling of blood Circulatory instability and loss of vasomotor tone Cerebral hypoxia Hyperventilation Inadequate acclimatization Infection	Weakness and fatigue Hypotension Increased venous compliance Blurred vision Pallor Syncope Elevated skin and deep body temperatures	Place supine and lower head Rest in cool environment Provide oral saline if conscious and resting	Ensure acclimatization Lighten work regimen with sudden rise in environmental temperature or humidity Avoid maintaining upright static work conditions
Water depletion and heat exhaustion	Heavy and prolonged sweating Inadequate fluid intake Polyuria or diarrhea	Reduced sweating, but excessive weight loss Elevated skin and deep body temperatures High hematocrit, serum protein, and sodium Dry tongue and mouth Excessive thirst Hyporexia Weak, disconsolate, uncoordinated, and mentally dull Concentrated urine	Bed rest in cool environment Replace fluids by intravenous drip if drinking is impaired. Increase fluids to 6–8 L/day Sponge with cool water Provide small quantities of semiliquid food Keep record of body weight, water and salt intake, and body temperature	Comment: predisposes to heat stroke Provide adequate water Provide opportunity for intermittent cooling and adequate rest
Salt depletion and heat exhaustion	Heavy and prolonged sweating Inadequate salt intake Inadequate acclimatization Vomiting or diarrhea	Headache, dizziness, and fatigue Hyporexia Nausea, vomiting, diarrhea Muscle cramps Syncope High hematocrit and serum protein, but low plasma volume Uremia and hypercalemia Low sodium and chloride in sweat and urine	Bed rest in cool environment Replace fluids and salt by intravenous saline drip if drinking is impaired Provide small quantities of semiliquid food Keep record of urinary osmolarity or specific gravity, blood pressure, pulse rate, hematocrit, blood urea, and serum/sodium/chloride Keep record of body weight, water and salt intake, and body temperature	Provide adequate salt and water; 10–15 g of salt per day may be necessary Provide opportunity for intermittent cooling and adequate rest Ensure acclimatization Comment: develops more slowly (3–5 days) than water depletion, heat exhaustion

Heat hyper-pyrexia lead-ing to heat stroke	Thermoregulatory failure of sudden onset	Lower body temperature to 38.9 C (102 F) within 1 hour with cold rinse or spray at 7.2 C (45 F). Use cool air fan or place in ice water bath. Use alcohol rinse if nothing else is available	Ensure acclimatization
	Generalized anhidrosis and dry skin	Use suction equipment to clear airway and perform tracheotomy if necessary	Adapt activities to environment
	Elevated skin and deep body temperatures frequently over 40.5 C (105 F) may have chills	Diazepam, 5–10 mg IM or IV for seizures	Screen participants with infection or past history of heat illness
	Irrational	Bed rest in a cool environment	
	Muscle flaccidity	Keep record of skin and deep body temperatures	
	Involuntary limb movements	Treat secondary disorders	
	Seizures and coma		
	Spotty cyanosis and ecchymosis		
	Vomiting and diarrhea frequently with blood		
	Tachycardia and tachypnea		
Skin lesions	Constantly wetted skin	Maintain shaded and dry skin	Dry skin when possible and keep shaded
	Overexposure to sun	Rest in cool environment	Examine skin regularly
	Erythematous papulovesicular rash		Provide opportunity for intermittent cooling and adequate sweat-free periods
	Itchy skin		
	Obstruction of sweat ducts		

Modified from Ryan, A., and Allman, F. 1974. *Sports medicine.* New York: Academic Press.

Bibliography

Grana, W., and Moretz, A. 1975. Ligamentous laxity in secondary school athletes. *J.A.M.A.* 240(18).

Knochel, T. 1975. Dog days and siriasis. *J.A.M.A.* 233(6):513.

Marshall, J., and Rubin, R. 1977. Knee ligament injuries—a diagnostic and therapeutic approach. *Orthoped. Clin. North Am.* 8(3):641.

Marshall, J., and Tischer, L. 1978. Screening for sports. *N.Y. State J. Med.* 78:243.

Murphy R., and Ashe, W. 1965. Prevention of heat illness in football players. *J.A.M.A.* 194(6):180.

Nicholas, J. 1976. Risk factors. Sports medicine and the orthopedic system; an overview. *Jul. Sports Med.* 3(5):243.

Nicholas, J. 1970. Injuries to knee ligaments. *J.A.M.A.* 212(13):2236.

O'Donoghue, D. 1976. *Treatment of injuries to athletes.* Philadelphia: W. B. Saunders Co.

Rang, M. *Children's fractures.* Philadelphia: J. B. Lippincott Co.

Rockwood, C., and Green, D. 1975. *Fractures.* Philadelphia: J. B. Lippincott Co.

Ryan, A., and Allman, F. 1974. *Sports medicine.* New York: Academic Press.

Salter, R., and Harris, R. 1963. Injuries including the epiphyseal plate. *J. Bone Joint Surg.* 45A(3):587.

Schaffer, T. 1973. The adolescent athlete. *Pediatr. Clin. North Am.* 20(4):837.

Scheurer, J., and Tipton, C. 1977. Cardiovascular adaptations to physical training. *Ann. Rev. Physiol.* 39:221.

Wilmore, J. 1977. The female athlete. *J. School Health*, p. 227.

-19-
Nutritional Issues in Adolescence

George J. Mellendick, M.D.

Recommended Dietary Intake for Adolescents
Recommended daily allowances □ An optimal diet for adolescents
Eating Patterns of Adolescents in the United States
Alternative and Special Diets
Quick weight loss diets □ Megavitamins □ High protein diets
"Natural" and organically grown foods □ Vegetarianism
Zen macrobiotic diet □ Yin-Yang foods
Management of Dietary Issues
Evaluation of Nutritional Status
Nutritional Disorders
Obesity □ Anorexia nervosa □ Other nutritional deprivation states
The thin adolescent who wants to gain weight

Recommended Dietary Intake for Adolescents

RECOMMENDED DAILY ALLOWANCES

Reviewed and revised every 5 years by the National Research Council of the National Academy of Sciences, Recommended Daily Allowances (RDA) for calories and various nutrients are generous estimates of what individuals should consume to avoid nutritional disease and remain in optimal nutritional health. It should be noted that RDAs for adolescents (Table 19-1) are only approximations. First they are based on age, rather than maturational stage, a much more relevant criterion (see Chapter 1). Second, RDAs for young people largely are extrapolated from data established for infants and adults. Third, even in the case of infants and adults, not all minimum requirements are well defined. Thus applying RDAs in assessing the adequacy of an adolescent's diet must be done with discrimination. Minimally these should be modified by considering the timing of the growth spurt along with such other factors as total body mass, general activity level, special

physical demands, strenuous physical conditioning, heredity, and climate.

Calories. Caloric needs are highly variable from one adolescent to the next. Short of assessing the amount of body fat through skin fold measurements (Chapter 2 and Appendix I) or a comparable method, it is difficult to ensure that calorie intake is optimal for growth and activity. In most instances, however, this question is moot for, excepting those conditions clearly associated with malnutrition, most adolescents have adequate caloric intakes and no special attentions are required to ensure sufficient amounts. Indeed, there is more justifiable concern for excessive caloric intake and obesity than for deprivation.

It should be noted that adolescent females need to increase their calories sooner than males and curtail them more sharply when grown due to the earlier onset of puberty and the lesser total body weight that ultimately needs to be sustained. Calories may also need to be varied in relation to seasonal changes in activity levels.

TABLE 19-1
FOOD AND NUTRITION BOARD, NATIONAL ACADEMY OF SCIENCES–NATIONAL RESEARCH COUNCIL, RECOMMENDED DAILY DIETARY ALLOWANCES (REVISED 1980)

	Age (years)	Energy (kCal)	Protein (g)	Ascorbic acid (mg)	Thiamine (mg)	Riboflavin (mg)	Niacin (mg)	Vitamin B (mg)	Vitamin B_{12} (pg)	Folacin (pg)
Males	11–14	2800	45	50	1.4	1.6	18	1.8	3.0	400
	15–18	3000	56	60	1.4	1.7	18	2.0	3.0	400
Females	11–14	2400	46	50	1.1	1.3	15	1.8	3.0	400
	15–18	2100	46	60	1.1	1.3	14	2.0	3.0	400
Pregnant		+300	+30	+20	+0.4	+0.3	+2	+0.6	+1.0	+400
Lactating		+500	+20	+40	+0.5	+0.5	+5	+0.5	+1.0	+100

Fat-soluble vitamins			Minerals						
	Vitamin A activity (U)	Vitamin D activity (IU)	Vitamin E activity (IU)	Calcium (mg)	Phosphorus (mg)	Iodine (mg)	Iron (mg)	Magnesium (mg)	Zinc (mg)	Fluoride (mg)
Males 11–14	1000	10	8	1200	1200	150	18	350	15	1.5–2.5
15–18	1000	10	10	1200	1200	150	18	400	15	1.5–2.5
Females 11–14	800	10	8	1200	1200	150	18	300	15	1.5–2.5
15–18	800	10	8	1200	1200	150	18	300	15	1.5–2.5
Pregnant	+200	+5	+2	+400	+400	+25	A*	+150	+5	
Lactating	+400	+5	+3	+400	+400	+50	A*	+150	+10	

*The increased requirement during pregnancy and lactation cannot be met by the iron content of habitual American diets nor by the existing iron stores of many women; therefore, the use of 30–60 mg of supplemental iron is recommended.

Protein. The growing individual is particularly vulnerable to protein deprivation and consequent interference with growth. The observation that contemporary adolescents initiate puberty sooner and achieve a taller final height than their ancestors is largely attributed to improved protein and caloric intake throughout their growth. There is little evidence of protein deficiency today among adolescents in the United States, this being more a problem for developing countries. Recommendations for protein consumption range between 50-55 g/day for adolescent girls and 55-60 g/day for boys. This should comprise between 10% and 15% of total calories.

Vitamins. Vitamin deficiency states also are rarely encountered in the average adolescent. RDAs for all but A and C generally are well met. However, there is little indication for supplementation with A and C in ordinary circumstances; adequate amounts can easily be achieved by attention to diet alone. Supplementation with B_{12}, however, may be needed by strict vegetarians. There is no indication that megavitamins, singly or severally, have any beneficial effects. Excessive intake of vitamins A and D may even be hazardous, each having a toxic potential.

Minerals. Calcium and iron are the two minerals with particular clinical significance for adolescents. Zinc intake in this age group also has been reported as below the RDA. Although zinc deficiency states have been recognized in children, they have not yet been identified in otherwise healthy teenagers.

Calcium is essential for rapid bone growth and finalization of dentition. RDAs during puberty range between 1.2-1.3 g for girls and 1.2-1.4 g for boys. This can be met by the daily intake of three glasses of milk. Some adolescents believe themselves too old to drink milk and no longer in need of it. They should be dissuaded from this assumption.

Iron deficiency anemia is the most commonly encountered nutritional disorder in the adolescent age group and affects boys as well as girls. Iron requirements of either sex are greater at this time of life than at any other stage due to the rapid expansion in body size, vascular space, and red blood cell mass. Boys have higher requirements than girls due to their relatively larger vascular space and their greater muscle mass, which increases the demand for myoglobin. Girls who have reached menarche need an extra 1.4 mg/day to compensate for menstrual blood loss. The RDA for iron for male and female adolescents is 18 mg/day during the growth spurt and 10 mg/day for males and 14 mg/day for females thereafter.

TABLE 19-2
MAJOR SOURCES OF ESSENTIAL NUTRIENTS

Protein
Meat (beef, veal, pork, lamb)
Poultry
Fish
Dairy products, eggs
Vegetarian: beans, cereal grains, nuts, seeds (see Table 19-5)

Vitamins
Vitamin A: liver, fortified margarine, butter, whole milk, yellow vegetables and fruits; some available in green leafy vegetables as well
Vitamin C: citrus fruits, tomatoes, strawberries, currants, lettuce, green leafy vegetables, broccoli, potatoes (diet source should be uncooked as vitamin C is heat-labile)
Vitamin D: sunlight, milk, egg yolk, canned fish
Vitamin B_{12}: milk, eggs, fish, fortified soymilk meals
Folacin: liver, navy beans, dark green leafy vegetables, nuts, fresh oranges, and whole wheat products
Thiamine: pork, beans, peas, nuts, enriched and whole grain wheat products

Minerals
Iron: lean meats, whole grain and fortified wheat products, eggs, dried beans and peas, green leafy vegetables, dried fruits and nuts
Calcium: milk, dairy products, dark green leafy vegetables, some nuts and legumes
Zinc: meats, nuts, beans, wheat germ, cheese

AN OPTIMAL DIET FOR ADOLESCENTS

Recommended daily allowances meeting the needs of growing young people of either sex will be amply met by the following:

1. Milk: 3 cups per day

2. Meat (or equivalent): two servings per day

3. Vegetables and fruits: four servings per day, including one serving each of a food containing vitamin A or C

4. Breads and cereals: four servings per day; whole grain or fortified products preferred

5. Other foods: as needed to make up caloric requirements.

A variety of foods are available in meeting protein, vitamin, and mineral requirements. All members of any group may be substituted for any other in the daily dietary plan (Table 19-2). No RDA for fats has been established. Most diets include ample sources for essential fatty acids.

Nutritional adequacy must be measured against the total intake over several days or weeks rather

TABLE 19-3
MEAN CALORIC INTAKE AND MEAN INTAKE PER 1000 CALORIES OF
SELECTED NUTRIENTS BY AGE, SEX, AND RACE: UNITED STATES, 1971–1974*

Sex and race	Mean caloric intake	Mean nutrient intake per 1000 calories							
		Protein (g)	Calcium (g)	Iron (mg)	Vitamin A (IU)	Vitamin C (mg)	Thiamine (mg)	Riboflavin (mg)	Preformed niacin (mg)
Ages 12–14									
Male									
White	2564	37.09	526.10	5.29	1877	34.64	0.62	1.03	7.11
Black	2253	35.20	388.45	6.12	1935	39.72	0.64	0.92	7.56
Female									
White	1918	38.14	523.43	5.38	2034	41.55	0.64	1.02	7.20
Black	1970	35.39	374.24	5.35	1763	42.45	0.65	0.85	6.84
Ages 15–17									
Male									
White	3057	38.07	479.83	5.47	1995	33.61	0.61	0.97	7.51
Black	2489	36.30	367.99	5.45	1403	32.95	0.60	0.81	7.43
Female									
White	1750	37.42	480.19	5.38	2077	41.46	0.61	0.97	7.24
Black	1802	37.18	381.04	5.57	1895	38.57	0.73	0.93	7.82
Ages 18–19									
Male									
White	3018	38.95	436.34	5.63	1987	40.89	0.59	0.93	7.88
Black	2627	34.69	323.41	5.15	1405	25.76	0.59	0.76	7.94
Female									
White	1756	39.07	431.92	5.78	2230	54.93	0.63	0.92	8.11
Black	1668	40.48	322.38	5.75	2730	46.96	0.62	0.79	8.33

*Adapted from Dietary Intake Findings: United States, 1971–1974, U.S. Dept. of Health, Education and Welfare, Series 11, No. 202, pp. 62–64.

than the regularity and consistency of each day. There is no well-established basis for preferring a three-meal-a-day plan, except for those with special dietary requirements. Healthy adolescents, as will be discussed further on, tend to eat in a highly irregular fashion without detriment.

Although considerable debate surrounds cholesterol limitation as a desirable dietary pattern for all individuals, until further research indicates firm evidence to the contrary, we do not recommend restriction for adolescents. Foods high in cholesterol also are important sources of protein and iron. Special precautions, however, are indicated for those with a genetic predisposition for the hyperlipidemias, as indicated by a history of these disorders or of an early heart attack in a close relative. Restrictions are mandatory in adolescents already identified as having hyperlipidemia.

Eating Patterns of Adolescents in the United States

Recent data from the ten-state nutritional survey (HANES) have given us a picture of the average dietary intake of American adolescents (Tables 19-3 and 19-4). Keeping in mind that RDAs exceed minimum requirements to a considerable degree and that in many instances these values are imprecise, teenagers have far better balanced nutrition than most adults would believe. Protein, caloric, vitamin, and mineral recommendations are closely approximated or exceeded with the exception of calcium, iron, zinc, and vitamins A and C. The clinical significance of these low intakes is obscure in all instances except iron. Deficiency states due to low calcium, zinc, or vitamin intake are rarely encountered (it should be noted that RDAs have no applicability in measuring nutritional status but simply designate amounts

TABLE 19-4
PERCENT DISTRIBUTION OF PERSONS AGED 12-17 YEARS BY FREQUENCY OF
INTAKE OF SELECTED FOOD GROUPS, ACCORDING TO RACE: UNITED STATES, 1971-1974*

Race and food group	Frequency of intake					
	4 times or more a day	3 times a day	2 times a day	Once a day	1-6 times a week	Seldom or never
White						
Whole milk	12.6	24.1	21.1	18.0	5.7	4.5
Meat and poultry	0.3	1.8	27.9	52.5	6.1	0.3
Fish and shellfish	0.0	0.0	0.1	0.8	54.1	45.0
Eggs	0.0	0.0	0.0	17.3	70.1	12.6
Fruits and vegetables (all kinds)	3.4	17.9	33.4	33.3	11.4	0.4
Cereals	0.0	0.3	1.7	29.9	60.1	8.2
Desserts	0.5	3.2	13.3	39.2	40.7	3.3
Salty snacks	0.1	0.0	2.7	15.8	67.9	13.6
Black						
Whole milk	4.6	9.9	32.1	30.6	12.8	5.4
Meat and poultry	0.3	4.1	36.7	48.9	8.7	0.7
Fish and shellfish	0.0	0.0	0.0	2.6	59.9	37.6
Eggs	0.0	0.3	0.8	16.8	59.9	18.6
Fruits and vegetables (all kinds)	2.5	21.8	33.7	32.9	9.2	0.0
Cereals	0.3	0.0	1.8	29.1	60.1	8.8
Desserts	0.0	2.1	12.5	44.3	39.7	1.5
Salty snacks	1.6	0.3	4.2	23.4	62.6	6.6

*Adapted from HANES Food Frequency Data. 1979. *Selected findings: food consumption profiles of white and black persons 1-74 years of age in the United States, 1971-74.* Advance data, U.S. Department of Health, Education and Welfare, Public Health Service, Number 21.

to be consumed that in all probability will preclude any deficiency).

On the other hand, iron deficiency anemia is common. Cycle III of the National Health Survey found between 36% and 41% of all teenagers falling in the fifth percentile or less for hematocrit values; more 16 and 17 year old males were at these low levels than females of any age. Some caution is needed in interpreting these data; they are probably artifactually high, as values were correlated with age rather than maturity rating and, as pointed out in Chapter 3, the latter is a much more significant correlate. In any event, it is probably safe to assume that at least 20% of the adolescent population is at risk of iron deficiency to some degree; this is the percentage of teenagers with intakes significantly less than the RDA.

With the exception of iron and, possibly, calcium, much of the public alarm about teenaged eating behavior is unfounded. Admittedly, few teenagers eat in a manner that conforms to dietary patterns perceived by parent or nutritionist as best, but there is little evidence of malnutrition in this age group. It must be concluded that teenage dietary

habits are not as deleterious as one might think. Parameters of typical adolescent food habits include the following and provide a norm against which the eating behavior of any one teenager should be measured.

1. Fifty percent of adolescents have no breakfast; a traditional three-meal-a-day pattern is rare in all teenagers and especially rare in black youths. Young people tend to be snackers and tend to snack with the most readily available foods.

2. Great nutritional variability and irregularity in dietary patterns is the rule. A single day's intake does not always reflect the actual degree of nutritional balance achieved over time. Adolescent food combinations, although seemingly bizarre, usually are nutritionally satisfactory with the exception of iron and calcium.

3. Lean girls have a higher intake of calories and nutrients than average and obese girls. But in boys it is those with average weight who have the highest intake. Boys tend to consume foods of better nutritional value than girls and tend to be more conscious of nutrition for health, whereas girls' concerns about diet emphasize its implications for weight.

4. Adolescents who eat fewer than three times a day (not necessarily standard meal times) generally have poorer diets from the nutritional standpoint; those who eat more frequently (including snacking) tend to have overall good diets. The highest correlation with dietary quality is found between the mean number of servings of food and the mean number of different food items, emphasizing the utility of variety. When caloric intake increases, protein, carbohydrates, vitamins, and minerals increase as well without particular attention to what foods are used to achieve this.

5. No relationship appears to exist between the quality of the diet or eating patterns and school performance.

6. About 50% of teenagers rate their diets as good; 15%–20% as excellent; 25%–30% as fair; and only 5% as poor. However, only 50% are able to identify the four essential food groups (milk and dairy products, meat and meat equivalents, vegetables and fruits, and cereals and grains).

7. Other factors that vary eating patterns include cultural and family traditions, as well as adolescent attempts to modify size and shape. The latter are often perceived in negative terms, objective assessment to the contrary.

Alternative and Special Diets

QUICK WEIGHT LOSS DIETS

Some quick weight loss diets may be harmful for any individual, as has been found with ketotic and liquid protein diets. Additional harm accrues to the adolescent by withholding protein and minerals at a time of heightened need. Even when nutritionally balanced, such diets are but snares and delusions. Weight loss is difficult for those who are obese to sustain even under the most disciplined circumstances; dietary management of obesity must be life-long, and quick loss programs are ineffective over the long run.

Dieting in adolescence requires an appropriate reduction of calories but with sufficient intake of other nutrients to ensure proper growth. Adolescents who are mildly overweight but not truly obese and who wish to lose a few pounds for cosmetic reasons should first establish a reasonable minimum weight consistent with their height, body build, stage of growth, and activity level; they should seek to achieve this loss through modest reduction in daily caloric intake over time—a month or two rather than in a few days. True obesity is discussed in more detail further on.

MEGAVITAMINS

Adolescents are likely to mimic their elders in the commitment to megadoses of vitamin C out of the fallacious belief that this will ward off colds and influenza. Most individuals appear to be able to take 1000 mg of vitamin C a day without harming anything more than their pocketbooks. On the other hand, this practice may not be entirely inconsequential. Studies have shown that excess levels of vitamin C alter copper and iron metabolism, may be associated with the formation of oxalate renal stones, and may precipitate uterine bleeding in pregnant women. Vitamin C also may interfere with the detection of melena in giving a false-negative stool guaiac test.

Megadoses of vitamin mixtures, sometimes resorted to by young athletes in the mistaken notion they will improve physical performance, have a definite potential for harm in introducing the possibility of hypervitaminosis A or D. The former is characterized by pseudotumor cerebri, hepatosplenomegaly, headache, irritability, nausea, hair loss, joint pain, and irregular menses. Hypervitaminosis D may result in hypercalcemia and hypercalciuria with the likelihood of renal or gallbladder stones and abnormal calcium deposits in the tissues.

HIGH PROTEIN DIETS

Many athletic training regimens include a high protein diet. Since the individual usually has an adequate intake of other foods as well, nutritional balance is achieved. Exclusive protein diets may be resorted to by some dieters. When the diet consists of natural foods there appears to be little harm provided vitamin and mineral requirements are met by supplementing with appropriate foods or pills. The only contraindications for such diets are in adolescents with renal disease, in whom the high nitrogen solute load may have an adverse effect, and in those at risk for the hyperlipidemias when protein predominantly comes from cholesterol-containing meats.

Commercial liquid protein as the exclusive source of nutrients may be harmful, and currently (1979) available preparations cannot be recommended. These may contain inadequate amounts of potassium, and deaths from hypokalemia have occurred. Correction of this deficit is underway and the potential benefits and risks of new preparations must be viewed with an open mind.

"NATURAL" AND ORGANICALLY GROWN FOODS

No hazards are posed by a diet using natural and organically grown foods. The only caution would be

TABLE 19-5
VEGETABLE SOURCES WITH HIGH TOTAL
PROTEIN CONTENT AND AVAILABILITY OF ESSENTIAL AMINO ACIDS

Vegetable sources	Essential amino acids							
	Tryptophan	Threonine	Isoleucine	Leucine	Lysine	Methionine (or cystine)	Phenylalanine	Valine
Soybeans: soymilk, tofu (bean curd), soy-enriched yogurt, tempeh	X	X	X	X	X	X	X	X
Grains, nuts, seeds: wheat, wheat germ, oats, sunflower seeds, buckwheat (kasha), rice, peanuts, pumpkin seeds, cashews	X/O*	X	X	X	O	X	X	X
Beans: red, white, and black beans, garbanzo beans, lentils	O	X	X	X	X	O	X	X
Nutritional yeast: Saccharomyces cerevisae; 2 tbsp. flakes or 1 tbsp. powder = 9 g; provides full RDA of all B vitamins except folic acid (29%)	X	X	X	X	X	X	X	X

From National Research Council, National Academy of Sciences, Food and Nutrition Board. 1974. *Recommended dietary allowances*, 8th ed. Washington, D.C., p. 4.

*Tryptophan present in most members of this group but may be absent in some seeds.

for those who restrict their intake to solely vegetarian sources (see Vegetarianism). Drinking large amounts of herbal teas, readily available in most natural food stores, warrants some caution as well. These are variable mixtures of assorted plant materials, some of which contain mild medicinal and psychoactive substances, including stimulants, sedatives, hallucinogens, and naturally occurring alkaloids. These drugs generally are so dilute that their effects are only modest, but occasionally they have produced significant toxicity.

VEGETARIANISM

Vegetarian diets can be divided into three types:

1. Lactovegetarian: includes plant foods complemented with milk and milk products.

2. Lacto-ovo-vegetarian: includes the above plus eggs.

3. Strict vegetarian, or vegan: includes only foods of plant origin. Lactovegetarians and lacto-ovo-vegetarians usually meet all RDAs satisfactorily in that milk and milk products offer excellent quality protein and plant foods can provide all other nutrients easily. The addition of eggs offers extra protein insurance, as well as a source of some iron. Adolescents pursuing such diets should be able to

obtain sufficient nutrients for growth with the possible exception of adequate amounts of iron; supplementation may be indicated by low serum iron and/or red blood cell indices indicative of iron deficiency (dose = 5 grains of ferrous sulfate or ferrous gluconate one to three times per day).

Strict vegetarianism presents more of a problem. With the exception of soybeans, no other plant source contains all essential amino acids. This deficiency can be overcome if two or more of the following groups are combined providing a complete protein source of reasonably high protein content:

1. Beans and other legumes: protein content is 20% of dry weight.

2. Cereal grains: protein content of whole grain forms is 10% of dry weight.

3. Nuts and seeds.

Meat analogs made with soybeans or wheat protein combined with peanuts or other nuts and made into meatlike steaks, patties, or loaves are complete in and of themselves.

Other nutritional inadequacies that may be encountered in the vegan diet include calcium, iron, and vitamin B_{12}. Vitamin B_{12} is generally lacking in the plant world, and supplementary doses are indicated for all vegans, either in fortified soymilk or pure tablet form (25 μ g twice a week). Iron (see preceding discussion) and calcium (1 g Ca gluconate or 2 g Ca lactate per day) are recommended supplements during growth and for pregnant or lactating females. Iron should be continued indefinitely for menstruating females even when growth is complete.

Adolescents should be discouraged from strict vegetarianism; but those committed to this course should at least include ample milk and milk products. Individuals who have followed an exclusive vegan diet all their lives tend to have a lower total caloric and B$_{12}$ intake than nonvegans. This is reflected in shorter adult height and lower vitamin B$_{12}$ levels than in nonvegan controls.

Regardless of which of the vegetarian diets a young person elects to follow, he or she should be strongly advised to purchase a responsible vegetarian cookbook that also reviews the specific nutritional value of various vegetables and fruits and discusses how to prepare a well-balanced meal. These young people also should be willing to do some cooking themselves. Few nonvegetarian mothers are willing to put two separate menus on the table each day, and there are few places offering vegetarian fast foods. Yogurt and lettuce are insufficient to the nutrient task.

ZEN MACROBIOTIC DIET

An essential element of the religious practices of certain Zen sects, the macrobiotic diet is comprised of ten stages, each requiring an increasingly restricted intake of fluids and foods in both type and amount. Although animal foods and a variety of fluids are allowed initially, the diet ultimately is limited to cereals and water, the latter only in amounts allowing for urination no more than once a day. This diet poses obvious hazards, not only for nutrition but also for renal function. All adherents should be screened for disturbed kidney function and evaluated for adequacy of caloric intake.

Growing adolescents certainly should not partake of this diet, but it is uncommonly seen in this age group. The propriety of such a selection by a young adult who has achieved majority is beyond the scope of this chapter, although we do advocate respect for individual freedom of choice in religious expression and life-style. This does not mean, however, that harmful dietary practices should be overlooked. The Zen dieter should be counseled appropriately and encouraged to ensure an adequate intake of fluid and nutrients or at least be advised that failing to take such steps can result in serious physical harm.

TABLE 19-6
EXAMPLES OF YIN AND YANG FOODS*

	Yin	Yang
Vegetables	Beans	Carrots
	Cabbage	Endive
	Corn	Lentils
	Lettuce	Onion
	Peas	Pumpkins
Fruits	Bananas	Apples
	Figs	Cherries
	Peaches	
	Oranges	
Nuts	Almonds	Chestnuts
	Peanuts	

*In general, yin foods have an alkaline ash residue and yang foods have an acid ash, but this is not true in all cases.

YIN-YANG FOODS

The basic Tao philosophy, which means the "way," or path, is to attain harmony, peace, and inner goodness. The Tao philosophy is the basis for many Chinese medical and scientific concepts, one of which is the yin-yang duality. Yin represents femaleness, introversion, passivity, and gentleness; yang represents maleness, extroversion, aggressiveness, and strength. In Tao, all foods have been designated as having either a yin or yang quality (Table 19-6). Although an alkaline residue ash closely parallels yin and an acid residue, yang, actual determinants are based on a complex system taking the five flavors (acid, salt, sweet, bitter, and pungent), the seasons of planting and harvesting, and other such matters into consideration. Inner harmony and health, according to Tao, depends in considerable measure upon a properly balanced intake of yin (passive) and yang (active) foods. Diseases may be treated by an appropriate formulation of yin and yang substances designed to counteract disease-related imbalance.

In the normal Tao diet, meat consumption is discouraged, and an optimal balance is perceived to come from a mixture of grains, nuts, vegetables, and fruits. In essence it is the vegan diet discussed above. Some additional nutritional problems may be encountered in that there is heavy reliance on expensive seeds, and the amount consumed by some adherents tends to be small because of cost. Additionally, the counterbalancing foods must also be consumed in reduced amounts to maintain proper yin-yang proportions. In consequence, there may be an inadequate intake of total calories and specific nutrients.

Management of Dietary Issues

In evaluating the nutritional adequacy of a teenager's diet, it should be kept in mind that adolescent eating behaviors rarely follow traditional adult concepts of what is best, yet few young people evidence specific nutritional deficiencies other than iron deficiency anemia. Aside from the latter, overnutrition is more problematic. We also wish to belie the myth of "empty" calories. There is no such thing as an empty calorie; a calorie is a measure of heat production when a food substance is burned—the nature of its source is irrelevant. Even under optimal circumstances most calories come from carbohydrates and fats; only 15% of total calories is recommended to come from protein. Moreover, the body makes little distinction between one carbohydrate source and another; they all end up in the bloodstream as glucose. Let us also challenge those who believe refined sugars (sucrose) have harmful effects. Sucrose is simply two molecules of glucose combined. Simple sugars do have deleterious effects on dentition, forming the substrate for bacterial growth and resultant caries. It is rational to restrict these substances on this count but difficult to defend such restriction on any other. There is rationale for focusing on reduced fat intake in those who are overweight; fats have particularly sneaky consequences in giving more bounce to the ounce (9 calories per gram compared to 4 calories for either carbohydrates and proteins). But aside from these well-proven and logical aspects, there is as much faddism among those who espouse strict eating patterns as among adolescents who belie them.

On the other hand, although there is exaggerated concern for adolescent eating behavior from the nutritional standpoint, there is merit in attempting to encourage a more consistent approach to nutrition. First, adolescents grow up to be adults and parents. The dietary habits they assume for themselves generally will be those they visit on their children as well. Young people should be prepared to provide their future offspring with appropriate nutrition for optimal growth. Secondly, many nutritional issues remain unresolved, such as the debate about the intake of cholesterol or food additives. Encouraging young people to inculcate some restraint on their dietary vagaries during their teenage years may facilitate the incorporation of appropriate modifi-

cations as future knowledge warrants. Third, it is true that many adolescents have an excessive caloric intake, largely through carbohydrates and fats, and thus become obese. Diminished intake of these substances is indicated for those with a tendency to overweight. Lastly, iron deficiency anemia is sufficiently ubiquitous to warrant specific nutritional modification on this count.

In assessing the adequacy of an adolescent's diet, the physician first must look at total intake over time, not just a single day, if dietary practices are irregular; second is an evaluation of the degree to which irregular and even bizarre eating patterns are nutritionally deficient or harmful. Of equal importance, the physician must be aware of the degree to which his or her own personal biases, dietary practices, folk beliefs, and maternal influences interfere with an objective appraisal.

To evaluate young people on fad or special diets the physician must first determine why such a diet was elected. In some instances the choice will be the legitimate consequence of moral or religious commitment. Barring specifically harmful practices, the young person's views should be respected. The physician's responsibility rests in assuring that the patient properly understands how to achieve balanced nutrition and that nutrients necessary for adolescent growth or likely to be sparse in general are taken in adequate amounts, either by consuming high-value foods or supplementation in pure form. Appropriate doses to this end are:

☐ Iron: 5 grains ferrous sulfate or gluconate one to three times per day
☐ Calcium: 1 g Ca gluconate or 2 g Ca lactate once a day
☐ B_{12}: 25 μg 2 times per week or a standard vitamin-mineral compound once a day

In some instances, deviant diets reflect something more than a moral commitment, desire to lose weight or misguided efforts to improve health, physical well-being, and athletic ability. They may be the outward manifestation of inner emotional stress. Food is one of our earliest symbols of love or rejection, reward, or punishment. We all resort to food, on occasion, as a substitute gratification. Some of us use it for psychologic defense or self-abuse through overeating and obesity or the pathologic dieting seen in anorexia nervosa (see section on anorexia nervosa). Without belaboring the issue, some evaluation of psychosocial factors is always indicated when an adolescent's diet varies from the norm and is unsupported by reasonable defense. Significant underlying stress should be dealt with accordingly.

Psychopathologic states aside, modifying any adolescent's diet must take into account two essential points. First is that any decision to change must be the young person's own. Such matters cannot be imposed or dictated; suggestions will fall on deaf ears. (Refer to the counseling approach detailed in Chapter 23.) Second is the importance of parental involvement unless the adolescent is fending for himself or herself. No dietary modification can be successful without the willing support of the family and, usually, some degree of modification of the family's diet as well.

Evaluation of Nutritional Status

The nutritional status of a healthy adolescent can be assessed and monitored adequately through the standard history, physical examination, and health maintenance plan as outlined in Chapters 2 and 3. The following are, however, particularly relevant factors in the history:

1. The patient's and parents' separate perceptions of the patient's dietary adequacy.

2. Any nutritional disorders or feeding problems in the past.

3. The patient's progress in height, weight, and pubertal events

a. As plotted on standard growth curves or compared with percentiles suitably modified to take the patient's time of pubertal onset into account

b. As genetically consistent by comparison with the same parameters in other family members

4. A 24-hour recall of the most recent "average" day or a record of 3 alternate days in those with highly variable intake patterns.

5. Parental history of weight, height, and pubertal events.

6. Signs or symptoms of any of the nutritional disorders.

Relevant points in the physical and laboratory evaluation are:

1. Height and weight in relation to the growth spurt and stage of sexual maturity (Tanner stage).

2. Triceps skin fold measurement or equivalent (simple observation of apparent fat—the "eyeball test"—and the less precise measure of skin fold thickness by holding same between the examiner's thumb and index finger is often an adequate screening technique; obesity is deemed present if such a fold measures more than 2.5 cm).

3. Clinical evidence of any of the vitamin deficiency diseases (as these are rare, signs and symptoms

are omitted here and the reader is referred to an appropriate reference text).

4. Hematocrit (plus red blood cell indices and serum iron and iron-binding capacity if below normal range; see Appendix I).

More detailed evaluation is indicated when there are signs and symptoms of illnesses that cause nutritional disorders or are secondary to them or as indicated by deviant growth (failure to thrive, short stature, obesity, excessive thinness). In such instances a more detailed dietary history should be obtained. The patient is asked to record in a notebook all food intake for 1 week (or longer if intake patterns vary enough to be inadequately reflected in the shorter time). This includes not only what foods were eaten but also the approximate amount and the time and circumstances of their consumption. It is important to assign this task to the adolescent alone and not to anyone else, particularly parents. It may be helpful to point out to the patient that the physician's sole goal is to obtain some idea of what is going on and that he or she has no intention of scolding, punishing, clucking, or otherwise indicating disapproval and that honesty and completeness are essential. When simple weight gain or loss in an otherwise healthy individual is the goal, it also can be helpful for the adolescent to purchase a booklet of caloric values and calculate caloric intake on each of the recorded days.

Special tests evaluating nutritional status in those suspected of malnutrition include examination of the hair root and shaft (a sensitive indicator of protein intake over time) and various serum levels of vitamins and their metabolites. These serum levels are most useful in suspected malabsorption syndromes together with nitrogen balance studies and the analysis of fat, carbohydrates, and proteins in stools collected under metabolically controlled circumstances. Reference should be made to a standard text in gastroenterology for details.

Nutritional Disorders

The most common nutritional problems occurring in adolescence, in descending order of frequency, are overnutrition and undernutrition, dental caries, iron deficiency anemia, anorexia nervosa, and dangerous forms of food faddism. Iodine-deficient goiters and trace mineral deficiencies may be encountered on rare occasion. Pregnant teenagers, drug or alcohol abusers, athletes, and young people with restricted diets due to poverty pose special nutritional problems as do certain diseases with particular dietary components to their management, such as diabetes, hyperlipidemia, inflammatory bowel disease, or peptic ulcer.

Although all of these issues are germane to this chapter's coverage, discussion here concerns obesity, anorexia nervosa, and simple underweight. Treatment of iron deficiency anemia is discussed in the chapter on hematologic disorders; comment on special dietary aspects of the management of specific diseases is found in the appropriate organ system chapter. Dietary management in alcoholism and drug abuse or for the young athlete is predicated upon a well-balanced diet with attention to increased caloric intake and vitamin and mineral supplementation when indicated. Consideration of the dietary vagaries encountered in many healthy adolescents, food faddism and alternative diets have already been discussed.

OBESITY

Obesity can be defined as the excessive deposition of fat resulting in an actual weight 20% or more above the ideal weight for height. Not all excessive weight, however, constitutes obesity, and a particularly large skeleton or increased muscle mass should be considered before ascribing this cause. Triceps skin fold measurements are the most reliable method of differentiation (see Appendix I). Measurements equal to or greater than 18.6 mm in boys or 25.1 mm in girls have been established as the arbitrary value determining obesity by the Ten State Nutritional Survey.

Approximately one in eight adolescents is obese; 98% of these were overweight as children and 80% will remain overweight as adults. It is a discouraging problem whose answer depends far more on early childhood prevention than on intervention once obesity has arrived.

Determinants of obesity are considerably more complex than too much food and too little will power. Genetics appears to play a major role; children of nonobese parents have only an 8%–9% probability of becoming overweight, whereas this probability escalates to 40% and 80%, respectively, when one or both parents are obese. The likelihood that more than family eating patterns alone are involved is indicated by the absence of such a correlation for adopted or foster children. Studies of obese adults suggest a possible override mechanism or specific abnormality of the hypothalamic appetite regulation center with an inability to perceive or respond to ordinary satiation cues. Other investigators have postulated disturbances in the metabolisms of fat with a one-way pump effect and it being easier to deposit fat than mobilize it. Once an individual becomes obese, significant metabolic abnormalities have been identified, predominantly in the area of glucose metabolism evidenced in a diabetic-type glucose tolerance curve.

Childhood-onset obesity brings additional dilemmas in that hypernutrition during growth produces an excess number of fat cells (hyperplasia) in addition to an increase in cell size (hypertrophy). Although one may reduce the amount of fat in any single cell, one cannot eliminate the cell itself. Further, homeostatic mechanisms appear to limit the degree to which a fat cell may shrink, with cell size a seeming mediator of starvation signals to the body. Increased insulin output results when fat cells diminish below a critical size. Failing a corrective response at this point, conservational steps somewhat paralleling hibernational states are triggered; metabolism is lowered and activity reduced. In many respects obesity qualifies as an addictive disease with specific physiologic changes in response to hypernutrition that in turn promote the continued intake of increased amounts of food for homeostasis.

Although considerable empathy is warranted for the obese adolescent and the difficult task of reducing, when all is said and done weight loss still can be accomplished only by shifting the caloric-intake-versus-caloric-output equation. This requires a salutary modification of eating and activity behavior. Thus some understanding of these behaviors in overweight teenagers will be helpful in evolving a therapeutic plan. Compared to adolescents of normal weight, those who are obese tend to have the following characteristics:

1. Have diets that are higher in carbohydrates and fats.

2. Snack less frequently and skip meals more often.

3. Consume fewer total calories per day but also tend to be less active.

4. Eat more food at a given sitting and eat more rapidly.

5. Overeat without being aware of the ordinary sensations of hunger and satiation.

6. Indulge in aberrant eating patterns such as night eating, binge eating, or eating without hunger or appetite.

7. Do less well in physical performance tests.

8. Have broader bone structure.

9. Be faster growing and earlier maturing if boys or slower growing and later maturing if girls.

The emotional dimensions of obesity are just as complex as metabolic and behavioral aspects and are as likely to be consequent to being obese as they are the primary cause. Usually obese as a child, the overweight teenager already has a life experience of being seen as different and devalued, particularly in cultural milieus where slimness is the ideal. This becomes heightened in adolescence and, although the characteristic intense preoccupation with appearance and attractiveness would seem sufficient motivation to prompt weight loss, being fat sometimes has self-protective aspects. The isolating and devaluating consequences of obesity can lead to an all-encompassing sense of inferiority and fear of rejection. Establishing a relationship with the opposite sex is perceived as fraught with the possibility of failure. Obesity is then invoked as a justifying reason for noninvolvement.

Although obesity has its own secondary self-fulfilling psychopathology, some individuals may invoke obesity as a defense against primary emotional distress. As already noted, food has symbolic significance in the life of the infant or child, its giving or withholding being indicative of the degree to which he or she is valued or devalued or the extent to which he or she has earned parental love or provoked their retribution. Overeating may be a response to feeling emotionally deprived and a means of seeking psychologic comfort in the intake of food. For others who have failed to resolve oedipal issues in childhood or adolescence, obesity may be a protective veneer against forbidden sexual feelings and fantasies. A third mechanism may be the outward confirmation of a pervasive sense of inner worthlessness. Sometimes obesity may be self-inflicted as a punishment for being "bad." Such defenses usually are unconsciously mediated and the patient is unaware of the degree to which being overweight and personality structure are interwoven.

Nothing is more difficult than helping an adolescent, obese since childhood, lose weight and maintain this loss. This is not to say one should abandon trying but rather to recognize the dimensions of the problem and the need for maximal support and a carefully orchestrated approach using a variety of resources. An effective management plan includes the following:

1. Motivation. An adolescent can lose weight effectively only when he or she is strongly motivated to do so. This depends on perceived benefits in relation to such matters as enhanced self-esteem, attractiveness, improved athletic ability, or wider availability of good-looking clothes. Weight loss desired by parents or proposed because of future health hazards has little perceived relevance or motivational force.

2. Nutritional assessment. Before any dietary modification the adolescent should record and calorically evaluate a 1-week history of intake and associated activities as described in the previous section on evaluation.

3. Realistic diet. The diet plan needs to be carefully constructed on an individual basis and be one the adolescent perceives he or she can follow. Handing out a standard diet sheet without taking the patient's and family's eating patterns into account invariably fails. A reasonable starting point is an initial decrease in total intake of about 300–400 calories per day, titrated subsequently to achieve a weight loss of 1–2 pounds a week. Alternatively, if the adolescent is still growing, simply stabilizing weight will reduce fat stores in favor of increased muscle and skeletal mass. Additional points include:

a. Ensuring an adequate intake of nutrients essential for adolescent growth. Use supplementation when necessary.

b. Deleting calories from fat where possible, and from carbohydrates for the remaining decrease.

c. Encouraging small frequent meals.

d. Providing for low-calorie snacks at usual snack times.

e. Discussing and planning for maintaining diet at school and social events.

f. Providing for periodic intake of modest amounts of favored foods even if high in calories.

g. Encouraging patient to purchase a low-calorie recipe book and make attractive low-calorie dishes the whole family can enjoy.

h. Encouraging the patient to maintain a food diary and keep tabs on total caloric intake.

i. Using other behavior modification techniques as given in Table 19-7.

4. Physician attitude. All of the injunctions against becoming a parental surrogate in adolescent health care (Chapter 2) are particularly applicable here. The physician also should avoid getting caught up in a professional or countertransference investment in the patient's success. This only prompts frustration, personal disappointment, anger, or even rejection when the patient is less than optimally compliant. The wise physician working with obese adolescents perceives weight loss to be the patient's responsibility and himself or herself as merely its facilitator. The physician is happy for the teenager who succeeds but continues to empathize and support the one who is having a more difficult time.

5. Frequency of visits. Visits initially should be at weekly intervals, tapering to monthly as progress warrants. The goals are (a) to review the therapeutic plan and revise troublesome aspects, (b) review and discuss other aspects of the adolescent's life, (c) provide encouragement and support, and (d) check weight. The fervor of initial commitment is difficult to maintain and the patient needs frequent reinforce-

TABLE 19-7
BEHAVIOR MODIFICATION TECHNIQUES FOR WEIGHT REDUCTION IN OBESITY

1. Identify and eliminate environmental food cues.
   a. Eliminate high-caloric food from household or place in a relatively inaccessible spot.
   b. Do not leave full serving dishes on the table.
   c. Do not watch TV food commercials if they trigger getting a snack.
   d. Change daily schedule to occupy usual snack times with involving activities.
   e. Change routes to and from school if passing by the bakery prompts stopping in for a jelly donut (or equivalent).
2. Change act of eating to promote satiation with less food.
   a. Lengthen meal time and eat more slowly.
   b. Take smaller bites and chew thoroughly.
   c. Put utensil down between each bite.
   d. Swallow each mouthful before taking up more food on utensil.
   e. Use smaller plates to make smaller portions appear larger.
   f. Leave a small amount of food behind at each meal.
   g. Prepare just enough food for one helping.
   h. Dispose of leftovers immediately.
3. Preplan meals and snacks. Define in advance exactly what will be eaten, when, and how much for each meal or snack for each day.
4. Change activity patterns.
   a. Increase energy expenditure in usual daily activities; use stairs rather than elevator; walk rather than ride; get off the bus one or several stops sooner than necessary and walk the rest of the way.
   b. Increase physical activity; walking, jogging, bicycle trips, after school athletics, programs at the Y, boys and girls clubs, and so on.

---

ment. A nurse, nurse practitioner, nutritionist, or social worker can be particularly helpful in providing such counsel.

6. Family. No diet will be effective unless parents help by modifying what is served at meal times and restricting the amount of high caloric foods in the ice box or pantry larder. As one or both parents also are apt to be overweight, modification of eating behavior can become a family activity. In any event, the adolescent should not feel that he or she is being selectively discriminated against, being served a stick of celery while the rest eat chocolate cake. Although family support and encouragement are essential, parents should be advised to leave dietary compliance to the adolescent in consultation with the physician or other involved professional and to assiduously avoid contests for control over food or making derogatory or humiliating remarks.

7. Activity. Increased physical and recreational activity has two advantages. First is increased energy expenditure. Second is keeping the mind off food and hands away from the cookie jar. Many obese adolescents spend a good bit of time at home alone with temptation rife. Community resources for such activity include after school programs, Boys' and Girls' Clubs, Y's, neighborhood community centers, churches, youth groups, and others.

8. Specific support groups. Weight loss without a support group can be a lonely and discouraging business. Alliance with such a group provides an approach toward obesity similar to that used successfully by Alcoholics Anonymous for alcoholism. Weight Watchers, Overeaters Anonymous, and TOPS (Take Off Pounds Sensibly) are national programs, and many branches have special sessions for teens. Some hospital clinics, schools, and those youth-oriented community resources mentioned in No. 7 also may have weight reduction support groups. Setting up rap group sessions in a private office also is feasible.

9. Opportunities for interpersonal success. Many obese adolescents have poor self-images and tend to isolate themselves. It is important that they have opportunities for normal peer congress and the pursuit of development tasks. This may be forthcoming from the specific activity and/or weight loss support programs mentioned previously. In other instances it may be helpful to involve the patient in age-specific rather than obesity-specific groups. Here again, various rap, social, and athletic programs in school and community can be employed.

10. Specific treatment modalities
   a. Behavior modification. In essence, the entire weight loss program employs various forms of behavior modification by altering eating patterns through negative and positive reinforcement. Some programs formalize this process and can be helpful.
   b. Hypnosis. The use of posthypnotic suggestion and/or self-hypnotic techniques is a field of growing significance in handling difficult behaviors and other adverse situations (for example, the self-management of pain). Provided this is supervised by a responsible and well-trained therapist, considerable benefit may accrue.
   c. Camps for overweight teens. These can be very helpful in that significant weight loss is usually achieved during the camp season, prov-

ing to the young person that he or she really can lose. Other aspects of the camping program are opportunities for success and self-esteem in activity accomplishments or improved interpersonal relationships. A successful summer, however, should be reinforced by the resumption of home, medical, and group support systems in the fall.

d. Starvation diets. Morbidly obese adolescents with serious medical complications such as marked hypertension or the Pickwickian syndrome (interference with respiration by obesity to the point of CO_2 retention and decreased oxygenation) or other illnesses adversely affected by overweight may warrant hospitalization and the institution of exceptionally low ($\geq$ 500 calories per day) or total starvation diets. Although such regimens do not offer a long-term answer, they will result in the rapid loss of weight necessary for physical reasons. Starvation diets of several weeks or months have been followed by adolescents without serious adverse physical effects provided vitamin and mineral supplementation and close medical supervision are provided.

Other approaches to managing obesity are more questionable:

1. Traditional psychoanalytic modalities have not been singularly effective in managing obesity. Assistance should not be looked for from this quarter except as warranted by concurrent emotional disability.

2. There is only the most limited place for anorexic agents such as amphetamines and their derivatives. Tolerance rapidly develops, and psychologic habituation is common. Most medical organizations have now eschewed their use in obesity management. Their use may have some justification, however, in helping an adolescent who has reached a discouraging plateau after losing some weight to get back on the track, but only for a week or two at the most.

3. Obesity "mills" and the various mixture of pills often handed out should be avoided. These programs are inadequate in support, and the medications can be harmful; they sometimes include digitalis, thyroid preparations, diuretics, laxatives, amphetamines, and cellulose fillers.

4. The patient should not indulge in crash diets, starvation diets, or diets advocating aberrant food sources, which risk protein and other nutrient deficiencies or pose specific metabolic harm.

5. There is little place for surgical approaches in adolescent obesity. Both intestinal bypass operations and the excision of body fat have significant risks. They should be considered only in the most exceptional circumstances.

The overall therapeutic plan should be realistic in terms the patient feels he or she can meet. Weight loss goals should be set in relatively small steps; it is easier to contemplate trying to lose 5–10 pounds than 50. When the smaller goal is reached, a new one can be established. Long-range expectancies also should be realistic. An adolescent overweight since childhood simply cannot end up with high fashion model proportions. Lastly, modified eating patterns established at this time will need to be followed for life.

ANOREXIA NERVOSA

Anorexia nervosa is characterized by uncontrolled dieting and rapid weight loss without apparent predisposing physical or psychiatric disturbance. The degree of starvation commonly is severe with a loss of 25% of total body weight within 2 or 3 months and a 5% mortality rate. Anorexia nervosa most often occurs in white middle and upper middle class adolescents and young people under the age of 25. Females outnumber males by 10 to 1. Sometimes there is a family history with a sibling or close relative also victim. Although the reported incidence a decade ago ranged between 0.16 and 0.24 per 100,000 population, more recent estimates suggest it is far more prevalent, occurring in 1 out of every 200 girls. Although this may represent a secular increase in absolute rate, an equally plausible explanation rests in improved diagnosis and recognition of partial forms.

The etiology of anorexia nervosa is obscure. Formerly thought to be exclusively psychiatric in origin, newer concepts include the possibility of hypothalamic malfunction as well. This is suggested by not only the marked metabolic changes that occur (see following discussion) but also the discrepancy between the severity of the disease and the considerably milder degree of premorbid psychologic problems evidenced by many patients and their families.

Psychodynamically, anorexia nervosa is thought to represent a pathologic struggle for independence in an adolescent who has no other way to become autonomous except through control of food intake. These young people commonly are bright, achieving, and conforming, often described as "perfect" children by their parents. The parents themselves frequently have rather rigid value systems and high behavioral and academic expectancies for their child, but such a dynamic structure has usually worked well and these families have been intact, competent, and happy until anorexia nervosa rather unexpectedly and suddenly strikes.

The disease typically starts in a mildly overweight or normal-weighted adolescent girl who initiates dieting following an idle comment about her chubbiness or other aspects of her appearance, watching a television commercial extolling thinness, or some other such trivial event. Dieting progresses beyond the stated weight loss goal to frank inanition. The patient is unable to put brakes on her food restriction or to perceive herself as other than unacceptably fat, even though an objective appraisal clearly belies such an assessment.

Other features include an overriding preoccupation with food, the patient often spending long hours preparing meals for others while maintaining strenuous self-imposed dietary restriction. Some patients attempt to speed up the weight loss process through excessive physical exercise, self-induced vomiting, or by taking frequent laxatives. These measures also may be resorted to in an effort to atone for intermittent binge eating. Increased physical activity may progress to a generalized hyperactivity, with the patient always on the go. School and social functions remain intact, although they may be compromised due to preoccupations with food and physical activity.

Anorexia nervosa should be suspected in any girl—or boy—who seems to fit this picture. Diagnostic criteria are cited in Table 19-8. Differential considerations include weight loss due to an underlying biologic cause and the so-called secondary anorexias associated with severe depression or schizophrenia and bizarre food delusions. In these instances, anorexia usually takes a slower course and has a more obvious underlying psychogenic cause.

A variety of physical and metabolic abnormalities are also common. Amenorrhea is particularly noteworthy, often occurring early in the course and sometimes even anteceding significant weight loss. Other findings are variable. Physical examination may reveal one or more of the following:

1. Dematologic abnormalities (lanugo hair, desquamation, scaling)
2. Hypothermia (rectal temperature below 96.6 F.)
3. Bradycardia (pulse rate less than 60/min)
4. Bradypnea (respiratory rate less than 14/min)
5. Hypotension (systolic blood pressure below 70 mm Hg)
6. Heart murmurs
7. Peripheral edema

TABLE 19-8
DIAGNOSTIC CRITERIA
OF ANOREXIA NERVOSA

1. Weight loss of approximately 25% of original body weight.
2. Onset before the age of 25.
3. Negative attitude toward eating.
4. No primary physical or psychiatric illness.
5. Four of the following:
   a. Distorted body image; perceiving self as fat even if obviously cachectic.
   b. Periods of excessive activity.
   c. Amenorrhea, usually early in course of disease (70%).
   d. History of mild-to-moderate overweight, often with onset of disease coincident with efforts at weight reduction; fear of obesity.
   e. Self-induced vomiting.
   f. Preoccupation with food.
   g. Denial of illness with failure to recognize nutritional needs.
   h. Apparent enjoyment in losing weight, even if looks malnourished to others.

Possible metabolic and laboratory abnormalities include the following.

1. Endocrine abnormalities:
   a. Decreased leuteinizing hormone (LH) and follicle-stimulating hormone (FSH); delayed release of LH and FSH after administration of gonadotrophin-releasing factor.
   b. Increased insulin binding; disturbed oral glucose tolerance test.
   c. Decreased serum thyroxine, iodine and triiodothyronine; delayed release of thyroid-stimulating hormone after administration of thyroid-releasing factor.
   d. Diabetes insipidus (occurs in 44%).
   e. Absent diurnal variation in cortisol secretion.
   f. Elevated growth hormone.
2. Cardiovascular abnormalities evident in electrocardiogram changes.
3. Hematologic abnormalities:
   a. Leukopenia.
   b. Bone marrow hypoplasia.
4. Renal abnormalities:
   a. Elevated blood urea nitrogen.
   b. Decrease in xylose excretion.
5. Nutritional abnormalities:
   a. Iron deficiency anemia.
   b. Hypercarotenemia.
   c. Hypovitaminosis A.
6. Hypothalamic abnormalities: disorders of thermoregulatory mechanisms.

The treatment of anorexia nervosa takes two directions: first, the medical correction of severe malnutrition and second, psychotherapeutic attention to modifying eating behavior and dealing with the underlying emotional dilemmas of patient and family. In accomplishing these goals, concordance between physician and psychiatrist is essential, with the former taking the lead in managing health care and weight maintenance while the latter attends to psychological dimensions. If the patient is hospitalized, care should be mediated through an interdisciplinary approach with the additional involvement of nurses, social workers, adolescent life workers (recreational therapists), nutritionists, and any others involved with the young person. Whether the advantages offered by such a team effort will be available on an ambulatory basis depends on the clinical setting in which the patient is being seen.

Some patients can be managed solely on an ambulatory basis. Others with severe malnutrition require an initial hospitalization. Tube feedings and/or vitamin and mineral supplementation may be necessary. A variety of pharmacologic agents also have been used, including chlorpromazine, amitriptyline, cyproheptadine, metoclorpramide, L-dopa, and phenytoin. It is our opinion, however, that these agents have little established therapeutic role.

Weight gain is best achieved through a behavior modification approach using the gain or loss of specified amounts as the criteria for gaining or losing specified privileges. Such an approach is often more easily implemented in the hospital than at home (Table 19-9). The focus is upon achieving weight milestones, not the amount eaten per se. A power struggle over what is and is not consumed should not be allowed to develop, and control should be handed over to the patient, it being her choice whether or not to achieve the requisite weight to gain the associated privilege.

Food should be served and trays removed without comment. Patient requests for between-meal snacks or alternate foods to the hospital fare are honored. Uneaten food or that thought to have been flushed down the toilet is ignored. The patient is weighed at more or less the same time of day but in an unpredictable manner (some caution should be taken against the patient filling up on water just before being weighed or inducing vomiting right after). Privileges are then meted out accordingly.

Ambulatory treatment involves much the same kind of approach, with weight maintenance being equated with staying out of the hospital and weight loss being associated with readmission and the possibility of tube feedings. Home privileges can be

TABLE 19-9
A BEHAVIOR MODIFICATION PLAN FOR ACHIEVING WEIGHT GAIN IN ANOREXIA NERVOSA

Weight (lbs)*	Privilege lost or gained
70	Hospitalize In room; full bed rest No telephone, television, radio, phonograph, and so on No books, school work, or craft materials No visitors
−3	Tube feeding
+¼	Bathroom privileges
+½	May have books, school work, craft materials
+1	May have radio
+1½	May have television
+2	May have brief visit with parents
+2½	May have telephone
+3	May go out of room
+3½	May have friends visit
+5	May go home
−5	Rehospitalize with all restrictions
−8	Reinstitute tube feedings

*Privileges should be accorded at ¼ lb gains in the beginning. Later they may be set at ½ lb intervals. This listing is only an example of one behavior modification approach.

worked out in a similar manner to those suggested for the hospital setting, but the physician rather than parents should continue to be the one who determines when privileges should be granted or withheld. Parents will need considerable support to reverse their former preoccupation with the patient's food consumption and to be persuaded that the physician will protect the adolescent from medical jeopardy.

Psychotherapy must proceed in conjunction with combined family and individual therapy, exploring not only issues contributing to the production of this disease, but also the effect it has upon all family members. Anorexia nervosa can be disrupting all around and usually poses a major crisis in the life of a family that formerly perceived itself as doing very well. Treatment goals are predicated on finding healthier ways for the patient to express her drives for independence and autonomy and in helping the family to accept and allow such steps. Occasionally, profound intrafamily disturbances or parents who are totally unable to accept the therapeutic plan may be encountered. Alternate living arrangements may be required in these circumstances, with the adolescent living with a relative or being placed in residential or foster home care.

OTHER NUTRITIONAL DEPRIVATION STATES

Malnutrition may be a causal factor in adolescents who are at less than the fifth percentile standard for height and/or weight when adjusted for constitutional delays in puberty (a late-maturing adolescent may be small in relation to standards predicated upon the inclusion of normal and early maturing youths but catch up with time). Weight loss also may be the first indication of intercurrent disease. Table 19-10 presents differential considerations in such instances.

THE THIN ADOLESCENT WHO WANTS TO GAIN WEIGHT

There are no significant health risks with simply being thin (not malnourished). It has cosmetic implications only. Of course this can be of singular importance to the adolescent; from a developmental perspective, physical appearance is closely interrelated with self-esteem during these years.

Rapidly growing teenagers may well be excessively thin as a component of the growth spurt. This is particularly apt to be the case in males who do not have the same predisposition for fat deposition as females. Acquisition of male muscle mass also is a late pubertal event. Such young people only need be reassured that they will fill out later on. A dietary history usually reveals ample intake of calories and nutrients.

Some adolescents are thin and wiry on a constitutional or genetic basis. It usually is as difficult for this group to gain weight as it is for obese teenagers to lose. Management focuses on dietary counseling and seeking ways of increasing caloric intake without inhibiting appetite; these individuals often give a history of relatively small meals. Planning capitalizes on this observation by using five to six eating periods per day, rather than the traditional three, with limited portions each time. A behavior modification plan, the reciprocal of that recommended for obesity, can be tried. It also may help to increase caloric concentration without increasing volume through adding extra margarine, butter, or sugar to a normal portion of food. Some caution is indicated in supplementing with fats in that they tend to slow gastric emptying time and decrease appetite further. Some thin adolescents have resorted to commercial preparations advertised for their weight-gaining benefits in extolling terms. These preparations are simply fat emulsions and, for the

TABLE 19-10
DIFFERENTIAL DIAGNOSIS
OF UNDERWEIGHT IN ADOLESCENCE

Chronic long-standing
☐ Constitutional or genetic thinness
☐ Growth disorders:
  Hypopituitarism
  Skeletal malformations
  Congenital metabolic disorders
  Rubella syndrome
  Severe brain injury and neuromuscular dysfunction
  Mongolism and certain other chromosomal anomalies
☐ Chronic debilitating disease
  Renal disease
  Cyanotic heart disease and/or chronic heart failure
  Pulmonary disorders
  Chronic gastrointestinal disease
  Malignancy and treatment of malignancy
☐ Chronic infections
☐ Scarcity of food

Recent onset
☐ Gastrointestinal disorders
  Inflammatory bowel disease
  Superior mesenteric artery syndrome
  Peptic ulcer
☐ Collagen disease
☐ Malignancy
  Hodgkin's disease
  Lymphoma
  Leukemia
☐ Intracranial lesion
☐ Anorexia nervosa
☐ Secondary anorexias
  Depression
  Schizophrenia
☐ Iatrogenic: effects of some medications
☐ Behavioral:
  Drug or alcohol abuse; heavy smoking
  Athletic
    Heavy training
    Weight loss requirements for making a given weight class
    Diuretic abuse in above situation
☐ Sociologic/cultural
  Political activism; hunger strike
  Religious fasts
  Fad and cultist diets
  Scarcity of food

same reasons cited for fats in general, have little benefit.

In many instances, efforts to gain weight are fruitless. Here the adolescent will need to be helped to accept his or her thinness without personal devaluation.

Bibliography

GENERAL

Daniel, W. Z. 1977. *Adolescents in health and disease*. St. Louis: C. V. Mosby Co.

Heald, F. P. 1975. Adolescent nutrition. *Med. Clin. North Am.* 59(6):1329-1336.

Heald, F. P.; Rosebrough, R. H.; and Jacobson, M. S. 1980. Nutrition and the adolescent: an update. *J. Adolescent Health Care* 1:142.

Huenemann, R. L.; Hampton, M. D.; Benke, A. R.; et al. 1974. *Teenage nutrition and physique*. Springfield, Ill.: Charles C Thomas, Publisher.

McKigney, J. I., and Munro, H. N., editors. 1976. *Nutrient requirements in adolescents*. Cambridge, Mass.: M.I.T. Press.

Meyer, H. 1980. The underweight adolescent: etiologic factors and a review. *Clin. Pediatr.* 19:819-823.

Smith, N. J. 1980. Excessive weight loss and food aversion in athletes simulating anorexia nervosa. *Pediatrics* 66:139-142.

Winick, M. 1978. Nutrition during adolescence. *Modern Med.* Jan. 15, 1978, pp. 58-60.

Winick, M., editor. 1977. *Nutritional disorders of American women*. New York: John Wiley & Sons.

Young, C. M. 1976. Adolescents and their nutrition. In *Medical care of the adolescent*, 3rd ed., editors, J. R. Gallagher; F. P. Heald; and D. C. Garell. New York: Appleton Century Crofts.

Zerfas, A. J.; Shorr, I. J.; and Neuman, C. G. 1977. Office assessment of nutritional status. *Pediatr. Clin. North Am.* 24(1):253-272.

INVENTORIES/SURVEYS

U.S. Department of Health, Education and Welfare, Public Health Service, Health Resources Administration. 1977. *Dietary intake findings, United States 1971-1974* (includes HANES Program Data), *Vital and Health Statistics*, Series 11, No. 202. Data from the National Health Survey. Hyattsville, Md.: National Center for Health Statistics.

U.S. Department of Health, Education and Welfare, Public Health Service, Health Resources Administration. 1977. Selected findings: food consumption profiles of white and black persons 1 to 74 years of age in the United States, 1971 to 1974. *Advance-data*. Rockville, Md.

U.S. Department of Health, Education and Welfare. 1974. Skin-fold thickness of youths 12 to 17 years: United States vital and health statistics. Data from the National Health Survey, Series 11, No. 132. Public Health Services, Health Resources Administration, National Center for Health Statistics, Rockville, Md.

U.S. Department of Health Education and Welfare. 1972. *Ten state nutrition survey*, 1968 to 1970, Publication (HSM) 72-8133.

VITAMINS, MINERALS, NUTRIENTS AND CHOLESTEROL

American Diabetic Association. 1978. *Vitamin-mineral safety, toxicity and misuse*. Consortium Report. Chicago, Ill.

Committee on Nutrition of the American Academy of Pediatrics. 1978. Calcium requirements in infancy and childhood. *Pediatrics* 62(5):826-834.

U.S. Department of Health, Education and Welfare; Public Health Service, Health Resources Administration, National Center for Health Statistics. 1976. *Total serum cholesterol values of youths 12 to 17 years*. United States Vital and Health Statistics Data from the National Health Survey, Series 11, No. 156. Rockville, Md.

OBESITY

Barnes, H. V., and Berger, R. 1975. An approach to the obese adolescent. *Med. Clin. North Am.* 59(6):1507-1516.

Beller, A. S. 1977. *Fat and thin: a natural history of obesity*. New York: Farrar, Straus, and Giroux.

Bruch, H. 1973. *Eating disorders: obesity, anorexia nervosa and the person within*. New York: Basic Books, Inc.

Carruth, B. R., and Iszler, J. 1981. Assessment and conservative management of the overfat adolescent. *J. Adolescent Health Care* 1:289-299.

Coates, T. J. 1978. Treating obesity in children and adolescents: a review. *Am. J. Public Health.* 68(2):143-172.

Fisher, M.; Nitkin, R.; Shenker, I. R.; et al. 1981. Long-term follow-up of obesity in adolescents. *J. Adolescent Health Care* 1:229-231.

Heald, F. P. 1975. Juvenile obesity. In *Childhood obesity*, editor M. Winick. New York: John Wiley & Sons.

Merritt, R. J.; Bistrian, B. R.; Blackburn, G. L.; et al. 1980. Consequences of modified fasting in obese pediatric and adolescent patients. I. Protein-sparing modified fast. *J. Pediatr.* 96:13-19.

Meyer, E. E., and Neumann, C. G. 1977. Management of the obese adolescent. *Pediatr. Clin. North Am.* 24(1):123-132.

ANOREXIA NERVOSA

Bruch, H. 1966. Anorexia nervosa and its differential diagnosis. *J. Nervous Mental Dis.* 141(5):555-566.

Casper, R. C.; Offer, D.; and Ostrov, E. 1981. The self-image of adolescents with acute anorexia nervosa. *J. Pediatr.* 98:656-661.

Minuchin, S.; Rosman, B. L.; and Baker, L. 1978. *Psychosomatic families: anorexia nervosa in context*. Cambridge, Mass.: Harvard University Press.

Silverman, J. A. 1977. Anorexia nervosa: clinical and metabolic observation in a successful treatment plan. In *Anorexia nervosa*, editor R. A. Vigersky, New York: Raven Press.

Vigersky, R., editor. 1977. Anorexia nervosa. New York: Raven Press.

FADS/VEGETARIANISM
Christoffel, K. 1981. A pediatric perspective on vegetarian nutrition. *Clin. Pediatr.* 20:632-643.

Nutrition misinformation and food faddism. 1974. *Nutrition Rev.* (Special Suppl.) July.

Robson, J. R. K. 1977. Food faddism. *Pediatr. Clin. North Am.* 24(1):189-202.

Vegetarian Information Service. P. O. Box 5888, Washington, D.C. 20014.

Vyhmeister, E. B.; Register, U. D.; and Sonnenberg, L. M. 1977. Safe vegetarian diets for children. *Pediatr. Clin. North Am.* 24(1):203-210.

-20-
Drug and Alcohol Use and Abuse: Medical and Psychologic Aspects

Adele D. Hofmann, M.D.

Medical and Pharmacologic Aspects
Definitions □ Factors contributing to a drug's effect
Classification of Drugs and Management of Addiction and Overdose
Narcotics □ Central nervous system depressants, group I
Central nervous system depressants, group II □ Central nervous system stimulants
Hallucinogens, group I □ Hallucinogens, group II □ Cannabis □ Atropinic drugs
Nitrites □ Laboratory diagnosis of drug use □ Medical detection of drug use in adolescence
Psychologic Aspects of Drug and Alcohol Abuse in Adolescence
Diagnosis □ Management □ Prognosis

Adolescents may use a variety of licit and illicit substances out of experimentation, recreation, habituation, addiction, or suicidal intent. This chapter reviews the medical and pharmacologic aspects of drug and alcohol use, overdose, withdrawal phenomena, and associated medical complications as well as the psychologic aspects of chronic substance abuse and its management.

Medical and Pharmacologic Aspects

DEFINITIONS

Addiction. Addiction is a predictable biologic response to the regular daily intake of certain drugs; metabolic processes are altered in adaptation with resultant *physical dependence*. Abstinence results in a *withdrawal syndrome*, a drug-specific complex of various symptoms and signs. Addiction is lost when

withdrawal is complete, a process usually taking from 5–14 days. Not all drugs are addicting, and this property has been clearly documented to occur only with narcotics and central nervous system (CNS) depressants; controversy exists in relation to CNS stimulants.

Habituation. Habituation is the compulsive emotional need for a drug's effects, or *psychological dependence*. All drugs may be habituating, but in most instances, the user must be vulnerable in the first place. There is only limited evidence that habituation will occur in an emotionally intact individual.

Tolerance. Tolerance is a biologic response to the regular daily administration of a given drug dose; the drug's effects gradually diminish in intensity and increasingly larger doses are required to produce the desired effect. Toxicity and lethality diminish in parallel. Tolerance is readily lost when the user abstains. This property occurs with many but not all drugs and does not necessarily go hand in hand with addiction.

Cross-tolerance. Cross-tolerance is the capacity of one drug to substitute for another in meeting requirements of physical dependence and preventing abstinence syndromes. Most members within each class have cross-tolerance for each other. This property forms the basis of methadone detoxification and maintenance in heroin addiction or the use of barbiturates in drying out the alcoholic.

FACTORS CONTRIBUTING TO A DRUG'S EFFECT

Purity. The results and/or consequences of a drug's administration are affected by (a) the amount of psychoactive material present in a given dose; (b) the irritant properties of the material with which the drug may be diluted or "cut" (starch, lactose, mannitol, talc, quinine, glucose, house dust); (c) bacterial or viral contamination; and (d) the possible substitution or addition of drugs other than as alleged. In the last instance, most pills and powders purporting to be mescaline, psilocybin, or tetrahydrocannabinol are in fact LSD, phencyclidine, or nothing at all. Atropinic drugs or CNS stimulants may be present as well. Increasingly, marijuana has been reported to be contaminated with phencyclidine.

Method of administration. Drugs may be taken by virtually any route: Intravenous or subcutaneous injection, orally, or inhaled, smoked, or sniffed. The rate of onset, degree, and duration of effect follow usual pharmacologic expectancies. Intravenous use, however, may produce results unobtainable by other routes; heroin, amphetamine, and cocaine injection are associated with an immediate, brief "rush"—a feeling described as akin to sexual orgasm.

Other variables. Frequency of administration and the total amount taken are obvious factors in determining effect. The expectations and past experience of the user and the environment in which the drug is taken also are reported to have significant impact; novice users are most apt to have unpleasant or minimal reactions the first few times out.

Classification of Drugs and Management of Addiction and Overdose

Table 20-1 indicates the class, street and trade names, appearance, and common methods of administration for various drugs. Table 20-2 summarizes selected properties, and Tables 20-3, 20-4, and 20-5 list signs and general management principles of overdose. It should be noted, however, that young people are ardent experimenters, and a variety of other substances may enjoy transient popularity. They rarely make their way onto the permanent list because of unacceptable side effects of minimal psychoactivity. Nonetheless, the practitioner should be alert to this possibility when encountering an unfamiliar toxic syndrome.

NARCOTICS

Prototypes. Heroin, morphine, meperedine, propoxyphene.

Properties. Narcotics are derived from the opium poppy and chemical manufacture; members of this class are analgesic and sedative. They relieve pain and anxiety, produce euphoria, suppress cough, and are constipating. Addiction and tolerance result within a few days of regular intake in even small amounts. Cross-tolerance exists among all members. Depressant effects are additive, with drugs from other classes having a similar property.

Although heroin is the drug most commonly involved in narcotic addiction, among adolescents propoxyphene (Darvon) should not be overlooked. Addiction can occur with a daily intake of 500–800 mg of propoxyphene hydrochloride or 800–1200 mg of the napsylate salt (8 to 12 capsules). Abuse of other members of this class is rarely encountered among adolescents.

Subjective effects. An immediate "rush" is experienced on intravenous injection. Administration by any route also produces euphoria, drowsiness, and a dreamy state free of anxiety and tension. Appetite and sexual drive diminish. Novice users may have dysphoric effects such as nausea, vomiting, and dizziness.

Objective signs. The user is oriented to reality but sedated, indifferent, and lethargic. Speech may be laconic, impoverished, and slurred; gait unsteady; pulse and respirations slowed. Pin point pupils are characteristic. There also may be evidence of recent intravenous or subcutaneous injection sites. Chronic users may demonstrate pigmented "needle tracks" over the veins of the arm, hands, or legs; subcutaneous use may result in punched-out ulcers in any reachable location.

Overdose. CNS depression predominates, and death can occur. Miosis and injection marks, when present,

TABLE 20-1
CLASSIFICATION OF PSYCHOTROPIC DRUGS

Class	Commonly used drugs	Street or trade name	Appearance	Usual method of administration
Narcotics	Heroin	H, horse, Harry, smack, dope	White powder	IV or SQ Sniffing
	Methadone	Meth	Pill, powder, liquid	IV or SQ
	Meperedine	Demerol	Per pharmaceutical manufacture: pills capsules, injectables, cough mixtures, etc.	IV, SQ, p.o.
	Codeine			
	Morphine			
	Propoxyphene	Darvon		
CNS depressants, group I	Barbiturates	Downers, goof balls	Per pharmaceutical manufacture	P.o., rarely IV
	Secobarbital	Reds, red devils, Seconal		
	Pentobarbital	Yellows, yellow jackets, Nebutal		
	Secobarbital and amobarbital	Blues, blue birds, Tuinal		
	Methaqualone	Quaalude, Sopors		
	Weak tranquilizers			
	Diazepam	Valium		P.o., rarely IV
	Chlordiazepoxide	Librium		
	Meprobamate	Equanil, Miltown		
	Ethanol	Alcohol	Beer, wine, hard liquor	P.o.
CNS depressants, group II	Commercial solvents		Glues, cleaning fluid, paint thinner, nail polish remover, lighter fluid, etc.	Inhalation of volatile vapors (called "sniffing")
	Toluene			
	Trichlororethylene			
	Acetone			
	Methanol			
	Ketones			
	Spray-can propellants	Freon	Aerosol spray cans	Inhalation of volatile vapors (called sniffing)
	Fluorinated hydrocarbons			
	Nitrous oxide			
	Gasoline (leaded and unleaded			Inhalation of volatile vapors (called sniffing)
CNS stimulants	Amphetamines	Uppers	White powder or per pharmaceutical manufacture (pill, capsule)	P.o. or IV (sometimes by serial injection)
	Methamphetamine	Meth, speed, crystal, methedrine		
	Amphetamine	Bennies, benzedrine		
	Dextroamphetamine	Dexies		
	Cocaine	Coke, snow, dust	White crystalline powder	Sniffing, IV
Hallucinogens, group I	Lysergic acid diethylamide	LSD	Pill, capsule, powder, liquid, sugar cube; adulterant of marijuana or cigarette papers	P.o., smoking
	Mescaline	Peyote, buttons	Pill, powder, dried cactus	P.o.
	Psilocybin		Pill, powder, dried mushroom	P.o.

Continued

TABLE 20-1
CLASSIFICATION OF PSYCHOTROPIC DRUGS (CONTINUED)

Class	Commonly used drugs	Street or trade name	Appearance	Usual method of administration
Hallucinogens, group II	Phencyclidine	PCP, angel dust, crystal, hog, peace, rocket fuel, cyclones	Pill, powder, liquid; adulterant of marijuana or cigarette papers	P.o.
Cannabis	Marijuana	Pot, weed, Mary Jane, grass	Dried plant material	Smoking, cooked in food
	Hashish	Hash	Brown resinous solid	Smoking
	Tetrahydrocannabinol	THC	Brown viscous liquid	P.o.
Atropinic drugs	Belladonna	Various pharmaceuticals and plant substances	White powder, pills, liquid	Smoking, p.o.
	Atropine	Jimson weed	Dried or fresh material	Smoking, p.o.
	Scopolamine	Sominex, deadly nightshade	Pill, plant material, liquid (ampule)	P.o., rarely IV
Nitrites	Amylnitrite		Liquid, ampule	Sniffing
	Isobutyl nitrite	Poppers, bolt, rush	Liquid, ampule, room odorizer	

are important signs differentiating narcotic overdose from that due to other depressant drugs. Table 20-4 details general management. Naloxone (Narcan) is a specific antagonist. An initial dose of 0.4–0.8 mg by slow intravenous push should produce an observable return toward consciousness within several minutes. This may be repeated several times over 20–30 minutes for a total dose of 3 mg. If no response occurs, a drug other than a narcotic probably is causative. Naloxone should be used only to alleviate respiratory depression in patients suspected of addiction; attempts to restore consciousness may overshoot the mark and precipitate serious withdrawal symptoms, including convulsions. The duration of antagonistic effect is considerably shorter than that of narcotics; the patient should be observed for a return of depression and the need for additional medication.

Pulmonary edema is an unpredictable and late event, occurring 24–36 hours after the overdose itself and unaffected by antagonist administration. This can be fatal, and all patients with a serious narcotic overdose should be watched over this period of time.

Propoxyphene overdose is becoming increasingly common and ranks second only to barbiturates as the most common prescription drug associated with drug fatalities (in all age groups). In most instances, overdose is motivated by suicidal intent, but inadvertent overdose can occur, particularly when abused in conjunction with other respiratory depressants such as alcohol.

Addiction and withdrawal. The narcotic addict experiences three states of consciousness over a span of 6–8 hours after taking a "fix" (dose); an initial "high" from the drug's psychotropic effects; being "straight" or physically comfortable but not intoxicated; and feeling "sick" or entering withdrawal. The withdrawal syndrome includes malaise, nervousness, jitteriness, anxiety, muscular aches and pains, abdominal cramps. diarrhea, piloerection, lacrimation, sweating and, in particularly severe instances, convulsions. The intensity of these symptoms is proportionate to the level of addiction and can vary from a mild flulike state to marked distress. Serious life-threatening consequences are rare, and full recovery can be expected within 7–10 days, even without intervention. At this time the patient is no longer addicted and has lost all tolerance. Overdose deaths among those who then return to their habit can easily occur due to miscalculation.

Medically supervised withdrawal is best carried out in a hospital setting by the substitution and

TABLE 20-2
PROPERTIES OF PSYCHOTROPIC DRUGS

Class	Addiction	Habituation	Tolerance	Risk of overdose death
Narcotics (heroin)	+	+	+	High
CNS depressants I (sedatives, tranquilizers, alcohol)	+*	+	±	High
CNS depressants II (volatile solvents, spray can propellants)	0	+	?	Variable[†]
CNS stimulants (cocaine, amphetamines)	+/0[‡]	+	+	Low
Hallucinogens I (LSD, mescaline, psilocybin)	0	+	+	Low [§]
Hallucinogens II (PCP)	0	+	+	Moderate [§]
Cannabis	0	+	+	Low/absent
Atropinic drugs	0	±	?	Low for adults
Nitrites	0	±	?	Low/absent[‖]

*When threshold dose exceeded.

[†] Significant toxicity with aerosol propellants (freon) only; individual may suffocate with any if plastic bag is used.

[‡] Controversial.

[§] May result in death due to reckless or violent acts while delusional.

[‖] May present significant risk to individual with cardiovascular disease but not to healthy person.

gradual tapering of another narcotic or, in mild cases, a tranquilizer. The patient experiences little if any discomfort. Methadone is the drug of choice in moderate to severe addictions (six to ten bags of heroin a day or more). It is long-acting and can be given by mouth. Sufficient amounts are given in the first 24 hours to alleviate withdrawal symptoms. An initial dose of 15–20 mg p.o. (or IM if vomiting) is followed by an additional 10–15 mg every 4 hours until the patient is stabilized. This total 24-hour amount is then reduced by 20% every day (or on alternate days if not tolerated) and given in two divided doses. Withdrawal will be completed within 5–10 days, depending on the schedule used.

Lesser degrees of addictions (three to five bags a day) can be effectively treated with diazepam (Valium), which renders mild withdrawal symptoms tolerable. A similar protocol to that with methadone employs an initial oral or IM dose of 10 mg followed by 5–10 mg more every 4 hours until the patient is comfortable. Tapering this total amount by 20% every day or on alternate days, given in three or four divided doses, follows accordingly.

Other complications. The major complications are consequent to injecting irritant adulterants and in-

fectious agents rather than to the drug itself. Hepatitis (all types have been reported, although type B predominates), tetanus, osteomyelitis, right-sided endocarditis, mycotic cerebral aneurysms, septicemia, local abscesses, cellulitis, pulmonary microemboli, and microinfarcts can occur.

CENTRAL NERVOUS SYSTEM DEPRESSANTS, GROUP I

Prototypes. Barbiturates, methaqualone, weak tranquilizers, alcohol.

Properties. These sedative drugs relieve anxiety, but do not have prominent analgesic or euphoric effects. Addiction occurs, but only if a minimum daily threshold is exceeded. This threshold is specific for each drug (secobarbital or pentobarbital, 400 mg; diazepam, 100 mg; meprobamate, 1600 to 2400 mg). Only limited tolerance results; after a moderate initial increase, the desired effect will be achieved without further dosage rise. Similarly, the lethal dose remains relatively unchanged. Cross-tolerance exists between all members, including alcohol.

Subjective effects. Low doses result in a pleasant sense of diminished tension, relaxation, and social

TABLE 20-3
ACUTE OVERDOSE REACTIONS: PHYSICAL SIGNS

Drug class	Mental status	Pulse rate	Respiratory rate	Blood pressure	Pupils	Temperature	Other
Narcotics	Lethargy → coma	↓	↓	No change	Pin point	No change	May have injection marks Responsive to naloxone
CNS depressants	"drunk" behavior → coma	↓	↓	No change	No change unless anoxic	No change	Nystagmus on lateral gaze Characteristic odor with alcohol
CNS stimulants	Agitation → paranoid psychosis	↑	↑	↑	Dilated (mild–moderate)	No change	Sometimes injection marks
Lysergic acid diethylamide	Detached → "bad trip"	↑	↑	↑	Dilated (mild–moderate)	No change	
Phencyclidine	Variable psychoses → coma	↑	↑ or ↓	↑; can be marked	Dilated (mild–moderate)	Elevated	Muscular rigidity, spasms; laryngeal stridor; rotatory nystagmus; ↓ perception of pain and touch; flushing; drooling
Atropinic drugs	Delirium → coma	↑	↓	No change or ↑	Dilated (marked)	Elevated	Marked flushing; dry hot skin; dry mucous membranes Responsive to physostigmine

facilitation. Slightly higher amounts decrease inhibitions; this is sometimes perceived as a "stimulant" effect, as the user becomes louder, more garrulous and impulsive, and exercises less than customary restraint. Moderate levels of intoxication produce sedation, drowsiness, stupor, and sleep; males will experience impotence. Large amounts can induce coma and death.

Objective signs. Objective signs parallel the amount taken; they vary from slurred speech, ataxia, impulsive behavior, and labile affect to stupor, semicoma, or coma. Pupils do not change unless the patient is anoxic; dilation may then occur. Sustained nystagmus on lateral gaze is characteristic. Alcohol ingestion may be differentiated by the typical breath odor.

Addiction and withdrawal. Addiction occurs when the threshold dose is exceeded on a daily basis. Withdrawal is potentially fatal and should be undertaken only in a hospital. If untreated, the withdrawal syndrome variably includes nervousness, jitteriness, agitation, insomnia, profuse perspiration, hallucinations, and toxic delirium (referred to as delirium tremens in the alcoholic). Severe forms can proceed

**TABLE 20-4
MANAGEMENT OF ACUTE
OVERDOSE REACTIONS: DEPRESSIVE**

Signs: Drowsiness, lethargy, stupor, semicoma, coma

Drugs that may be involved:
Narcotics
CNS depressants
Phencyclidine
Atropinic drugs

Immediate management
1. Check pulse and respirations.
2. Establish airway; detain accompanying persons.
3. Ensure ventilation; intubate and bag if necessary.
4. Establish IV line.
5. Gastric lavage.
6. Send blood, urine, gastric contents for toxicologic testing.*
7. Inquire of accompanying persons:
   a. What drug was taken? If not known, what is currently on the "street"?
   b. Are samples available?
   c. If suicidal o.d., are residual pills or container available?
   d. What was patient's immediate past behavior? Any definitive signs of what drug might have been used?
8. Examine for specific drug signs (see Table 20-3 and text).
9. Trial of specific therapy as indicated.
   Narcotics: naloxone.
   Phencyclidine: gastric drainage and acidification of urine; cool if fever marked.
   Atropinic drugs: Physostigmine; cool if fever marked.
10. Biologic supports until conscious.
11. If suicidal o.d., institute appropriate precautions.

---

*Note: Routine drug screen generally includes narcotics, stimulants, and depressants only. Test for atropine should be specifically requested. THC, LSD and PCP detection may be limited in availability.

---

to convulsions, fever, tachycardia, exhaustion, cardiovascular collapse, and death.

Detoxification is accomplished by substituting a barbiturate, regardless of the addicting agent. An initial oral dose of 200 mg of pentobarbital should be followed by a similar or adjusted dose every 6 hours in amounts sufficient to produce mild intoxication as evidenced by slurred speech, ataxia, and nystagmus on lateral gaze. Stabilization is maintained for the second 24 hours by repeating the total amount given the first day in four divided

doses. This is then decreased by 100 mg on each successive or alternate day as tolerated until the patient is fully withdrawn and drug free, a process taking between 10 and 21 days.

Overdose. Serious coma is most commonly encountered with sedatives and tranquilizers; it occurs less often with alcohol, although it may be a significant factor when taken simultaneously with other depressants. Preventing anoxia is the most urgent matter in managing severe overdose, followed by other steps as outlined in Table 20-4. Provided that the patient has not been hypoxic for an excessive period of time and is without irreversible brain damage before treatment, adequate ventilation, maintaining fluid and electrolyte balance, and other supportive measures should be sufficient to preserve normal functioning until metabolic processes clear the drug and consciousness returns. There are no specific antidotes of notable benefit. Dialysis has been employed in the most obtunded, but the evidence is scant that this significantly alters outcome.

Other complications. Oral intake of sedatives and tranquilizers is singularly devoid of other complications. An occasional report of bullous skin lesions has appeared. Alcohol has its own pathologic constellation with prolonged chronic use, but such complications are uncommonly seen in the adolescent; early cirrhosis may be encountered in the older youth who began drinking heavily at an early age. Users who employ intravenous routes of administration risk the same range of problems relative to contaminants and infections seen with narcotics. The major hazard of this class of drugs for adolescents is in the greatly enhanced potential for automotive accidents when driving while intoxicated.

CENTRAL NERVOUS SYSTEM DEPRESSANTS, GROUP II

Prototypes. Toluene (glue), trichloroethylene (cleaning fluids), fluorinated hydrocarbons and nitrous oxide (aerosol sprays), gasoline (leaded and unleaded).

Properties. Virtually any commercial product containing a psychoactive volatile substance has been sniffed at one time or another. Yet despite their diverse chemical nature, these substances have remarkably similar effects, producing CNS depression and varying levels of sedation. The major differences between group I and group II CNS depressants rest, first, in the method of administration; second in the brevity of the drug effect, group II being quickly excreted through the lungs; and, third, in the hallucinatory experiences reported by some users of group II drugs. Convincing evidence of tolerance or addiction has not been reported.

Subjective effects. Group II CNS depressants cause subjective effects similar to those of group I, with the additional occurrence in some but not all users of visual distortions, heightened visual imagery, and delusions.

Objective signs. Drowsiness, lethargy, ataxia, slurred speech, and characteristic odor to the breath are objective signs of group II use. Profound sedation is unlikely in that it is difficult to achieve and sustain sufficiently high concentrations for this to occur. A nonspecific rhinitis and bronchial irritation may be present.

Overdose. Coma or semicoma is seldom encountered. However, an idiosyncratic reaction to aerosol propellants containing fluoridinated hydrocarbons has resulted in sudden death and poses the greatest hazard in this class. The mechanism is thought to be similar to sudden anesthetic deaths, with anoxia and a myocardial sensitizing agent combining to produce ventricular fibrillation. Deaths also have resulted from suffocation when the plastic bag used for sniffing becomes sealed around the mouth and nose and the user fails to appreciate his or her impending anoxia. Sniffing from paper bags, balloons, or solvent-soaked cloths does not create a closed-circuit seal and will not produce this result. Some sniffers have also suffered serious and fatal injuries consequent to reckless acts while delusional.

Other complications. The use of trichlorethylene and related halogenated hydrocarbons, most often found in cleaning fluids, has been associated with hepatic and renal toxicity with organ failure on rare occasion; supportive measures generally result in full recovery. The sniffing of other commercial solvents has been singularly devoid of significant side effects except as mentioned for aerosols. All may produce transient nonspecific bronchial and nasal irritation. Toluene has produced a temporary mild proteinuria and increase in urinary RBCs and WBCs. Gasoline sniffing poses its greatest hazard when leaded; plumbism can occur. More hazardous solvents such as benzene and carbon tetrachloride have not been used commercially for a number of years and would not be encountered today.

CENTRAL NERVOUS SYSTEM STIMULANTS

Prototypes. Amphetamines, cocaine.

TABLE 20-5
MANAGEMENT OF ACUTE
OVERDOSE REACTIONS: PSYCHOTOMIMETIC

Signs: Agitation, restlessness, disorientation, detachment, hallucinations, delusions, paranoia, catatonia.

Drugs that may be involved
LSD, mescaline, psilocybin (rarely the latter two)
Phencyclidine
Atropinic drugs
CNS stimulants
Withdrawal from alcohol or barbiturate addiction
(rare in adolescents)

Immediate management
1. Place in quiet room with subdued lighting; detain accompanying friends.
2. Attempt to calm by reassuring verbal and tactile contact.
3. Avoid restraints and rapid, sudden movement if possible, but dangerous behavior must be contained.
4. Inquire of accompanying friends:
   a. What drug was taken? If not known, what is currently on the street?
   b. Are samples available?
   c. What was patient's immediate past behavior? Any definitive signs of what drug might have been used?
5. Examine for specific drug signs (see Table 20-3 and text).
6. Gastric lavage.
7. Send blood, urine, gastric contents for toxicologic testing.*
8. Trial of specific therapy as indicated.
   LSD: chlorpromazine, haloperidol.
   Phencyclidine: gastric drainage and acidification of urine; cool if fever marked.
   Atropinic drugs: Physostigmine; cool if fever marked.
   CNS stimulants: Chlorpromazine, haloperidol.
Note: Avoid phenothiazides if atropinic drugs may be involved. Use diazepam when in doubt.
9. Continue supportive and specific therapy until rational.

---

*Note: Routine drug screen generally will include narcotics, depressants, and stimulants only. Testing for atropine should be specifically requested. THC, LSD and PCP detection may be limited in availability.

Properties. CNS stimulants create generalized sympathomimetic activity and stimulate the central nervous system. The effects of cocaine are brief, a single dose lasting approximately 20 minutes compared to an hour or more for methamphetamine. Cocaine also is a local anesthetic and vasoconstricting agent. Tolerance regularly results with even small daily doses. Whether addiction occurs is unclear; some feel it does not, whereas others view the prolonged period of depression and lassitude often following an episode of protracted use to constitute addiction.

Subjective effects. Low to moderate doses produce a sense of well-being, alertness, increased energy, and enhanced powers of concentration, Appetite and fatigue are reduced. Sexual powers are purported to be enhanced. If the drug is injected intravenously, these feelings are introduced by a "rush." Higher drug concentrations, often achieved by serial injections, produce a sense of omnipotence, extraordinary mental powers, and unlimited inner energy.

Objective signs. Restlessness, agitation, garrulousness, emotional lability, and grandiose flights of ideas are common. Contact with reality is maintained, but feelings of omnipotence may appear as delusions. Physical signs include tremors, increased motor activity, a rise in blood pressure, tachycardia, and moderate pupillary dilation.

Overdose. Excessive amphetamine intake can result in a toxic paranoid psychosis. In most instances this clears in a few days. In some users, however, this reaction is prolonged or persistent. Because it generally presents as a psychiatric emergency, some caution needs to be exercised, as with hallucinogenic drugs, against misdiagnosis. Table 20-5 outlines management. Sedation through the use of strong tranquilizers is useful, although, here, as elsewhere, phenothiazines are contraindicated if atropinic drugs also might be present, as both possess anticholinergic activity, a combination that has resulted in cardiovascular collapse and death. Diazepam, 5–15 mg IM or IV, is a useful alternative. Caution also needs to be exercised in individuals who have sustained drug intoxication over several days. Upon cessation, the user commonly experiences a "crash." Initially, he or she is overwhelmed by sleep and, on awakening, is ravenously hungry. This is followed by a variable period of lassitude and depression that may be of sufficient magnitude to prompt suicidal behavior. Overdose deaths from amphetamines or cocaine are extremely rare, although convulsions, exhaustion, and cardiovascular collapse leading to death have been reported. Lethality may be enhanced when used in combination with other drugs.

Other complications. Persistent psychoses have followed toxic psychoses and represent a significant hazard. Administration by injection bears the same risk of contaminant effects as with narcotics. An early report of necrotizing angiitis among youthful polydrug users (with amphetamines predominating) has not been verified by others. Cocaine sniffing classically is associated with nasal perforation but is seldom seen among adolescents today, although nonspecific nasal irritation may readily occur. Otherwise the use of this class of drugs appears to be relatively devoid of serious medical consequences.

HALLUCINOGENS, GROUP I

Prototype. Lysergic acid diethylamide (LSD), mescaline (peyote), psilocybin.

Properties. Although primarily hallucinogenic, this group of drugs also possesses sympathomimetic properties. It should also be noted that drugs purporting to be mescaline or psilocybin are far more likely to be LSD or phencyclidine (PCP). Various other hallucinogens appear on the street from time to time and are alleged to produce a new and better "high." In some instances these are new compounds; in others they may be mixtures of substances already known (for example, LSD has been combined with amphetamines, atropinic drugs or both). The psychoactive results often fail to satisfy because they are too mild, unpredictable, or extended, and their popularity is usually short lived. But the possibility of substitution or adulteration always must be kept in mind in managing an adverse reaction. Tolerance readily occurs with frequent use but is easily lost upon 4–5 days' abstinence. Addiction has not been reported and withdrawal symptoms are not encountered.

Subjective effects. Feelings of depersonalization and derealization; distortion of visual imagery with heightened colors and shifting form; sensory distortions in "hearing" colors and "seeing" sounds; fluid and introspective mental processes, often assuming a mystical quality are common subjective effects. Delusions are also common and may result in serious injury. Outright visual hallucinations sometimes occur. Such sensations are usually experienced as pleasurable and desirable, the user being aware that he is in a drug-induced state and able to reestablish contact with reality at will (an important differential point between LSD and phencyclidine intoxication).

Objective signs. Mental status varies, with the user drifting in and out of the hallucinatory state, seemingly off in his or her own world at one moment and relating coherently to the observer the next, able to recount what he or she is seeing and thinking on request. Speech may be slurred and gait unsteady, but not invariably. Tachycardia, mild elevation of blood pressure, and mild to moderate mydriasis are evidence of sympathomimetic activity. Restlessness and agitation are less common, being countered by psychotomimetic self-preoccupations.

Overdose. True overdose reactions are rare. Some users have ingested enormous amounts with few untoward reactions beyond an extended intoxicated state. The most frequently encountered adverse effect is the idiosyncratic "bad trip," a state lasting from several hours to a day or more in which the perception of drug induction is lost and hallucinatory components become terrifying. Treatment consists of "talking down" the patient. He or she is placed in a quiet room with subdued lighting and continually reassured by an accompanying person (staff member, relative, or friend) that everything is all right, he is having a bad trip, it will pass, and someone will always be near to keep him safe. Gastric lavage may be indicated. The use of phenothiazides also can be helpful, but caution must be exercised against the possibility of coexisting atropinic drugs. When uncertain, diazepam is safe. Regardless of what tranquilizing agent is used, the amount should be adequate to the situation; low dosage may only inhibit available rational control and exacerbate hallucinations. A reasonable starting point would be 10–15 mg of diazepam or 100 mg of chlorpromazine three to four times a day, given p.o. or IM as best tolerated. (Also see Table 20-5.)

Other complications. The most commonly encountered adverse effect is that of flashbacks. Fragments of a previous drug experience will suddenly and unpredictably recur, lasting seconds to minutes each time. Sometimes flashbacks may be induced inadvertently by the use of another substance, commonly marijuana; in other instances they are spontaneous. Frequency varies from several times a day to once a week or less, usually tapering off and disappearing with time. The nature of the "flashback" may be pleasurable or the recapitulation of a "bad trip." They tend to occur most frequently in the novice user, although those who are more experienced are not immune. Treatment consists of supportive counseling and avoiding precipitating agents such as marijuana. Sedatives or tranquilizers are not particularly helpful due to the intermittent and relatively brief nature of each episode.

Considerable controversy surrounds the issue of genetic damage. Studies have shown LSD capable of producing mutagenesis in animals and leukocyte changes in humans, but the precise clinical significance is unknown. Reported consequences to infants born of LSD-using mothers vary, with some indicating a higher incidence of congenital abnormalities, others not. However, the weight of evidence now available suggests that persistent chromosomal damage or mutagenesis is not a major risk.

The question of permanent chemical alteration of mental processes also is under debate. Many heavy polydrug users, often with hallucinogens predominating, have certain personality traits in common. They care little about achievement, are passive and pacifistic, and often have a high investment in meditational religious alternatives and communal lifestyles—characteristics that have been termed the "amotivational syndrome." But the tendency toward these characteristics usually antecedes drug taking, suggesting that substance abuse is a result rather than cause. In addition to the possibility of self-harm while intoxicated, the most serious consequence of hallucinogenic use is the possibility of extended or persistent psychotic states. Although the consensus is that LSD usually has simply unmasked an underlying predisposition, a few apparently emotionally intact individuals have succumbed.

HALLUCINOGENS, GROUP II
Prototype. Phencyclidine (PCP).

Properties. Originally investigated for use in humans as an anesthetic agent (closely related to ketamine), PCP was soon abandoned because of unacceptable psychologic side effects. It continues to be legitimately manufactured for use in veterinary medicine but also can be easily made in underground laboratories. The major action of PCP appears to be a blockage of the perception, processing, and integration of external sensory stimuli. The user is limited in the ability to test and relate to reality, experiencing dissolution of ego boundaries and sensory isolation. The drug also possesses sympathomimetic activity and, in high doses, has an analeptic, strychninelike effect. Although primarily a CNS stimulant, exceedingly large amounts of PCP can depress respirations and produce coma. One of the more complicated aspects of this drug is the unpredictability and multiplicity of its effects and variability in manifestations, many of which can be severe. Veteran users seem to develop tolerance, requiring 50–75 mg to achieve the effect obtained with around 5 mg for most others. The capacity for addiction is as yet unknown.

Subjective effects. Low doses (1–5 mg) tend to produce a floating euphoria, sometimes associated with numbness, release of inhibitions, and emotional lability. Increased amounts (5–15 mg) gradually isolate the user from external stimuli and produce an excited, confused state in which the body is perceived in distorted form; sensations of pain and touch are markedly reduced and verbal communications are impaired. The individual feels suspended and isolated in empty space. At the 10 mg level and above, highly variable psychotic reactions emerge, appearing as either catatonia, manic catatonia, paranoia, or simple schizophrenia. These reactions tend to be more pronounced and more prolonged than with other hallucinogens, sometimes lasting days, weeks, or even months and may be indistinguishable from a nontoxic psychosis if the sometimes subtle physical signs are overlooked.

Objective signs. Observable signs relative to the patient's mental state parallel the subjective effects as previously described. Fever, drooling, rotatory nystagmus, diminished response to pain and touch, and sympathomimetic effects also may be seen in variable combination. The user commonly is agitated and restless, experiencing difficulty in establishing contact with others. He or she may become combative or assaultive or, alternatively, unresponsive and remote. Manifestations of intoxication are rather unpredictable and no single set of signs consistently predominate.

Overdose. Adverse reactions take one of two directions: a toxic psychosis or coma (although the former may progress to the latter over time with sufficient drug ingestion). In the first instance, any of a variety of psychotic behaviors, usually of an agitated nature, are evident. Sympathomimetic signs consequent to drug effect may not be singularly helpful to the diagnosis in that tachycardia, mildly elevated blood pressure, and mydriasis could be equally due to the patient's excitation. Rotatory nystagmus and fever, however, are almost pathognomonic signs if present. Muscular hyperreactivity consequent to PCP's analeptic action also can be a significant finding.

Higher PCP dosage may result in coma, with respiratory depression, laryngeal stridor, and increased muscle tone bordering on opisthotonous. Convulsions and severe muscle contractions can occur. This hyperreactivity is a significant finding in differentiating from coma due to other drugs. Hyperpyrexia also may be evident. Hypertensive crises with intracerebral hemorrhage or hypertensive encephalopathy have been reported. Death may result from respiratory arrest.

The vigor of treatment (see also Tables 20-4 and 20-5) in either form of overdose depends on the severity of the symptoms. In instances of agitated psychotic reactions and marked muscular hyperreactivity, external stimuli should be eliminated to the degree possible by placing the patient in a quiet and dimly lighted room and avoiding restraints and unnecessary procedures; ear plugs may be helpful.

The use of tranquilizers is controversial. Diazepam, 5–15 mg p.o., IM or IV, has been beneficial in some cases. Haloperidol, 3–5 mg p.o. or IM, also may be used, although its antipsychotic effect may be minimal. Caution should be exercised in using any tranquilizer in serious overdose situations where coma and respiratory depression is possible. It also needs to be kept in mind that strong tranquilizers are relatively ineffective in assisting the patient to reorganize his or her mental processes as they do in non-drug-related psychoses. Failure to improve on medication may be misinterpreted as a particularly unresponsive schizophrenic break and even larger doses given. This is particularly true of the phenothiazides, which do not lead to mental reorganization and may even exacerbate the situation, making the toxic psychosis worse. (This outcome thus contraindicates their use.) It is highly likely that a number of adolescents have been misdiagnosed in this manner and institutionalized as schizophrenics. The increasing availability of laboratory testing for PCP and physician alertness to this possibility should preclude such mistakes. A blood specimen for hallucinogen analysis should always be drawn in any psychotic state: this should include tetrahydrocannabinol (THC) and lysergic acid diethylamide (LSD) as well as PCP.

Metabolic clearance of the drug should be promoted by capitalizing on the pharmacokinetics of PCP; it is secreted in considerable amounts by gastric mucosa and recycled through intestinal absorption; it is also excreted in large amounts in an acid urine. In serious overdose reactions, gastric lavage should be performed, followed by the instillation of a saline laxative (15 g sodium sulfate) and, after 1 hour to allow for its action, continuous gastric drainage until conscious. Urine should be acidified with ammonium chloride (2.75 mEq/kg/dose) administered in 60 ml of saline through the nasogastric tube, waiting 1 hour for absorption before resuming suction, and with ascorbic acid given intravenously (2 g/500 ml IV fluid); this schedule should be repeated every 6 hours as necessary to achieve and maintain a urinary pH below 5. Diuresis is encouraged through the use of furosemide (20–40 mg IM or IV). Attention also needs to be given to fluid and electrolyte balance and replacement of drainage loss. Improvement of the patient's mental state should be quickly apparent if one is on the right track. Premature discontinuation of therapy should be avoided lest coma recur as PCP is released from storage sites. Urinary acidification with cranberry juice and p.o. ascorbic acid should be continued throughout the patient's hospital stay. Milder forms of intoxication can be treated with gastric lavage, p.o. ascorbic acid, cranberry juice, laxatives, and copious fluids alone.

Other complications. Serious personal injury to self or others can occur. Some users have remained in extended psychotic states. Here again the question of permanent drug effect versus preexisting vulnerability is raised; most favor the latter cause. No other complications have as yet been identified, although the appearance of PCP on the drug scene is sufficiently recent to preclude long-term observations. Various psychiatric manifestations mark the chronic user, including anxiety, agitated states, severe depression, and paranoia.

CANNABIS

Prototypes. Marijuana, hashish, tetrahydrocannabinol (THC).

Properties. Delta-9-tetrahydrocannabinol (THC) is the psychoactive compound present in all members of this class. It is a component of the resin secreted by flowering tops of the plant *Cannabis sativa*. The resin drips onto the upper leaves, which are harvested, dried, and marketed as marijuana. Pure resin scraped from the leaves and formed into solid brown blocks of material is hashish, or "hash"; small flakes are pared off and most commonly smoked in a pipe. Pure THC is a brown viscous liquid prepared from hashish. Production is complicated and costly. Street drugs alleged to be pure THC are either "hash oil," a relatively recent introduction consisting of a concentrated extract of marijuana, some other hallucinogen such as LSD or PCP, or wholly inert. It also is common to adulterate marijuana or the paper in which it is rolled with other substances to enhance the user's experience. Here again, PCP or LSD are most frequently encountered, although atropine, formaldehyde, and a wide range of other substances have been reported. If atypical or unusually profound reactions are encountered, a dual drug effect should be considered.

All cannabis preparations are potentially hallucinogenic, although common usage falls short of this

mark. Marked variation in the drug experience also is introduced by the unpredictable and highly variable potency of the preparation used. Street marijuana, however, has increased markedly in strength over the past few years. In 1975 few samples exceeded 1% THC concentration. Currently, 5% is not uncommon. Hash oil commonly contains 15%–20% THC, with as much as 28% reported in some samples. Sufficient amounts of pure THC can produce a response indistinguishable from that produced by LSD. All forms also are mildly sympathomimetic. Tolerance rapidly develops but is quickly lost on abstention. Addiction does not occur.

Subjective effects. Highly dependent on the conditions under which the plant was grown (determining the amount of psychoactive material produced) and on the experience and expectations of the user, marijuana may produce little more than nausea and dizziness in the novice to a happier experience in those who are more accomplished. In the latter instance there is a vivid and pleasurable alteration of perception and an intensification of visual imagery. All sensory modalities are heightened. Time perception slows, limbs feel light, and mood is euphoric, often manifesting in silliness and outbursts of uncontrollable laughter. Lower doses potentiate social interaction, whereas higher amounts tend to make the user more introspective. Hashish produces similar but more intense effects.

Objective signs. Physical signs are minimal. A dose-related tachycardia and conjunctival injection may be the only findings of note. However, verbal output, short-term memory, reading comprehension, abstract concept formation, counting, and color discrimination may all be impaired, counseling against even casual use on school days. A significant increase in braking time and delayed recovery from headlight glare at night are definitive contraindications for driving while intoxicated. Motor performance is also compromised; the contents of one-half to one marijuana cigarette produce about the same degree of impairment as three bottles of beer or 3 ounces of 100-proof whiskey.

Overdose and adverse reactions. The most common adverse reaction is an acute anxiety episode, sometimes to the point of panic. This usually is associated with the consumption of unexpectedly strong material. Individuals with preexisting serious psychiatric problems may experience exacerbation of this difficulty. Those who have previously had bad trips or flashbacks with LSD may reexperience them, with marijuana acting as a triggering agent. Hash oil or hashish of sufficient THC concentration may produce bad trips or flashbacks in and of itself.

Serious reactions, however, are rare. Marked toxicity or death attributed to marijuana is more likely to be consequent to adulterants as previously noted. The user commonly is ignorant of contamination with other drugs; if coma or toxic delirium is encountered, the examiner should look for signs of other agents as well as THC. Samples of blood and, if available, marijuana and cigarette paper from the implicated batch should be sent for laboratory analysis. Testing for all drugs, including the hallucinogens, is increasingly available today.

Medical complications. Occasional use of fewer than one to two joints of marijuana per week probably has few risks, but increasing evidence points to significant hazards when consumption is on a regular basis. The clearest risk is to pulmonary function; the consequences are similar to those caused by smoking tobacco. Consequences may be even greater in heavy users, because the absence of filtration and the practice of deep, prolonged inhalations to promote absorption of psychoactive material also promote deposition of tars and other particulate material in the lungs. The consumption of less than one joint a day has been noted to reduce vital capacity to the same degree as smoking 16 cigarettes per day. Chronic laryngitis, cough, hoarseness, bronchitis, and other symptoms marking the heavy cigarette smoker have been noted in marijuana users as well.

Evidence for deleterious effects on the male and female reproductive tract is less clear. A modest reduction in total sperm count, impaired motility, and abnormal sperm morphology have been reported among males during chronic use. These changes reverse to normal after several weeks of absention. Women smoking marijuana three times a week or more for at least 6 months have been noted to have a higher frequency of anovulatory menstrual cycles and lower prolactin levels than normal. Other drug use and life-style factors, however, also may have been contributory or even causal. These findings suggest that heavy marijuana smoking may interfere with fertility or fetal normalcy. To date this is purely conjectural. There are no reports suggesting a higher rate of infertility among marijuana users intending pregnancy or a greater incidence of congenital abnormalities among their offspring. Studies on marijuana-induced chromosomal abnormalities are contradictory and of questionable clinical significance.

Other reported effects, including the observation that high concentrations of THC suppress the immune response in laboratory animals, also are uncertain in their practical application. Reports of such effects in humans, however, are much more contradictory, and clinical implications remain in doubt. No epidemiologic studies have been carried out to establish whether there is a higher incidence of infections or other diseases attributable to marijuana use. THC also has been noted to inhibit DNA, RNA, and protein synthesis in tissue cell culture. Here again there is no evidence that this has significance for human use, and any such conjectures are speculative at best.

A 1971 report from Great Britain implicating cannabis with brain atrophy in a small group of poly-drug-using youths was faulty on a number of grounds and has not been borne out by further studies. Not only is there no gross evidence of any permanent brain effect, but detailed testing has failed to detect any lasting impairment of neuropsychologic performance or electroencephalographic abnormality.

In summary, the primary medical risks of marijuana use as recognized today (1982) relate to the respiratory tract with consequences similar to those of smoking tobacco. The true clinical implications or other reported consequences remain unconfirmed or obscure. Most significantly, no irreversible effects on neuropsychologic performance have been noted. Although the amotivational syndrome (a controversial entity) frequently has been attributed to heavy cannabis use, most of the evidence points to the prior existence of such characteristics predisposing the youth to habituation.

ATROPINIC DRUGS
Prototypes. Scopolamine, atropine.

Properties. These alkaloids are available either in pure chemical form, obtained from pharmaceutical sources, or as natural plant material, primarily deadly nightshade and jimson weed. The latter is ubiquitous in the southwest United States. Effects are achieved through smoking or ingestion. All members of this class inhibit parasympathetic autonomic effectors by antagonizing the muscarinic action of acetylcholine. Toxic doses first stimulate and then depress the central nervous system. Tolerance and addiction are not factors in use.

Subjective effects. Taken primarily for their hallucinogenic and excitatory effects, atropinic drugs also produce sensations of giddiness, disorientation, and confusion. The propensity for disorientation and confusion in combination with pronounced systemic effects (palpitations, blurred vision, headache, dry and hot skin, dry mouth, difficulty in urination) tend to preclude widespread or chronic use.

Objective signs. Excitation, confusion, and restlessness regularly occur. Characteristic signs are tachycardia, extreme mydriasis unresponsive to light, marked flushing, fever, and dry skin and mucous membranes. Muscular incoordination, weakness, and slurred speech may be evident.

Overdose. Excessive intake most often presents as a toxic delirium, sometimes with convulsions. A misdiagnosis of schizophrenia may be made, but the associated anticholinergic effects should be an effective tipoff if looked for. Larger amounts can produce CNS depression, falling blood pressure, paralysis, respiratory failure, and coma. Death has been encountered among children but is rare among adolescents and adults.

Management of milder forms of intoxication are simply supportive. Ice packs and alcohol rubs can be used for hyperpyrexia. Toxic delirium or CNS depression is rapidly improved by the use of physostigmine (1-4 mg in adults and 0.5-1.0 mg in children given by slow intravenous injection). As atropinic drugs are singularly long-acting and physostigmine particularly short-acting, repeated dosage may be necessary every 1-2 hours until improvement is sustained. (Also see Tables 20-4 and 20-5.)

In patients exhibiting excitation, agitation, or convulsions, IM or IV diazepam, 5-10 mg, also can be used. Large or repeated doses should be used with great caution lest their effects coincide with progression of the toxic state to CNS depression. Phenothiazides should *never* be used. Their muscarinic action will intensify the overdose effect and can precipitate coma, respiratory collapse, and even death.

Other complications. No other complications have been identified, and complete recovery from a toxic overdose can be expected if the patient has not been anoxic overlong. Chronic, repeated use is rarely encountered and consequences unknown.

NITRITES
Prototypes. Amylnitrite, isobutyl nitrite.

Properties. Nitrites produce nonspecific relaxation of all smooth muscles and pronounced cardiovascular effects. Hypotension can be marked consequent to a decrease in both central venous and systemic arterial pressures. An initial increase in cardiac output is followed by a precipitous fall. Relatively small doses produce syncope when the individual is in an upright position.

Subjective effects. Subjective effects closely parallel those sensations encountered in fainting. Users of nitrites describe a sudden and brief, pleasurable tingling—a jolt, high, or rush. Associated feelings of bursting chest and pounding heart are common. Some also report a sense of impending doom, others of exhilaration. Many users experience a prolonged, severe headache as well.

Overdose. Overdose has not been reported, although the severe headache and distressing cardiac sensations may be perceived as such by the user.

Other complications. No serious complications are known. The only significant hazard is among those with preexisting heart disease, in whom sudden alterations in cardiac output and arterial pressure could have adverse effects.

LABORATORY DIAGNOSIS OF DRUG USE
Laboratory testing is frequently regarded as a source of definitive diagnosis; however, some caution should be exercised in employing this resource and interpreting results. First, one must know what the laboratory will be testing for. "Routine drug screens," usually performed by thin layer chromatography, may be limited to narcotics, CNS stimulants, and CNS depressants. Commonly, quinine is included as this is a common diluent of heroin and may be present when the narcotic itself is undetectable. Hallucinogens (lysergic acid diethylamide (LSD)), phencyclidine (PCP), and tetrahydrocannabinol (THC) are present in body fluids in very small amounts and require specialized gas chromatographic techniques for detection; these may be available only in selected laboratories, although recent technical advances have facilitated the detection of these substances and analysis is more widely available today than heretofore. Specific inquiry should be made as to what drugs the laboratory can test for and, in any event, some indication should be given as to the class of drugs under clinical suspicion.

Secondly, testing results must be interpreted in light of the suspected patterns of use. Detecting a drug obviously depends upon the length of time between administration of the last dose and obtaining the specimen to be tested. Sufficient clearance will have been accomplished for most drugs after only 3–5 days' abstinence, rendering detection impossible. Further, the presence of a drug on such a screen means only that the user had that particular substance in his or her system at one point in time; it says nothing about the amount or duration of use or the possible consumption of other drugs. Nor can testing differentiate between the one-time experimenter or confirmed, chronic abuser.

Urine, blood, and gastric contents are all suitable materials for testing.

MEDICAL DETECTION OF DRUG USE IN ADOLESCENCE

Physicians may well be presented with an adolescent suspected of using drugs by parents and police or school authorities and asked to examine the youth to determine the true state of affairs. This is a perilous business. First, to accede to such a request places the physician in the unacceptable position of being a policeman, making it difficult to gain the youngster's confidence and trust so essential to effecting a constructive therapeutic alliance. Second, it is an impossible task. Few physical signs are evident unless the individual actually is intoxicated, and adolescents rarely present themselves to the physician's office in this state. In the absence of concurrent intoxication, the physical examination is singularly unrewarding. Only regular users of injection methods reveal puncture sites, needle tracks, or skin popping ulcers, and these are not common findings among teenagers today. The reddened conjunctivae seen with marijuana use are non-specific as are the nasal and bronchial irritation seen with the smoking, sniffing, or inhaling of any drug; perforation of the nasal septum consequent to cocaine is rare. Psychosocial evaluation may indeed reveal a youth who could be vulnerable to drug abuse, but this does not necessarily mean drugs actually are involved.

The limitation of toxicologic investigation through laboratory means has already been commented on. Few other laboratory tests are particularly revealing. Some liver enzymes, particularly serum γ-glutamyl transpeptidase (SGPT), may be elevated in chronic heroin users; proteinuria sometimes is present in those who sniff glue. Elevated SGPT levels also have been found in adolescents who consume six drinks of alcohol or more each day.

Psychologic Aspects of Drug and Alcohol Abuse in Adolescence

The use of drugs or alcohol that extends beyond experimental, social, or recreational motivations to the point of abuse is not a disease in and of itself but rather is symptomatic of some basic emotional problem. Drug abuse rarely stands alone, and a variety of other dysfunctional behaviors usually coexist, including delinquency, acting-out, promiscuous sexual activity, running away, or truancy. Excepting opportunity, peer group use, and drug availability, few indicators are predictive of drug abuse exclusively. Rather there is a constellation of factors suggestive of an adolescent at risk for any of a number of behavioral problems, drug abuse being but one. It is, however, a particularly seductive option in providing instant and passive surcease from anxiety.

The incidence of significant drug abuse is considerably less than the news media and the emotionalism surrounding this issue would lead us to believe. Although some 70% of adolescents drink socially by their senior year in high school and 40% have tried marijuana, with 5%–10% using it on a regular basis, fewer than 10% have used other substances to any significant degree and fewer than 1% of all adolescents develop definitive habituation. Use is ubiquitous; abuse considerably more contained.

Casual use of any substance does not in and of itself lead to abuse; this is a rare event in youngsters who have little predisposing risk. Low-risk adolescents usually can experiment with impunity and parental alarms can be put to rest except for three concerns. First is the serious problem of automotive safety in driving while intoxicated with alcohol or drugs. Second is the significant potential for serious adverse effects with even the one-time use of strong hallucinogens, LSD and phencyclidine in particular. Third is the conjectural argument that anything more than very occasional use (once a month or less) may be to any teenager's developmental disadvantage. Normal maturation involves the cyclical build up and resolution of tension between the security of well-known and practiced childhood dependency responses, on the one hand, and drives for moving on to new, but as yet poorly perceived and untested levels of function on the other hand. Healthy resolution rests in taking on this new challenge despite its associated uncertainties and progressing to a more advanced degree of maturity. Regular weekly intoxication, even if only on a social or recreational basis, bears a potential for ablating this tension and blunting the maturational drive. The consequences could be persistent immaturity and childish behavior at a time when its surrender is critical to growing up.

High-risk adolescents not only are vulnerable to the same problems previously cited, but to abuse, habituation, and/or addiction as well. The particular pattern of substance use depends on what is in vogue, what is available, how much it costs, and the youth's own drug preferences. A good number of youngsters, particularly those with major emotional problems, become polydrug users, taking anything and everything that comes their way.

Although alcohol use among adolescents is widespread, alcoholism is not commonly seen. It takes between 5 and 7 years of committed drinking for alcoholism to result, and a youngster would have to start a heavy habit at an early age for manifestations to appear before the teen years are completed. On the other hand, a number of reports indicate singularly vulnerable individuals can succumb to alcoholism in a considerably shorter period of time; some persons are said to be at risk with even a single drink. The precise etiology of this unique predisposition is unknown but is believed to relate to genetically determined, metabolic factors. Adolescents in this category theoretically are as vulnerable as adults, although no specific studies have been carried out.

Barbiturate addiction also is relatively uncommon in teenage years in that a rather large threshold dose must be exceeded on a daily basis over a number of weeks—an infrequent pattern of intake for teenagers. However, the use and abuse of sedatives and tranquilizers to a point short of addiction is common. Easy availability, low cost, and the frequent use by parents and other adult role models makes this class of drugs acceptable and attractive. It also appears that the effects of central nervous system depressants, whether sedatives, tranquilizers, or alcohol, tend to be preferred. Although many drug fads come and go, young people always seem to return to those which simply ablate anxiety and inhibit superego control without dysphoric or dissociative effects.

Narcotic addiction occurs with relatively short periods of low-dose intake. The production of euphoria as well as anxiety ablation is a compelling motivation. However, the well-advertised problems of addiction and the difficulty of obtaining a supply of heroin that has not been excessively cut at an affordable price have dramatically decreased the number of youthful addicts in recent years.

DIAGNOSIS

The primary care health provider may encounter a possible drug problem in a number of circumstances: as a discovery during a routine health maintenance evaluation, as a suspicion raised by parents or school, as a companion to other dysfunctional behaviors, as the confidential confession of the youth who wishes help, or as the underlying problem of an adolescent presenting to the emergency room with an overdose.

**TABLE 20-6
SIGNIFICANT RISK FACTORS
PREDICTIVE OF DRUG OR
ALCOHOL ABUSE IN ADOLESCENTS**

1. Peer group members known to use drugs and/or alcohol excessively.
2. A member of an ethnic group in which alcohol plays a significant cultural role among adults.
3. Family history of alcoholism, drug abuse, and/or addiction.
4. Family history of *strict* teetotalism.
5. Evidence of other dysfunctional behaviors, school problems, and/or home conflict.
6. Mood or affect chronically depressed, anxious, or angry.
7. Past history of poor adaptation to stress; ineffective coping mechanisms.
8. Poor self-esteem; sense of hopelessness and futility about future; no perception of what will be doing or wants to do 5-10 years hence.
9. Realistically few future options; for example, an inner city youth with inadequate education, lacking job skills, and facing high unemployment rates.
10. Ready availability of drugs and/or alcohol in community.

Any adolescent should be assessed for risk (Table 20-5) as a part of regular health care. Suggestive findings from the standard psychosocial evaluation will make possible more discriminating inquiry. But a word of caution. Of all adolescent behavior patterns, drug use is the least likely to be revealed readily. Denial is common even with the most skilled interviewing until trust is absolute.

Peer patterns of drug use are much more easily discussed and offer a good place to start, particularly in light of the high correlation between the patient's own behavior and that of his or her peer group. Specifically the interviewer might ask if any of the patient's friends use drugs, what ones, how much, and how often; do any of his or her friends have a drug problem and what does the patient think of this; are drugs going around in the school and/or neighborhood and would he or she be able to purchase them if he or she wished? The adolescent who has close friends who use drugs, perceives drug use as prevalent in school, knows where to obtain them, and does not perceive the drug use by others as a problem, either has used drugs or soon will. Table 20-7 cites more definitive indicators that a drug problem may exist.

The interviewer can then begin direct questioning about the patient's own level of involvement, starting with marijuana. Here the special interviewing techniques discussed in Chapter 23 are essential.

TABLE 20-7
INDICATORS THAT AN ADOLESCENT
MAY BE ABUSING DRUGS OR ALCOHOL

1. The presence of any of the risk factors cited in Table 20-6.
2. Increasingly poor adjustment and deterioration of function at home, school, and/or among peers.
3. Increasing emotional lability with rapid mood swings from excessive gaity to rage, but an undercurrent of increasing depression, irritability, and restlessness.
4. Increasingly secret behavior; longer periods of time spent in own room; locking of bedroom door if not a previous pattern; longer periods away from home with refusal to be accountable.
5. Deterioration in personal hygiene and dress.
6. Alteration of usual schedule; sleeping longer, staying up well after parents in bed, increasing tardiness in getting to places, episodic truancy from school.
7. Episodes of suspicious behavior suggesting intoxication associated with vigorous denial: slurred speech, unsteady gait, inappropriate silliness or giggling, unusual drowsiness or excessive daydreaming, flights of grandiose ideas and philosophic musings, garrulousness, restlessness and unusual energy, bizarre behavior of any sort.
8. The finding of any drug paraphernalia such as needles or syringes, usually secreted in some private place in the patient's room; unexplained pills, powders, or glassine bags (as used for postage stamp collecting); beer/whiskey bottles or cans secreted in patient's room; lowering levels of contents of family liquor supply.
9. Disappearing family money or valuables; unusual amounts of money in the patient's possession (he or she may be pushing drugs to provide own source of supply).

TABLE 20-8
DIAGNOSTIC CRITERIA OF ALCOHOLISM

1. Physiologic dependence (addiction) as manifested by the appearance of withdrawal symptoms somewhere between the first and third day of abstinence.
2. Evidence of tolerance. Some alcoholics defy pharmacologic principles of depressant drugs and are capable of ingesting large amounts with little apparent effect; the consumption of one-fifth of a gallon of whiskey or equivalent without evidence of intoxication is virtually diagnostic.
3. Alcoholic "blackouts" (failure to remember what happened while intoxicated).
4. Continued drinking despite strong social contraindications such as loss of job, expulsion from educational program, arrest, harm to family members due to drinking.
5. Continued drinking despite strong medical contraindications.
6. The presence of one or more associated medical conditions such as alcoholic hepatitis or cirrhosis, chronic gastritis, nutritional deficiency diseases (anemia, neuritis, etc.), alcoholic psychosis.
7. Subjective feelings by the individual that he has lost control of drinking.
8. Characteristic behavior patterns: gulping drinks, surreptitious drinking, morning drinking, repeated episodes of remorse and attempts at abstinence, frequent excuses from school or work on false medical excuses, loss of interest in other activities, frequent accidents, emotional lability.
9. Blatant indiscriminate use of alcohol with deterioration in all social functions: slovenly dress, poor hygiene, skid-row existence with or without signs of psychosis are advanced signs.

Patients must feel that the physician will fully respect their confidentiality and that the sole intent is to assess whether they need help. "Most young people today try out marijuana at least once. Where do you stand on this issue?" can be a productive introduction to the topic. Once patients perceive that marijuana use will be accepted nonjudgmentally, they usually feel sufficiently trusting to discuss this and other drug intake patterns in some detail.

Drinking behavior is far easier to ascertain. There is little secretiveness in that alcohol does not have the same connotation of illegality as illicit drugs; it even has assumed cultural validation as a rite of pubertal passage. Here, too, the primary care physician should establish if an adolescent drinks, when, how often, how much, and whether any of the signs of abuse or alcoholism are present (Tables 20-7 and 20-8).

Parents often bring an adolescent to the physician with the suspicion that he or she has a drug problem. They may have found pills, marijuana, or other drug materials in the patient's room or clothing, may be concerned because his or her close friends are known to use drugs, or may have noticed some sort of suggestive change in the adolescent. These mothers and fathers usually fear the worst and are verging on panic. They expect the physician to confirm their fears and look to him or her to persuade the patient to stop. It is essential not to get caught up in being detective and judge. Although the parents may want the physician to play such a role, the adolescent will perceive the doctor who does so only as an adversary, a parental ally, and an agent of societal retribution. No therapeutic rela-

TABLE 20-9
SIGNIFICANT FACTORS IN DIFFERENTIATING BETWEEN
SUBSTANCE USE, ABUSE, AND HABITUATION IN ADOLESCENCE*

	Use	Abuse	Habituation
Setting	Social groups	Social groups and/or alone	Social groups and/or alone
Time	Evenings, weekends	Anytime	Anytime including before and during school
Drugs used	Alcohol and marijuana predominantly; some minimal experimentation with other drugs if in vogue (e.g., cocaine, CNS depressants)	All substances possible; polydrug use common	Commitment to one particular substance; unable to function without intake. May supplement with other substances.
Frequency	Intermittent; less than 1 time per week	Regular; weekly or more often	Daily
Amount	Same as friends; one to two drinks or marijuana joints of an evening	More than friends; significant level of intoxication sought each time	Sufficient to maintain a constant level of drug effect (in intent, if not in actuality, due to limiting environmental factors).
Purpose	Socialization, relaxation, experimentation, recreation	To achieve intoxication, relieve anxiety	To maintain intoxication, relieve escalation of tension on abstinence, relieve anxiety from other sources
Complications†	Unintentional excessive intoxication.	Blackouts/passing out with alcohol, habituation, addiction, overdose	As for abuse

*Not all factors need to be present for a pattern to qualify under any one of the three categories of consumption, but a dominant theme usually emerges.

†Any use, regardless of category, poses certain risks; for example, untoward reactions with strong hallucinations, medical complications if administered by the intravenous or subcutaneous route, impaired judgment and reaction time when intoxicated with particular hazards for driving a car.

tionship can be established under these circumstances. This needs to be clearly stated to parents and confidentiality rules firmly laid down.

Regardless of presentation, once the possibility or actuality of substance abuse has been raised, subsequent action depends upon the following assessment:

1. Is the patient in the significant risk category (Table 20-6)?

2. Does he or she use alcohol or drugs. What is the pattern of intake: heavy user, abuser, or habituated (Table 20-9)?

3. If the patient is at risk but denies use, does he or she exhibit any suggestive behaviors (Table 20-7)?

4. Is there evidence of narcotic or barbiturate addiction or of alcoholism (Table 20-8 and as suggested in the previous section on pharmacologic aspects)?

Keep in mind that there are few distinctive physical signs unless the patient is intoxicated at the time of examination or evidences such specific findings as needle marks, related infections, or adverse side effects such as flashback phenomena. Also remember that drug screens of blood or urine are not always revealing; the substance in question must have been taken within the previous few days and be a type the laboratory is equipped to detect.

In any event, laboratory detection has its primary role in diagnosing and managing a drug overdose or monitoring individuals in a drug-free therapeutic community. It has a lesser place in the diagnosis of drug-abusing behavior in that it tends to introduce compromising confrontation and mistrust into the therapeutic relationship. If an abusing adolescent initially denies having a problem, the truth only can come through establishing sufficient trust to encourage voluntary honesty. A coercively

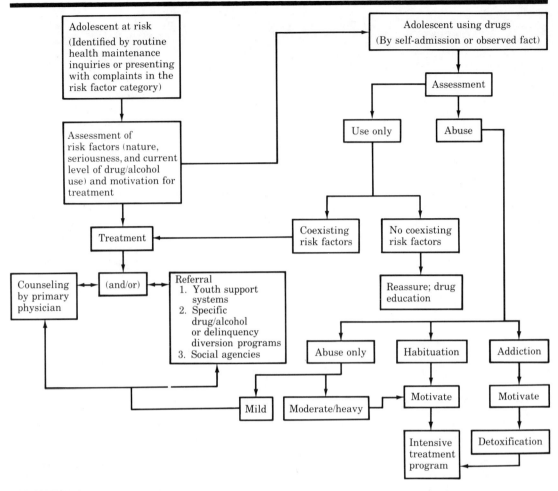

FIGURE 20-1
MANAGING DRUG OR ALCOHOL ABUSE IN ADOLESCENCE

or surreptitiously obtained urine test is not particularly helpful to this end. Even if test results are positive, the adolescent may well still deny intake or attribute this to a one-time experiment and the physician is back at ground zero.

MANAGEMENT

Figure 20-1 presents the management approach. An adolescent who proves to be a user but without significant risk factors should be reassured as to his or her emotional health and provided appropriate drug counseling and education. All young people should be aware of the legal prohibitions against marijuana possession and of drinking under age, as well as the great dangers of driving while intoxicated or riding

as a passenger with an intoxicated driver, whether the intoxication is due to alcohol or marijuana. They also should have honest, unbiased facts about the effects of drugs and alcohol as currently known. Younger adolescents in particular would be well advised to abstain from any mind-altering substances; they need all of their faculties unimpaired and a clear head for optimal maturation. Older adolescents who feel they cannot make a commitment to abstain until adulthood should consider limiting themselves to no more than monthly intake and this in modest amounts.

The management plan for an adolescent at risk begins with counseling and educational measures for minimal involvement and is expanded through the use of various community resources as seriousness increases. Any plan, however, must take the following into account:

1. The underlying psychologic problem(s) that gave rise to abuse in the first place.

2. The frequency of patient denial and the youth's perception that he or she can stop using drugs at will.

3. The common absence of patient motivation for treatment.

4. The possible complications of habituation and/or addiction.

5. Possible medical complications when injection routes are used.

6. Possible idiosyncratic responses to strong hallucinogens, for example, "flashbacks," "bad trips," and persistent psychoses.

Adolescents at risk or those in the early stages of abuse who are not habituated or addicted (Table 20-9) may benefit from programs similar to those recommended for predelinquent and early delinquent behavior (see Chapter 24). Specific drug diversion programs often offered by schools and various youth-serving agencies can be particularly helpful. Information may be obtained from local boards of education, school guidance offices and psychologists, Boys' and Girls' Clubs, YMCAs and YWCAs, city and state departments of health and mental health, and/or offices of drug addiction or narcotics control. Regional residential treatment programs for serious drug abuse specifically or mental health problems in general also may have suitable community outreach or day programs.

Alcoholics Anonymous has branches in most communities and can advise about resources for alcohol abuse. AA also offers a support system for young people with alcoholic parents through Alateen or for a spouse in Alanon. Regional councils on alcoholism as well as the resources listed previously for drug abuse also may have useful information.

Well-established abuse, particularly if complicated by habituation or committed polydrug use, is best treated in drug-free residential or intensive daycare programs. Odyssey House and Daytop Village are national prototypes, but any community where drug addiction has been a problem probably will have a variety of such resources. Long-term methadone maintenance for narcotic addiction is not a treatment option for adolescents.

Residential programs offer particular benefit by insulating the youth from environmental influences while providing a well-defined treatment plan, usually lasting from 12–24 months. Although traditional psychotherapy using the analytic approach has proven of little help in drug abuse, the highly structured program combining behavior modification principles with encounter group therapy offered by these centers has been found effective. The latter consists of regular weekly or semiweekly sessions in which group members let their feelings "all hang out" about the behavior of one particular member selected as target, either in rotation or because of particular need. The one under scrutiny then has a chance to put forth his or her views. Finally, the group spells out just how the individual could do better, and he or she is offered the love, encouragement, and support of all participants.

The overall program usually is divided into three different stages: induction, an introductory period of about 2 months; treatment, lasting a year or more; and reentry, consisting of several months of increasing community involvement and making specific plans for the future. Each stage has a particular set of goals that slowly move the individual up a well-defined ladder of increasing responsibility and privileges. At any point, failure to meet responsibility may be dealt with by encounter group process, the withdrawal of various privileges, and specific punishments. Some programs use humiliating techniques such as making the culprit wear a dunce cap, hanging a sign marking the transgression around his or her neck, or shaving the head. No program has locked doors, and a resident is free to elope at any time. Indeed, half of all who enter drop out in the first few months, finding the discipline, structure, isolation from family and past friends, and absence of drugs intolerable. Although many of these dropouts ultimately return, it often takes a "bottoming out" experience for effective motivation. This could be getting into trouble with the law and facing residential treatment or jail, a serious overdose experience, the death of a friend from an overdose, or harm to another or self because of intoxication. Once a resident has endured for 3–4 months, the outlook for a good rehabilitative outcome becomes promising.

Residential treatment programs vary greatly in their level of competence and should be checked out before referral. Those with trained mental health staff in addition to staff coming from the ranks of former residents (a common occurrence) are best equipped to cope with the difficult, multiproblemed adolescent.

Youths who are addicted or alcoholic will need to be detoxified before entering a treatment program. This is best accomplished in a hospital, preferably on a ward devoted to this purpose. If none is available, detoxification can be accomplished on an adolescent psychiatric or medical floor. Therapy through tapered replacement (specific regimens will be found in the first section) keeps the patient quite comfortable, and he or she poses little danger to self or others. However, particular care is warranted as the drug-free state is approached lest the patient obtains drugs from outside or hospital supplies.

PROGNOSIS

The future of any drug-abusing youth is a highly individual matter dependent upon the nature and extent of the habit, the coexistence of other dysfunctional behaviors, motivation for treatment, and the seriousness of underlying psychopathology. A number of characteristic patterns, however, have been identified. "Typical" narcotic addicts take their first dose of heroin at age 15, are addicted by the end of their teens or early twenties, and continue the habit a number of years. They may be societal dropouts or remain capable of normal function to a considerable degree. Commonly the addiction becomes "burned out" by age 35; emotional and behavioral problems may persist or other substances may enter the pictures, but narcotics are no longer craved.

Alcoholism has a somewhat later onset and persists for life. The alcoholic generally does not "drop out" but attempts to continue usual life patterns with variable degrees of success. Alcoholism is a problem for adults in all economic strata, as is the abuse of other central nervous system depressants. This is in contrast to narcotic addiction, which is more of an inner city dilemma. Whether the increasingly heavy use of alcohol by adolescents in recent years will result in a higher rate of alcoholism as they become adults remains to be seen.

Many youthful polydrug abusers or heavy marijuana smokers return to a productive life with appropriate treatment but may have missed important educational and developmental steps that cannot be made up. Those more resistant to treatment often progress to what has been termed the amotivational syndrome. Although heavy abuse usually abates to a considerable degree or is rejected entirely, these youths become rather passive individuals with some drifting about in alternative life-styles; others may seek the more structured and programmed experiences of religious cults or look to Eastern meditational philosophies. Of course this is somewhat of a chicken-and-egg situation. We do not know whether amotivation causes drug abuse, is the result, or is the combinant effect of both possibilities.

Bibliography

MEDICAL AND PHARMACOLOGIC ASPECTS

Alper, K., and Cohen, S. 1980. Pulmonary effects of marijuana. *Drug Abuse Alcoholism Rev.* 3:1-13.

Aronow, R., and Done, A. R. 1978. Phencyclidine overdose: an emerging concept of management. *J. Am. College Emerg. Phys.* 7(2):56.

Aronow, R.; Miceli, J. N.; and Done, A. K. 1980. A therapeutic approach to the acutely overdosed PCP patient. *J. Psychedelic Drugs* 12(3-4):259-266.

Baerg, R. D., and Kimberg, D. V. 1970. Centrilobular hepatic necrosis and acute renal failure in "solvent sniffers." *Ann. Intern. Med.* 73:713.

Barnes, H. V. 1980. Cannabis: an important issue for adolescent health care professionals. *J. Adolescent Health Care* 1:159-160.

Boeck, R. L.; Postl, B.; and Coodin, J. 1977. Gasoline sniffing and tetraethyl lead poisoning in children. *Pediatrics* 60:140.

Co, B. T.; Goodwin. D. W.; Gado, M.; et al. 1977. Absence of cerebral atrophy in chronic cannabis users. *J.A.M.A.* 237:1229.

Cohen, S. 1977. Angel dust. *J.A.M.A.* 238:515.

Dole, V. P. 1977. Narcotic addiction, physical dependence and relapse. *N. Engl. J. Med.* 286:988-992.

Harris, W. S. 1973. Toxic effects of aerosol propellants in the heart. *Arch. Intern. Med.* 131:162.

Hayden, J. W.; Comstock, E. G.; and Comstock, R. S. 1976. The clinical toxicology of solvent abuse. *Clin. Toxicol.* 9:169.

Hofmann, F. G. (in collaboration with Hofmann, A. D.). 1975. *A handbook on drug and alcohol abuse.* New York: Oxford University Press.

Goodman, L. S., and Gilman, A. 1975. *The pharmacologic basis of therapeutics,* 5th ed. New York: Macmillan Pub. Co.

Litt, I. F.; Cohen, M. I.; Schonberg, S. K.; et al. 1972. Liver disease in the drug-using adolescent. *J. Pediatr.* 81:238.

Litt, I. F.; Colli, A. S.; and Cohen, M. I. 1971. Diazepam in the management of heroin withdrawal in adolescents. *J. Pediatr.* 78:692-696.

National Council on Alcoholism. Criteria Committee. 1972. Criteria for the diagnosis of alcoholism. *Ann. Intern. Med.* 77:249.

National Institute on Drug Abuse. 1980. *Marijuana Research Findings: 1980* (Research Monograph 31). Washington, D.C.: U.S. Government Printing Office.

Richter, R., editor. 1975. *Medical aspects of drug abuse.* Hagerstown, Md.: Harper & Row.

Sellers, E. M., and Kalant, H. 1976. Drug therapy: alcohol intoxication and withdrawal. *N. Engl. J. Med.* 294:757.

Smith, D. E., and Wesson, D. R. 1971. Phenobarbital technique for the treatment of barbiturate dependence. *Arch. Gen. Psychiatr.* 24:56.

Solursh, L., and Clement, W. 1968. Hallucinogenic drug abuse: manifestations and management. *Can. Med. Assoc. J.* 98:407.

Thienes, C. H., and Haley, T. J. 1972. *Clinical toxicology*, 5th ed. Philadelphia: Lea & Febiger.

PSYCHOLOGICAL ASPECTS OF DRUG AND ALCOHOL ABUSE

AMA Council on Scientific Affairs. 1978. Clinical aspects of amphetamine abuse. *J.A.M.A.* 240:2317.

Bachman, J. G.; Johnston, L. D.; and O'Malley, P. M. 1981. Smoking, drinking, and drug use among American high school students: correlates and trends, 1975-1979. *Am. J. Public Health* 71:59-69.

Baldwin, B. A.; Liptzin, M. B.; and Goldstein, B. B., Jr. 1973. Youth services: a multifaceted community approach to drug abuse. *Hosp. Commun. Psychiatr.* 24:695-697.

Bosma, W. G. 1975. Alcoholism and teenagers. *Maryland State Med. J.* 24:62.

Biener, K. J. 1975. The influence of health education on the use of alcohol and tobacco in adolescents. *Prevent. Med.* 4:252.

Easson, W. M. 1976. Understanding teenage drug abuse. *Postgrad. Med.* 59:173.

Hofmann, A. D. 1978. Alcohol and the adolescent girl. *The Female Patient* 3:19 (July).

Jessor, R.; Chase, J. A.; and Donovan, J. E. 1980. Psychosocial correlates of marijuana use and problem drinking in a national sample of adolescents. *Am. J. Public Health* 70:604-613.

Joe, G. W., and Hudiberg, R. A. 1978. Behavioral correlates of age at first marijuana use. *Int. J. Addict.* 13:627.

Kandel, D., and Faust, R.   Sequence and stages in patterns of adolescent drug use. *Arch. Gen. Psychiatr.* 32:923.

MacKenzie, R. 1973. A practical approach to the drug-using adolescent and young adult. *Pediatr. Clin. North Am.* 20:1035.

McAlister, A.; Perry, C.; Killen, J.; et al. 1980. Pilot study of smoking, alcohol and drug abuse prevention. *Am. J. Public Health* 70:719-727.

Mendelson, J. H.; Rossi, A. M.; and Meyer, R. E., editors. 1975. *The use of marijuana, a psychological and physiological inquiry.* New York: Plenum Press.

Miller, L. L., editor. 1974. *Marijuana: effects on human behavior.* New York: Academic Press.

Paton, S. M., and Kandel, D. B. 1978. Psychological factors and adolescent illicit drug use: ethnicity and sex differences. *Adolescence* 13:187.

–21–
Managing Chronic Illness

H. Paul Gabriel, M.D.
Adele D. Hofmann, M.D.

Impact Issues
Psychosocial development □ Intellectual development
Nature of the condition □ Parents □ Siblings
Potential Behavior
General Principles of Management
Phase I: engagement □ Phase II: contract □ Phase III: short-term adaptation
Phase IV: intermediate adaptation □ Phase V: long-term adaptation
Variations on a Theme
Preadolescent onset □ Serious illness □ The persistently disturbed adolescent
Other problem situations □ The dying adolescent

Managing chronic illness in adolescence is founded on understanding and responding to its interaction with the developmental issues characteristic of these years. Failure to do so can result in an unwarranted degree of poor compliance, maladaptive behaviors, reactive psychopathology, and even maturational arrest. Although no guarantee can be given against such consequences occurring to some degree, much can be done to moderate them by introducing a developmental dimension into the therapeutic plan. To this end, this chapter reviews the variable issues that need to be taken into account and applies them in a prototypical approach.

Impact Issues
PSYCHOSOCIAL DEVELOPMENT
Illness and physical handicaps directly challenge virtually all adolescent developmental tasks, including emancipation, identity, and functional role (Table 21-1). Various aspects of these tasks assume preeminence, depending on the patient's maturational stage (Chapter 1; Table 21-2). Very young adolescents require options primarily for mastery and control, physical mobility, and reassurance over

body image integrity in face of their rapid pubertal growth. Plans for older youths need to emphasize concerns surrounding functional role, autonomy, and intimacy. Dependence-independence conflicts and sexual identity issues assume preeminence in midadolescence and are best responded to by providing opportunities for self-determination, the exercise of choice (a choice always can be given, even if within narrow limits), and appropriate gender identity behaviors.

One often overlooked matter of particular concern to both mid and late adolescents is specific sexual function. Worry in this quarter does not necessarily mean that such a youth is sexually active, although this may be the case. But all teenagers who perceive themselves as less than whole, regardless of the nature of the condition, are fearful about the possible compromise of sexual performance or reproductive competence or both.

INTELLECTUAL DEVELOPMENT
The emergence of abstract thought, roughly between the ages of 12 and 15 years, increasingly permits the adolescent to perceive his or her situation in future

TABLE 21-1
IMPACT OF CHRONIC ILLNESS OR HANDICAP ON ADOLESCENT DEVELOPMENT

Developmental task	Maturational goal	Potential impact of illness/handicap
Emancipation (arena: home)	Resolve dependence-independence conflict	Enforced continued dependence and need to rely on parents for care
	Acquire mastery and control of self and environment	Impaired competence in mastery and control
	Achieve self-reliance and autonomy	Limitation of capacity for autonomy
Identity (arena: peers)	Establish sound sense of body integrity	Direct damage to body image, real or perceived
	Finalize gender role definition	Impairment of gender role definition through altered appearance or limits on determinant activity
	Develop capacity for reciprocity in interpersonal relationships	Isolation from peer group
	Develop capacity for intimacy in heterosexual relationships	Isolation from "dating" options; impairment of specific sexual function
	Gain self-esteem	Compromised self-esteem; devaluation
Functional role (arena: school, work)	Complete education/training	Delay/cessation of education
	Plan for career, job	Alteration of career/job plans
	Plan for marriage/family	Impairment of capacity for marriage/household management/sexual function/procreation/child-rearing; genetic implications
	Establish recreational interests and skills	Limitation of recreational alternatives
	Establish adult life-style	Limitation of life-style options

as well as present terms. But, at the same time he or she has a proclivity for engaging in abundant fantasy and can easily distort or misinterpret even the most carefully conveyed information. Cognitive advance permits the teenaged patient to become a competent participant in care decisions and assume self-management responsibilities. But this also needs to be supported by periodic review of the adolescent's understanding to minimize distortion and revise it appropriately for his or her expanding intellectual capacity and shifting developmental concerns.

From a different perspective, intellectual ability often needs to be carefully nurtured and enhanced. This can be a critical asset in achieving adult autonomy for the youngster facing life-long physical disability.

NATURE OF THE CONDITION

Age of onset. As a general rule, the younger the patient when first affected by illness, the less psychologically disruptive the illness will be. With the exception of blindness and deafness, congenital or very early childhood-onset conditions usually are incorporated into the ego structure and adaptation is good. So too are conditions initiating at times of relative developmental stability, such as between

7 and 12 years or after the age of 20. But when the onset is in adolescence, a period of active intrapsychic reorganization, the additional stress can overwhelm integrative functions already maximally at work. Reactive behaviors tend to occur much more frequently than at other times, and persistent psychologic injury is more likely.

Visibility. Directly visible conditions have particular impact on adolescent body image concepts, prompting a sense of personal devaluation and diminished self-esteem. Consequently, there is a tendency for self-protective isolation or overcompensation and provocative acting-out. Compliance with regimens that produce observable and significant improvement is less likely to be a problem, whereas therapies that seem to be ineffective will be easily abandoned.

Nonvisible conditions are difficult for the patient to appreciate in direct, concrete terms, and factual distortion is likely to occur. The nature of the lesion may be perceived to be much more serious than it actually is (the fantasy of impending death inevitably being an unspoken attendant fear). This can result in regression, but denial and the associated tendency for poor compliance have greater likelihood in the adolescent who needs to see him-

TABLE 21-2
RELATIVE IMPACT OF CHRONIC ILLNESS OR HANDICAP
UPON DEVELOPMENTAL ISSUES BY DEVELOPMENTAL STAGE

	Early adolescence (12–14 years)	Mid adolescence (14–17 years)	Late adolescence (17–20 years)
Mastery and control	+++	++	+
Physical mobility	+++	++	+
Body image integrity	+++	+++	+
Sexual self-concept	++	+++	+
Peer interrelationships	++	+++	+
Emancipation drives	+	+++	++
Mutuality, intimacy	±	++	+++
Autonomy, self-reliance	±	++	+++
Education/vocational training	±	++	+++
Career plans·	±	+	+++
Marriage/family plans (child-bearing, genetics)	±	+	+++

self or herself in "normal" terms. When the nature of the situation cannot be ignored, nonvisible conditions may prompt acting-out or be put to the service of secondary gain; parents often share the same uncertainties as well as a sense of causal guilt and can be easily manipulated.

Degree of impairment. Immobilizing handicaps and handicaps that impose unavoidable restriction obviously require more emotional reorganization than handicaps that are not significantly disabling. The patient has indeed suffered a serious loss and inevitably goes through a mourning process. Depression and/or acting-out behaviors are commonly encountered as initial, if not long-term, responses. This may be particularly marked in the midadolescent.

Course. Conditions that result in chronic, unremitting invalidism produce a stable situation and tend to produce consistency in adaptive modes, for better or worse. Those that oscillate between remission and exacerbation are considerably more unsettling and require constant revision of self-perceptions and psychologic responses. Consequently, wide swings in behavior and mood can result. The increased attention paid by others to an exacerbation and its sometimes crisis nature result in the patient's manipulative use of the disease for secondary gain unless the consequent gratification can be minimized.

Resolution of childhood conditions in adolescence, as may occur in the natural course of some diseases such as asthma or juvenile rheumatoid arthritis or as a result of surgical correction, may not always be as welcome as one might think. Patients who have incorporated a "sick role" into their self-concept since early years may encounter considerable difficulty in adapting to being well. If resolution occurs late in adolescence, it is entirely possible that this compromised self-image cannot be wholly revised.

PARENTS

Parents often experience a variety of conflicting feelings that need to be understood with empathy but dealt with directly when counterproductive. In addition to altruistic concern, these include the following:

1. Irrational guilt over the belief that they have caused the condition in some way.

2. Heightened ambivalence over the adolescent's impending separation.

3. Fear over their own competence in managing the disease.

4. Overwhelmed inner resources and feelings of anger, resentment, and frustration.

Whereas many parents are able to handle these emotions and function in a highly supportive way, others will not be so successful. Less constructive responses may vary from overprotection and overindulgence to outright rejection. Commonly, parents and patient become hopelessly embroiled in power struggles over just who is in control of the disease and responsible for its therapy.

SIBLINGS

Any care plan for adolescents must also take siblings into account, ensuring that they do not feel slighted

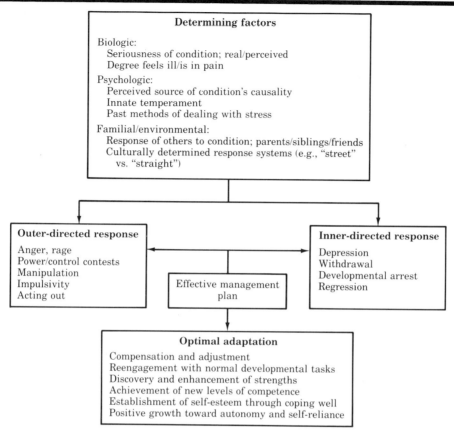

Determining factors

Biologic:
  Seriousness of condition; real/perceived
  Degree feels ill/is in pain
Psychologic:
  Perceived source of condition's causality
  Innate temperament
  Past methods of dealing with stress
Familial/environmental:
  Response of others to condition; parents/siblings/friends
  Culturally determined response systems (e.g., "street"
    vs. "straight")

Outer-directed response

Anger, rage
Power/control contests
Manipulation
Impulsivity
Acting out

Effective management
plan

Inner-directed response

Depression
Withdrawal
Developmental arrest
Regression

Optimal adaptation

Compensation and adjustment
Reengagement with normal developmental tasks
Discovery and enhancement of strengths
Achievement of new levels of competence
Establishment of self-esteem through coping well
Positive growth toward autonomy and self-reliance

FIGURE 21-1
BEHAVIORAL OPTIONS IN RESPONSE TO CHRONIC ILLNESS OR HANDICAPS

and that their needs are being met. Younger children in particular can come to feel devalued and somehow to blame for the situation through misinterpreting the genesis of increased parental attentions to the patient and withdrawal of attention from themselves. Older siblings, although usually more perceptive, still can come to resent the special privileges accorded the one who is ill if they are extended indefinitely. Either group may become moody or act-out, increasing intrafamily tension even more.

Potential Behavior

How a given adolescent will react to an illness or handicap is a vector of all the foregoing plus his or her inherent temperament. To some degree, past methods of responding to adversity may be predictive, although serious conditions often impose unprecedented stress and elicit behaviors not previously

seen. This is particularly true during the initial period of adjustment to a new situation.

As indicated in Figure 21-1, patterns of behavior can be divided into those that are outer-directed, engaging persons surrounding the patient in the process, and those that are inner-directed in a regressive, insulating, and isolating mode. Patients who are acutely ill, seriously debilitated, or in significant pain often adapt by isolating themselves, as do those who perceive causality as coming from within themselves. Outer-directed behaviors are more characteristic of adolescents who face physical compromise without feeling unwell or who tend to perceive any problem as emanating from the external world. Cultural factors may also play a role; young people in inner city ghettos often have had to learn to be aggressive and outer-directed simply to survive and do not abandon such techniques easily.

General Principles of Management

An optimal management plan begins with identifying significant illness factors on the one hand and the patient's specific developmental needs and behavioral potentials on the other hand. These are combined into a "prescriptive" approach designed to achieve the following goals to the degree the condition permits:

1. Optimal medical control
2. Patient autonomy in management
3. Patient and parent understanding of the condition and adaptation to it
4. Realization of full functional, educational, recreational, and activity potential
5. Attainment of self-esteem and self-confidence
6. Completion of adolescent developmental tasks
7. Attainment of autonomous adulthood, an independent life-style, and a rewarding vocation or career

Such an approach is most likely to promote effective adaptation and minimize inappropriate responses. It also has the distinct potential for turning the experience of illness to the advantage of personal growth. It should always be kept in mind that some degree of anger, frustration, depression, denial, and/or acting-out are inevitable accompaniments to serious chronic disease, particularly in the beginning.

We have devised a prototypical approach for an adolescent with onset of a chronic illness or disability in the early teen years. This is comprised of five stages, taking the young person and his or her family from initial awareness through adolescence into adulthood. Each of these stages has its own constellation of concerns and behavioral responses and a set of specific management recommendations that are outlined in the following discussion.

PHASE I: ENGAGEMENT

Extending from the first few days through the first week after onset, the engagement period is one of initial disbelief and shock, during which the care provider seeks to keep unrealistic fears and fantasies from getting out of hand. The goal is to achieve the patient's and parents' commitment to reality and engage them in a therapeutic alliance. This is accomplished by providing concrete information about the disease, exploring immediate concerns, correcting misunderstanding, and diffusing anxiety through a highly supportive and directive mode. The family as a whole is primary, and discussions take place with parents and patient both alone and together.

The patient's concerns at this time generally include worry over his or her health and its immediate implications, anxiety over being relatively helpless and having lost control, together with more unconscious fears of possible devaluation and loss of esteem. Denial, depression, regression, anger, and/or withdrawal are commonly seen. Management accepts the behavior as an inevitable initial response, reassures about the current situation, provides considerable detail about diagnostic and therapeutic procedures, and affords opportunity to discuss any broader concerns or questions that the patient may have.

Parental concerns usually relate to immediate fears for the patient's health, unconscious guilt, a sense of loss, and diffuse contemplation about the short- and long-range effects. Variably, they may deny and withdraw from the situation or become highly overprotective, infantilizing the patient and not wishing him or her to have any control or information. They also often evidence disregard for family continuity, home functions and needs. Here too management is accepting of this behavior but tempers extremes through considerable support and direction.

Siblings usually are genuinely worried about the patient and accepting of his or her primacy. They also may experience anxiety over family disruption, irrational guilt, or both. Management ensures that there is competent alternate care provision if needed, that siblings are kept informed about what is going on, and that their contact with the patient is maintained through visits or telephone calls.

PHASE II: CONTRACT

From approximately the second week through the first month the goal is to establish a trusting relationship among all concerned and to set the care contract by defining and delegating therapeutic responsibilities. The patient should be given as much control as possible; which aspects of care are the patient's alone, parent's alone, or shared should be clearly delineated. This is also a time of providing continued information about the disease and revising initial misperceptions. The patient assumes a more primary position in the relationship, being seen alone for part of each contact whether in hospital or office. Parents should be less dominant but still actively involved. They usually will come with the patient for visits and be the ones to call about problems and make appointments.

The patient tends to be most concerned about personal and physical integrity, independence, peer relationships, self-esteem, body image, and sexual identity, that is, those issues of primacy in adolescence in general. He or she also may have fears over competence in carrying out the contract. Regression, resistance to assuming responsibility, and reluctance to reengage with peers together with anger and frustration are common behaviors. Management accepts the patient's distress, but firmly encourages his or her assumption of responsibilities. This may take time, and efforts should not be abandoned. Opportunities for reassuring peer support and relationships also should be provided through continued contact with friends through visits or telephone.

Continuing to experience diffuse anxiety, guilt, and mourning, parents are often ambivalent over whether they are their adolescent's emancipator or protector. Concern for their own competence in management and doubting the patient's competence are common. The parents can be inconsistent and vacillating in carrying out the contract and may find it difficult to give up overprotection and insulation in order to allow the patient to do his or her part. The physician's efforts to promote patient autonomy may be resented, being perceived as direct competition for and challenge to parental control. Management consists of offering parents empathy and the opportunity to discuss their ambivalence, uncertainty, and sadness while continuing to reinforce the contract. Introducing flexibility into the medical protocol can simplify this task by relieving the family of the burden of rigid control for the sake of patient autonomy and avoiding patient-parent power struggles. It may be necessary to compromise some nonmandatory, albeit desirable, aspects. (For example, does the urine of a diabetic really need to be tested three times a day? Do the physical limitations imposed upon a youth with cardiac disease really need to be so stringent?)

Siblings usually continue to be accepting of the patient's primacy, but become increasingly more curious about the nature of the condition and its implication for themselves: Will they "get" it? Did they cause it in any way? Management is as for the previous phase, along with providing age-appropriate information and reassurance over their irrational fears.

PHASE III:
SHORT-TERM ADAPTATION

Generally extending over the second and third months after onset, short-term adaptation consists of stabilizing a consistent and mutually acceptable treatment program, promoting competence in carrying out management tasks, restoring intrafamily balance, and initiating the patient's reentry into normal adolescent developmental pursuits. At this time the patient becomes primary in the physician-family relationship, coming alone to most office visits, making appointments, and instituting most calls

about problems unless still quite young or seriously ill. Parents need to be helped to take more of a back seat but still need regular planned opportunities for independent discussion and periodic joint review with patient and physician together.

Patients now tend to experience an amalgam of real and fantasied worries about the present and future implications of their condition. They also continue to question their competence in management and are greatly concerned about reentering the mainstream of life, fearing devaluation and rejection. Behaviors vary from unrealistic optimism and denial to depression and avoidance of usual activities or anger and acting-out in testing the parameters of their altered life-style and compromised independence. They may centralize the disease and its management as a symbol of and focus for emancipation conflicts and rebel against its requirements. Management includes providing the patient with an honest but hopeful appraisal of his or her health status and honest answers to any questions. Return to school and peer activities must be insisted upon. Testing and acting-out behaviors usually are transient and should be tolerated unless they pose major health risks. The physician needs to be readily available over the telephone, and visits should be scheduled at fairly frequent intervals for support even if not medically required. If asked, patients usually will indicate themselves how often they would like to be seen.

Parents commonly continue to be uncertain about the patient's ability to handle the situation. Normal ambivalence about separation may be heightened and the disease invoked as an excuse to maintain control. They may exhibit premonitory hovering and be unrealistically pessimistic about the ability of the patient to reenter a normal life. Parents will try to follow the contract, generally being more comfortable in their own management skills and more accepting of the situation, but tend to be hesitant and uncommitted to the patient's part and readily take over if he or she falters. They easily succumb to the use of the disease as a focus for power struggles or other secondary gain. Management here also requires the availability of the physician and his or her empathy, reassurance, and support while continuing to reinforce the contract, patient autonomy, and return to normal activities.

By now, siblings wish for stability in the household and a return to their place in parental affections. Decreasing tolerance for disruptions and increasing resentment over the patient's continuing primacy may be evident, as will continuation of earlier fears. Tension on the home front can evidence in the siblings' depression, acting-out, or avoidance. Every effort should be made to resume intrafamily balance and encourage parents to express their understanding and appreciation of the siblings' help.

PHASE IV:
INTERMEDIATE ADAPTATION

Extending from several months after onset through midadolescence, the intermediate adaptation phase focuses on securing patient autonomy in management and completing developmental tasks through sustained participation in normal peer and educational pursuits. Most aspects of management are handed over to the patient exclusively and reinforced by periodic review of his or her understanding about the disease. The patient is primary, making his or her own appointments, coming to medical visits alone, calling the physician about intercurrent problems, and being an active partner in all care decisions. Parents are secondary and seen less often, but contact should be maintained through intermittent visits or telephone calls.

By this time, the patient's perceptions about the disease should be relatively reality based. His or her concerns primarily focus on the real impact of the condition on sexual identity, peer activity, autonomy, and other developmental issues. He or she may begin early contemplation of possible effects on the future. In the earlier part of this stage, the patient frequently exhibits fluctuating behaviors, including periodic testing of the system, acting-out, denial, anger, and/or depression. Later, the patient usually initiates constructive coping and adaptive skills with reintegration into normal activities, provided he or she is not severely disabled or disfigured or has not converted the situation into one of secondary gain. The disease may continue to be a focus of intergenerational conflict to the degree that this was allowed to happen previously. Management consists of continued reinforcement of autonomy and competence, and the substitution of compensatory activities for those that may be lost (particularly focusing on methods by which the patient can gain mastery, control, and self-esteem). The physician maintains a neutral supportive position vis-à-vis intrafamily dynamics, although relating to the patient as the primary person involved. Direct discussion with the patient about the disease and its present and future impacts should be initiated. Obvious adolescent concerns, including sexual function and adequacy, must be raised deliberately even if not first spoken of by the patient.

Parental concerns vary and respond directly to the patient's evident capacity for effective manage-ment and compliance. They generally return to normal preillness responses toward their adolescent when the situation is stable but tend to react with overindulgence or overprotection at times of exacerbation. If the future appears significantly compromised, parents may continue to experience mourning and depression. They may also feel overwhelmed, resentful, and angry, often displacing these feelings onto the patient, spouse, siblings, or physician. Management is essentially an extension of the previous stage in reinforcing the contract and ensuring the patient's return to adolescent affairs but within a framework of empathy and support. At this time it may be helpful to parents to review normal parenting modalities for adolescents and encourage their following this path (that is, the conveying of guided and graduating independence together with appropriate limit setting).

PHASE V:
LONG-TERM ADAPTATION

Extending from late adolescence through young adulthood, the final stage, long-term adaptation, focuses on the patient's attainment of adult autonomy and optimal emotional and functional adaptation to the condition. All management is handed over to the patient. Parents are seen on an as needed basis only. Information about the disease expands to include issues of relevance to marriage, childbearing, genetics, life expectancy, etc. Resources are invoked as necessary to secure independent living skills.

Patients generally achieve good adaptation if earlier conflicts have been resolved and the disease is not seriously disabling. Otherwise, arrested development, maladaptive behaviors, isolation, and/or poor interpersonal relationships may be evident. Management supports realistic interpersonal career and life-style goals and the acquisition of autonomy. Psychotherapeutic referral may be indicated for significant maturational lag or maladaptation (also at any prior point when matters are not proceeding in reasonable tune with this protocol).

Parents are primarily concerned for the patient's future but will have major emotional investment in the implication for themselves if the condition mandates continued dependency and care. They are usually supportive of the patient's autonomy but may demonstrate inappropriate responses if earlier conflicts have not been resolved. Preillness patient-parent problems may persist unchanged or be exacerbated by the experience. Marital problems may now surface once the illness no longer is a continuous pressing and primary concern; a chronically ill child in the family can take its toll in many ways. Management consists of continued support for the patient's autonomy and ultimate departure from home (if medically possible) and referral of parents for psychiatric or marital therapy if indicated.

Variations on a Theme
PREADOLESCENT ONSET

When chronic illness has its onset in childhood there is a tendency to overlook the need to anticipate and plan for adolescence. The consequence is either a crisis-ridden midadolescence and poor medical control or continued dependence resulting in an unemancipated young adult incapable of autonomy. Anticipating adolescence begins around 6-10 years of age, giving the child some management responsibilities of his or her own even if minor. The patient should also begin to contribute to the interval history, even though a parent will usually provide most of the information. At about age 10-12 he or she should be the primary historian and also should be seen alone for part of each visit. Information about the disease should be given the patient in relatively concrete age-appropriate terms and all questions fully explored. This is also a good time to begin to involve the patient in deciding about management issues. Although the child's wishes may not necessarily be determining, he or she should at least sit in on planning sessions and be consulted about the acceptability of recommended plans. The stage of *intermediate adaptation* can then be introduced at about age 13.

SERIOUS ILLNESS

Some chronic illnesses or handicaps clearly impose major limitations on the acquisition of autonomy and normal adulthood. In attempting to minimize the impact, the following points should be considered:

1. It may be necessary to compromise an ideal medical plan to allow for developmental tasks. Curtailments upon activity, therapies that interrupt a normal day, limitations upon school attendance, and so on should be closely questioned to determine whether they are truly critical or merely advantageous to maintaining a stable state.

2. When possible, surgical interventions should not take place during midadolescence (roughly 14-17 years). The preteens, early adolescence, or young adulthood is preferable. Normatively heightened body image and identity issues make it particularly difficult for midadolescents to adapt to disruption of their biological continuity. Surgical procedures aimed at significantly improving function or appearance, however, can be done at any time—the sooner the better. Particularly mutilative procedures, such as colectomy to prevent malignant degeneration of bowel disease, should be deferred as long as possible, preferably to young adulthood. Insofar as possible surgery also should be timed to avoid missing important schooling and other events.

3. The reality of the situation may require extended, life-long dependency on others for care and modification of predisability expectations, as in the instance of spinal cord injury. Honesty with all concerned is essential, and the true state of affairs should not be hidden from the patient. The delivery of such information, however, needs to be sensitive, properly timed, and offered within a framework of realistic hope.

4. Compensation is particularly important for the seriously disabled youth. Every effort should be made to provide substitutive activities and avoid isolation.

5. Knowledge of resources is essential, either through the physician's own information or through the use of a skilled social worker or referral agency. Special programs can be critical to the optimal adaptation of a seriously handicapped youth and the family; every effort must be made to ensure that he or she has access to all available resources and is not simply sequestered away. Resources include special programs for education, rehabilitation, vocational training, recreation, and socialization as well as specific disease support groups. Laws for both children and adults pertaining to equal education, nondiscrimination in employment, social security eligibility, and aid to crippled children and the handicapped can also be looked to for assistance. Specific information often can be obtained from local and state boards of education; national and local disease-related organizations; local and state departments of health, mental health, and social service; local social service agencies; institutes of rehabilitation; and local service groups (Shriners, Junior League, women's clubs, Kiwanis, etc.).

THE PERSISTENTLY DISTURBED ADOLESCENT

Despite all that may be done, some chronically ill adolescents simply do not adapt well. This may derive out of the realistically overwhelming nature of the condition itself, premorbid psychologic problems, a chronic illness that has been poorly managed for some time, parental adjustment problems, or out of innate temperament that renders the adolescent unable to cope effectively with a major life stress. Indicators that all is not going well include the following:

1. Unmodified and unremitting acting-out behaviors interfering with disease management or normal maturation at any time.

2. Isolation and refusal to reengage with peers or school past the *short-term adaptation* stage.

3. Persistent regression or depression or both past the *early adaptation* phase.

4. Poor school performance relative to the pre-illness state (provided catch up tutoring has been carried out and the patient is not simply hopelessly behind).

5. Inappropriate levels of dependence in *intermediate* or *long-term adaptation*.

In any of these instances the following steps may be helpful:

1. Review the existing management protocol to ensure the adolescent's developmental needs have been taken into consideration.

2. Review the contract with patient and parents, together and alone, assessing the degree to which this lacks clarity or is being sabotaged.

3. Explore with adolescent and parents (together and individually) whether there is any specific provocation (for example, school problems, peer rejection, sabotage of autonomy, misunderstandings). Alleviate the problem if it exists and reassess in 6 months. Be alert to the presence of a deeper seated problem if none is found.

4. Referral for psychotherapy is indicated when any deviant behavior persists for 6 months despite attempts to institute change or *at any time* if there is no apparent environmental cause and an optimal management plan has been incepted throughout. Do not delay such consultation or referral in the belief that the adolescent will "grow out of it." This is rarely the case.

OTHER PROBLEM SITUATIONS

1. *The maladapting adolescent who has been chronically ill as a child with failure to incept an advance plan for adolescence.* In this instance the physician should return to the guidelines for managing the adolescent and start from phase I, reviewing the patient's and parents' understanding of the disease and the therapeutic plan. Establishing the contract requires particularly careful attention to exploring and revising past practices. This can be difficult as it is hard to shift old, well-entrenched patterns. The liaison psychiatrist can be of distinct benefit here.

2. *Onset of illness in midadolescence.* This age youngster is particularly apt to have a difficult time adjusting to serious handicapping or disfiguring conditions that threaten to compromise independence, body image, gender role, and other identity issues. Psychiatric consultation is an important preventive step unless the physician feels comfortable and is experienced with this developmental stage.

3. *Conditions whose management falls primarily to the organ or surgical specialist.* "problem behaviors" will be encountered frequently in teenaged patients managed solely through a traditional medical or surgical approach. It is essential that the primary care physician become the patient's advocate, ensuring that the developmental approach is not ignored.

THE DYING ADOLESCENT

Adolescents who face fatal diseases pose difficult problems for all concerned. In the early stages, when the possibility of a favorable outcome still exists, management is as for any serious chronic illness in that optimism generally prevails. The only particular modifying issue relates to the patient's essential need to know his or her situation in candid but hopeful detail. The worst possible tack one can take in this situation is to engage in a conspiracy of silence; the adolescent always intuits the true state of affairs, yet is denied any opportunity to talk about them and to adapt to them in his or her own best way.

If the course takes a downhill turn and death becomes inevitable, openness and honesty again are essential. Younger adolescents may not yet perceive the true implications of death, but those who have progressed into abstract thinking will. Most terminally ill adolescents and their families progress through Kübler-Ross's stages of dying, and the physician can be guided accordingly. *The Hospitalized Adolescent* (Hofmann et al., 1976; see Bibliography) also discusses this issue in considerable detail.

Bibliography

Belfer, M. L.; Harrison, A. M.; and Murray, J. E. 1979. Body image and the process of reconstructive surgery. *Am. J. Dis. Child.* 133:532-535.

Boyle, I. R.; diSant'Agnese, P. A.; Sack, S.; et al. 1976. Emotional adjustment of adolescents and young adults with cystic fibrosis. *J. Pediatr.* 88:318-326.

Breslau, N.; Weitzman, M.; and Messenger, K. 1981. Psychologic functioning of siblings of disabled children. *Pediatrics* 67:344-353.

Cogan, S. J.; Becker, R. D.; and Hofmann, A. D. 1975. Human figure drawing in adolescent males with congenital urogenital anomalies. *J. Youth Adolescence* 4:359-365.

Drotar, D.; Doershuk, C. F.; Stern, R. C.; et al. 1981. Psychosocial functioning of children with cystic fibrosis. *Pediatrics* 67:338-342.

Garson, A., Jr.; Williams, R. B., Jr.; and Reckless, J. 1974. Long-term follow-up of patients with tetralogy of Fallot: physical health and psychopathology. *J. Pediatr.* 85:429-433.

Geller, B., and Greydanus, D. E. 1979. Psychological management of acute paraplegia in adolescence. *Pediatrics* 63:562-564.

Gordis, L.; Markowitz, M.; and Lilienfeld, A. M. 1969. Why patients don't follow medical advice: a study of children on long-term antistreptococcal prophylaxis. *J. Pediatr.* 75:957-968.

Greydanus, D. E., and Hofmann, A. D. 1979. Psychological factors in diabetes mellitus. *Am. J. Dis. Child.* 133:1061-1066.

Hofmann, A. D.; Becker, R. D.; and Gabriel, H. P. 1976. *The hospitalized adolescent: a guide to management of ill and injured youth.* New York: The Free Press.

Hofmann, A. D., and Becker, R. D. 1973. Psychotherapeutic approaches to the physically ill adolescent. *Int. J. Child. Psychother.* 2:492-512.

Hofmann, A. D. 1975. The impact of illness in adolescence and coping behavior. *Acta Paediatr. Scand. (Suppl).* 256:29.

Hodgman, C. H.; McAnarney, E. R.; Myers, G. J.; et al. 1979. Emotional complications of adolescent grand mal epilepsy. *J. Pediatr.* 95:309-312.

Kim, S. P.; Ferrara, A.; and Chess, S. 1980. Temperament of asthmatic children. *J. Pediatr.* 97:483.

Kellerman, J.; Zeltzer, L.; Ellenberg, L.; et al. 1980. Psychological effects of illness in adolescence. I. Anxiety, self-esteem, and perception of control. *J. Pediatr.* 97:126.

Kumar, S.; Powars, D.; Allen, J.; et al. 1976. Anxiety, self-concept and personal and social adjustments in children with sickle cell anemia. *J. Pediatr.* 88:859-863.

Miller, J. J.; Spitz, P. W.; Simpson, U.; et al. 1982. The social function of young adults who had arthritis in childhood. *J. Pediatrics* 100:378-382.

Millstein, S. G.; Adler, N. E.; and Irwin, C. E., Jr. 1981. Conceptions of illness in young adolescents. *Pediatrics* 68:834-839.

Passero, M. A.; Remor, B.; and Salomon, J. 1981. Patient-reported compliance with cystic fibrosis therapy. *Clin. Pediatr.* 20:264-267.

-22-
Legal Issues in Adolescent Medicine

Adele D. Hofmann, M.D.

Consent and Confidentiality
The mature minor rule □ Emancipation □ Venereal disease □ Contraception
Pregnancy □ Abortion □ Sterilization □ Rape, incest, and sexual abuse
Statutory rape □ Substance abuse □ Mental health □ Emergency care □ Confidentiality
Physician Protection in Treating Minors on Their Own Consent
Health Record Privacy
Payment Issues
Research

As a basic developmental principle, any adolescent benefits most from concerned and caring parental guidance. There are, however, exceptions to every rule. In some circumstances, mandatory parental involvement can significantly jeopardize a minor's health. In other situations it is unresponsive to growing societal acceptance of minors' rights. In either instance, the issue of consent and confidentiality is a constant dilemma in the delivery of adolescent health care. Teenagers frequently are involved in personal and private behaviors bearing significant medical risks and would rather deny an associated health need than have parents know. The fear of rejection or retribution is a potent force.

This chapter reviews the major legal trends pertaining to consent and confidentiality as they affect the physician-minor-parent axis in relation to emancipation, sexuality, substance abuse, mental health, and emergencies. All are situations in which parental consent requirements can impose significant psychologic and pragmatic barriers upon an adolescent's obtaining needed, timely care.

The question of consent, however, is but the tip of the confidentiality iceberg. This question cuts across the health care system and also includes patient privilege (versus parental notification), health record privacy rights, payment practices, and re-

search. Unfortunately, there may be little statutory continuity between any one of these issues and another. For example, a girl clearly may be legally entitled to consent for contraceptive services on her own, yet at the same time her parents may possess the right to be notified of services rendered or to review her health record. Inadvertent advisement also may come about in connection with confidential services paid for by a family health insurance policy and notification of the head of household of payments made. Hopefully this lack of consistency will be corrected in the future. But this seems a distant goal in light of current (1982) legal and legislative controversies surrounding confidential adolescent care in federally subsidized family planning programs.

Further complicating matters, some legal precedents have national applicability, since they are derived from federal legislation and case and constitutional law; others are more variably defined in state statutes. More specific local direction can be obtained from consultation with an attorney or from one or more of the following:

1. City and state bar associations
2. County and state medical societies
3. State and city departments of health or social service

4. State attorneys general

5. Planned Parenthood and other family planning programs

6. The Children's Rights Project of the American Civil Liberties Union

7. Attorneys for hospitals and/or malpractice carriers.

Consent and Confidentiality

Two basic questions are involved; one relates to access to care and the capacity to consent,* the other to confidentiality and patient privacy versus parental knowledge. Although clearly interrelated, they reflect separate points. Minors' consent laws often include confidentiality implicitly or explicitly, but this is not invariably so. A number of statutes may permit an adolescent to consent to certain services but also require parental notification, particularly for abortions. Currently proposed (April, 1982) federal administrative regulations governing use of Title X family planning grants also would require parental notification of adolescents of 17 years or less receiving prescription contraceptives. The constitutionality of such provisions for at least mature minors, however, is in serious question. This is a rapidly evolving situation with final denouement unlikely before the publication of this book. Implications and a bit of crystal ball gazing will be dealt with in more detail in appropriate sections to follow.

THE MATURE MINOR RULE

The law surrounding minors' consent and confidentiality is a rather complex amalgam of state and federal statutes, governmental funding regulations, case law (court decisions), and constitutional rulings. Considerably broader possibilities exist than are defined by state statute alone. This situation has been of sufficient magnitude to give rise to the "mature minor rule." Even in the absence of specific statutory permission, there is firm legal support and minimal risk of liability for the treatment of minors on their own consent and in confidence when they are mature enough to give an informed consent and

*Note: Under common law tradition, minors may not make contracts of their own; only a parent can do this for them. To treat any patient without a valid contract (consent) is to commit an unauthorized touching, or assault and battery. Negligence is not involved. This position has never been absolute, and the courts regularly have upheld the capacity of some minors to consent to health care on their own. The governing principle in such decisions has been the minor's maturity and capacity to give an informed consent, not age or economic status.

the treatment is for their benefit. The United States Supreme Court clearly has upheld this position in relation to abortions (*Baird* v. *Bellotti*). Although the mature minor doctrine only confers probable, not axiomatic, immunity, the total absence of litigation seeking *damages* from physicians for providing minor adolescent's sexuality and drug-related health care on the minor's own consent should be highly reassuring. Virtually all court action has been of a civil nature simply seeking an *injunction* against certain practices.

Specific commentary on the permissory trends in the United States as of 1979 is offered in the following discussion, although the answers for each state are not always clear. When issues are ambiguous or not addressed in a given state, the physician still will be in a strong defensive position if he or she follows the mature minor rule. Moreover, as of this writing, no case has been discovered in which damages have been awarded against a physician for treating a minor over 15 years of age on the minor's own consent for any purpose or for rendering fertility-related services to a minor of any age.

EMANCIPATION

The following categories of minors may qualify as emancipated for health care purposes in general, although special considerations surrounding sterilization may override (see following sections):

1. Persons of a specific age; by state statute in all states. These either emancipate the minor for health care purposes alone or establish majority in toto. In most instances this is at age 18, but one only need be 14 in Alabama, 15 in Oregon, or 16—excluding operations—in South Carolina to consent for care. On the other hand, a minimum age of 19 obtains in Alaska, Nebraska, and Wyoming.

2. Minors who are or have been married; by statute in two-thirds of the states.

3. Minors who are parents; by statute in one-fourth of the states. These laws are not operative until after delivery and may or may not include permission for the minor to consent for her child's health care as well.

4. Minors who are:

a. Simply away from home and managing their own financial affairs; in some states. This may be by health care statute alone, usually with little additional qualification (for example, source of income or parental permission is not at question, in contrast to item b, although in some instances a minimum age of 15 may apply). Alternatively, the minor may qualify under a new legislative trend defining a more general emancipation status. Such statutes now exist in several states and are somewhat more demanding in their criteria than those addressing health care alone, usually requiring a minimum time away from home, a minimum age, and a court decree.

b. Minors away from home with parental permission, employed, and earning their own support; by common law tradition in all locales. Such adolescents would have to be 16 years or more and no longer subject to compulsory school laws.

c. Minors living at home but working and contributing to their own support. Although not addressed statutorily and somewhat less clear than previous categories, case law precedent suggests these individuals might well also qualify as emancipated.

5. Minors in the armed forces; by statute in some states. This group also would probably qualify under common law emancipation definitions in any locale.

6. Minors who are high school graduates; by statute in Alabama, Montana, and Pennsylvania.

7. Minors who, in the judgment of the treating physician, are deemed sufficiently mature (or "intelligent") as to be able to understand the nature of the proposed services; by statute in Arkansas, Kansas, Ohio, and Mississippi (viz., the mature minor rule).

VENEREAL DISEASE

All states have statutes permitting minors to consent to the diagnosis, treatment, and prevention of venereal disease. In some instances, this may include all communicable diseases. A minimum age of 12 (California, Delaware, Illinois, Oregon, and Vermont) or 14 (Hawaii, Idaho, New Hampshire, North Dakota, and Washington) may apply. Hawaii requires parental notification when possible. In Massachusetts such services can only be provided in public health facilities. Connecticut extends this provider limitation to include private voluntary clinics and hospitals as well.

CONTRACEPTION

Nonemancipated minors may consent to contraceptive services (excluding abortion and sterilization) under a variety of permissions:

1. A number of states have enabling statutes variably addressing minors who are sexually active; or for the diagnosis, treatment, and prevention of pregnancy; or if referred by a clergyman, physician, or social agency, and so on.

2. In any state through programs receiving federal funds under Titles XIX and XX of the Social Security Act per antidiscrimination requirements of DHEW funding regulations. State mandates for parental consent were ruled impermissable in these circumstances by the United States Supreme Court (*Jones et al.* v. *T. H. et al.*).

3. Statutes and social service regulations in some states that:

a. Mandate family planning services be made available to any sexually active minor already receiving public assistance (AFDC or SSI) who wishes them

and/or

b. Permit minors who could become public assistance recipients to obtain family planning services (as might occur to any adolescent were she to bear a child). Although the question of who is to consent in these instances usually is not mentioned (parent or minor), many interpretations have held that access through the minor's consent alone is implicit by virtue of this omission.

4. Any minor may purchase nonprescription contraceptives in a drugstore by United States Supreme Court decision (*Carey* v. *Population Services International*).

Federal Title X appropriations legislation for fiscal year 1981–1982 include an amendment directing grantees to *encourage* parental involvement when rendering services to minor adolescents on their own consent. The administration has carried this one step further in *mandating* parental notification in currently proposed federal regulations and has given every indication that it intends to put this into force. The only exception would be if the provider believed such notification would result in physical harm to the adolescent. Moreover, these regulations would supercede any less restrictive state laws or regulations. Substantial legal opinion, however, suggests that converting the legislative intent of encouraging parental involvement to a mandate is unconstitutional. The mature minor rule would add further support for this perspective for those who would qualify. Even if put into force, it is certain that this issue will make its way through the courts. In any event, these regulations apply only to Title X grantees and not to adolescent health services rendered under Titles V, XIX, or XX. And they certainly are not applicable to services paid for by nonfederal sources.

PREGNANCY

Many state statutes permit minors to consent to the diagnosis and treatment of pregnancy, usually excluding abortion and sterilization. Even when there is no statutory direction, the early institution of prenatal care is so clearly beneficial to the pregnant adolescent and the fetus that it would seem quite defensible to initiate such treatment in confidence, with the intention of involving parents as soon as possible (and so noting in the chart). Any girl who is not emancipated and plans to carry her pregnancy to term obviously must advise her family sooner or later. Most such patients want this to occur but simply do not know how to go about it. With supportive counseling over a visit or two, the girl usually will tell parents herself or is willing for the physician to do so.

ABORTION

Minors have been no less subject to the abortion controversy than adults, and the law in this area is in flux. At present (1982), emancipated minors usually may secure abortion services as adults, although those who are under 18 and neither married nor a parent may face special qualifications for this procedure in some states.

Under two landmark decisions, *Planned Parenthood of Central Missouri* v. *Danforth* and *Bellotti* v. *Baird*, the United States Supreme Court established the right of all minors, including those who are unemancipated, to obtain abortions without parental consent. However, the Court in *Bellotti* did establish that minors who were not mature could be subject to special protections and concluded that although it is permissible for states to encourage parental involvement by requiring parental consent in most cases, a minor must be given the alternative of going directly to court without first involving her parents. Once in court, the minor must be given the right to abortion services as an adult if she can show that she is mature. If she is not found mature, the judge must authorize a confidential abortion if this is felt to be in her best interests. Many states have enacted statutes attempting to meet the requirements of *Bellotti*, but not all have succeeded. Laws in Massachusetts and Missouri are examples of those that have been upheld and are now in operation. Concerned health providers will need to check with local authorities periodically in determining their particular jurisdictional status.

In further seeking to contain an adolescent's access to confidential abortion, a number of states passed by the consent issue but mandated parental notification. In March of 1981 in *H-L* v. *Matheson*, the Supreme Court ruled on a class action suit from Utah claiming to represent all minors. The Court upheld the right of Utah to require parental notification, ruling that this was an appropriate protection for minors who were still dependent and immature and pointing to the fact that the plaintiff made no distinction between this group and those who were mature. The Court went on to suggest that it might rule differently for mature minors. The process of enacting state statutes that comply with *H-L* v. *Matheson* are underway in many states. On the other side, a number of cases seeking to invalidate notification requirements for mature minors also are in progress with the expectancy that one of them sooner or later will make its way to the Supreme Court and the further confirmation of the right to unqualified and confidential abortion by those who can demonstrate their maturity. Here too, specific inquiry needs to be made as to local provisions due to the rapidly changing situation.

From another perspective, case law consistently has held that no one, including parents, may force a minor to have an abortion against her will. And, in a corollary issue, a minor mother can neither be forced to place her child for adoption nor to keep it. The decision is hers alone.

STERILIZATION

Recent trends in sterilization law espouse the principle that elective termination of reproductive capacity can only be performed with the patient's voluntary and fully informed consent. (Although still existent in about half the states, old compulsory sterilization laws for the mentally incompetent are no longer enforced.) Minors generally are not eligible for this procedure no matter who consents or what the minor's mental status might be. Even sterilization of young people who reach majority at age 18 but are less than 21 may not be entirely in the clear, at least for federal funding—genetic or medical considerations notwithstanding. Department of Health and Human Services (DHHS) regulations prohibit the use of federal funds for the sterilization of anyone under 21 without exception. Although theoretically 18 to 21 year olds are as entitled to consent to sterilization as to any other medical procedure, there is widespread ethical and psychologic controversy over whether anyone who has neither borne children nor reached a sufficient age to have had full opportunity to do so ever can rationally elect to terminate fertility.

More common and problematic is the question of sterilization in mentally retarded adolescents, for whom personal freedom and education may be curtailed seriously by problems surrounding sexual indiscretion and/or menstrual hygiene. A court order for this procedure may be sought by parents. It has been difficult, however, to obtain judicial permission, and such applications often have been denied.

But the lack of precedent does not mean that the courts may not review their position and become willing to consider the relative needs and rights of such handicapped adolescents in more balanced measure. A recent (1979) landmark New Jersey decision granting parents the right to make a decision for sterilization of their retarded, adult daughter is a case in point.

RAPE, INCEST, AND SEXUAL ABUSE

An increasing number of states are enacting statutes permitting minors to obtain care following rape and sexual abuse as if an adult. Emergency provisions also would apply (see section on emergency care).

In addition, it should be remembered that persons under age 18 are subject to child abuse laws. If the sexual abuse is by a family member (incest) or otherwise reflects harmful parental practices, the situation must be reported to the proper authorities as would be the case for the physical abuse of a younger child.

STATUTORY RAPE

Statutory rape is a charge against a male for having sexual intercourse with a female below a state-stipulated age on the presumption that she is unable to give an effective consent to this act by virtue of her immaturity. This age is quite variable from one jurisdiction to another and may be as young as age 12 or as old as age 18.

These laws have been all but ignored in recent years, and few such charges have been made except in instances of child abuse. However, some have recently expressed interest in seeing statutory rape laws as one way in which to control the sexual behavior of the young or at least to inform parents of their offsprings' activity. Thus California enacted a law requiring physicians identifying a minor female as sexually active to report this to the Child Protective Services; under these circumstances she was held to be the victim of child abuse and in need of protection. Subsequent furor over just how to enforce this law and the probability that many adolescents would not seek important medical assistance in this situation resulted in the law's repeal.

Challenges to the validity of statutory rape laws have also recently come to the attention of the courts. The United States Supreme Court in 1981 upheld the legitimate interest of states to protect minor females in this manner and discarded invalidity on the basis of sex discrimination and the fact that these laws do not apply to males. The Court stated that the fact of possible pregnancy made sex discrimination appropriate in this instance.

Just how further actions in relation to statutory rape will affect medical practice for adolescents remains to be seen. This is a relatively new issue on the judicial horizon.

SUBSTANCE ABUSE

More than half the states permit minors to consent for treatment for drug and alcohol abuse. In states not having such legislation, DHHS regulations permit federally funded programs to provide confidential care for the first visit but require both the minor's and parent's consent thereafter. When no legal permission is clearly defined, a practice similar to that outlined for pregnancy would be appropriate, viz. catching the young person up in health care for a visit or two and then helping him or her to tell his parents.

MENTAL HEALTH

A number of states permit minors to obtain mental health services on their own. Massachusetts also permits emergency care for minors without parental consent in instances of "health and *mental health risk.*" In the absence of enabling statutes, it would be appropriate to initiate care for a disturbed adolescent, planning to involve parents as soon as this could be accomplished without alienating the patient from care—an approach similar to that suggested for pregnancy and substance abuse.

An unresolved problem occurs when no enabling statutes exist and the minor wishes psychiatric assistance but parents refuse. This probably is a set of circumstances that only a court order can resolve, although in some instances the mature minor rule could be invoked.

In a related manner, the United States Supreme Court has recently ruled that parents do have the right to voluntarily commit their minor child to a mental hospital even if the minor does not agree. Charges that a few parents act out of self-serving interests in sequestering a troublesome offspring were ruled insufficient to justify invading the family unit and abrogating the controlling rights of most parents who act out of benevolence rather than malice (*J. L. and J. R.* v. *Parham*).

EMERGENCY CARE

Many states have relatively broad statutes permitting emergency measures beyond simply those required to save life and limb. Usually these provide for treatment in any situation in which the time it would take to contact parents could increase the risk to the minor's life *and health.* What constitutes such a health risk is left to the physician's judgment. The following criteria should be helpful in making this determination:

1. Denial or delay of care bears significant risk of producing greater health harm than if treatment is promptly instituted.

2. The treatment is life and limb saving or clearly beneficial and without major risk of serious side effects.

3. The minor appears to be sufficiently mature to be able to give informed consent (unless comatose or confused and life or limb is endangered, in which case no consent is required).

4. Reasonable efforts to contact parents have been unavailing or their whereabouts unknown and provision for their ultimate notification has been taken (for example, sending a statement home with the patient about what was done and asking the parent to call; sending a telegram; sending the police; calling at a later time).

5. Additional weight is added if delayed treatment is likely to cause the patient to suffer unnecessary pain, to become unduly emotionally upset, or to leave the premises untreated and fail to return for timely treatment at a later date.

In some instances, states have resolved the problem by permitting another adult such as a teacher, adult relative, or parent of a friend to act in loco parentis.

CONFIDENTIALITY

When no comment is made about notification in a given minor's consent statute, it probably can be assumed that confidentiality is implicit and need not be broken unless warranted by overriding circumstances. The law aside, good medical practice demands that parents be notified when failing to do so puts the minor at significantly greater health risk. Many minors' consent statutes confirm this view by including such permission. An example would be the adolescent intending suicide or a pregnant minor bent on an illegal abortion.

Physician Protection in Treating Minors on Their Own Consent

Unless the law is quite clear or the physician is working in a health facility with well-defined policies, it is a good idea to document in the record the decision to treat confidentially on the minor's own consent. This documentation should include:

1. A statement that the minor was deemed mature enough to give an informed consent, together with the factors leading to this judgment.

2. Notation as to what information was provided in obtaining an informed consent and that the

patient did, in fact, give it, including a signed consent form. (The latter, of course, is indicated in any circumstance.)

3. A comment on the potential for health harm through denial or delay of care and the likelihood of this outcome were parental consent or notification insisted upon.

4. A statement as to the action taken by the physician in encouraging the minor to involve his or her parents.

In situations where treatment bears more than modest risks, additional protection can be obtained by securing and documenting a second physician's concurring opinion.

Health Record Privacy

An increasing number of state and federal initiatives are beginning to define and institute patient health record privacy rights. For the most part, these closely follow the recommendations of the Federal Privacy Protection Study Commission (PPSC) report issued in 1976 and provide for the patient to (a) give his or her *informed* consent for disclosure of information to third parties; (b) have opportunity to see his or her record should he or she so wish; (c) seek adjustment or expungement of any information deemed incorrect or unfair or insert his or her own rebuttal statement if expungement is refused.

The recommendations also address a number of obvious problems and conflicts. Direct review may be denied if thought potentially harmful to the patient, but the patient may then ask any other person of his or her choice to view it in his or her stead. No patient authorization is necessary in a number of instances, such as for training, audit, and research (provided patient identification goes no further) or as mandated by public health law or court subpoena.

The PPSC report, however, did not address the special needs of minors. It is difficult to say whether the traditional position of parental representation invariably would apply or whether exception would be made for minors consenting to their own care. In light of minors' consent law and the mature minor rule, this ambiguity makes for considerable confusion. It is unlikely that this matter will be soon clarified due to the abatement of interest in health record privacy in general, at least at the federal level.

Some direction however, does exist in DHHS regulations issued pursuant to the Federal Privacy Act of 1974 and before the publication of PPSC report. In relation to eligible medical records (viz. those maintained by DHHS or by programs receiving DHHS funds), minors have rights of access as an adult; they may know whether a record exists and have it sent to any person of their choice but not view it directly. Parents may not gain access to their minor's record nor even know whether it exists, but they may designate a nonfamily member health professional to receive any record that *might* exist. The designate is to consider the impact upon the minor and family in deciding how much to reveal. In addition, the minor is to be notified of his or her parents' request. DHHS regulations for records in federally funded drug and alcohol treatment programs are somewhat different. Minors may exercise all privacy rights in relation to the first visit (viz. review through a designate, informed consent for disclosure, and options for correction of misinformation). Minors and parents together exercise them thereafter.

Physicians who send records to schools should also be aware of the Family Privacy in Education Act of 1975. This act and its DHHS regulations provide parents with the right to give informed consent for information release from schools to a third party, to see their child's educational record on request, and to challenge any of its content and seek expungement if they so wish. This right devolves on the student when he or she reaches age 18. The "educational record" encompasses all data that affect the student's educational course in any way or is available to teachers or school administrators—anything from a full medical and psychologic evaluation of a developmentally disabled youngster to a gym excuse. University student health records that are available to treating professionals only (not educators or administrators) are exempt. The status of similar records at the primary and secondary school level is not mentioned and therefore is unclear. The essential implication for the physician is that parents can read any document that he or she may have sent to schools, as may students themselves if 18 years of age or more. Students under 18 do not have such rights themselves, but there is nothing to contravene such a policy at the local level.

Payment Issues

If all other aspects of care are confidential, privacy still can be breached if parents are made aware through payment practices. This probably is the most difficult aspect of the confidentiality issue. Legally, the person contracting for a service is financially responsible as well. In contemporary law this applies as much to minors as adults. Many minors' consent statutes spell this out, specifically relieving parents of any obligations to pay, but this still does not answer the pragmatic question of where the dollars are to come from. There are, however, a variety of options, all of which have been used to resolve this dilemma at one time or another.

1. Payment arrangements can be established with parents in advance. As is customary in psychiatric care, parents pay unitemized bills, no questions asked. It is unclear whether a parent who pays has the de facto right to know what it was for, particularly when the minor is entitled to consent to the care at issue. This is a thorny question that is best avoided. When a trust relationship exists between parent and physician and when they see each other as collaborators in the business of helping the minor to become responsible and grow up well, this is an effective system and the matter of parents' wishing to know what they paid for does not arise.

2. Many minors, given reasonable opportunity, often can pay at least part if not all of the fee out of allowance or personal earnings. They may not be as indigent as one might think.

3. The minor can be referred to low- or no-cost clinics. A variety of such programs exist. Planned Parenthood and other family planning programs, some regional adolescent medical clinics, free clinics (a few are left), children and youth programs, and maternal and child health clinics may have special payment practices for minors needing confidential care. Admittedly, these resources are often limited to large cities; young people in small towns and rural areas may have no such option.

4. Third-party payment systems can be used when the patient is eligible (see following discussion).

5. The physician can do what he or she long has done for the financially indigent and render care free.

Third-party payment systems may offer some help, particularly in the instance of Medicaid, which does not require a parental signature on the claim form. However, the family policy number is required, and the minor must be able to supply this and other appropriate qualifying evidence. He or she may be able to produce the family's card or if previously registered with the health provider, this already will be known. In most instances Medicaid payment systems preserve individual privacy. At one point about 11 states sent notice of claims made and paid for any family member to the head of household as an accountability measure. The potential for privacy violation, however, became recognized, and these rules have all been reversed.

Private third-party payment systems generally are not available to minors in confidence. With rare exception, the parent policy holder not only must sign the claim form but also receives notice of the claim's disposition. Only if the minor is employed and has health insurance benefits will he or she be likely to have a policy of his or her own. In any event, excepting abortion, most services recompensed by private third-party insurers are unlikely to fall into the confidential category unless the minor is seeking care under an emancipated status.

Future directions in National Health Insurance are unclear overall, much less in relation to minors. Hopefully, if some form of NHI is enacted, appropriate provisions for adolescents will be made. One such option now exists in Canada, where any NHI claim form needs only to be marked confidential by the physician and privacy automatically will be preserved.

Research

The 1977 report of the National Commission for the Protection of Human Subjects in Biomedical Research established a number of recommendations for children. The following are those of particular pertinence to adolescents and the issue of consent.

1. As a general rule, minors 7 years of age or more are to "assent" and their parents to give "permission." Assent implies concurrence and allows the minor to agree or not to agree to participation but does not require the capacity to give an informed consent.

2. Waiver of parental permission requirements and endowment of the minor with sole consent rights may be made by the Institutional Review Board upon application by the investigator when:

a. "The research is designed to identify factors related to the incidence of treatment of certain conditions in adolescents for which, in certain jurisdictions, they legally receive treatment without parental consent"

or b. "The research involves subjects who are 'mature minors' and the procedures involved entail essentially no more than minimal risk that such individuals might reasonably assume on their own"

or c. "The research is designed to understand and meet the needs of neglected or abused children, or children designated by their parents as 'in need of supervision.'"

The recommendations further add that there is no single mechanism that can substitute for parental permission in every instance. In some cases the consent of mature minors should be sufficient. In other cases, court approval may be necessary. In any event the Institutional Review Board is to ensure that the research protocol seeking waiver of parental permission provides an appropriate alternative mechanism for protecting minor subjects.

Bibliography

Alan Guttmacher Institute. 1982. *Family planning, teenagers and government. Issues in brief,* Vol. 2., No. 2.

American Civil Liberties Union. 1977. *The rights of young people.* New York: Avon Books.

Hofmann, A. D. 1980. A rational policy toward consent and confidentiality in adolescent health care. *J. Adolescent Health Care* 1:9.

Hofmann, A. D. 1978. Legal issues in pediatrics. In *Principles of pediatrics,* editors R. A. Hoekelman et al. New York: McGraw-Hill Book Co.

Hofmann, A. D. 1976. Consent and confidentiality and their legal and ethical implications for adolescent medicine. In *Medical care of the adolescent,* 3rd ed., editors, J. R. Gallagher; F. P. Heald; and D. C. Garell. New York: Appleton-Century-Crofts.

Holder, A. 1977. *Legal issues in pediatrics and adolescent medicine.* New York: John Wiley & Sons.

Paul, E. W., and Pilpel, H. F. 1979. Teenagers and pregnancy: the law in 1979. *Family Planning Perspectives* 11:297-302.

Paul, E. W., and Wasserman, R. 1982. Teenagers and reproductive health care: the law through 1981. *Transitions* 5(1):4-8.

National Commission on Confidentiality of Health Records. 1978. *Report of the National Conference on the Health Records Dilemma.* NCCHR 1978. Washington, D.C.

Silber, T. J. 1980. Physician-adolescent patient relationships; the ethical dimension. *Clin. Pediatr.* 19:50-55.

FEDERAL REGISTER, RELEVANT LEGISLATIVE REPORTS, AND DHEW IMPLEMENTING REGULATIONS: Confidentiality of alcohol and drug abuse patient records. 1975. *Regulations* 40:27802-27821 (July 1).

Education for all handicapped children. 1977. *Regulations* 42:42474-42518 (Aug. 23).

Implementation of Executive Order 11914. 1978. *Nondiscrimination on the basis of handicap in federally assisted programs* 43:2132-2139 (Jan. 13).

Privacy Act of 1974. 1975. *Regulations pertaining to medical records* 40:47406–47415 (Oct. 8).

Privacy rights of students. 1976. *Regulations* 41:24662–24675 (June 17).

Report and recommendations on research involving children of the National Commission for the Protection of Human Subjects of Biomedical and Behavioral Research 43:2084–2114 (Jan. 13) 1978.

Requirements applicable to projects for family planning services; proposed rule (pertaining to Title X services to unemancipated minors and parental notification requirements) Vol. 47, No. 35 (Feb. 22) 1982.

NATIONAL RESOURCES FOR LEGAL INFORMATION:

The American Civil Liberties Union, Children's Rights Project, 22 East 40th St., New York, N.Y. 10016.

Children's Defense Fund of The Washington Research Project, Inc., 1520 New Hampshire Ave., N.W., Washington, D.C. 20036.

Legal Services Division. Planned Parenthood Federation of America, 810 Seventh Avenue, New York, N.Y. 10019.

Mental Health Law Project, Suite 300, 1220 19th Street, N.W., Washington, D.C.

PART FOUR

PSYCHOSOCIAL ISSUES IN ADOLESCENT MEDICINE

Adele D. Hofmann
H. Paul Gabriel

CHAPTER 23
Principles of Psychosocial Evaluation and Counseling

CHAPTER 24
Behavioral Problems

CHAPTER 25
Emotional Problems with Physical Manifestations

CHAPTER 26
Depression, Suicide, Out-of-Control Reactions, and Psychoses

Introduction

It is difficult to classify the various emotional and behavioral problems the primary care physician may encounter. Generally considerable overlap exists between one set of problems and another. Some issues, such as a school problem, may simply be the outward signs of inner turmoil from a quite unrelated cause. How a problem manifests itself is also a matter of the adolescent's own unique style combined with past learned coping mechanisms. One young person may respond to a given situation in an outer-directed, acting-out mode, while the next may deal with precisely the same circumstances by withdrawal and insulation in an inner-directed manner. All possible combinations and permutations cannot be taken into consideration. In Chapter 23, however, we have tried to give direction for an overall approach to any troubled youth. Subsequent chapters have categorized problems according to the most common presenting complaint based on the authors' experience in a general adolescent medicine setting.

Bibliographies for each chapter comprise articles specific to the subjects treated therein. We also offer a more generalized bibliography with this introduction. Many of these books also have material of particular significance for topical issues in each chapter and should be considered resources for further information in any instance.

A. D. H.
H. P. G.

Bibliography

ADOLESCENT PSYCHOLOGY: NORMAL DEVELOPMENTAL ISSUES

Adelson, J., editor. 1980. *Adolescent psychology: normal developmental issues.* New York: John Wiley & Sons.

Blos, P. 1962. *On adolescence.* New York: Free Press.

Blos. P. 1970. *The young adolescent.* New York: Free Press.

Erikson, E. H. 1963. *Childhood and society,* 2nd ed. New York: W. W. Norton.

Erikson, E. H. 1968. *Identity: youth and crisis.* New York: W. W. Norton.

Esman, A. H., editor. 1975. *The psychology of adolescence: essential readings.* New York: International Universities Press.

Freud, A. 1958. Adolescence, *Psychoan. Study Child* 13:255.

Grinder, R. E., editor. 1975. *Studies in adolescence,* 3rd ed. New York: MacMillan Pub. Co.

Group for the Advancement of Psychiatry. 1968. *Normal adolescence.* New York: G.A.P. (G.A.P., Publications Office, 419 Park Avenue South, New York, NY 10016).

Josselyn, I. M. 1972. *The adolescent and his world,* 2nd ed. New York: Family Service Association.

Stone, L. J., and Church, J. 1968. *Childhood and adolescence: a psychology of the growing person,* 2nd ed. New York: Random House.

ADOLESCENT PSYCHOPATHOLOGY: THE TROUBLED YOUTH

Chapman, A. H. 1965. *Management of emotional problems of children and adolescents.* Philadelphia: J. B. Lippincott.

Gallagher, J. R., and Harris, H. I. 1972. *Emotional problems of adolescents,* 3rd ed. New York: McGraw-Hill Book Co.

Kalogerakis, M. G., editor. 1973. *The emotionally troubled adolescent and the family physician.* Springfield, Ill.: Charles C Thomas, Publisher.

Miller, D. 1974. *Adolescence: psychology, psychopathology and psychotherapy.* New York: Jason Aronson.

Schoolar, J. C., editor. 1973. *Current issues in adolescent psychiatry.* New York: Brunner/Mazel.

Usdin, G. L., editor. 1967. *Adolescence: care and counseling.* Philadelphia: J. B. Lippincott.

Weiner, I. B., and DelGaudio, A. C. 1976. Psychopathology in adolescence. *Arch. Gen. Psychiatr.* 33:187.

Wolman, B. B., editor. 1972. *Manual of child psychopathology.* New York: McGraw-Hill Book Co.

-23-
Principles of Psychosocial Evaluation and Counseling

The Therapeutic Relationship
The setting □ Fees □ Approach □ Confidentiality □ Interviewing options
Problem Definition and Evaluation
The psychosocial data base □ General problem indicators
Mental status assessment
Referral Versus Treatment by the Primary Care Physician
Implementing referral □ Referral resources
Principles of Counseling
The counseling sequence
Psychotropic Medication

The primary care physician frequently is the first port of call for an emotional problem of an adolescent. The situation may present as (a) the complaint of parents or other adults (schools, police); (b) the patient's own concerns, overtly stated or covertly masked by a screen complaint about some other and usually innocuous need; (c) the physician's own discovery consequent to routine inquiries during a visit for some other purpose; or (d) an implicit element of specific medical problems such as a drug overdose, psychosomatic symptoms, chronic illness, or pregnancy.

The derivation of such problems is equally diverse and runs the gamut from normal adolescent testing and experimenting behavior to temporary overloading of stress tolerance circuits (or an adjustment reaction) to the insidious onset of a psychosis. In each instance, the task is to identify and define the problem, determine its seriousness, and initiate treatment by direct management or referral (Figure 23-1).

The Therapeutic Relationship

From the beginning, patient contacts need to be carried out within the context of the "therapeutic relationship." This sets the tone for effective data gathering and forms the cornerstone of trust that is essential to the treatment process.

THE SETTING

Interviewing and counseling are best conducted in a relaxed and informal setting. Sitting in several easy chairs grouped in the corner of the office is far better than standard methods of having the desk intervene. Sufficient time should be allowed to eliminate the impression of being pressured or rushed. The adolescent is highly sensitive to the examiner's tone and resents being given short shrift. He or she also may misperceive this as disinterest or impatience—not a particularly good start. When a problem is identified during an extremely busy time, it is best to be open about your situation; tell the patient you do not have all the time you would like to have and reschedule a longer appointment within the next few days (the sooner the better). It can be helpful to set aside an afternoon or evening exclusively for 30–45 minute counseling sessions.

FEES

Payment should be appropriate to the time involved. Counseling is a valuable professional service and should not be a "loss leader." Inadequate recom-

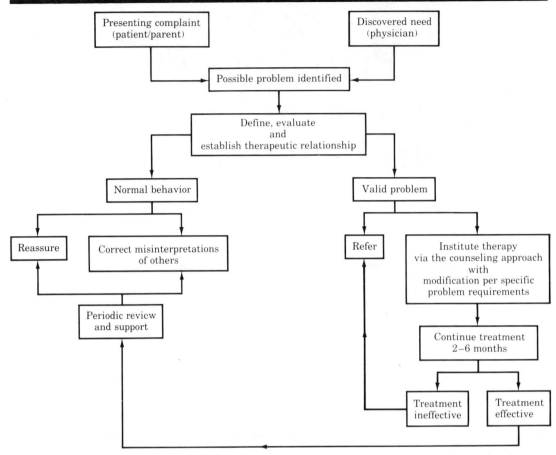

FIGURE 23-1
MANAGEMENT SEQUENCE FOR EMOTIONAL AND BEHAVIORAL PROBLEMS IN ADOLESCENCE

pense over time inevitably influences the physician's effectiveness through associated feelings of exploitation and resentment. Most parents understand that psychological problems simply cannot be managed according to the traditional primary care perspective of high volume, low cost.

APPROACH

Counseling and psychotherapeutic intervention require much the same orientation as does adolescent health care in general (Chapter 2). Respect, empathy, and comfortable exchange in a shared collaborative approach are essential. Paternalism and parentalism should be avoided. This dependency relationship is precisely what adolescents are divesting themselves of and the physician who assumes such a role will fail to secure the patient's full trust.

The use of coaxing, cajoling, threats, and various overt and covert coercions is also unavailing; such tactics are akin to waving a red flag at a bull and merely set the stage for a power struggle that no one will win. Rather, the physician's legitimacy and authority stem from the patient's perception of his or her knowledge, expertise, justice, fairness, and concern.

Overidentification is at the opposite end of the spectrum from a power-based paternalistic approach. It is equally problematic. If the physician confuses empathy (being sensitive to and in tune with the patient's plight) with overidentification (or taking on the adolescent's problems as if they were his or her own), he or she cannot respond without bias. This inevitably interferes with accurate understanding of the situation and puts the physician in league with the adolescent against the perceived parental adversary. If overidentification occurs in relation to intrafamily conflict, the physician becomes party to the problem; parents hardly appreciate being seen as the enemy and may well terminate the physician's services. The reciprocal can be even more fatal; the therapeutic process becomes impossible if the doctor perceives the patient's behavior as outrageous or immoral and identifies with the parents instead.

Discussions should be straightforward, open, and honest with give and take on both sides. The physician should also be true to his or her own style and vocabulary, excepting the avoidance of terminology the patient may not understand. The adoption of teenage jargon, dress, or mannerisms, if alien to personal style, will be perceived readily as artifice and will not promote trust.

CONFIDENTIALITY

An effective relationship also requires respect for confidentiality. Adolescents are heavily invested in establishing their own separate world from parents and are unlikely to share highly personal feelings, thoughts, and clandestine behaviors if they believe the physician will tell "all" to parents or other adults without their permission. Both the patient and parents must understand this essential rule.

But there also must be an "out" for those relatively rare instances where the failure to advise parents and invoke their protection can result in genuine harm to the patient. For the most part such situations are limited to suicidal ideation of a significant degree. Plans to run away or commit an illegal act also might qualify. Young people usually accept such exceptions if they know they will be told beforehand.

Other less urgent situations occur, about which parents must eventually be informed. Examples are pregnancy going to term or significant drug or alcohol abuse; in these cases, treatment and planning inevitably are a family matter. In addition, most adolescents in such circumstances do want their parents to be involved but fear the consequences of revelation and do not know how to proceed. While preserving confidentiality, and thereby trust, it usually is not difficult to work with the patient toward this goal. After several visits the youngster usually will agree. The method of accomplishing parental advisement then can be worked out—by the youth alone or in the physician's presence, or by the doctor alone.

Parental confidences also need to be preserved, but the physician needs to discriminate between matters that are personal and private for the parents themselves and those that reflect worries, concerns, and ambivalences about their offspring. Although privacy is appropriate for some matters and for the initial interview, parental feelings about the adolescent (as well as the adolescent's feelings about the parents) ultimately are best brought out into the open and shared in the interest of mutual understanding. In such instances, the physician may need to become mediator to keep conflict and tempers down to manageable levels and to maintain open lines of communication.

INTERVIEWING OPTIONS

Various interviewing options exist and all have their role. They include:

1. Patient alone. No intervention is effective without most interaction taking place with the patient alone. Much of the initial visit should be conducted in this manner, permitting the patient to get "first crack" at stating his or her views.

2. Parents alone (mother or father alone or both together). It is difficult for parents initially to speak of and explore their disappointments, fears, hurts, and angers about the patient in his or her presence. It also is often necessary to discuss matters parents will perceive as private for themselves, such as the marital relationship. It is neither necessary nor appropriate for the patient to know these issues in full detail.

3. Patient and parent(s) together. This arrangement is helpful in the data gathering stage and later therapeutic stages. Initially, much can be learned by observing intrafamily interactions. Later, solutions often involve enhancing intrafamily communication and mutual understanding or the working out of various compromises, agreements, and household rules.

The sequence of these options varies according to circumstances but is always subject to two provisos. First, the patient is always primary and must perceive the physician as his or her advocate. Although this emphasis is not always appreciated by parents, it can be pointed out that this position is essential to establishing the patient's trust; without trust no progress can be made, and this position best serves the interests of the family in the adolescent's return to health. Second, parents should not be interviewed alone for any extended period of time when the patient must stay in the waiting room. He or she will only worry excessively about what is being said behind closed doors, feeling cheated of rebuttal opportunities and resentful of the physician's interviewing priorities.

Problem Definition and Evaluation

THE PSYCHOSOCIAL DATA BASE

The identification and evaluation of any psychosocial problem is predicated upon obtaining an appropriate psychosocial data base (Tables 23-1 and 23-2). If the physician has known the patient since infancy, much of this information should be available from the record. Noting current developmental and behavioral progress in a sentence or two at each regular visit for an infant or child can be invaluable at adolescence. With a new patient, one obviously must start from scratch.

In obtaining information, it is as important to look for strengths as vulnerabilities, avoiding the common pitfall of exclusive problem orientation. Intervention builds far more on what the young person has going for him or her than in attempting analytic ego reconstruction. In many respects, adolescence is a time of affirmative emotional growth. When positive developmental forces are supported and encouraged, the less healthy aspects often simply fall by the wayside with time.

GENERAL PROBLEM INDICATORS

It can be difficult to determine when a behavioral or emotional manifestation is truly dysfunctional. Normal adolescent behavior can be moody and provocative at times. Age-appropriate challenging of adult behavior may be misperceived as an impulse disorder; casual drug or alcohol experimentation may be misinterpreted as abuse. On the other side of the coin, a shy and retiring young person may be seen as pleasantly compliant when in fact he or she is significantly depressed. Table 23-3 lists various common indicators of potentially deviant behaviors, but pathologic significance must be measured against the norm (Chapter 1) and tested for seriousness by qualifying in two or more of the following categories.

1. Intensity. Symptoms are clearly demarcated from the premorbid state or comprise an inappropriate and exaggerated response to ordinary provocations (for example, intense rage reactions with property damage or assaultive behavior in contrast to simply angry mutterings and epithets and the occasional slamming of doors in response to parental limit setting).

2. Inconsistency. The symptoms are inconsistent with those concerns appropriate to the adolescent's developmental stage. Intrafamily contests over control are normal for the midadolescent but inappropriate if they persist into young adulthood. Lack of interest in dating is not of concern in early teen years, but should raise a question if it persists. The absence of friends and being a "loner" at any time

TABLE 23-1
PARENT-DERIVED
PSYCHOSOCIAL DATA BASE

Developmental stage	Data to be obtained
Prenatal and perinatal	1. Medical aspects of pregnancy/birth 2. Parental feelings toward pregnancy, delivery, infant
Early years (birth to age 4 years)	1. Progression of developmental steps 2. Status of feeding, sleeping, play, health, temperament, and general adjustment
Primary school years (ages 4–11 years)	1. Ability to separate from home 2. Home, peer, teacher relationships 3. School performance, behavior 4. Eating, sleeping, play, health, temperament, and general adjustment 5. Fine and gross motor control
Adolescence (ages 12 years +)	1. Shifts in home, peer, school relationships 2. School performance, behavior 3. Activities and interests 4. Successes/problems and outcomes
Intrafamily dynamics	1. Composition of family, ages, occupations 2. Emotional, physical, and functional status of patient, other members 3. Status of parent-parent, parent-patient, patient-sibling relationships; general household tone
Current status of patient	1. Parental perception of how patient is doing; areas of strength/vulnerability; satisfied/dissatisfied with progress; particular concerns 2. Parental hopes for patient's future 3. Parents' perception of own competence in parenting and areas of concern (e.g., communication, confidence, limit setting, sex education)
Sociological	1. Financial status (comfortable/hardship) 2. Housing adequacy; sleeping arrangements

TABLE 23-2
PATIENT-DERIVED
PSYCHOSOCIAL DATA BASE

Functional sphere	Data to be obtained
School/work function	1. Feelings about school/work; likes and dislikes 2. Relationship with teachers/classmates; ability to get along; special problems 3. Behavior; perceives self as adaptive or disruptive 4. Performance; best/worst subjects and marks 5. Educational/vocational plans
Peer relationships	1. Prefers to be with friends or alone 2. How many friends; close/casual; when sees; what do together; best friend(s) and level of confidence
Sexuality	1. Dating partner(s); current/past; nature of and comfort with relationship 2. Extent of physical involvement and comfort level; ever had intercourse; contraceptive use; ever pregnant and outcome; ever had sexually transmitted disease 3. Sexual problems/worries 4. Gender orientation/preference 5. Masturbation and feelings about 6. Sexual abuse (rape, incest, molestation)
Parent relationships and sibling	1. Major points of support/conflict; feelings toward parents/siblings 2. Level of communication and confidance; tells everything/reserves some information and what 3. Perceived strengths/problems of parents and siblings
Activities and interests	1. Use of leisure time; hobbies; jobs
Religion	1. Traditional/Eastern/cult; place in life
Future plans	1. Imminent and long-range; educational; vocational; marriage; family; life-style
Self-assessment	1. What likes most/least about self; strengths/liabilities 2. How would describe self to others 3. Prevailing mood; happy/sad/suicidal thoughts; optimistic/pessimistic/helpless and hopeless 4. Major problems and concerns

is inconsistent with developmental demands for peer group affiliation.

3. Frequency and chronicity. To be classified as abnormal, symptoms must be present for more than 4–6 weeks and occur at a frequency in excess of peer group norms (drinking more than friends) or persistent and unmitigated by counterbalancing trends (always sad without periodic upward mood swings). In some instances, early indicators of chronicity may be missed until forced into the open by an acute event such as a suicidal attempt or running away.

4. Dysfunctionality. Symptoms interfere with developmental progress, interpersonal relationships, and/or participation in school and other normal adolescent activities. This may be through depression, withdrawal, and isolation or acting-out and antisocial behaviors (more than simply nonconforming), and/or incapacitating anxiety. Such patients usually perceive that they are in emotional pain and not performing as they would like.

MENTAL STATUS ASSESSMENT

Appropriate evaluation of the patient's mental status can give important information. In many respects, the physician begins to make such assessment from the moment the patient walks in the room and he or she should be sensitive to various clues given by the patient during the course of the history and medical examination. These intuited clues are later translated into an assessment of mood, affect, and intelligence. Although such a random and unstructured approach is valid in many instances, the physician should always have some specific informational objectives in mind. In other instances, such as in head trauma, drug toxicity, suspected psychosis or learning disorder, the conduct of a formal mental status examination is indicated (Table 23-4). If the physician is concerned about asking seemingly stupid questions, the topic can be introduced by saying, "I know some of these questions may sound silly to you, but they are just routine and necessary to ensure we are being thorough in finding out just what is going on."

TABLE 23-3
SPECIFIC INDICATORS IN PSYCHOSOCIAL
DATA BASE OF POSSIBLE BEHAVIORAL
OR EMOTIONAL PROBLEMS IN ADOLESCENCE

Area affected	Indicators
School	1. Loss of interest; deteriorating or chronically underachieving performance 2. Recurrent truancy; refusal to attend entirely 3. Disruptive behavior; inability to get along with teachers/classmates in general (not just one or two individuals)
Home	1. Continual disagreement plus acting-out (running away, recurrent staying out late, repeated rages, abusive language, assaultive threats, flagrant and persistent disregard for family operational rules) 2. Pronounced increase in secretiveness and isolation
Peers	1. Lack of involvement; inability to make friends or dropping of former friends 2. No dating or evident interest from midadolescence on 3. Active member of a peer group known to be involved in dysocial behaviors
Functional	1. Chronic sleep disturbances (more than going to bed late and reluctant waking up) 2. Major shifts in eating patterns; rapid weight loss or gain 3. Psychosomatic and/or hypochondriacal complaints (more than normal preoccupations with body and body image)
Appearance	1. Deterioration in dress and personal hygiene
Mood	1. Chronic depression; poor self-esteem; self-deprecation; suicide ruminations/proclamations/attempt 2. Chronic and unmitigated anger/hostility; recurrent out-of-control rages 3. Chronic anxiety or "nervousness"; fearfulness; refusal to engage in new situations 4. Recurrent "hysterical" outbursts; recurrent episodes of hyperventilation and palpitations
Substance abuse	1. Use of strong hallucinogens or narcotics to any degree 2. Consumption of any drug or alcohol weekly or more often in amounts more than used by friends; at inappropriate times (morning, school, alone); to cope with anxiety; preference for being "high" to "straight"
Antisocial behavior	1. Delinquency; in trouble with police
Sexual	1. Promiscuity (multiple partners) 2. Pregnancy 3. Sexual abuse (incest, rape, molestation) 4. Gender identity and orientation problems (homosexuality, transexualism, transvestitism, general confusion)
Medical	1. Chronic illness or handicap 2. Any illness resulting in prolonged absence from school and/or isolation from peer group

The "draw a person" test can be particularly useful. Although not suitable for assessing an adolescent's intelligence quotient unless retardation is suspected (calibrated scoring in the Goodenough "Draw a Man" scale is not particularly sensitive or discriminating past 10 years of age), it can given important insights into the patient's body image concepts. Give the patient a plain sheet of paper and pencil; then simply ask him or her to "draw a whole person in the best way you can," offering no further commentary other than reassurance that you are not looking for artistic skill or handing out marks. If only a head or stick figure is forthcoming, ask the patient to try again. Then request a second drawing of the opposite sex. The patient may be asked to elaborate on who these persons are and something about them, but unless needed to help clarify obscure aspects of the drawings themselves, this usually is not as productive as with younger children. The significance rests in the pictures themselves and the usually clear evidence of the patient's self-concepts and perception of others.

Other simple methods of assessing intellectual competence are having the patient bring in some of his or her school books and written work in English and mathematics, inquiring about what books he or she likes to read, having the patient read from something appropriate at hand, writing several sentences on a specific subject such as what he or she did the previous weekend, and solving various mathematical problems, including simple fractions and long division. These approaches are particularly useful in the preliminary assessment of a youngster with a school

---

TABLE 23-4
AN OUTLINE FOR THE PERFORMANCE
OF A MENTAL STATUS EXAMINATION

---

1. Appearance: Compared to patients' own subcultural and peer group standards
2. Behavior: Conduct; facial expression; motor activity; posture; mannerisms
3. Affect (emotional state or "feeling tone"):
   a. Objective: anger; irritability; elation; depression; agitation; indifference; inappropriateness; flatness; impoverishment, and so on
   b. Subjective: patient views about his or her own feelings, suicidal ideas
4. Stream of mental activity (quality and content of speech production): logical and coherent vs. overproductive, rambling, disconnected, impoverished, delayed
5. Though content: hallucinations; delusions; compulsions; phobias; ideas of unreality and depersonalization; fantasies; disordered body image
6. Orientation: for time, place, person, situation
7. Memory:
   a. Remote: date of birth; names of schools attended and teachers; past illnesses/injuries; important past events
   b. Recent: events surrounding onset of present illness/injury; own address and telephone number; names and ages of siblings; present school name and location
   c. Retention and recall: immediate recall of 4-7 digits (forward and backward); 5-minute delayed recall of words, name, street address
8. Intellectual function:
   a. General information: presidents; cities; capitals; recent news/sports items
   b. Counting and calculation: count 1-20; serial subtraction from 100 (7s, 5s or 2s depending on educational status); simple addition and subtraction
   c. Reading, writing, speech: aphasia; dyslexia; speech defects; perception problems
   d. Abstracting: proverbs; similarities
9. Judgment: ability to make a reasoned decision on how to act in a given situation (what would you do if you saw a house on fire, found a stamped, addressed envelope?)
10. Insight: awareness of why visiting physician? Any understanding of dynamics of emotional conflicts?

---

problem and can often differentiate between borderline retardation, learning disability, and simple emotional disturbance. Patients who have a sixth grade or better reading level, can write sentences effectively, and can contend with fractions and long division probably are neither dyslexic nor retarded.

Although formal psychologic testing will be required in such instances for definitive answers, these preliminary measures together with a thorough neurological examination can be invaluable in setting up a well-organized plan of evaluation and treatment. Too often such youngsters get sent from one consultant to another with no one person seemingly in charge or coordinating results.

Referral Versus Treatment
by the Primary Care Physician

Following assessment, the physician needs to decide if treatment is within his or her scope or whether to refer. There are no hard and fast rules, but the following considerations offer guidance.

1. Duration of symptoms. Referral usually is indicated when the patient's symptoms have been present since preadolescent years. These tend to be well entrenched, resistant to modification, and require more intense therapy than the primary care physician usually is equipped to give.

2. Seriousness. Symptoms and behaviors that bear the potential for serious harm (such as a suicide attempt); are known to be particularly recalcitrant to treatment (drug addiction, major delinquency); or of psychotic proportions (schizophrenia or affective psychosis) should always be referred.

3. Persistence. Referral is usually indicated in any dysfunctional situation that is unresponsive to the efforts of the primary care physician over 4-6 months.

4. Special problems. A number of conditions require highly specialized and comprehensive services, or at least the use of adjunctive resources complementing the primary care physician's own treatment plan. These include such matters as pregnancy, learning disabilities, and retardation.

5. Patient acceptance. Many troubled adolescents are suspicious of psychiatry and resist referral. Some believe mental health professionals have special methods for reading their minds and can discover thoughts they would not wish to reveal. Others perceive that taking such a step implies they are "crazy" and reject such labeling. Yet others may be reluctant to give up a valued relationship with the primary care physician for one that is an unknown quantity. Regardless of other considerations, referral cannot be effected without a willing youth.

6. Physician comfort and skill. Managing psychosocial problems in adolescence requires willingness to make a commitment of interest and time to the patient. It also requires a certain level of comfort and skill. These factors are ones that each primary care physician needs to assess for himself or herself. Referral, or at least psychiatric consultation, is the

appropriate course when in doubt of one's own competence, unsure as to the seriousness of the problem at hand, or simply not inclined to take on these issues by virtue of personal interest or time factors.

IMPLEMENTING REFERRAL

If referral is decided upon, patient (and parent) motivation is critical. As noted above in point No. 5, it is futile to attempt to refer a recalcitrant youth. Unless the situation is serious and acute, warranting possible emergency hospitalization (commitment to suicide, acute decompensation, a schizophrenic break), a little time and several visits may be needed to help the patient and family agree. Steps in motivation include:

1. Reassurance that the patient is not "crazy" but does have problems that he or she might like to straighten out. The physician should point out (a) that this can be difficult to do alone and it could be useful to have someone help him or her gain better understanding; (b) the primary care physician is not properly trained for this purpose; and (c) the patient deserves the very best in care and the services of a specialist.

2. Reassurance that a psychiatrist has no magic tricks or crystal ball and can only know as much as the patient wishes to reveal. Psychotherapy is the holding up of a mirror in which the patient may come to see himself or herself more clearly, make more effective decisions, and come to better self-control and control over his or her environment.

3. You, the primary care physician, will remain the patient's regular doctor, will continue to be very much interested in his or her well-being, will continue to see him or her from time to time, and will be available to talk whenever he or she might wish.

4. Sometimes it is necessary to create or aggravate psychic pain in overcoming resistance to referral. This is accomplished by reviewing problem areas in close detail and pointing out quite bluntly, but empathically, how it really must hurt a lot to be missing out on so much, to be embroiled in continuing emotional conflict, always to be feeling sad and lonely, etc.

REFERRAL RESOURCES

Although we have spoken exclusively of referral to a psychiatrist for the sake of simplicity, in reality, a variety of options exist as cited in Table 23-5. These can be invoked singly or severally, depending on the patient's needs and financial resources.

TABLE 23-5
REFERRAL RESOURCES FOR PSYCHOSOCIAL PROBLEMS*

Private practitioners	Psychiatrists Psychologists Social workers
Mental health clinics	Free standing Associated with general and psychiatric hospitals (private, city, county, state)
Adolescent comprehensive health clinics	General hospitals Free clinics
Social agencies	Jewish Family Service Catholic Charities Local private and governmental agencies
Youth-oriented programs†	Boys' clubs/Girls' clubs Big Brothers and Sisters YMCA, YWCA, YMHA, YWHA
Schools	Guidance counselors School psychologists "Rap" groups Peer leadership programs Special education for handicapped
Special problem programs	Drug abuse; day care and residential centers Alcoholics Anonymous; Alateen Weight Watchers; Overeaters Anonymous, etc. Lighthouse for the Blind City and state associations for brain-injured children BOSES (Bureau of Special Educational Services) or equivalent in all school districts Reading clinics (should be evaluated; Orton Society has good reputation) Teenage pregnancy programs in clinics and schools Teen-oriented family planning programs and "rap" groups

*Can be identified through national organizations; professional affiliations; professional societies; general and/or psychiatric hospitals; regional special purpose associations such as for mental health, and social service. (Also see Appendix II.)

†Usually focus on preventive mental health; special drug and delinquency diversion programs.

Principles of Counseling

In many instances, the primary care physician can manage behavioral and emotional problems most effectively. This is accomplished through combining the therapeutic relationship with the counseling approach. Patient and physician work together to clarify the problem, examine options, and implement solutions. This process employs a wide variety of communicative and interpretive methods and resource options. These are applied in a definitive sequence (Table 23-6) predicated upon the following concepts:

1. Adolescence is a time of revising earlier dependency-based ego developmental issues into new autonomous terms. Although manifested in considerable emotional intensity, vulnerability, and fluctuation, this process also offers opportunity for undoing old maladaptive patterns and discovering new and more constructive ways. Adolescence often is referred to as a second chance.

2. Given support and encouragement, developmental forces favor adaptive rather than maladaptive solutions to conflict or stress. Troubled adolescents generally do want to do better if they can overcome intrinsic and extrinsic barriers to the contrary.

3. Counseling is based as much on identifying and building on strengths as it is in undoing problems. The patient is helped to use his or her assets in constructive ways to achieve success as measured by enhanced self-esteem, mastery, and control. Success then breeds success.

4. The physician's role is to help the adolescent discover his or her own best way. Although the physician obviously must have a clear sense of what is going on and possess skills to help the patient clarify these issues and come to understand his or her full range of options, ultimately it is the patient's own actions that effect change and not professional ministrations.

THE COUNSELING SEQUENCE

Ventilation. Most troubled adolescents have a good bit of pent up tension and free-floating anxiety surrounding their emotional problem. This tends to dominate the picture and block a more rational and considered approach. Encouraging the patient to freely express feelings of anger, sadness, injustice, or exploitation clears the air, helps organize thinking, and sometimes enables him or her to see a solution rather quickly. Although ventilation is the primary goal in initiating treatment, it is not an answer in and of itself. Anxiety will reaccumulate quickly until the fundamental conflict resolves. Additional oppor-

---

TABLE 23-6
THE COUNSELING SEQUENCE

1. Ventilation
2. Problem exploration
3. Problem definition
4. Interpretation
5. Definition of options
6. Option choice
7. Option motivation
8. Option implementation
9. Ongoing support

---

tunities for ventilation should be made available at the beginning of any session.

Not all adolescents take to this process easily. Those who are not particularly verbal or introspective or who are depressed and withdrawn may find it difficult to speak of their feelings. These patients may be encouraged by several specific techniques. Ventilation is introduced most naturally at the beginning of the session with such nondirective questions as "Why don't you tell me about the problem from your point of view?" or "What's been happening since I saw you last time?" Vague answers such as, "I don't know" or "Nothing much" can be followed up in a more directive manner. These methods not only are useful here but also at any point when issues need to be brought out into the open more. They can be particularly helpful in problem exploration and problem definition.

1. Projective technique. The physician makes some assumptions about how the patient must feel based on experience and sensitivity to the particular situation. These are then offered to the patient, who is asked to test them for truth. "If I were in your situation, I think I would feel this way...." When the physician is on target, the patient appreciates his or her perceptiveness, often acknowledging this with a smile, a nod, relaxation of anxiety, or direct verbal affirmation and often picks up and carries the conversation from here. Nothing is lost if the patient says, "It's not that way at all." The clear rejoinder is, "Why don't you tell me how it is for you?"

2. Third-party displacement. Some adolescents find it difficult to tell of their own feelings and behaviors directly but are less threatened when the issues are one step removed, that is, displaced onto someone else or framed in generalized terms. "What feelings do you think young people your age experience when...?" "What do teenagers do in this situation?" "What's going on in your school, peer group

about...(sex, drugs, etc)?" As adolescents tend to project their own range of experience when answering, responses are strongly, albeit not absolutely, indicative of how they have felt or behaved in similar circumstances. In addition to reflecting projection, peer group behavior in and of itself is a strong indicator of the patient's own current or future behavior.

3. Permission. Reluctance may be encountered in discussions over controversial behaviors when the patient fears he or she may be embarrassed or suffer devaluation, rejection, or punishment. These concerns often may be diffused if the physician indicates he or she is aware and accepting of such behaviors, will not judge or devalue the patient because of them, and has no interest in seeking atonement or retribution. Such an attitude is implicit in such statements as, "Many young people your age smoke pot (have sex) today. Where do you stand on this issue?" It should be noted that acceptance does not imply that any particular behavior is necessarily desirable or to be condoned. But exploration of the direct implications for the patient and actual or potential harm is best deferred until the interpretive or option choice stage. A premature negative commentary may well be interpreted as judgmental and will only confirm the adolescent's initial fears.

Problem exploration. Problem exploration consists of rounding out preliminary information with additional details and completes the psychosocial history. Close attention should be paid to behavioral patterns, feelings, and attitudes surrounding the problem, providing the physician with a good idea about what is going on in situational and dynamic terms. Data gathering is best carried out in a give and take manner, avoiding rapid-fire, cross-examination type inquisitions, which inevitably pressure the patient, who then may become defensive rather than opening up. It may be necessary to take somewhat more time than usual in hearing out various digressions, and matters may not always proceed in an orderly sequence. But time well spent at this point will pay off in the end. It also should be noted that problem exploration often goes on throughout the counseling process as the patient gains in confidence and becomes increasingly capable of exploring his or her problems in greater depth.

It is also wise to avoid being judgmental at this or at any time. The adolescent in trouble has already experienced—and resisted—more than ample adult preachments and admonition. If the physician also takes such a stance, he or she only introduces similar conflict into the therapeutic relationship. This breeds resistance rather than change.

Problem definition and evaluation. Problem definition and evaluation are the natural result of earlier stages. Sufficient evidence should now be at hand to permit definition and evaluation of the problem with reasonable clarity. It is essential to gain such understanding before proceeding further. (If in doubt, assistance may be forthcoming from a psychiatric consultation.) In general terms, the physician now should be able to assign the problem to one of the following categories:

1. A relatively acute adjustment reaction to a situational (environmental) crisis or change and not necessarily an inappropriate reaction (the breakup of an important relationship, moving to a new community, entering or graduating from high school, being mugged or raped, prolonged absence from school due to illness).

2. An inappropriate response of the environment to normal adolescent development and needs (parental attempts to maintain the youth in a childhood dependency status; an unresponsive, chaotic school situation; an inappropriate school placement).

3. A persistent maladaptive response carried over from childhood with no clear current situational conflict (an impulse disorder and the failure to internalize external controls in childhood).

4. No clear situational conflict and earlier unresolved but suppressed issues now surfacing consequent to developmental arousal (conversion hysteria; the genesis usually rests in unresolved childhood sexual conflict).

5. Situational conflict responded to in an exaggerated and/or inappropriate manner consequent to poor development of effective coping mechanisms or constitutional proclivities (prolonged depression following a personal loss or suicidal attempt on going to college; acting-out behavior in face of a chaotic home situation).

It should be kept in mind, however, that the nature of the problem often will shift and change as therapy advances; periodic reevaluation is therefore a continuing process.

Interpretation. The physician now offers the patient a definition of the problem (or problems) and issues involved as he or she sees them, allowing for feedback, exchange, and modification from the patient's perspective. Both then arrive at a mutual agreement on the problem's nature and extent. This is the time to comment on inappropriate behavior but always from the perspective of the patient and the ways in which his or her actions do him or her harm. If the situation involves a moral issue, determination of "harm" derives from the patient's own conflict over values, not from the physician's imposed judgment. Avoiding judgmentalism is essential because taking such a stance simply recapitulates the adolescent's past and often troubled relationships with other adults. It only sets conflict and power struggles into motion and can well result in a therapeutic impasse. It is quite legitimate, however, for the physician to express his or her own views and attempt persuasion through debate but not to impose them. Exception, of course, would be made for a youth, often sociopathic, who has little perception of right and wrong and is involved in highly questionable activities. The message that such behavior is unacceptable needs to be given loud and clear but in a manner that does not imply rejection or devaluation of the youth or suggest that the physician will abandon the patient if he or she does not change.

Defining options. The physician and patient together should identify and review various alternatives to change the situation. This includes the entire spectrum from the ridiculous to the sublime to no change at all. It is important that the adolescent perceive the full range of options and be able to realistically appraise the probable outcomes and consequences of each. Only in this way will he or she have sufficient information on which to base the most rational possible choice. The physician may need to give considerable guidance at this point, as the still concrete or as yet imperfectly formed abstractive thinking processes of adolescents can make it difficult for them to fully appreciate consequences and future implications. Their orientation tends to be more existential than futuristic, at least during the early and midadolescent years.

Options vary greatly; they may range from various methods of handling conflicts in interpersonal relationships; altering problematic environments by changing classes, teachers, or schools; invoking supportive resources such as Boys and Girls Clubs, family planning clinics, Weight Watchers; or specific treatment resources such as the primary care physician, psychiatrist, or therapeutic residence. Sometimes options are few and far between, and the most that can be offered is the primary care physician's continued empathy and support until the passage of time, further maturation, or the patient's age open up a broader range of possibilities.

Option choice. Choosing a course of action involves the patient's (and often the parents') exploration of the acceptability and nonacceptability and the ultimate selection of a realistic course. This requires more than recourse to a simple check-off list and includes mutual exploration of feasibility, ambivalence, barriers, and preferences. The ultimate decision—and commitment—must be the patient's own if he or she is to be effectively motivated. Although the physician may suggest, recommend, and even express distress over a poor choice, the old adage, "you can lead a horse to water but you can't make him drink" still obtains. If an effective trust relationship has been established, it can be assumed that the patient values the physician's views but may need to save face and maintain some sense of control in accepting them. It can be helpful to set things up so that the patient can take the physician's choice while preserving independence ("I could do X, but I'll take your suggestion and do Y," with Y usually the preferred course) or incorporating one of the physician's views, which then emerges as the patient's own "new" idea.

It is also important to base encouragement to take one course rather than another on the perception of what would best promote the adolescent's return to normal developmental tasks and the acquisition of self-esteem. This may not always coincide with societal norms or the physician's own value system. Pressures to conform based solely on such external determinants constitute judgmentalism and are to be avoided: it is not necessarily incompatible with normalcy for a teenager to engage in a sexual relationship, smoke marijuana recreationally, go to a commune, or pursue Eastern meditational religions. This does not mean that such options are always appropriate, but that their measure is based on what best serves the needs of the patient, not those of the physician or other adults.

A last aspect of option choice is that the patient may not always take a better course from the beginning. He or she may engage in a period of testing-out the physician or be unable to shift gears easily because of entrenched past patterns. Tolerance and patience are essential while the adolescent's elected course is periodically reviewed and revision encouraged. It is essential that the physician not succumb to frustration and impatience, taking a coercive course or hinting at rejection in exasperation. It is, however, legitimate and useful to calmly advise of such feelings ("I understand why you are so angry. But when you bring this into the office it sometimes makes me feel angry too. Can we talk about this, as it really is getting in the way of our working together and helping you feel better?") or to make other adverse commentary by dissociating valuation of the adolescent as a person from his or her behavior: ("I think you really are a good person, but what you are doing is very destructive for you. I know you can do better if we work at it together").

Option motivation. Basically an extension of the previous step, option motivation employs the same processes as the previous step in helping the patient consolidate his or her choice into a commitment. Founded on the trust relationship, this usually involves establishing a "contract" defining certain expectancies of the patient on the one side and the physician's support on the other. The latter should include promises (which must be kept) of ready availability for discussion at any time and the willingness to smooth pathways or otherwise function as a protective intermediary or advocate.

Option implementation. Option implementation involves taking whatever steps are necessary to put the contract into motion. Generally these fall into one or more of the following categories:

1. Helping the patient modify his or her behavioral response systems through discussion, increasing self-awareness, and rehearsal of how to cope with difficult or conflictual situations more effectively.

2. Modifying the environment in a more responsive manner (for example, working out a mutually acceptable home behavioral code in family sessions or effecting a more appropriate school situation.

3. Identifying and arranging for the marshalling of supportive resources, such as recreational options, peer support and/or "rap" groups, remedial education, weight loss programs etc.

A word of caution when using outside resources: it is important that the physician arrange for personalized contact and a specific appointment. The adolescent should be given the time of the appointment, the name of the contact individual, and specific directions as to where to go in written form along with a note of introduction. The patient should also be asked to call the physician the day after the first appointment and report on how things went. If the patient does not call, the physician should take the initiative instead. Young people frequently find institutionalism and bureaucracy overwhelming. They also easily succumb to denial when faced with having to take a new and unfamiliar step. An excellent plan can fail due to inadequate attention to the foregoing details. The physician may have to do a good bit of the footwork in the beginning, but it is useful therapeutically for the patient to explore and implement certain aspects on his or her own after gaining sufficient self-confidence.

Ongoing support. The need for a plan of continuing contact is self-evident. This plan should provide for regularly scheduled visits and interim telephone or drop-in contact as needed. Initially the patient should be seen on a weekly basis until there is evidence of positive change and the patient feels he or she need not come so frequently. This may require only several weeks for an acute adjustment reaction or environmental problem with easy solution or from 6–8 weeks or more in instances such as major intrafamily conflict. Visits may then be tapered to monthly intervals until symptoms are well controlled or cleared and the patient feels more confident that he or she can manage things on his or her own. The goals here are to stabilize progress to date, promote further advance, and defend against such threats as may be encountered in the progression of developmental tasks (for example, a young troubled teenager faces new stresses when he advances to midadolescence and may have difficulty sustaining earlier therapeutic progress). This period may last anywhere from 2–3 months to a year or more depending on the intensity, chronicity, and seriousness of the problem and the degree to which the patient can consolidate and maintain his or her gains. Once this point has been reached, it is still well to continue to see the patient semiannually and on an as-needed basis.

In many respects, ongoing support is an abbreviated recapitulation of the entire counseling process at each visit, focusing on different aspects as the current situation warrants. Ventilation often takes on new dimensions in self-awareness; problem perception becomes increasingly reality based and old problems emerge in new terms. If counseling is effective, each cycle will carry understanding to greater depths, opening up new and better options, consolidating gains, and giving the patient an increasing sense of being able to cope well.

The initiative for terminating treatment usually will be taken by the adolescent. Normal emancipating drives inevitably promote surrender of dependence upon the physician, and there need be little fear that this dependency will continue indefinitely. Visits then can be placed wholly on an as-needed basis.

Some degree of continuing support also is indicated even if the patient is referred to another resource. This is primarily to ensure that the referral "takes." Not all are successful. An institutional referral may break down in the course of inherent red tape or patient and parent confusion over how to negotiate the system. A recommended psychiatrist may simply not be a particular adolescent's "cup of tea." It is a useful and simple matter to have the patient check back after the first referral visit to find out how things went. If all went well, the primary physician may well continue to be involved for medical care. No more than this is necessary or advisable, as it is important not to perpetuate the primacy of the physician-patient relationship to a degree that interferes with the youth's transference of his or her therapeutic allegiance to another. Of course, if the referral does not work out initially or at a later time, continued contact of some degree will ensure that an alternative plan will be made and incepted.

Psychotropic Medication

We hold the optimistic view that psychotropic drugs are not necessary for most emotionally distressed adolescents and that normal drives toward healthy adaptation, when supported by appropriate psychotherapeutic management, are sufficient unto themselves. We are adamant in our conviction that psychotropic medication is not an answer per se and should never be used without psychotherapeutic intervention as well. We particularly feel such agents have only a minimal role in instances of intrafamily conflict, school problems, psychosomatic disorders, dysfunctional social behaviors, and acting out.

In some situations, however, medication is an important adjunct in giving the patient a better sense of control and promoting more integrative and adaptive behavior. These include the following:

1. Initial management of diffuse acute anxiety reactions (minor tranquilizers).

2. Support during transient high-stress situations over which the adolescent has little control. Immobilization in traction for fracture of a leg or the conduct of painful medical procedures are examples (minor tranquilizers, sedatives and analgesics as indicated).

3. Long-term impulse disorders (major or minor tranquilizers).

4. Emergency management of out-of-control reactions such as panic or rage (major or minor tranquilizers depending on intensity and effectiveness).

5. Psychoses and dissociative reactions (major tranquilizers).

6. Depressive reactions when the patient is unable to function adequately (minor tranquilizers if associated with agitation, sedatives for sleep, mood elevators—although mood elevators are less clearly effective in adolescents than in adults).

Many agents are available, each with its own set of attributes as propounded by manufacturers' claims. This multiplicity of drugs can be confusing, and we recommend the primary care physician limit his or her repertoire to one or two agents from each class and become familiar with their use (Table 23-7). We have been content with diazepam, chlorpromazine, and haloperidol but do not exclude other choices if the situation warrants; Stelazine or Mellaril may be better tolerated in chronic administration than chlorpromazine in that sedative effects are less pronounced, although haloperidol also meets this criterion. We do not subscribe, however, to the use of antihistamines (hydroxyzines) even as very mild agents due to their generally poor effectiveness in adolescents. If a mood elevator is indicated, imipramine or amitriptyline are preferred due to their wide margin of safety. Monoamine oxidase inhibitors are contraindicated due to the dietary restrictions that must be observed in avoiding complications. Few adolescents can be depended upon to remember these injunctions.

Whatever agent is selected, it should be given in sufficient dosage to achieve the desired effect (Table 23-7). Intramuscular routes should be reserved for particularly agitated patients and dosage should be higher than for those who are less distressed. Emergency sedation can be achieved with the use of 5-10 mg of diazepam by slow intravenous push and repeated once as needed, the size of the dose being dependent on both the patient's size and degree of disturbance.

Unfortunately, all tranquilizers also have a sedative effect and, excepting at bedtime, most adolescents dislike feeling sleepy or groggy. The timing of administration and the amount given should be titrated accordingly. Major tranquilizers can produce extrapyramidal tract signs, and the patient should be warned about these symptoms. Major tranquilizers—Mellaril in particular—also may result in impotence in males, an important advisement at the time of initiating such treatment.

Another complicating factor to be considered in prescribing medication is suicide risk. When suicidal intentions are in the least suspected, agents with wide margins of safety in overdose situations such as diazepam should be used and the number of tablets given at any one time strictly limited. Specific directions should be given to the pharmacist not to refill the prescription more often than indicated by the instructions for use. Parents may need to keep the pills in their possession, dispensing one at a time as needed and otherwise ensuring that the patient is not storing up or has access to a lethal supply.

The use of psychotropic agents, as has been implied, is limited to those situations in which adolescents are acutely or chronically unable to function

TABLE 23-7
SELECTED PSYCHOTHERAPEUTIC AGENTS AND DOSAGES SUITABLE FOR ADOLESCENTS*

Generic name	Trade name	Selected dosage forms	Initial single p.o. dose (mg)	Single IM dose (mg)	Usual range p.o. daily dose (mg)
Minor tranquilizers (sedative-antianxiety)					
Chlordiazepoxide	Librium	5, 10, 25 mg caps 100 mg amps	5-10	10-15	20-40
Diazepam	Valium	2, 5, 10 mg caps 10 mg/2 ml amps	2-5	10	5-20
Major tranquilizers (antipsychotic)					
Chlorpromazine	Thorazine	10, 25, 50, 100, 200 mg tabs 25 mg/ml, 50 mg/2 ml amps	25-50	25	75-150 anti-anxiety 200-800 anti-psychotic
Thioridazine	Mellaril	10, 25, 50, 100, 150, 200 mg tabs	10-25		100-600
Trifluoperazine	Stelazine	1, 2, 5, 10 mg tabs	1-2		4-15
Haloperidol	Haldol	0.5, 1, 2, 5, mg tabs 5 mg/ml amps	0.5-1	3-5	2-6
Tricyclic antidepressants					
Doxepin hydrochloride	Sinequan	10, 25, 50 mg caps	25-50		75-300
Imipramine	Tofranil, Presamine	10, 25, 50 mg tabs	25-100		75-300
Amitriptyline	Elavil	10, 25, 50 mg tabs	25-100		75-300

*Dosage should be adjusted downward accordingly for adolescents who have not yet achieved 75% or more of anticipated adult growth (Tanner stage 3 or less).

in an adequate manner and unresponsive to other therapeutic measures or at significant risk of irreparable harm. This would include the depressed adolescent who is falling hopelessly behind at school or is suicidal. Impulsive adolescents also may be helped to contain their outbursts more effectively. Those who are responding to situational crises in highly maladaptive ways also may be helped to cope more effectively. The timing of drug therapy, therefore, is a highly individual matter largely based on the patient's degree of dysfunction and availability to other treatment measures.

Medication should not be continued longer than necessary. It may be needed for only a few days in situational crises. In more chronic circumstances, the drug may be tapered after several months' improvement in function and mood, observing the consequences, and whether discontinuance may proceed or reinstitution is necessary. Some adolescents, however, may need medication indefinitely, primarily those with psychotic or impulsive tendencies. It is fair to say, however, if psychotropic drugs are needed for more than 6-8 weeks, the patient belongs in the hands of a psychiatrist.

Bibliography*

Bird, B. 1955. *Talking with patients.* New York: J. B. Lippincott.

Hofmann, A. D.; Becker, R. D.; and Gabriel, H. P. 1976. *The hospitalized adolescent.* New York: The Free Press.

Hofmann, A. D. 1979. Counseling the adolescent patient. In *The clinical practice of adolescent medicine,* editor, J. T. Y. Shen. New York: Appleton-Century-Crofts.

Meeks, J. 1982. *The fragile alliance.* 2nd ed. Baltimore: Williams and Wilkins.

Miller, D. 1974. *Adolescence; psychology, psychopathology and psychotherapy.* New York: Jason Aronson.

Schneiders, A. A., editor. 1967. *Counseling the adolescent.* San Francisco: Chandler.

Walen, S.; Hauserman, N.; and Lavin, P. 1977. *Clinical guide to behavior therapy.* Baltimore: Williams and Wilkins.

*Note: Other useful references will be found in the introductory bibliography and those of subsequent chapters.

-24-
Behavioral Problems*

Intrafamily Conflict
Parenting normal adolescents □ Problematic adolescent-parent conflict
Battering and abuse □ Running away □ Siblings
School Problems
Evaluation □ Mild and borderline retardation □ Learning disabilities
Maturational cognitive delay □ Deficient schooling
Intraschool psychologic stress □ Psychologic problems with extraschool derivations
School problems external to patient involvement
Predelinquent and Delinquent Behaviors
Overview □ The juvenile justice system

The previous chapter offers guidelines for assessing psychosocial problems in general. The next three chapters examine specific symptom complexes as classified in Table 24-1. Sexuality-related problems, (including incest), drug and alcohol abuse, and chronic illness, are discussed in separate chapters. Anorexia nervosa and obesity are discussed in the chapter on nutrition.

Intrafamily Conflict

Some degree of distancing and testing vis-à-vis parents is a normal adolescent phenomenon, generally occurring sometime between the fourteenth and seventeenth years and lasting from 6–12 months. The absence of any such signs and the perpetuation of dependency are as concerning as is florid challenge of parental authority. Severing earlier childhood ties through emotional separation is essential for the achievement of autonomous adulthood. The intensity of this process varies greatly from one individual to another, reflecting the combined effect of the adolescent's own temperament, parental attitudes, and various social and cultural factors. Emancipating behavior can be deemed deviant only when the consequences are harmful to the adolescent, not solely

*Note: See Chapter 17 for sexuality issues, Chapter 19 for obesity and anorexia nervosa, Chapter 20 for drug and alcohol abuse.

because they are distressing to parents nor fully in line with societal expectancies.

PARENTING NORMAL ADOLESCENTS

The teen years may be made somewhat easier all around if it is recognized that the adolescent is not a child and requires a different set of parenting modalities. Parents should be introduced to these concepts as a part of preventive mental health counseling before adolescence begins, gradually putting them into action when the adolescent is between ages 12 and 14. It is far easier to incept this approach before the period of midadolescent conflict than after its arrival.

Parental self-awareness. Mothers and fathers often have their own hidden agendas, which can interfere with parenting effectiveness. These include the following dilemmas:

1. The adolescent's growing up signals the end of the parenting role. Parents who are heavily invested in child-rearing may experience significant threats to their own identity.

2. Accustomed to perceiving themselves in a nurturing relationship with a dependent child, parents may encounter problems in surrendering a protective stance, in coming to perceive their adolescent is competent in some measure to conduct

TABLE 24-1
CLASSIFICATION OF BEHAVIORAL AND
EMOTIONAL PROBLEMS IN ADOLESCENCE

A. Intrafamilial
  1. Patient-parents
    a. Hostility, alienation, loss of parental control
    b. Values conflict
    c. Acting-out, physical abuse of parents, running away
    d. Physical or sexual abuse by parents; incest
  2. Patient-siblings
    a. Conflict
    b. Physical abuse, incest
    c. Resentment in caring for younger sibling
    d. Illness in sibling
B. School
  1. Underachievement
  2. Classroom disruption, poor teacher and/or classmate relationships
  3. Refusal to attend, truancy
  4. Inadequate performance
    a. Learning disability
    b. Mild to moderate retardation
C. Dysfunctional social behaviors
  1. Predelinquent or delinquent behaviors
  2. Drug/alcohol abuse
  3. Sexual promiscuity, prostitution, gender deviations, homosexuality
  4. Runaways
D. Emotional problems
  1. Psychosomatic complaints
  2. Hysterical conversion
  3. Hysteria, hyperventilation syndrome, and globus hystericus
  4. Out-of-control behaviors
    a. Panic
    b. Rage
    c. Impulse control disorder
  5. Depression, suicide
  6. Psychosis
    a. Toxic brain syndrome
    b. Cyclical affective disorders
    c. Schizophrenia
E. Combined emotional-physical
  1. Anorexia nervosa
  2. Obesity
  3. Chronic illness or physical handicap

his or her own affairs, and to accord him or her increased independence.

3. Adolescent emancipating behavior may be difficult for adults to tolerate. First, in order to be different teenage culture of necessity is alien. Second, the withdrawal of affection and closeness can be painful and bewildering to parents who have not changed their loving ways; they may perceive this withdrawal as unprovoked and unfair.

4. Adolescents are experimenting by nature in finding their identity and securing independence. It is hard for parents to stand by and let the young person take risks, make mistakes, and learn to stand on his or her own two feet.

5. To some degree, all parents perceive their children as extensions of themselves and invest them with their own hopes and dreams. It can be difficult to accept the possibility that a child may well grow up to hold different values and aspirations than they may have wished and that there will be little they can do.

6. The rise of the young inevitably presages the downfall of the old, inherently threatening the dominance of adults. The generation in charge is about to be deposed by insurgence and takeover. This is singularly manifested in contemporary American culture with the marked valuation of youth evidenced in the media and consumer markets.

Parents must test their response to adolescent provocations against issues such as these. Is the behavior truly detrimental for the youth or simply an emancipating challenge? Can parents live with it a while without feeling devalued or threatened? Is there not some basis for trusting their offspring's own judgment, even if nonconforming? Unless prepared to assume a new relationship with their adolescent at considerable variance from that appropriate to a child, they may find themselves with few effective controls other than instituting 24-hour-a-day surveillance! Otherwise there is ample opportunity for a determined 15-year-old to do whatever he or she wants, and few sanctions can coerce the teenager into unwilling compliance.

The parent-adolescent relationship. Considerable freedom and mobility are accorded contemporary American adolescents. In many situations, the ultimate behavioral choice perforce falls to the adolescent alone. A young person will best meet this challenge if equipped with knowledge and skill through prior review of alternatives, discussion of what choice he or she would like to make, and a collaborative exploration of ways in which he or she can adhere to this choice and not succumb to contrary pressures. Parents have an essential responsibility in this process in providing guidance and support, in teaching values, and in establishing the standards by which young persons are expected to live, at least during their minority. But inevitably parents are also handicapped in supervising the entirety of the adolescent's life consequent to the emancipating, distancing process. A fair amount of activity may be going on that they know nothing about. This is a disability that is uniquely the parent's own.

The degree of distancing, however, can be significantly modified by guidance derived from a willingness to listen and compromise rather than from arbitrary dictates and deaf ears. In a calm moment, after the heat of a confrontational disagreement has died down, values and concerns should be discussed, and the parents should actively solicit the adolescent's views: "You know, Dad (Mother) and I had a rather different upbringing about X (whatever the concern may be). We find ourselves very confused about how young people see this today. Could you help us to better understand and tell us your views?" Parents can then offer their thoughts and encourage a give-and-take discussion, sharing perspectives in a collaborative manner. Various options and their consequences can then be reviewed in a particular situation and a joint decision arrived at about how the young person wishes to act. Role playing and rehearsal also can be used to good advantage.

Even under optimal circumstances, parents should not expect to be told "all." The emancipating teenagers always will keep certain matters private simply because they are his or her own and symbolize separation. Parents need to respect this developmental fact, yet they can be confident that what they have to say is valued and will be heard.

As tempting as succumbing to intemperate exasperation may sometimes be, it is always wise to try to avoid heated confrontation. This only sets up a contest over just who is in control, a contest that neither side wins. Adolescents often further respond by protecting their tenuous hold on independence in proving that they, not the parents, are in charge of their own affairs. Obviously, this is best accomplished by doing the exact opposite of what parents wish. It is a wise adult who understands that helping an adolescent gain self-control rests in the degree to which that adult can surrender the need to control in a directive manner, offering rather than imposing wisdom and experience.

Limit setting. Adolescents do need to have clear boundaries set in terms of adult expectancies. Indeed, they want them even though they may violently protest. Moreover, parents do have rights of their own in expecting certain things of their teenager at home. Accountability as to where a young person is going and when he or she expects to return, curfews, allowance, household chores, per-

sonal dress, manners, limits on sexual behavior, drug and alcohol use and the like are matters that require discussion and agreement about reasonable rules. These rules should be realistic in terms of community social norms and ordinary good judgment and be tempered by flexibility. Expecting a teenager to be home by 9:00 PM when an appropriately supervised social event is not over until midnight is unnecessarily restrictive, although this might be a reasonable school night hour for one who never seems to get homework done or for a young person who lives in a high crime area. Long hair, blue jeans, and hanging shirttails may need to be tolerated, but slovenly hygiene or offensive habits need not. Acceptance of a messy room does not mean that it should become a public health hazard or that anyone but the adolescent has to clean or pick it up. Although sexual intimacy outside the home may not be controllable, "making out" in an upstairs bedroom does not have to be condoned.

Behavioral expectancies are based on a mutually agreed upon code. If the code is worked out calmly and cooperatively, most adolescents will agree to parental limits, particularly if accompanied by reasonable explanation: "I am concerned about the possible harm to you if you do X because ...." or "What do you think would be an appropriate hour for you to be home on weekends? ... We think your suggestion a little late. Would ___ PM be a reasonable compromise?" or "We really get very worried about you when you are late and don't call. Would you let us know the next time?"

The consequences of code violations also need to be negotiated and carefully spelled out but in terms the parents can enforce. Sanctions usually are best related to parentally controlled issues such as transportation and finance. It is not helpful to tell an adolescent he is "grounded" because of curfew violations if he will flaunt the restriction and walk out of the house anyway. The application of sanctions also needs to be consistently but fairly imposed. Unenforceable penalties or those that are inconsistently or unfairly applied only promote manipulative behavior and aggravate contests over control.

PROBLEMATIC ADOLESCENT-PARENT CONFLICT

Problematic intrafamily conflict goes beyond challenging behavior to the point of dysfunctionality. Most often this is manifested in acting-out behaviors such as verbal or physical abuse, provocative or promiscuous sexuality, running away, frequent rages with breakage or banging fists or head into walls and

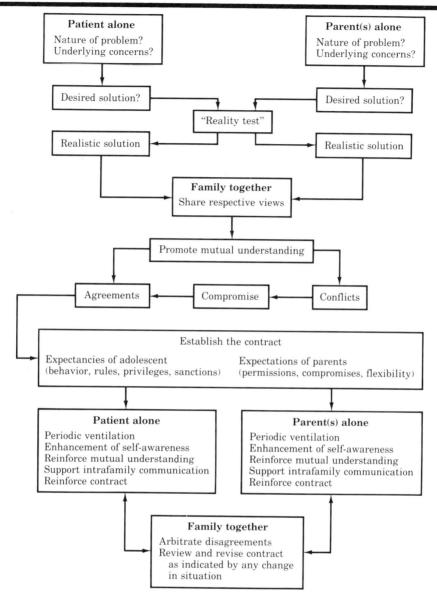

FIGURE 24-1
A MANAGEMENT SEQUENCE FOR INTRAFAMILY CONFLICT

windows, or stealing from home. Other symptoms may include deteriorating school performance, increasing drug or alcohol use, increasing isolation, and depression or a suicidal act.

Management follows the counseling approach outlined in the previous chapter, but the physician takes a more active role as arbitrator and mediator.

More emphasis is placed on family sessions in improving communication and understanding with the goal of working out a mutually agreed upon contract (Figure 24-1).

Other serious intrafamily problems should be looked for as well. The serious failure of parent and adolescent communication usually does not stand alone. Parental alcoholism, depression, disappointment with life, and marital discord are not uncommon as husband and wife approach midlife and identity reappraisal.

Particularly tempestuous midadolescent crises also may be encountered in families in which parents have imposed singularly rigid and confining rules in excess of community norms. As these usually derive from committed beliefs about proper child-rearing practices, often with a religious base, achieving a more flexible position may be impossible. The only feasible option may be for the teenager to go along with parental demands in the best way he or she can until reaching majority. Periodic visits with the physician can be helpful for ventilation and working out ways of contending with parental restrictions in a constructive manner. Arranging for the adolescent to get out of the home frequently can help relieve pressure, but these arrangements must be acceptable to parents and usually will need to be highly structured and supervised situations (church, school, relatives and, sometimes, a hospital's junior volunteer program).

We also are encountering an increasing number of instances in which significant mother-daughter alienation and running away behavior may be associated with incest. Although this is not the most commonly reported pattern, physicians encountering such a combination should at least consider this possibility in their differential diagnosis. (Incest is reviewed in Chapter 17.)

Although the management of adolescent-parent conflict seeks solutions that keep the family intact, placement with another relative or in a group home sometimes is necessary. These situations may include (a) the youth whose acting-out behavior is so out of control that it poses a real danger to self or others; (b) those cases in which no possibility of negotiation exists and the patient is unable to modify his or her own approach; (c) the absence of significant improvement after treatment for 4-6 months; or (d) the presence of other family problems of such magnitude as to make meeting the adolescent's needs impossible. Another important issue in considering alternative living arrangements is willingness. The physician may think this helpful but find neither adolescent nor parent agree. Only when the probability of serious physical or emotional harm is great can removal from the home be entertained without at least the patient's concurrence. Placement may last from a few weeks or months to a more permanent arrangement, depending on the potential for significant improvement in the family situation or the adolescent's ability to adapt.

BATTERING AND ABUSE

The use of physical force by parents upon an adolescent occurs with considerably greater frequency than is usually recognized. Although physical punishment is sometimes a reasoned disciplinary measure, it is more apt to be an impulsive act stemming from anger and frustration at perceived loss of control or in displacing other frustrations onto the adolescent. Not infrequently, parental alcoholism, poor impulse control, or psychosis is a concomitant.

Physical abuse of adolescents may be more difficult to define than for little children. Puritan concepts of "spare the rod and spoil the child" tend to be quite acceptable when applied to older children and youth, particularly if a boy is wayward and unruly or a girl suspected of sexual laxity. Our own view is that corporal punishment has no legitimate place in adolescent discipline, but in any case considered spankings should be differentiated from intemperate expressions of parental rage. Although few adolescents are seriously harmed by physical abuse, it rarely solves a problem and is more likely to provoke even greater dysfunctionality. It also is symptomatic of a significant breakdown in intrafamily interaction.

Child abuse laws usually cover all minors up to their eighteenth birthday, and the physician is required to report accordingly. However, systems set up to protect children are not always responsive to teenagers. There may be need for continuing support of the adolescent and consultation with the social service agency handling abuse in making appropriate plans.

RUNNING AWAY

Running away simply is a symptom, albeit a dramatic one, that all may not be going well at home. An increasing phenomenon since the mid 1960s, this is one avenue an adolescent may take in attempting to cope with an intrafamily dilemma. The physician may encounter this problem when parents seek help after their offspring has gone or when a patient proclaims intent to run away or presents as a runaway with a medical need. A wide variety of motivations exists and management depends on which one is underlying:

1. Normal testing and experimenting behavior. Young people in communities bordering on old hippie/flower children enclaves such as New York's Lower East Side or San Francisco's Haight-Ashbury or newer centers of residual youth culture devotees such as New Orleans may spend several days away from home seeking adventure and testing parents. Evaluation usually reveals rather marked midadoles-

cent distancing coupled with a fairly strict and directive parental attitude but a basically loving and intact family structure and a patient with little evidence of dysfunctionality in other aspects of his or her life. Usually the teenager returns voluntarily and, if this gesture results in constructive realignment of the parents' response more in keeping with their offspring's age, he or she will not run away again.

2. A cry for help. In this instance, running away may vary from going to the home of a nearby friend to distant travel. In many respects it has the same impulsive, unplanned quality and precipitating factors as a suicide gesture or an impulsive act of any kind. Frequently the teenager stays away until forcibly returned by police or until an intervening agency negotiates a reconciliation. A major complication in this and the subsequent category is the involvement of boys and girls in prostitution. In the last few years there has been a rather tragic pattern of young adolescents, girls in particular, running from smaller cities and towns to New York. On arrival, without funds, friends, or a place to stay, they are picked up and befriended by pimps. For many this is simply a means for economic survival. For others it is a more deliberate component of psychopathology.

Evaluation inevitably reveals escalating parent-adolescent conflict of a significant degree, an abusive situation, or a youngster who always has dealt with stress through avoidance. Management seeks to negotiate a more viable home situation and introduce the adolescent to more effective coping modalities through individual and family therapy. An initial period of separation for cooling off and promoting reasoned rather than heated communication may be indicated. Usually, referral to a mental health professional for long-term therapy is required. Special youth programs may be useful in addition to more traditional treatment forms. Youth-serving social agencies can be helpful in defining these alternatives. Also see the referral resource list in the previous chapter.

3. Escape from a "hopeless" situation. Here the adolescent has carefully considered his or her options and elected to leave home as a permanent solution to a perceived irreconcilable conflict or an insoluble home problem. This may include (a) abusive and/or chaotic homes possibly complicated by alcoholism, (b) rigid, austere, and punitive parents who impose extreme limits on the adolescent's mobility, or (c) families so preoccupied with other issues that the teenager feels cut off from any affective relationship. Usually, repeated unsuccessful efforts to establish contact and elicit understanding have been made by the youth who has come to perceive himself or herself as unwanted and unloved. The teenager also may have become the family scapegoat and have been told he or she is the root of all their problems. Guilt, despair, and futility escalate. Feelings of devaluation and rejection finally culminate in the decision to leave home. Some may become involved in prostitution. Others manage to live by their wits on the street or wander aimlessly from city to city. Some find sanctuary in a communal setting or turn up at runaway centers. The primary care physician usually encounters this group of young people in various clinic settings where they go for medical help or in emergency rooms following an injury.

Management depends on the degree to which the family situation can be salvaged and the degree to which the adolescent is willing to live under some form of structure and rules. Young people who have been on the streets for some time become used to the totally self-directed existence and may not easily return to a more disciplined life. Residential placement may be necessary for fairly extended periods of time, although adolescents may escape from these settings as well and remain on the streets, in communes, or other retreats indefinitely. In any event, treatment generally requires a multidisciplinary approach and referral to a mental health resource familiar with alienated youth.

4. Institutional escapees. A significant number of runaways are psychologically disturbed to a major degree. They frequently have histories of recurrent psychiatric hospitalizations or residential placements and other psychotherapeutic efforts, usually to little avail. Often schizophrenic, sociopathic, or impulse-disordered, they have poor interpersonal relationships at best and escape societal demands by becoming "lost" in the quicksilver life of the streets. Treatment depends on the degree to which some one person can convey sufficient concern and caring to catch this youngster up in a relationship he or she values, thereby motivating him or her to stay in touch. Only then can any rehabilitative process begin, usually through an alternative youth program rather than traditional techniques.

5. Amotivational youth. Running away is a sometime solution for an amotivational youth. Characteristically this is a chronic school underachiever with little self-direction, drive, or ambition. He or she may be heavily invested in the youth and drug cultures or meditational Eastern religions and religious cults, often moving from the former to the latter. By virtue of inability or personal philosophical choice they have elected not to contend with a

competitive society in traditional terms. The emphasis is placed on interpersonal relationships, albeit often superficial, in the low-pressure setting of street, commune, or cult. Traditional psychotherapy has been helpful for only a few; more often the solution rests in finding alternative but structured life-style patterns. Communes may be an option for some, the more legitimate religious cults for others. Parents may need to be helped to give up their investment in what they would like their adolescent to become if the youth can find a sense of belonging, personal integrity, and self-realization in such settings.

6. Abandoned youth. Largely a phenomenon of inner cities, an unknown number of older children and adolescents roam the ghetto, moving between the homes of friends or relatives, the streets, and abandoned buildings. In New York City alone it has been estimated that some 10,000 youngsters fall in this category. Usually victims of poverty and overburdened single parent homes beseiged by continual economic, social, and emotional crises, these teenagers have had little opportunity to gain any sense of security or loving discipline or to have vision of a hopeful future. Often predelinquent, delinquent, or impulsive, their acting-out behaviors usually cause parents to feel that efforts to control their offspring are futile and to abandon trying. Not infrequently, such parents literally lock out the youth or simply pick up and leave for an unknown destination while he or she is out. Solutions rest not only in residential or foster care placement but also in linking the youngster up with a youth program that can provide, through effective role models, peer leadership training, success options and the like, opportunities to gain self-esteem and the perception that hope is possible.

In the event that an adolescent has run away and parents seek advice about what to do, the following steps can be recommended:

1. Contact the adolescent's friends, favored relatives, or other persons of meaning in his or her life. Most runaways seek such refuge rather than more risky and unknown options.

2. If the preceding is unavailing, call the police. All local precincts have hookups with major city runaway units.

3. Call the National Runaway Switchboard (800-621-4000) and leave word that the parents are interested in getting in touch.

4. Leave word with nationally known runaway centers such as New York City's Covenant House and at runaway centers in nearby cities. The Switchboard or police can usually help identify these facilities.

5. Be willing to invest substantially in introspec-

tion and compromise in intrafamily relationships and expectations when the youth returns. Family therapy may be indicated.

Parents may be reassured that most younger runaways ultimately return home if the home has anything at all to offer. This outcome, however, may not be true for the older youth who may have taken this step for full emancipation.

SIBLINGS

Normal adolescence brings a heightening of feeling tone in sibling relationships, particularly between those who are of the same sex and within 2 years of each other. Initial closeness becomes closer. Those who never got along well may move into open warfare until young adulthood brings peaceful coexistence or even filial closeness. Relationships between siblings more disparate in age or of opposite sexes ordinarily do not change to this marked degree. We offer the following rules of thumb in assessing the seriousness of complaints and implementing management.

1. Variable degrees of sibling conflict are inevitable and largely need to be tolerated as long as they remain at the verbal level. It is appropriate, however, to set limits on extremes but with fair and equitable distribution of responsibility for maintaining the peace and in parental arbitration and sanctions. It usually is futile to attempt to establish fault, the truth being undiscoverable amidst self-justifying accusations launched from both sides.

2. Repeated physical assault (other than roughhousing) or sexual acting out usually is outside the norm and should be evaluated as for any dysfunctional behavior as to seriousness and the need for treatment.

3. Patient complaints of exploitation in household chores, "baby sitting" younger siblings, or taking care of chronically ill family members need to be tested against reality. A reasonable amount of responsibility for home affairs is an appropriate requirement that contributes to self-esteem and healthy maturation, but such demands become inappropriate when they interfere with the adolescent's pursuit of developmental tasks in relation to school and peers. Perceived unfairness in this regard may prompt anger and acting out or exacerbate depression and withdrawal. Management rests in family and patient counseling in bringing about a mutually acceptable situation.

School Problems
EVALUATION
School problems may present in one or more of a number of ways, including inadequate performance,

TABLE 24-2
DIFFERENTIAL DIAGNOSIS OF SCHOOL PROBLEMS IN ADOLESCENCE

Primary conflict	Diagnostic category	Etiologic considerations
I. Patient: academic	A. Information processing	1. Learning disability 2. Mild retardation 3. Maturational lag
	B. Deficient schooling	1. Inadequate preparation for secondary school 2. Missed schooling due to illness
II. Patient: school environment	A. Psychologic stress	1. Personality conflict with teacher 2. Personality conflict with student
	B. Adjustment reaction	1. New school 2. Shift to junior or senior high school
	C. Anxiety reaction	1. Fear of significant tests 2. Fear of graduation
III. Patient: extraschool psychologic stress	A. Adjustment reaction	1. Withdrawal of energy for other developmental tasks 2. Home/peer problems 3. Recent loss/breakup of important relationship 4. Moved to new community
	B. Anxiety reaction	1. Pubertal delay 2. Disfigurements/handicaps 3. Fear of pregnancy
	C. Chronic emotional problems	1. Poor impulse control 2. Chronic depression 3. Chronic acting-out 4. Drug/alcohol abuse 5. Childhood autism
	D. Psychotic break	
IV. Patient: physical	A. Sensory disorder	1. Myopia 2. Hearing loss
	B. Systemic illness	1. Acute: mononucleosis, hepatitis 2. Chronic illness
	C. CNS disorder	1. Epilepsy 2. Brain tumor
V. Extrapatient:	A. Poor educational program	1. Large class size 2. Poor teachers 3. Budget cuts
	B. Diversion of academic primacy to other concerns	1. Integration conflict 2. Budget crises 3. Teacher crises
	C. Disaffected student body	1. High percent of impulse-disordered youths; chaotic classrooms 2. High percent of acting-out and predelinquent youths; potential for acts of violence and petty crime very real 3. Alienated youth from philosophical/political base 4. Amotivational syndrome youth
	D. Inappropriate placement	1. Vocational vs. academic programs 2. Too advanced class section 3. Too easy, unchallenging class section

poor attention, daydreaming, and insufficient participation; classroom disruption; frequent truancy or complete refusal to attend; and drug or alcohol use during school hours. Any one of a number of causal factors may be at work and symptoms may be present singly or in combination (Table 24-2). Careful assessment is necessary to tease out the significant issues.

Minimally, the primary care physician should establish a provisional diagnosis and set a comprehensive diagnostic and treatment plan into motion, even if he or she will not be the continuing therapist. Immediate referrals to psychologist, neurologist, or psychiatrist may be tempting, but such early dispatch to system specialists all too often results in missing some important need or overlooking the simplest and most straightforward solution. School problems can only be seen in holistic terms, as school itself is a major milieu for many life experiences and occupies a dominant place in the adolescent's world.

In addition to the usual medical and psychosocial evaluation outlined in Chapters 2 and 23, more detailed information should be obtained from the patient, parents, and school about the range of manifestations and the perceptions of each separately as to the nature of the problem (Table 24-3). An examination of the student's records from first grade to the current year is particularly helpful in differentiating between chronic and acute difficulty. A modest degree of retardation or learning disability may be missed early on but be evidenced upon a collective review of past academic performance. This review should include the level of classroom accomplishment in various subjects, standard achievement tests, and teacher comments on classroom behavior. Most schools are willing to collate such information upon parent authorization. If any problems are encountered, parents should know they have the full legal right to see their offspring's educational records and obtain a full copy at any time under the Family Privacy in Education Act of 1974, which governs all schools receiving federal funds. This right devolves on the student at age 18.

When information-processing deficits or longstanding emotional difficulties are significant possibilities, either psychologic testing or psychiatric consultation or both are indicated. Neurologic consultation is less likely to offer help. In any event, the primary care physician should encounter no difficulty in appropriately assessing neurologic functions, including the "soft signs" commonly found in minimal brain dysfunction or, as now called, attention deficit disorder.

The electroencephalogram rarely helps in the assessment of school problems unless a seizure disorder is suspected. The presence or absence of abnormal patterns and foci has no diagnostic significance in learning disabilities. Skull roentgenograms and computerized axial tomography also are unrevealing and need not be performed unless there is some other indication for them.

Full assessment of a learning problem can be expensive. It should be noted that under Public Law 94-142 schools receiving federal funds are now required to fully evaluate such problems themselves or to pay for independent evaluation. Such evaluation includes medical, neurologic, psychologic, and psychiatric evaluation as well as specific educational assessment. Students with any form of learning difficulty, from the organic to purely emotional, are covered and family income is not an eligibility factor. Physicians and parents of adolescents with such problems should advocate the provision or payment of these federally mandated services with local school districts.

MILD AND BORDERLINE RETARDATION

Theoretically, even modest degrees of retardation should have been recognized in the patient's early years. However, relatively mild deficits (intelligent quotients in the 70-85 range) often are missed until made evident by the greater academic demands of secondary school. They may continue to be overlooked by the primary care physician as a cause of school problems in that developmental progress in psychosocial and motor skill spheres may be little affected. These youngsters often are wholly adolescent in their orientation, interests, and behavior—particularly in the early teens when many normal classmates still have concrete thought operations. It is only later when abstractive thinking is increasingly prevalent in the class as a whole that the retarded youth comes to stand out.

The frequency of secondary emotional problems further obfuscates the true diagnosis. A retarded adolescent who defensively acts out in class, is truant, or exhibits other dysfunctional behaviors may be thought disturbed on a primary basis. Some of these youths may even get caught up in delinquency. The street gang may be the only accepting peer group, the relatively defenseless retarded youth becoming pawn and scapegoat to gang functions and gang leader's ego. Others in this category remain isolated and depressed when their deficit is sufficient to prevent keeping up with any peer group expectancies.

TABLE 24-3
EVALUATION FOR SCHOOL PROBLEMS IN ADOLESCENCE

History
1. Chief complaint (from perspective of patient, parents, and school individually)
   a. Nature of problem: academic failure, classroom behavior, truancy, others
   b. Manifestations: specific description, duration, effects, precipitating factors
   c. Causality: perceptions, contributing factors
2. Academic performance
   a. Current: present grade, appropriateness for age, reasons for any repeated grades; current marks for each course taken
   b. Past: classroom marks and national test scores in all years; comparison of present with previous year's function
3. School administration competency
   a. Average reading level of students in patient's grade
   b. Drop-out rate
   c. General teacher competency; specific teacher competency in relation to patient's classes
   d. Capacity of school to control disruptive students
   e. Incidence of assault, vandalism, and theft
4. Acute adjustment-reactive factors
   a. Recent change: first year in junior or senior high school, new school with or without change in geographic location
   b. Recent loss: parental divorce, death of parent or other important person in adolescent's life, breakup of a significant relationship
   c. Personal crisis: illness in parent or sibling, pregnancy
   d. Missed schooling due to illness: infectious mononucleosis, hepatitis, appendicitis, accident, surgery, others
5. Chronic psychosocial problems
   a. Home: intrafamily conflict, parental alcoholism, physical abuse, and so on
   b. Peers: problems in establishing interpersonal relationships
   c. Characterological: impulse disorder, sociopathic behavior
   d. Acting-out behavior (other than characterological): consequent to school, peer, home problems
   e. Depression: consequent to school, peer, home problems
   f. Substance abuse: usually associated with

underlying acute reactive or chronic psychosocial problems
   g. Psychosis: early signs may first manifest as school problem usually with isolating, withdrawn behavior

Physical evaluation
1. General health, vision, hearing
2. Neurologic: gross and fine motor control, visual-motor coordination, balance, speech, extraocular muscle balance, handedness, restlessness/activity level, attention span, concentration, distractibility

Intellectual/mental evaluation
(preliminary screening)
1. Draw-a-person test (Chapter 23); observe for:
   a. Evidence of self-concepts as reflected in figure image
   b. Evidence of retardation (Goodenough scoring techniques give rough index of IQ up through early adolescence)
   c. Evidence of perceptual disorder in disturbed body part relationships
2. Mental status examination (Table 23-3): observe for cognitive capacity, possible thought disorder
3. Spatial-perceptual function: should be able to satisfactorily copy various shapes, demonstrating appreciation of and capacity to replicate spatial relationships between two forms; e.g., circle in a triangle, a 3-dimensional box, abutting triangles or hexagons, etc. (formal psychological testing employs the Bender-Gestalt)
4. Reading and writing skills: secondary school students should be able to:
   a. Read a section from the state driver's manual (6th-grade reading level) and answer related questions in the model test section
   b. Write two or three sentences with grossly correct grammar, spelling, and letter formation about some concrete, non-anxiety-producing topic (what he/she plans to do on leaving the office/next weekend/next summer)
5. Arithmetic skills: secondary school students should be able to perform all standard functions (addition, subtraction, multiplication, long division) at the 3-digit level plus basic fractions. They may well be able to do more, but performance at the above level indicates intellectual competence in this sphere.

Carefully asking the youth about his or her own feelings and perceptions may produce important diagnostic information. A significant number of these patients report that they simply find the school work too hard and cannot seem to keep up.

Although this is by no means a universal complaint, when present it does differentiate between those with learning difficulties and those with school problems of other cause; in the latter instance, complaints rarely include comments about problems in

TABLE 24-4
SIGNIFICANT FINDINGS IN MAJOR CATEGORIES OF SCHOOL PROBLEMS IN ADOLESCENTS

Diagnosis	School performance	Behavior	Family problems	Peer problems	Evaluation	Comments
Learning disability	Poor; long-standing related to reading	Variable; reactive	Absent	Variable; reactive	Significant; in intellectual function primarily	May have history and neurologic findings of minimum attention deficit disorder. May have abstractive skills in cognition.
Mild retardation	Poor; long-standing, related to all subjects	Variable; reactive	Absent	Variable; reactive	Significant; in intellectual function primarily	Physical and neurologic evaluations normal; only concrete cognitive skills.
Acute adjustment reaction	Satisfactory or recent deterioration	Problems common; either acting-out or withdrawal	Common; usually situational crisis	Uncommon	Normal except for specific causal factors	Recent change/loss, crisis, or missed schooling due to illness evident in history.
Chronic emotional problem	Satisfactory or deterioration at time of problem onset	As above	Common	Common	As above	History reveals significant psychosocial problems; intrafamily difficulties predominate.
Health problem	Poor; onset related to timing and consequences of illness	Withdrawal or depression common	Absent	Absent; low energy level may isolate to some degree	Significant; in physical examination and medical history	Evident by past history and current findings.
Sensory deficit (myopia, hearing loss)	Poor; timing related to onset of deficit	Commonly normal; may have reactive withdrawal	Absent	Absent	Vision or hearing tests significant	Myopia commonly first appears during adolescent growth spurt; mild hearing deficits of congenital origin may not be detected until large classroom size exacerbates problem.
School/teacher deficits	Satisfactory until enters school in question; then deterioration	Acting-out common	Absent	Absent	Normal	Assessment of school itself reveals serious deficiencies.

comprehension. Retarded adolescents also may openly state that they know they are just plain "dumb" and usually experience the pain and isolation of this handicap just as much as if it were a physical disability. One should never lose sight of the singular discrepancy between emotional integrity and intellectual impairment. These young people often have exquisitely sensitive feelings and a startling degree of self-awareness.

Definitive diagnosis is established by psychologic testing and the finding of below average scores equitably distributed among all subtest units.

Treatment requires the combination of an educational program consonant with the patient's ability and supportive counseling aimed at finding and building on strengths, providing options for success in even the smallest of ways, and promoting self-esteem. Few if any retarded youths develop abstract thinking; many remain relatively immature. Educational planning should focus on concrete, structured, and vocationally oriented goals with early entry into work-study programs or sheltered workshops. Additional attention may be needed in learning life skills such as negotiating public transportation, budgeting money, making wise food and clothing purchases, or applying for jobs.

A variety of programs, funded by federal or state sources, are available in most communities. Information can be obtained from schools and their bureaus of special educational services, city and state associations for brain-injured children, city and state programs for vocational rehabilitation, and programs for handicapped children and adults. State and local departments of mental health and boards of education can be helpful in identifying regional resources as well. Broad federal mandates governing eligibility of local school programs for federal funds now demand that all children under 18 receive an education appropriate to their needs under the Education for All Handicapped Children Act. Despite the more prevalent therapeutic opportunities for the retarded than for many other afflictions, adolescents are still not as well served as younger children and the physician may need to institute vigorous advocacy on their behalf simply to secure that to which they are legally entitled.

These young people also need enrichment of their lives and psychologic support in other ways. They often function well and gain considerable benefit from participation in structured youth programs in such resources as Boys' and Girls' Clubs, YMCAs, YWCAs and Big Brothers and Big Sisters.

LEARNING DISABILITIES

Although dyslexia and other specific learning disorders increasingly are being identified in childhood, a significant number escape early detection only to emerge under the greater academic demands of junior and senior high school. Not all children with minimal brain dysfunction (or attention deficit disorder) grow out of this with time; although some may have simple developmental lags, others have permanent disabilities. It has been estimated that half of all adolescents labeled as chronic school underachievers have impaired learning functions. Although true that significant improvement in some of the more obvious signs seen in early childhood (hyperactivity, "childish" behavior, enuresis, clumsiness) occurs by puberty, subtle evidence in the areas of fine motor control, spatial relationships, and other perceptual difficulties may well remain in addition to dyslexia. In other instances dyslexia alone persists.

In addition to chronic learning problems, historical clues include ambidexterity or left-handedness beyond age 6, clumsiness and poor coordination, poor attention span, distractibility, hyperkinesis, prematurity or perinatal insults such as anoxia or infection, and being of the male sex (male to female ratio = 5:1). The full range of childhood symptoms that have been associated with this disorder is cited in Table 24-5. However, not all signs appear in all affected children; anywhere from one to a multiplicity may be present.

Further indication is found in a discrepancy between reading or writing skills and verbal process in a basically bright youngster. Learning-disabled adolescents do acquire abstract cognitive function and have normal or better intellectual capacity, but they perform far better in oral than written classroom work. In that academic progress is marked far more by the latter, these young people may have been labeled as slow for a long time. The response of the environment may be quite discrepant with their true ability, and the resultant psychologic reaction may be more dominant and provocative of attention than the underlying true cause. Acting-out behaviors, depression, and poor interpersonal relationships may all occur.

A proper diagnosis can only be achieved with careful psychoeducational testing and evaluation, but the possibility of disability should be raised with any adolescent doing poorly in school who has a history of any of the childhood symptoms, who seems to be normal in verbal processes but fails in written work or reading or reports he or she has poor or absent reading comprehension, or who takes forever to complete a reading assignment. Additional developmental screening techniques are offered in the previous chapter.

Management requires special educational programs—something more than tutoring or makeup classes. Unfortunately, although resources for learning-disabled children have rapidly expanded in recent years, those for adolescents may be few and far between. But as noted for retarded adolescents, the Education for All Handicapped Children Act provides a basis for demanding that federally funded school programs rise to meet this need. Seriously dyslexic youths may require the physician's further advocacy in colleges as well as schools in arranging for various audiovisual educational supports and oral rather than written examinations. Here, too, there is considerable legal and legislative support for such requests in antidiscrimination provisions and the Rehabilitation Act of 1976, applicable to older adolescents and adults.

Management also requires attention to such reactive emotional problems as may exist. Learning-disabled adolescents often are capable of considerable insight and may do well in traditional psychotherapy. Others may be highly responsive to the primary care physician's counseling. Opportunities for success and the gaining of self-esteem are also essential and often can be found in various youth programs, rap groups, or community service.

MATURATIONAL COGNITIVE DELAY

As in any other aspect of adolescent growth and development, abstractive ability can make its normal appearance at any time during a broad age range. On the average, the shift from concrete thought begins about age 12 and is complete by age 15, but some normal young people may be delayed in this function for several years, and 30% of the populace never achieve it at all. (Educational influences appear to be as significant for this process as innate ability.) As secondary school learning requires abstractive competence in a number of areas (algebra, interpretation of social studies, English literature), adolescents who are at the lower end of the normal distribution curve may do less well at this time compared to their peers than they did in earlier grades when all students were concrete thinkers. Some of these young people will shortly catch up. Others may not, being in that one-third of the population whose thinking is persistently concrete; although these individuals usually can "make it" through high

TABLE 24-5
COMMON SIGNS AND SYMPTOMS OF ATTENTION DEFICIT DISORDER (MINIMAL BRAIN DYSFUNCTION) IN CHILDHOOD

Motor behavior	Hyperactivity (hyperkinesis) Restlessness Impaired coordination; clumsiness Speech problems Left-handedness; persistent ambidexterity Enuresis and/or encopresis
Attention and perceptual-cognitive function	Short attention span; poor concentration; distractibility Poor perception of spatial relationships
Learning ability	Dyslexia; letter/word/sentence reversals Poor handwriting Chronic underachievement with normal or better IQ
Impulse control	Low frustration tolerance Impulsive antisocial behavior Poor planning and judgment
Interpersonal relations	Resistance to socialization demands Increased drive for "doing it myself" Extroversion
Emotional	Lability of mood Increased aggressiveness Heightened reactivity to stimuli Dysphoric response to pleasant situations
Reactive, secondary emotional response	Decreased self-esteem Increased negativism and hostility Acting-out and/or depression
Neurologic signs	Poor fine motor control Impaired visual-motor coordination Poor balance Clumsiness Poor speech Strabismus
Psychologic testing	Discrepancy between WISC IQ scores in motor and verbal subtests Impaired perception on Bender-Gestalt Reading and writing reversals Short-term memory impairment Overall normal or above normal intelligence

school, they would be well advised to pursue a vocational program rather than college.

Diagnostic points include a history of satisfactory educational progress in elementary school years and a relative decrease in performance around the eighth or ninth grade (often first manifested with the introduction of algebra), the absence of any signs or symptoms of minimal brain dysfunction, and generally good psychosocial functioning up to this time.

Management consists of recognizing this developmental variation and modifying the ordinary school program to allow the young person to encounter success rather than failure. Taking basic rather than advanced courses, supplemental tutoring, parental assistance with homework, and summer review courses can help. At all costs, the student should not be subjected to parental and teacher rejoinders that he or she simply is being lazy, needs to shape up, or other demeaning and pejorative experiences.

DEFICIENT SCHOOLING

Inadequate preparation and poor learning skills acquired at the elementary school level lead to poor performance in secondary years. This is most apt to be seen in large inner-city school systems where low reading scores are ubiquitous or in adolescents moved from school to school because of frequent business transfers of parents. We do not propose solutions for either of these complex problems but simply point out that academic underachievement must be measured against the academic opportunities proffered in the first place.

A more remediable problem rests in those adolescents who become academically compromised by illness. Some students encounter exceptional difficulty in catching up after an absence of even 2 weeks. The one who ordinarily is struggling along in the lower half of the class is particularly vulnerable. It can be overwhelming when makeup work must be done on top of each day's regular assignment, particularly when the student has missed a significant amount of explanatory classroom work. The problem is often compounded by teachers who see the matter solely in relation to their particular subject, each pressuring the youngster separately under the threat of being given a failing or incomplete mark. The student increasingly feels it a hopeless task to make up and keep up at the same time. This "Catch-22" situation has caused more than one adolescent to drop out of school.

Management consists of the early recognition of this potential hazard in any adolescent whose illness will result in more than a few days' absence and ensuring that he or she receives homework and tutoring to the degree tolerated. Followup after the illness should always include inquiry about school progress and remedial needs. Medically required limitations in school attendance should be lifted as soon as possible or home teaching provided for. When transportation is a problem, many school districts have provisions for special bus service taking the student from door to door.

An overwhelming situation may require modification of the student's schedule to take off pressure, coupled with advocacy in securing the empathy and understanding of all teachers involved. It may be far better to drop a single particularly difficult course and make it up later than to do miserably in all classes and fail an entire term. Such recommendations are well within the primary care physician's province to make. It should not be assumed that schools always are as aware of the problem as one might think they should be. Parents also should be encouraged to meet with the school guidance counselor or psychologist to make appropriate arrangements. The student will be the best guide in advising when academic demands have again assumed manageable proportions.

INTRASCHOOL PSYCHOLOGIC STRESS

Just as all people do not get along with each other in the world in general, not all students get along with all other students or all teachers. It is also true that not all teachers are effective pedagogically or in interpersonal relationships. Although the student who fails or causes classroom disruption usually is accused of being at fault, this is not always true. Complaints of inattention or underachievement require examination of the school's role as well as the student's. The student's view of teacher incompetency or personality deficit may be correct, or the two simply may bring out the worst in each other in their interactions. Management in this instance includes empathy with the student's predicament, a realistic appraisal of the situation, and changing teachers or helping the student to cope more effectively and make the best of a bad bargain (there are better ways for an adolescent to contend with a difficult teacher than through confrontation, power struggles, and self-justification). Usually these problems are relatively isolated and relate to no more than one or two teachers. When failure or conflict is present in all classes, another cause should be looked for and probably signals student maladaptation.

Intrastudent conflict can also cause problems.

Two students may not get along as a matter of course, and changing seats or classrooms may be all that is needed. In other instances, the school may be dominated by disruptive, bullying students who do indeed extort money and property from others or are randomly abusive and even assaultive. In this instance, the patient will not be the only one experiencing anxiety or refusing to attend. Such responses have a certain legitimacy, and a school change may be indicated.

It is a different matter if trouble-makers do not dominate, and the patient has set himself or herself up as scapegoat, selectively becoming the butt of cruel teasing and other persecutions. Causality usually lies within the youth. Although a school change may or may not be indicated, change alone is an inadequate solution. Attention to the patient's psychopathology, either by counseling or suitable referral, is necessary to avoid recapitulating the old problem in a new setting.

PSYCHOLOGIC PROBLEMS WITH EXTRASCHOOL DERIVATIONS

The most common cause of difficulty in school is a psychologic problem derived from conflict in some other venue. Any source of stress can give rise to deteriorating academic performance, acting-out or withdrawal, and isolation in the school setting. Educational progress is apt to be the first of all adolescent pursuits to become compromised when emotional resources are overburdened for any reason and psychic energy must be borrowed for other more pressing matters. Pervasive emotional problems also are more likely to be noticed in the classroom than in other settings. The greater demands for social conformity make deviant behavior stand out like a sore thumb.

Diagnosis is based on a thorough psychosocial evaluation and the ruling out of other school-related causes. Home conflict is particularly common and becomes evident in a careful history. Other issues may be the breakup of an important relationship, the death of a family member or close friend, concerns about homosexual feelings, childhood impulse disorders, illness in self or family member, a psychotic break, and so on. Virtually any conflict, maladaptation, or developmental failure can manifest as a school problem first. Particular attention should be given to differentiating between acute and chronic difficulty in that the first is relatively easy to manage and often well within the province of the primary care physician; the latter usually requires referral and the use of multiple resources.

Management obviously depends on the causal stress, seriousness, chronicity, and the like as discussed in Chapter 23 and elsewhere, but several points are worthy of special note here.

1. Young people with pubertal delay, physical handicaps, or disfigurements, or those with medically mandated special regimens invariably feel uncomfortably "different" in the school setting. Unable to conform to peer norm expectancies in appearance, activities, or both, they greatly fear rejection and isolation and often respond by depression, withdrawal, acting-out, or overcompensation. To some degree such fears are reality-based. These adolescents also encounter particular difficulty in resolving issues of sexual identity or in achieving emancipation if their condition provokes the continued enforcement of dependency. Attention to minimizing the psychologic impact of these conditions is as important as the medical regimen or ensuring an education. Specific details will be found in the chapter on chronic illness.

2. Not all young people look to high school graduation with joy. Some have escalating anxiety about embarking on an unknown future and consciously or unconsciously seek to remain in familiar territory for a while longer. This dilemma usually manifests in some form of symptomatology during the junior or senior year. Management rests in helping the young person recognize the problem and gradually work out plans for the future. Vocational testing and career planning resources may be helpful. The problem usually resolves when the course ahead presents specific options that are compatible with the youth's interests, and definition emerges out of amorphous haze. In some instances, when clarity is not easily forthcoming, it may be well for such young persons to take a year out and work at a job, even a menial one. This can provide opportunity for them to get their bearings and see what the work-a-day world is all about.

In other instances, these symptoms reflect a more fundamental failure in achieving emancipation. Evidence will emerge from an examination of patient-parent relationships and persistence of the early or midadolescent state. Look for an inappropriate degree of dependence upon parents for decision-making or nonresolution of the distancing process with continued conflict and challenge over who is in control. Counseling by the primary care physician often is effective for problems of relatively recent onset. Psychiatric referral is indicated when dysfunctionality has been a long-standing and pervasive theme or when counseling and vocational planning have been ineffective after a 4–6 month trial.

3. Not all acute-onset underachievement reflects deviancy. Many adolescents temporarily may redirect energy from school performance into other developmental affairs. This perfectly normal response is most apt to be seen in midadolescence with its heightened preoccupation with a multiplicity of issues—experimenting with new-found independence, exploring same sex and opposite sex relationships through active socialization, and the like. Patience and forebearance are the treatment of choice. An emotionally intact youngster with solid past school performance and good family support usually gets back on the academic track after a term or two. Rarely are these adolescents failing, rather they are simply squeaking by; compromised performance to the point of having to repeat a term is uncommon.

4. Long-standing emotional problems such as depression, poor impulse control, or acting-out may not come to professional attention until forced by secondary school demands for socialization, conformity, and self-control and the decreased tolerance for "making waves." Although such problems should have been identified and remediated in childhood, often they are not, and it is not until the teen years that parents, teachers, and other adults must face the situation and realize that the symptoms will not go away.

5. Chronic problems in impulse control, although previously recognized, may take on crisis proportions in school settings when adolescent physical and psychologic maturation makes control more problematic for adults and the behaviors become more provocative and threatening. It is one thing for a 5-year-old to flail out in rage, quite another when the student is age 15. The primary physician's task here is to discern whether such behaviors stand alone or are in association with learning deficit disorders and then refer for appropriate treatment. It is unlikely that such long-standing problems are amenable to the counseling approach alone.

6. The diametrically opposite situation may occur with some adolescents who are chronically depressed and manifest this in quiet seclusion. They may be totally ignored and their basic problem, as well as relative academic underachievement, go wholly unnoticed. They tend to sit in the back of the classroom, are obedient and compliant, and make little trouble. Usually passive by nature, they are welcome members of those classes more marked by unruly disobedience and overt aggression. Teachers tend to see them as pleasant but not particularly bright and are little challenged to promote intellectual curiosity. As depression is an all too common

phenomenon in adolescence, it should be a consideration in the routine evaluation of any patient who is normally bright but gives evidence of depression as described in Chapter 26. One cannot depend on the school to make such identification.

SCHOOL PROBLEMS EXTERNAL TO PATIENT INVOLVEMENT

A variety of school-based problems may present as a patient problem instead, even though the patient is blameless and probably normal in evidencing reactive behaviors or underachievement in situations where all students receive an inferior education or in schools beset by financial problems, teacher strikes, integration strife, student alienation, and the like. Whether the student can be helped to cope with these problems more effectively and without academic disadvantage or whether a school change is indicated (or possible) is an individual matter.

Predelinquent and Delinquent Behaviors

OVERVIEW

The single strongest indicator of an adolescent at risk of delinquency rests in his or her peer associations and the peer group's behavior as a whole. Peers, however, are not the fundamental cause of delinquency, although they may provide opportunity. In any community a variety of options exists in choosing friends, from the most conforming to those who flagrantly act out. Any teenager tends to be drawn to that group that seems most likely to support his or her own orientation. Being in with a "bad crowd" is predictive of possible trouble ahead, trouble the young person might not have gotten into otherwise, but the choice to run with a particular pack was affirmatively made.

Other predisposing factors are significant as well. These include major home conflicts, problems in interpersonal relationships, school difficulties, poor or absent role models, and other indicators of a rather chaotic and undisciplined life and few opportunities to gain a sense of stability or self-worth. Predelinquent adolescents tend to have strong undercurrents of anger and hostility toward authority and feelings of futility that anything they can do will affect their lives in a positive way. They expect to be "put down" regularly by adults or to be exploited and abused by them. The family often is one of rigid and punitive control with little warmth or one of ineffective parenting with ultimate abdication from a parenting role.

Delinquent behavior itself often begins with minor peer group incidents such as cutting classes, truancy, "hanging out," and minor theft. It then tends to escalate into drug activity, stealing more major items, or joy riding in stolen cars. Some discrimination is needed, however, between antisocial and simply experimental behavior. Many normal adolescents experiment with minor illegal acts. Smoking marijuana or drinking alcohol are ubiquitous, petty shoplifting a sometime occurrence. This pattern may take on the dimensions of delinquency if the police become involved. Discrimination rests in examining other functions in the adolescent's life. Hopefully, normal youths will have learned their lesson and will exercise more discretion in the future. If restitution is made, the police and juvenile courts are usually lenient.

Early intervention for predelinquent or delinquent youth is based on providing alternative, more constructive role models (often young adults from the same community who have been in trouble but have found a way out) plus supportive and empathic interpersonal activities that promote a sense of personal control and self-esteem. This plan is mediated through family counseling, structured group activities as offered by Boys' and Girls' Clubs, YWCAs and YMCAs, Big Brothers and Big Sisters, and school peer leadership projects. Many communities where juvenile delinquency has been a problem have a number of delinquency diversion programs. A call to one or more local youth-serving agencies may be of help. The physician's own relationship with the adolescent often can be important as well; he or she may be the only nonjudgmental person on the scene. The supervision of a probation officer, even for a first offense, sometimes can be a useful deterrent force.

More confirmed delinquent patterns are difficult to deal with at best and usually require a more intensive therapeutic approach through residential or day-care programs. Drug abuse programs also may be helpful in that many have expanded to include troubled, acting-out young people even when drugs are not involved.

If the police have entered the picture, therapeutic options may be limited by the decisions of a probation officer or juvenile court judge. The physician's advocacy, however, may have significant impact unless the juvenile is a repeat offender or has committed a major crime. The courts are overburdened and usually welcome the recommendations of an objective professional who knows the youth, particularly if accompanied by a rational and realistic treatment proposal. Dismissal of charges or avoiding significant penalty, however, is not always feasible when a serious crime has been committed.

THE JUVENILE JUSTICE SYSTEM

Young people may be subject to the law from a number of perspectives. It may be helpful to review the various categories of petitions and their implications.

Juvenile delinquent. A juvenile delinquent is a minor of more than 7 years and less than 17 who has committed a criminal act. He is subject to juvenile or family court process with the goal of being rehabilitated rather than punished. Proceedings are secret in an effort to avoid public identification of the youngster, giving him or her a chance for a fresh start. The options of the court range from dismissal of charges and a cautionary word, to a period of time under the supervision of a probation officer, to the ordering of various diagnostic and/or therapeutic measures, to incarceration in a state training school for months or years. Increasingly, minors accused of particularly serious crimes are being tried in the criminal courts. The disposition of these cases, however, differs somewhat from that for adult criminals.

Person, child, juvenile, minor in need of supervision. Colloquially known as PINS, CHINS, JINS, or MINS, depending on a given state's terminology, minors (also from 7 through 16 years) in this category are those who have committed "status crimes," or acts that would not be illegal if committed by adults. Examples include truancy, running away, staying out late, and other such "unruly, wayward, or incorrigible" behavior. Also subject to the juvenile or family court system, these youngsters are similarly approached from a secret, rehabilitative perspective. The same range of dispositional options exists as for the juvenile delinquent. In many states, PINS youngsters may end up being incarcerated with the latter, but in an increasing number of instances they are being separated. There is a growing movement to take status crimes out of the court system altogether because experience indicates that this process too often is inappropriately punitive as well as ineffective rather than rehabilitative. An effective alternative system, however, has yet to be developed.

Youthful offender. As a rule, persons between 16 and 21 who commit illegal acts are regarded as adults and tried from a punitive perspective in the criminal courts, although they may be separated from adults in serving sentence. But if the crime is not serious and the adolescent deemed worthy, he or she may be remanded to the juvenile or family court for secret process and rehabilitation as for one of younger years. In this event, he is called a "youthful offender."

Neglect and abuse petitions. The shoe of culpability is placed on the parental foot when a minor is adjudicated "neglected" or "abused." Neglect is more difficult to prove and less commonly invoked than abuse; it generally is applied to such matters as failing to send a child to school, improper or absent supervision, teaching the child to perform criminal acts, and the like. Abuse generally encompasses any action that results in physical harm—from outright starvation or locking the child up in a room or closet to specific assaults. To the adolescent, whether he or she comes to the attention of the court under a neglect or abuse petition or as a person in need of supervision sometimes seems irrational. But this distinction can have significant consequences. The PINS youngster often finds it difficult to escape pejorative labeling as culprit, whereas the one under an abuse or neglect petition is usually seen more as victim in need of protection.

Bibliography*

INTRAFAMILY ISSUES
Blum, R. W., and Runyan, C. 1980. Adolescent abuse: the dimension of the problem. *J. Adolescent Health Care* 1:121-126.

Group for the Advancement of Psychiatry. 1973. *The joys and sorrows of parenthood.* New York: G.A.P.

Kearsky, R. B.; Snider, M.; and Eaton, A. 1964. A practical, quantitative method for recognizing behavioral illness in boys 9 to 14 years of age. *J. Pediatr.* 65:256.

Smilkstein, G. 1975. The family in trouble—how to tell. *J. Family Practice* 2:19.

Steinberg, L. D. 1980. *Understanding families with young adolescents*, Center for Early Adolescence. Carrboro, N.C.

Williams, F. S. 1977. Parenting the adolescent. *Pediatr. Ann.* 6:647.

RUNNING AWAY
Deisher, R. W. 1975. Runaways: a growing social and family problem *J. Family Practice* 2:255.

Gordon, J. S. 1979. Running away: reaction or revolution. In *Adolescent psychiatry*, Vol. VII, editors S. C. Feinstein and P. L. Giovaccini.

SCHOOL PROBLEMS
Boder, E. 1976. School failure—evaluation and treatment. *Pediatrics* 58:394.

Cannon, I. P., and Compton, C. L. 1980. School dysfunction in the adolescent. *Pediatr. Clin. North Am.* 27:79.

Faigel, H. 1973. The adolescent with a learning problem. *Clin. Pediatr.* 12:577.

Hammar, S. L., and Barnard, K. E. 1966. The mentally retarded adolescent. *Pediatrics* 30:845.

Huessy, H. R., and Cohen, A. H. 1976. Hyperkinetic behaviors and learning disabilities followed over seven years. *Pediatrics* 57:4.

Levine, M. S.; Rauh, J. L.; Levine, C. W.; et al. 1975. Adolescents with developmental disabilities. *Clin. Pediatr.* 14:25.

Mendelson, W.; Johnson, N.; and Stewart, M. A. 1971. Hyperactive children as teenagers: a follow-up study. *J. Nerv. Ment. Dis.* 153:273.

McGrath, M. S. 1978. A practical approach to school problems in adolescents. *Pediatr. Ann.* 7:643.

Pincus, J. H., and Glaser, G. H. 1966. The syndrome of "minimal brain damage" in childhood. *N. Engl. J. Med.* 275:27.

Rafferty, F. T. 1978. Functional learning disorders. *Pediatr. Ann.* 7:314.

JUVENILE DELINQUENCY
Brown, B. S., and Courtless, T. F. 1971. *The mentally retarded offender.* DHEW pub. no. (ADM) 74-37, Rockville, Md.: NIMH Center for Studies of Crime and Delinquency.

Marohn, R. C., editor. 1979. Legal and psychiatric perspectives on delinquency and acting out, Part V. In *Adolescent psychiatry*, Vol. VII, editors S. C. Feinstein and P. L. Giovaccini.

Weiner, I. 1975. Juvenile delinquency. *Pediatr. Clin. North Am.* 22:673.

*Note: Also see other bibliographies in Part IV.

-25-
Emotional Problems with Physical Manifestations

Psychogenic Disorders
Psychosomatic Complaints
Diagnosis □ Management
Hysterical Conversion
Hyperventilation Syndrome and Acute Anxiety Attacks

Psychosomatic complaints such as headache, abdominal pain, dizziness, or chronic fatigue are among the most ubiquitous presented to the primary care physician, particularly among adolescent patients. Preoccupation with physical change and identity issues, so often reflected in physical appearance and function, make somatization exceptionally commonplace during these years. Also common are the psychogenic components of more specific conditions such as asthma, migraine, or peptic ulcer. Acute anxiety attacks also are frequent events in light of the complexity of developmental demands and the pervasiveness of major psychologic stress. The hyperventilation syndrome and true hysterical conversion, although less frequent than the others, are encountered sufficiently often to demand differential consideration in many instances. All these problems are among the most challenging the primary care physician will face, both because of the frequency with which they are encountered and the sometime difficulty posed by their diagnosis and management.

Diagnostically, the nagging doubt always exists that some serious condition has been overlooked. There also is the frequent problem of patient and parent disbelief and their rejection of a psychologic explanation for symptoms perceived as alarmingly real. This disbelief often leads the physician to fruitless recycling through extensive tests and procedures, even to the point of surgical exploration and to what some have called the "thick chart syndrome." Alternatively, the patient and parents, dissatisfied with an "inadequate workup," take off on a medical shopping spree, convinced that each new

physician is even less competent, less discerning, and less appreciative of the problem than the last.

The goal of this chapter is to provide direction for the evaluation, diagnosis, and management of psychogenically induced disorders in a manner that avoids unnecessary, extensive testing or patient and parent alienation and promotes a rational solution. In doing so, we wish to emphasize that this chapter cannot stand in isolation from other chapters and should be seen as an extension and modification of information provided in Chapter 23 and of appropriate sections in Part II. The principles elucidated there are basic foundations to what follows.

Psychogenic Disorders

Although possessing some common denominators and often coexisting in the same patient, psychosomatic complaints, hysterical conversion, hyperventilation syndrome, and acute anxiety attacks stand as somewhat separate entities. Their genesis, implications, and management differ in significant respects. Table 25-1 cites differential considerations.

Psychosomatic Complaints
DIAGNOSIS
Psychosomatic complaints can present in:

1. Vague aches and discomforts affecting one or more organ systems. Or,

2. Specific symptom complexes (for example, asthma, migraine, and some gastrointestinal disorders) in which there is an unconscious replication of earlier, organically derived symptomatology for secondary gain.

The first category is ubiquitous in adolescence and is one of the most common causes of physical complaints in this age group. The heightened attention to and awareness of bodily functions provoked by the rapid changes of puberty makes somatization virtually the first line of psychological defense. Frequent symptoms, presenting singly or severally, are headaches (with or without dizziness), abdominal pain, muscle and joint aches and pains, fatigue, and general malaise. They occur more commonly in females, although males are not exempt. Often there is a relationship to current stress situations. Anxiety symptoms such as hyperventilation or palpitations sometimes may be associated but are not part of the psychosomatic picture per se. The following are helpful diagnostic points:

1. Vagueness and variability of symptoms: Pain and discomfort are poorly described, inconsistent in nature, location, severity, and frequency.

2. Lack of replicability: Symptoms tend to occur at all times of day, but rarely during sleep, and lack association with any particular precipitants (such as a correlation of abdominal pain with meals).

3. Multiplicity of systems involved: Although a single system symptom such as headache or abdominal pain is most common, a plethora of complaints, sometimes involving every bodily function, may be encountered. Indeed, the more systems involved, the higher the index of suspicion of psychosomatic origin.

4. Pain and discomfort usually are not severe: Symptoms are not singularly disabling, although they may be complained of bitterly, produce an exaggerated response or both. Abdominal pain may be an exception, sometimes presenting with the severity of an acute abdominal condition but without clear evidence of peritoneal irritation, fever, an elevated white blood count, elevated erythrocyte sedimentation rate, or other confirmatory findings.

Patients with organic illness almost always evidence some other historical, physical, or simple laboratory evidence of their underlying process. Table 25-2, which offers selected discriminating features, focuses on those conditions that are most commonly encountered in this age group; it is not intended to be exhaustive, nor is it guaranteed to wholly rule out organic pathology. But a patient who (a) appears well, (b) is able to complete most daily activities (particularly if of a pleasant and recreational nature), (c) has no significant fever or weight loss and is advancing through puberty normally, (d) has a negative physical examination (including pelvic and rectal examinations for abdominal pain), and (e) has negative simple, low-cost, screening

test results (CBC, ESR, urinalysis, tuberculin skin test, liver enzymes, "mono spot" test, stool guaiac) is unlikely to have an organic disorder regardless of the severity or frequency of the patient's complaints. It is also safe to say that even if an organic disorder is present, despite a negative evaluation, there is no substantive risk to the patient by simply observing him or her until the picture becomes more consolidated. Conversely, a medical fishing expedition including invasive tests and radiologic procedures, which are discomforting, costly, and not without risks, is unlikely to serve such a patient well.

Specific system complexes (such as peptic ulcer, migraine, asthma), although less commonly seen, are still a frequent occurrence. They are less apt to have a predilection for the female sex, being more equally distributed between boys and girls. These conditions are particularly problematic. It can be difficult to sort out organic and emotional components, both often operating at the same time, reinforcing each other in resonance. Further, these conditions tend to be chronically remitting and exacerbating in an unpredictable manner, prompting heightened parental attentions, concern, and overprotection. The patient feels unsure of his or her body and its dysfunction and is subject to all the vulnerabilities of the chronically ill. A particularly careful analysis of all factors is necessary to discriminate between organic and emotional causal factors.

Psychosomatic disease is a diagnosis of exclusion, but judicious restraint is indicated in the extent of the medical evaluation. Although it obviously is important not to miss an organic condition and although a convincing assessment is necessary to allay patient and parent fears, there needs to be a rational limit. Figure 25-1 offers a logical approach.

MANAGEMENT

Treatment of psychosomatic disorders depends on the underlying cause. In most instances, symptoms are related to current stress. Three basic patterns can be identified:

1. Normal adolescent developmental concerns.

2. A temporary adjustment reaction to a new stress situation (entering high school or moving to a new community) or transient high stress (school examinations, job interviews).

3. A significant dysfunctional response to chronic stress.

In the first instance, heightened awareness of the body is a normal event in early adolescence and midadolescence when growth is at its most rapid. The various minor discomforts we all experience are

TABLE
DIFFERENTIAL DIAGNOSIS BETWEEN ORGANIC
HYSTERICAL CONVERSION SYNDROME AND ACUTE

	Organic illness	Psychosomatic disorders*
Symptoms	Specific symptom complex consistent with patho-physiologic and anatomic principles	a. Vague symptoms, including abdominal pain; headaches; muscle, joint, and back pain; fatigue, malaise; singly or severally b. Specific symptom complexes (asthma, migraine, certain bowel disorders, etc.); psychosomatic and biologically mediated elements difficult to distinguish from each other in parameters cited below
Replicability of symptoms	Consistent pattern; may vary in severity	a. Often vague, shifting, ill-defined; inconsistent from one episode to another
Nature and location of pain	Consistent; perceived as distressing	a. Highly inconsistent and variable; may or may not be perceived as distressing
Responds to medical treatment specific for symptoms	Yes	a. Variable; fair to good initial response with diminishing effect over time common
Responds to hypnosis or amytal test	No	a. Variable; not diagnostically significant as no clear end point in an essentially subjective set of complaints b. Suggestion may ameliorate but not clear symptoms and signs from either organic or psychosomatic cause
Wakes at night	Sometimes	a. Rarely
Associated current stress	No	a. and b. Usually
Effect on daily functions	Directly proportionate to severity of symptoms	a. Usually able to continue with daily affairs; interferes with function less than other groups b. As per organic illness
Duration of symptoms before help sought	Usually sought promptly if alarming	a. Usually 2–6 months b. As for organic illness
Level of patient concern	High	a. High concern but may be reluctant to relinquish symptoms; compliance with treatment recommendations may be poorer than in other groups b. High
Awareness of relationship to stress	——	a. Variable b. Rarely
Etiology	Organic	a. and b. Current acute and chronic stress factors; may be new events or carryover from childhood; may be real or perceived

greatly magnified at this time. The intensified perception of physical sensations or preoccupations with the body may be interpreted as pain, or the pain threshold may be significantly lower than at other times. Various vague complaints in a rapidly growing adolescent who otherwise is doing well can be attributed to such cause. Treatment consists of careful and thorough physical examination with a running commentary as to the normalcy of each part and the subsequent discussion of pubertal concerns. This discussion should not overlook such matters as penile size or gynecomastia in boys, breast development in girls, delayed puberty, variations from the median in height or weight, or sexual

25-1
ILLNESS, PSYCHOSOMATIC DISORDERS, ANXIETY ATTACKS/HYPERVENTILATION SYNDROME

Hysterical conversion	Acute anxiety attacks/hyperventilation syndrome
Specific symptom complex often inconsistent with pathophysiologic principles; paralysis and tics most common but may mimic any disease	Sympathetic and parasympathetic nervous system symptoms; e.g., hyperventilation, palpitations, tachycardia, nervousness, dizziness, vasovagal faints, blurred vision, nausea, vomiting, diarrhea; tachypnea predominates in hyperventilation syndrome; may alter blood gases and exhibit pseudoseizures, with or without carpopedal spasm
Consistent; usually persistent and unchanging	Consistent, episodic
Consistent, but patient often indifferent	Sensations dominated by nervousness, dysphoria; pain usually not experienced
Variable; may respond if R̸ accompanied by strong suggestion, but a new symptom may then emerge	No, but will respond to strong or adequate doses of weak tranquilizers, unlike other categories
Yes; particularly useful diagnostic tool	Sodium amytal will abort attack (nature of symptoms precludes hypnosis) but is inappropriate to situation, as diagnosis should be clear from other signs and symptoms
Variable	Rarely
No	Yes
Always disabling to some degree; particularly disabling in relation to trigger factors, permitting avoidance unconsciously	Highly disabling during episode only; feels well between attacks
Shortly after onset; parents may bring patient to hospital as an emergency	Variable; may present as an emergency if state of consciousness altered (faint, pseudoseizure) or patient out-of-control. Less severe symptoms may be present for weeks or several months before R̸
Degree of unconcern often marked and inappropriate to the severity of the symptoms; may be more concerned by tics on a social basis rather than worry about self	High
Never until after extended treatment	Frequently
Unresolved early childhood developmental issue or conflict suppressed until triggered by resurgence of issue in adolescence	Current stress situation; real or perceived

fears and masturbation in young people of either sex. Although the adolescent may appear normal to any adult, he or she often may well have irrational but quite normal preoccupations about any of the foregoing. Initial evaluation and reassurance of patient and parent should be followed by periodic visits every 3–4 months for continued support until the youth feels secure in his or her body image. This may not be until growth is complete.

Somatic complaints may also be a response to normal situational stress. Symptomatology in these instances usually is limited to one or two organ systems and is relatively consistent in manifestation. Precipitating factors tend to be readily identifiable.

TABLE 25-2
CLINICAL FEATURES DIFFERENTIATING
PSYCHOSOMATIC CAUSES FROM THE COMMON CAUSES OF ORGANIC DISEASE

Complaint/condition	Clinical features
Abdominal pain (see Chapter 8) Psychosomatic	1. Symptoms suggestive of spastic bowel syndrome; or nonspecific, vague, ill-defined, variable in nature and location; or recurrent episodes mimicking an acute abdominal condition 2. Physical examination negative except possibly mild-moderate tenderness on deep palpation; latter may disappear if patient distracted 3. No significant weight loss, appetite normal (although may be reported as decreased with or without vomiting); caloric intake normal 4. Screening tests all negative (ESR, CBC, urinalysis, stool guaiac, liver enzymes, "mono spot" test, tuberculin skin test)
Chronic gastritis, peptic ulcer (may have psychogenic component)	1. Pain dominantly epigastric; exacerbated on starvation or ingestion of acid/high roughage foods; relieved by intake of bland foods, antacids (clinical trial) 2. Physical examination negative except for possible epigastric tenderness 3. Weight loss and anorexia variable—not necessarily a dominant feature; may have vomiting with hematemesis 4. Screening tests may reveal melena; remainder normal
Hepatitis (viral, infectious mononucleosis)	1. Pain dominantly RUQ; may be exacerbated on ingestion of fatty foods; not relieved by ingestion of other foods or related to starvation 2. Physical examination usually reveals RUQ tenderness, liver variably enlarged; spleen sometimes enlarged with mononucleosis 3. Anorexia common; weight loss common with degree related to duration of disease; vomiting sometimes seen but without hematemesis 4. Screening tests may reveal ↑ WBC, ↑ ESR, ↑ liver enzymes (SGOT, SGPT); "mono spot" may be positive in mononucleosis; antigen and antibody tests may be positive in viral hepatitis
Chronic bowel disease	1. History may be similar to that of psychosomatic disease; or dull crampy pain or severe crampy pain with or without diarrhea 2. Physical examination commonly reveals patient to appear ill and debilitated; abdomen commonly tender throughout or in any quadrant 3. Anorexia and/or significant weight loss frequent 4. Screening tests commonly reveal ↑ ESR, melena
Constipation	1. Crampy abdominal pain, often LLQ and LUQ; may be severe, causing patient to double up 2. History of hard stools at infrequent intervals; may have blood streaking on stool or on wiping from fissure or hemorrhoid 3. Relief of pain with relief of constipation 4. Screening tests normal
Pelvic inflammatory disease	1. Lower abdominal and/or pelvic pain; variable in description; may have many features of psychosomatic types 2. Abdominal examination variable, with lower abdominal tenderness common; pelvic examination will reveal adnexal tenderness; tubal swelling and/or abscess may be present as well 3. No significant weight loss, anorexia, etc., unless patient toxic from infection with fever, acute pain 4. Screening tests variably may reveal ↑ WBC, ↑ ESR; cervical cultures variably positive for gonococcus, chlamydia
Headache (see Chapter 10) Psychosomatic	1. Characteristic features of tension or vascular headaches 2. Neurological examination normal 3. Screening tests normal

Continued

TABLE 25-2
CLINICAL FEATURES DIFFERENTIATING
PSYCHOSOMATIC CAUSES FROM THE COMMON CAUSES OF ORGANIC DISEASE (CONTINUED)

Complaint/condition	Clinical features
Headache (continued) Migraine (may have psychogenic component)	1. Classic symptomatology 2. Neurological examination normal during headache-free periods; commonly normal even when headache present but sometimes abnormal when ischemic phase results in motor or sensory symptoms and signs 3. Screening tests normal
Space-occupying lesions	1. Severe headache, exceptionally debilitating; vomiting common 2. Neurological evaluation significant; significant signs and symptoms common 3. Screening tests normal; visual fields may be abnormal
Joint pains (see Chapter 11) Psychosomatic	1. Pains may be specific to several joints or vague and migratory; involvement of large and small joints, back, and/or assorted muscle groups common; specificity of location, type of pain, and exacerbating or relieving factors (other than rest) notably absent 2. May give history of joint swelling but never documented by outside observer; never redness, although may be some tenderness on palpation or movement, which may disappear if patient distracted 3. General health excellent; negative physical examination results 4. Screening tests negative
Juvenile rheumatoid arthritis	1. Migratory pains usually involving large joints (one or more) and/or joints of hands or feet; back and muscle groups rarely involved 2. History of joint swelling confirmed by outside observer almost essential to diagnosis 3. Physical examination negative except for joints, which commonly evidence pain on motion, limited motion, swelling, and tenderness with or without erythema 4. Screening tests usually reveal ↑ ESR; absence of this finding tends to rule out active disease
Specific adolescent orthopedic conditions (Osgood-Schlatter's syndrome, chondromalacia patellae, slipped femoral epiphysis)	1. Specific historic features per Chapter 11 2. Pain limited to affected joint with specific clinical findings 3. Exacerbated by exercise, relieved on rest 4. Screening tests normal
Traumatic injury with inadequate rehabilitation; chronic muscle strain	1. May have chronic pain for extended period following a specific injury; usually related to injured part exclusively; also may be due to chronic strain from postural problems (e.g., poor supporting mattress, platform shoes, spike-heeled shoes, poor working conditions, improperly sized school desk) or exercise exceeding conditioning (moving heavy furniture, lifting weights); here back pain most common symptom 2. Physical examination correlates with injury 3. Screening tests normal
Fatigue/malaise Psychosomatic	1. Isolated phenomenon or in association with other typical psychosomatic complaints 2. Physical examination negative; patient in apparently good health 3. Screening tests normal
Organic	1. Almost invariably presents in combination with other features strongly suggestive of organic disease; infectious mononucleosis or hepatitis may be an exception when present in milder forms 2. Physical examination should be revealing

Continued

TABLE 25-2
CLINICAL FEATURES DIFFERENTIATING
PSYCHOSOMATIC CAUSES FROM THE COMMON CAUSES OF ORGANIC DISEASE (CONTINUED)

Complaint/condition	Clinical features
Fatigue/malaise (continued)	
Organic (continued)	3. Screening tests commonly positive, particularly ↑ ESR if significant or serious disease present (collagen vascular disorder, malignancy, chronic infection)
Dizziness	
Psychosomatic	1. Commonly in association with palpitations, tachycardia, tachypnea, and other signs of anxiety. May complain of transient blurred vision/ blackness as associated with vasovagal syncope; also may be hyperventilation syndrome
	2. Physical examination negative when not symptomatic; may evidence changes in vital signs consistent with vasovagal syncope or hyperventilation syndrome during an episode
	3. Screening tests normal
Organic	As for organic-derived fatigue

The emotional concomitants to shifts in environment, the breakup of an important relationship, major school examinations, times of significant decision, and the like frequently are dealt with by transient somatization. It usually is an easy matter for the patient to perceive the relationship between the stress and his or her symptoms, if he or she has not already made such a deduction (as is often the case). Once such an association has been made, little more is necessary beyond proffering continued encouragement and support at an appropriate frequency. These adolescents have pursued a normal developmental course and do not exhibit dysfunctionality in other areas. They generally soon adapt to new situations or learn to accommodate to a proclivity for tension headaches or butterflies in the stomach. Those who are more distressed than the average may find benefit in relaxation exercises, meditation, or self-hypnosis techniques.

Dysfunctional psychosomatic complaints are quite a different matter. Some instances of type a complaints (vague aches and discomforts) and all instances of type b (specific system complexes such as asthma or migraine) fall in this category. Symptoms represent a chronic maladaptive response to stress. They are not worked through with time and are significantly disabling. Psychosocial investigation commonly reveals significant problems at home, in school, or among peers. This group is also apt to exhibit chronic depression, acute anxiety attacks, and/or the hyperventilation syndrome. Type a complaints are particularly likely to involve multiple organ systems. The combination of a wide variety of

vague, ill-defined symptoms, depressed mood and affect, and psychosocial conflict beyond the norm is almost pathognomonic. There need not be clear cause and effect between symptoms and the stress itself.

The first step in management is to help the adolescent (and parents) accept the emotional genesis of the symptoms. Frequently this explanation is denied and great umbrage taken if the physician offers such an observation too precipitously. At all points it must be kept in mind that somatic displacement of emotional distress is an unconsciously mediated phenomenon and the pain or discomfort is very real—the patient is not malingering. Complaints must be taken seriously and not sloughed off or belittled. Recognition of the patient's genuine physical discomfort should be offered while working toward an association with the psychologic genesis. "You know, our minds and bodies are all of one part. It's in our language in such sayings as, 'you give me a pain in the neck,' 'I have butterflies in my stomach,' or 'that breaks my heart.' What kinds of physical feelings do you get when worried, upset, angry?" Most adolescents experience physical discomfort in these circumstances and can readily describe them. The physician can carry this one step further through permissive or projective techniques (see Chapter 23). "I bet when your parents get angry at you (or whatever is thought to be the probable provocation of the symptoms), you sometimes feel .... (describing symptoms)." Or "When I'm in a tense situation, I sometimes feel .... (describing some organic discomfort). Has this ever happened to

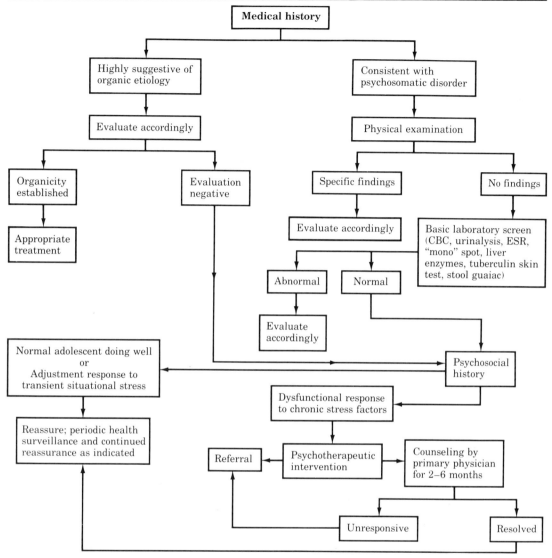

FIGURE 25-1
FLOW CHART FOR DIAGNOSIS AND MANAGEMENT OF A PSYCHOSOMATIC DISORDER

you?" Such statements frequently strike a responsive cord, reflected in a nod, smile of acknowledgement, or relaxation of reserve. Once even a slight association has been made, the counseling process can begin (Chapter 23).

When these measures are unsuccessful and denial of association persists, continued efforts at securing insight tend to be unfruitful and alienating. They should be dropped for the time being. This frequent-

ly happens in type b consolidated symptom complexes, particularly those productive of considerable secondary gain. It also is apt to occur when a number of physicians have been consulted previously and the problem dealt with solely from a biologic perspective, to little avail. The resultant frustration and enhanced worry of the patient and family that he or she has a mysterious, unrecognizable, and untreatable disease make for singular resistance to appreciating the true state of affairs. A full, but rational, medical evaluation is indicated, followed by reassurance to the effect that "Whatever is going on is not serious. If it were, tests X, Y, and Z would be positive or I would have found something in your physical examination. I am not worried about you, but we will continue to work together and see if we can't find some answers."

With either acceptance or denial of the psychogenic base, treatment proceeds with the counseling approach. When the patient has insight, this follows naturally. When absent, counseling is introduced in parallel with continued medical surveillance and reassuring examination at appropriate intervals. This approach can be initiated by some such comment as, "While we will continue to work toward finding the cause of your symptoms, I am also concerned about .... (whatever the suspected stress situation may be as identified in the psychosocial evaluation). I bet you are too and we should talk about this as well." If on the right track, symptoms should begin to improve as the patient becomes better able to deal with the conflict. Usually such improvement becomes evident after four to five weekly visits. If no results are forthcoming over this time, psychiatric consultation may be indicated. This is particularly likely to be the case when the psychosomatic complaints are long-standing, well-entrenched response patterns and/or accompanied by chronic depression.

We do not feel tranquilizers have a significant role in psychosomatic disorders, but relief of pain and other discomforts is indicated. Weak analgesics may be helpful for headaches or muscle aches; antacids or antispasmotics for abdominal pain, often associated with increased secretion of hydrochloric acid and/or intestinal spasm. Medication will be only transiently effective until the underlying cause is worked out, but even temporary relief of symptoms is appropriate to the situation and helpful in establishing trust and the patient's perception that the physician takes the problem seriously.

Hysterical Conversion

Hysterical conversion, a syndrome that occurs throughout adolescence, is more common during the midteen years. Females are considerably more vulnerable than males. The symptom complex represents a specific physical expression of repressed psychologic conflict; the patient usually is quite unaware of the emotional content of the symptoms and perceives them as biologically engendered.

Although paralysis of various extremities and simple motor tics are the most common manifestations of conversion reactions, symptoms may mimic any disease but often are illogical from the pathophysiologic perspective (for example, paralysis or paresthesias are not consistent with nerve distribution pathways). Conversion tics particularly need to be differentiated from those associated with Gilles de la Tourette syndrome, in which they are combined with compulsive, explosive sounds and words, often of an obscene nature.

The underlying cause may be difficult to discover, as it commonly relates to the resurgence of unresolved earlier childhood conflicts. Often these are sexual, raised to the surface by pubertal and adolescent developmental drives. There may be no clear stress situation associated with the onset of symptoms; rather it is the patient's unconscious perception of ordinary events as overwhelming. A case in point is that of a 16-year-old girl, raised in a particularly strict, religious home, who experienced the paralysis of one leg after dancing for the first time at her brother's wedding. The patient with serious conversion symptoms probably should be referred to a psychiatrist as resolution often requires special techniques, such as an extended analytic approach, hypnotherapy, behavior modification, and the like.

The primary care physician's major task rests in motivating the youth and parents to accept psychiatric treatment. They both may be highly resistant, denying the possibility of emotional origin. The physician may need to continue seeing the patient for awhile until the need for referral becomes acceptable. Treatment solely from a medical perspective, including the use of placebos, should be avoided. Such treatment risks further fixating the patient on an organic cause. (Although appropriate rehabilitative measures may be necessary to preserve function and avoid muscle wasting or contractures.) Moreover, if a strictly medical or placebo approach manages to relieve the presenting symptoms, the underlying conflict remains, and a new set of manifestations will likely emerge.

Milder, short-term conversion reactions are more apt to be related to current stress situations but with a past conflictual base. The degree of psychopathology is considerably less, and it takes a definitively provocative situation to precipitate a response. There often is a normal developmental element as well, for example, the young pubertal adolescent who experiences homosexual anxiety in the locker room or the boy with gynecomastia. Psychosocial assessment and counseling should seek to identify the conflict and bring about an association between cause and effect in the patient's mind, as with psychosomatic complaints. Simply exploring the meaning of the symptoms in relation to the generative stress and considering possible solutions often are all that is needed. In other instances, some sort of modest modification of the environment may be required as well. Usually this involves temporary insulation from the precipitating stress for several months. This might be as simple as a gym excuse for the previously mentioned boys.

Hyperventilation Syndrome and Acute Anxiety Attacks

The hyperventilation syndrome and acute anxiety attacks differ from each other primarily in degree. Both are due to the response of the sympathetic and parasympathetic nervous systems to conscious or unconscious fear. Feelings of nervousness, tachypnea, palpitations, and tachycardia predominate.

In the hyperventilation syndrome, tachypnea predominates even to the point of producing significant respiratory alkalosis. In turn, this may alter the state of consciousness, and the symptoms may be collectively perceived as a "seizure" by parents or other observers. This sequence often results in the patient presenting as an emergency in a seemingly postictal state. Frequently it is necessary to admit the patient to rule out a seizure disorder; once on the ward this usually becomes clear. The picture often is replicable by having the patient breathe deeply and rapidly; relief or the blocking of symptoms is afforded by repeating the maneuver while breathing into a paper bag. Feelings of nervousness dominate anxiety attacks. In addition to the symptoms mentioned in the introductory paragraph, the patient also may experience dizziness, faintness, blurred vision (everything going all "black" or seeming out of focus), nausea, vomiting, and/or diarrhea. When loss of consciousness does occur, it is the typical vasovagal faint.

Either syndrome is a direct physiologic response to a real or perceived stress. This stress may be similar to that seen in conversion hysteria, in which earlier unresolved childhood issues resurface upon the advent of puberty and adolescence; or it may relate to a clear current provocation. The response may be appropriate to the situation in mild degrees and is similar to mild psychosomatic symptoms in the face of such matters as school examinations, oral presentations before the class, starting a new school, and so on.

In more marked degree, these syndromes are likely to have a pathopsychologic base. Evidence of poor past coping is usually evident. Recurrent episodes or chronic anxiety can be quite disabling, the patient usually being fearful of entering new situations and tending to stay close to home in a rather dependent state. Parents may not perceive such an adolescent as in trouble unless reflected in loss of consciousness from hyperventilation or deteriorating school performance. Usually girls, these patients tend to be obedient and compliant and rarely are confrontational or cause other provocative concerns typical of the mid-adolescent period.

Treatment is as for any disorder consisting of biologic manifestations of psychologic stress. Mild forms associated with specific current anxiety-producing situations generally respond to changing the environment in a manner that will reduce or eliminate the provocative stress together with patient and family counseling. The goal is to achieve self-awareness and more adaptive coping methods. If an anxiety-producing situation is unavoidable (as may be the case for marital arguments between parents, school examinations, a troublemaker in school, or entering a new situation), symptoms may be aborted or at least minimized by various relaxation exercises, meditation or, with hyperventilation, by breathing slowly into a paper bag. More chronic and disabling symptoms usually require referral for psychotherapy.

Bibliography*

Asnes, R. S.; Santulli, R.; and Bemporad, J. R. 1981. Psychogenic chest pain in children. *Clin. Pediatr.* 20:788-791.

Friedman, S. B. 1973. Conversion symptoms in adolescence. *Pediatr. Clin. North Am.* 20:873.

Herman, S. P.; Stickler, G. B.; and Lucas, A. R. 1981. Hyperventilation syndrome in children and adolescents: long-term follow-up. *Pediatrics* 67:183.

Joorabchi, B. 1977. Expressions of the hyperventilation syndrome in childhood. *Clin. Pediatr.* 16:1110.

Lazare, A. 1981. Conversion symptoms. *N. Engl. J. Med.* 305:745-748.

Mahoney, M. J. 1980. Diagnosing hysterical conversion reactions in children. *J. Pediatr.* 97:1016-1020.

Marks, I., and Lader, M. 1973. Anxiety states (anxiety neurosis): a review. *J. Nerv. Ment. Dis.* 156:3.

Rock, N. L. 1971. Conversion reactions in childhood: a clinical study on childhood neuroses. *J. Amer. Acad. Child. Psychiatr.* 10:65.

Schonfeld, W. 1963. Body image in adolescence. *Pediatrics* 35:845.

Teicher, J. D. 1973. Psychosomatic problems in adolescence. In *The emotionally troubled adolescent and the family physician*, editor M. G. Kalogerakis. Springfield, Ill.: Charles C Thomas, Publisher.

*See general psychologic and psychiatric references following the introduction to Part IV. Most have substantial information of relevance to this chapter. Also see bibliographies in other chapters in Part IV.

-26-
Depression, Suicide, Out-of-Control Reactions and Psychoses

Depression
Diagnosis □ Management
Suicide
Assessment of risk □ Management
Rage, Panic, and Hysterical Outbursts
Evaluation and management
Impulse Disorders
Psychoses
Organic psychoses □ Cyclical disease □ Schizophrenia

Depression

Depression in adolescence can be divided into three types: normal (developmental), reactive, and constitutional (Table 26-1). In the first instance, some degree of depression is a common component of the adolescent experience—"blue" periods alternating with ones of more optimistic outlook. The developmental process of emancipation implies loss as much as acquisition; the loss of secure and comforting dependency ties as independence is gained, and the loss of parents as primary love objects to be replaced by appropriate age-mates. Although such surrender is an essential prerequisite to the assumption of adulthood, it is not without occasional regret. Such a response is recognizable by the absence or transience of dysfunctionality in school performance or in home and peer relationships. When dysfunctionality does exist, it should not last longer than 2–3 months to qualify as being within the normal range.

Reactive depressions of some degree are experienced by most of us at one time or another and run the gamut from mild to severe. Depression in this category may be based on long-standing or recent deprivations, chronic or circumscribed stress, real or perceived loss, or failure to achieve desired goals. Adolescence is a particularly vulnerable time for such a response consequent to the intensity and uncertainty of interpersonal relationships, the as yet tentative nature of self-esteem, and the inevitable loss of the *child*-parent relationship inherent in emancipation. The teenage years are well marked by stress, loss, and fear of failure. Significant factors in assessing whether a reactive depression is transient and appropriate to the situation, primarily to be managed with empathy and support, or of pathologic dimensions requiring definitive psychotherapeutic intervention include (a) the severity and chronicity of the precipitant, (b) the nature, intensity, and duration of the response, and (c) the degree of functional impairment or maturational impedance.

The third category, believed to be constitutionally and genetically derived, is manifested in a singular vulnerability to minimal provocations that most of us would weather well. Such individuals often have a family history of depressive responses and suicidal acts. Some degree of chronic impairment is inevitable, and support may be needed indefinitely. Constitutional depression is pathologic by definition.

DIAGNOSIS
Depressive symptomatology in adolescence, regardless of etiology, often varies with that seen in adults,

TABLE 26-1
OVERVIEW OF DEPRESSION IN ADOLESCENCE

Classification	Etiologic factors	Manifestations	Management
Normal depression	Normal developmental separation issues	Transient "down mood" or heightened irritability Less than 3 months in duration Minimum impact on function	Empathy and support on p.r.n. basis
Reactive depression Early adolescence	Long-standing stress, deprivation Family disruption Chronic illness/handicap	Irritability, anger Provocative behavior or withdrawal and infantile behavior	Counseling Alteration and enrichment of environment
Midadolescence	As for early adolescent Loss, impairment of current relationships Absence of options for gaining self-esteem	"Acting-out" behaviors Drug/alcohol abuse and/or adult-type depression	As above plus attention to possible suicide risk
Late adolescence	Situational stress or loss Failure to negotiate emancipation Failure to achieve academic, social, or personal goals	Classic adult type; vegetative signs, sleep disorders, preoccupation with guilt, agitation, etc.	As above
Constitutional depression	Exaggerated response to mild stress or loss	Appearance in mid to late adolescence Positive family history common Adult type symptoms	As above plus plan for chronic long-term treatment

particularly in the earlier years. The physician should not be fooled when such classic adult signs and symptoms as preoccupation with guilt, psychomotor apathy, agitation, insomnia, anorexia, constipation, and the like are not evident. More frequently, depression is masked by disruptive and disquieting behaviors; misdiagnosis is common. On the other hand, one should not make the error of calling all maladaptive behaviors depressive; they have a variety of derivations, and diagnosis must look beyond the behavior itself.

Early adolescents tend to evidence depression through irritability, easy anger, and various provocations or through regressive, whining, infantile behavior. Although there is no gender exclusivity, depressed males are more likely to engage in the former pattern and females in the latter. Early adolescent depression tends to be reactive and chronic, deriving from long-standing childhood stress. Important historical data include disorganized or deprived family situations, parental child-rearing attitudes far at one or the other end of the restrictive-permissive spectrum, child abuse, chronic illness in the family, parental alcoholism, and

physical or mental handicaps in the patient affecting body image and self-esteem.

Significant depression in midadolescence also is dominantly reactive, but constitutional forms now begin to appear. In any instance, manifestations are closer to those seen in depressed adults, but classic features can be masked by various behavioral outlets. School failure, truancy, running away, drug or alcohol abuse, sexual promiscuity, pregnancy, and juvenile delinquency may have depressive components. In other instances, withdrawal and isolation may be more prominent features because of the inability to tolerate increasing pressures for commitment to the peer group and for establishing heterosexual relationships. The arrival of abstract thought and the capacity to perceive the future implications of current events further complicate the situation. The earlier, more immediate, and circumscribed sense of deprivation and loss of the concrete thinker now takes on a new futuristic dimension in the bleak prospect of continuing indefinitely. In these circumstances, suicidal thinking and action (see next section) become more prevalent. Points of historic importance include those noted for the early adolescent and more current events pertaining to midadolescent developmental issues, for example, emancipation and sexual identity. In addition, a family history of depression or suicide now becomes significant.

Classic symptomatology and constitutional forms of depression become more common in late adolescence and, concomitantly, the suicidal potential increases. Separating from home and going to college is a frequent precipitating event for a vulnerable youth. Other provocative stresses may be the failure of academic achievement at the level of parental expectation, the failure to achieve vocational or personal goals, an inability to feel comfortable in adult society, or a sense of personal isolation and difficulty in establishing peer relationships. Although inquiry along lines similar to those for early and midadolescents may be revealing, constitutional depression in this older age group may have few readily apparent antecedents and may present with little warning. This is apt to be the case in a vulnerable individual who overtly has been conforming, achieving, and dutiful in earlier years, a model adolescent in his or per parents' eyes. In fact, such young people have never negotiated emancipation successfully nor have come to feel they have achieved the level of success expected of them. The prospect of becoming autonomous becomes untenable, resulting in depression with a high suicide potential.

MANAGEMENT
Therapy depends on the cause of the depression, its seriousness, chronicity, and degree of dysfunctionality. Figure 26-1 provides direction. The following points also should be considered:

1. A simple willingness to listen, coupled with concrete suggestions for solving current problems and continuing support can improve the patient's self-esteem significantly by giving him or her a greater sense of being in effective control.

2. Environmental enrichment and the use of special programs for adolescents such as camp, Girls' and Boys' Clubs, YMCA and YWCA activities, peer leadership programs, and the like may provide opportunities for success, promote supportive adult and peer relationships, and otherwise enhance self-esteem.

3. Family counseling, with and without the patient present (but in the latter instance always with the patient's knowledge and permission), is beneficial to examine intrafamily conflicts, create greater mutual understanding, and define more effective methods of resolving conflict.

The patient should be referred for more intensive psychotherapy when (a) the preceding interventions have produced only minimal results after 1 month; (b) there is moderate to serious suicidal risk at any time; (c) the depression is linked with significant drug or alcohol abuse and/or predelinquent or delinquent behavior; or (d) the depression appears to be constitutional.

Suicide
The third leading cause of death among young people aged 15–24 years and rising in total numbers and rate, suicide obviously is a dominant and critical concern. Three primary types of suicidal acts may be identified. First, an impulsive, acting-out rage response to punish or manipulate a loved person perceived as withdrawing that love (usually parents or a serious dating partner). Second, a gesture serving as a desperate cry for help in an adolescent who otherwise feels helpless. And third, a definitive self-destructive act. Various psychodynamic motivations have been ascribed to the latter instance, including a displacement of anger and the wish for death of another onto the self or seeing death as the only way to stop intolerable emotional pain.

Regardless of intention or motivation, *any suicidal ideation or attempt must be taken seriously* and promptly evaluated. Swallowing a handful of aspirin may appear impulsive and relatively innocuous, but it is apt to become a repetitive pattern; subsequent efforts may produce far more disastrous consequences out of miscalculation.

ASSESSMENT OF RISK
In practice it can be difficult to discriminate clearly between gesture and intent, and we do not recommend that the management course be based on this distinction. Rather we urge that a variety of factors be considered when assessing the overall risk. A gesturer may inadvertently succeed, or one simply thinking about suicide, even in vague terms, may progress to take active steps. Table 26-2 offers a basis for such discrimination.

MANAGEMENT
We obviously are unable to help those whose depression has not been identified and whose attempt succeeds. Males are more apt to fall in this category in that they generally employ more lethal methods: knives, guns, automobiles, and jumping from high places. Ingesting pills or slashing wrists is more common among females.

In any unsuccessful instance, identification and protection of those at risk, male or female, may be

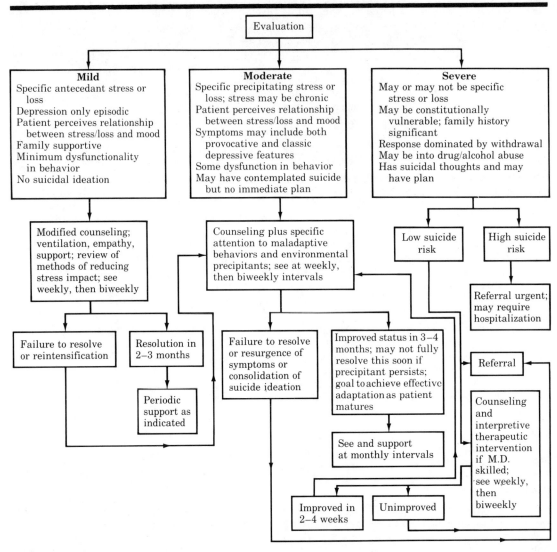

FIGURE 26-1
FLOW CHART FOR MANAGEMENT OF DEPRESSION IN ADOLESCENCE

afforded by observing the plan offered in Figure 26-2 and by the following rules:

1. Evaluation for suicide risk should be made in any adolescent who evidences depressive symptomatology of any sort, who appears "down" during the course of a routine health contact, who seems to be having more trouble than most accomplishing developmental tasks, or who has a history of depression or suicide in family members.

2. Initiating such inquiries should be direct:

"You seem somewhat sad/troubled/upset to me. Have you ever thought about suicide?" Indirection and hinting only confuse and can be misunderstood. Forthright questions usually produce forthright answers. Suicide is not an issue adolescents lie about when questioned, but they rarely reveal such concerns unless asked. Those who have had such thoughts are usually most relieved to be able to talk and to have someone step in to protect them. Suicide-prone young people also may have a history of

TABLE 26-2
SUICIDE ATTEMPTS AND PROCLAMATIONS: RISK ASSESSMENT FACTORS*†

	Low risk	Moderate risk	High risk
Precipitating event (What made you do this?" "Why do you want to do this?")	Argument with friend, teacher	Fight with close friend School failure Difficult home situation	Breakup of important relationship Parental rejection; thrown out of home Discovery of pregnancy plus family crisis and/or rejection by boyfriend Death of close relative/friend Thinking disorder; wishes to join deceased person; hear voices telling him/her to kill self
Intended purpose of act ("Why did you do this?" "Why do you want to do this?")	Does not know; impulsive, unreasoned act	Remorse over fight Can't face shame of failure To escape poor home situation To punish family/friend To call attention to own need	Wants to join deceased person Wants to be dead; no purpose in living
Plan, method, and perceived lethality ("Did/do you think this would/will kill you?")	Small amount of pills perceived of low toxicity (aspirin, antibiotics, random medicine cabinet selections)	Small/moderate amount of pills perceived as toxic (sedatives, tranquilizers) Slashing wrists	Violent method (jumping out window, gun, knife) Large amounts of pills/entire bottle of pills or substance perceived as toxic
Plan: real lethality	Relatively innocuous	Moderately harmful but high probability of recovery	Significant possibility of death
Plan: specificity (In proclamation only; "How would you go about suicide?")	No solid plan; a number of vague possibilities No method seen as really available	Specific plan, but not rehearsed Several specific alternatives, but no choice yet made Method easily available	One method chosen and steps for accomplishment defined Has been rehearsed (has taken pills/gun in hand and contemplated) Tentative implementation (taken a small number of pills, started to step in front of car)
Plan: discovery potential (In act only; as apparent in history, not necessarily consciously recognized by patient)	Someone in house Announces intent prior to act	Someone expected home soon Telephones friend/goes to friend's home after act Climbs to highly visible location and does not immediately jump	Commits act in isolated situation Tells no one before or after act (but may leave note) Did not expect anyone home Goes to a deserted, isolated location to commit act
Other stress factors in life ("Have you any other problems going on in your life?")	None or only perceived as of minimal significance	Environmental change (friend moved away, family relocated in new community, new school) Physical/body image problems (delayed puberty, chronic illness/handicap) Failure to achieve specific goals in school, job, personal life As cited under "precipitating event"	As cited under "precipitating event"

Continued

TABLE 26-2
SUICIDE ATTEMPTS AND PROCLAMATIONS: RISK ASSESSMENT FACTORS (CONTINUED)

	Low risk	Moderate risk	High risk
Mood/affect/behavior; psychosocial developmental status ("How are things going at home/school/with friends?" "How do you usually feel about life?")	Optimistic Performs well at school High level of ability to confide in parents Has many friends Relates well to interviewer	Depressed, but mood lightens after act or ventilation Anger/rage at parents Variable school problems One friend; somewhat isolated Poor ability to confide in parents Relates well to interviewer	Marked persistent depression, no relief after act or ventilation Feelings of hopelessness, helplessness, isolation Flat, distant affect Relates poorly to parents No friends; no confidant Deteriorating school function Difficult for interviewer to make emotional contact; patient remains remote, distant, sad
Past coping skills	Effective reality testing Usually is competent in handling environmental stress Uses support systems (parents, friends, church) Appropriate ventilation, e.g., has a good cry	Distorts reality Efforts to change situation often abortive or ineffective Poor use of support systems, e.g., locks self in room Impulsive outbursts; low frustration tolerance (temper tantrums/rages common) Is able to be reflective and think about situation	Loses reality boundaries Withdraws and isolates self No use of support systems Sees self as totally helpless and victim of fate
Past mental health	Generally has been well	Some depression, but seeks/accepts help Frequent mood swings from rage to depression Periodic abuse of drugs/alcohol	Chronic depression; rejects help Chronic drug/alcohol abuse Past suicide attempts Past psychiatric hospitalizations Affective thinking disorder; psychosis
Future plans	Has definite goals Can give good picture of how sees self in 5–10 years	Wants to be "somebody" but no definite plans Vague, stereotypic description of future	No plans for future Cannot imagine what will be doing in 5–10 years in any terms Alienated from mainstream of society
Family structure and mental health	Two-parent family Effective coping skills, competent Closeness among family members Extended family/ friends support system Not overburdened with stresses of poverty, illness No prior history of depression, suicide, alcoholism, drug abuse and/or addiction Parents flexible toward children; limit-setting mediated through open communication	Overburdened family, but usually able to cope effectively Occasional episodes of disorganization Tenuous, although maintained, stability Rigid and inflexible toward children; degree of control variable Tries to communicate but on parental terms	Overburdened family, copes poorly Generally disorganized and unstable No outside support system Previous mental hospitalization, depressive episodes, suicide or attempts, drug/alcohol abuse Rigid and inflexible toward children but no real control No efforts at communication No adult in home; adolescent alone due to parental death or abandonment

*Developed by Ilene Miner, A.C.S.W., and Adele D. Hofmann, M.D.

†Note: One or more of the listed examples and/or other examples of a similar intensity may be operative in any category.

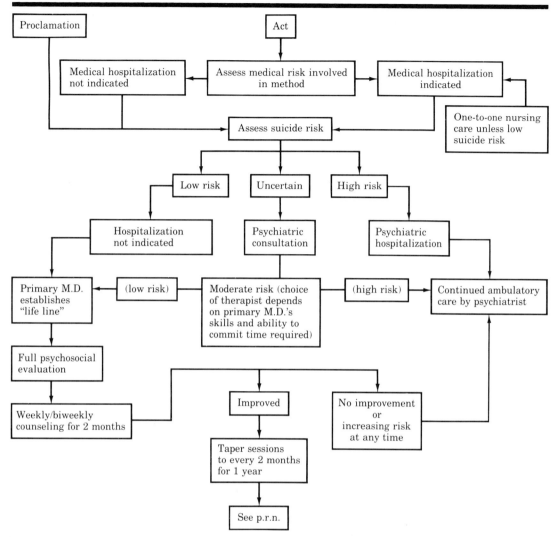

FIGURE 26-2
FLOW CHART FOR MANAGEMENT OF A SUICIDAL ACT OR PROCLAMATION IN ADOLESCENCE

one or more past episodes, sometimes only known to themselves. This should be looked for specifically as a significant risk factor.

3. Any adolescent involved in a clear or possible suicide proclamation or act should be thoroughly evaluated as to degree of risk without delay.

4. Management in every instance must include immediate, close supervision and the option of contacting a trusted professional *at any time* (what we call a "life-line").

5. Some experts recommend at least brief hospitalization for evaluation of any suicidal act,

regardless of apparent risk. We do not; this is an exceptionally common phenomenon in our clinic population and we are experienced in making competent discrimination between those who are at significant risk and need hospitalization and those who do not. Physicians who feel less than comfortable in making such a decision, however, should err on the side of conservatism and hospitalize in every instance or obtain immediate psychiatric consultation.

6. High-risk adolescents always should be hospitalized and managed by a psychiatrist.

7. Physicians who plan to treat a youth at mod-

erate or even low risk on their own must be prepared to

> a. Take sufficient time to establish the therapeutic relationship immediately.
>
> b. Be available to the adolescent by telephone or "drop in" 24 hours a day for at least the first month. Provide a home telephone number if the answering service is not wholly dependable or if it will be difficult to reach you otherwise on nights and weekends off. Most of these patients only call at times of real need and do not make pests of themselves.
>
> c. Establish a written or verbal contract with the adolescent that he or she will not do anything harmful without calling and talking about it first; most teenagers who can be managed on an ambulatory basis will accept and follow such a contract well and can be dissuaded from harmful actions once contact has been made, looking to the physician to shore up their self-esteem and impose superego control.

After the initial interview and establishment of the above therapeutic base, patients in moderate to low risk should evidence a lightening of their depressive mood, even smiling or joking a bit, convey the feeling that a tie has been made, and reverse the suicide commitment, at least temporarily. Adolescents at serious risk remain persistently depressed and continue to have active suicidal thoughts. In this instance hospitalization is indicated. The general rule of confidentiality in adolescent health care does *not* obtain when suicidal thoughts are present. Parents must be notified promptly and their protection enlisted, regardless of the degree of assessed risk.

Rage, Panic, and Hysterical Outbursts

Uncontrolled rage, panic, or hysterical outbursts represent an acute response to a major threat, real or perceived, and comprise a "flight, fright, fight" reaction of the most primitive sort. Any human being will succumb to one or another of these behaviors if sufficiently stressed, but the point of loss of control varies greatly, depending on individual factors such as resourcefulness in coping, adaptiveness, self-control, and stress threshold.

Adolescents generally are more prone to out-of-control responses than others because of the normally higher internal and external pressures and the fact that defense (coping) mechanisms have not yet been consolidated in a mature form; a boiler with poorly welded seams and working under a high head of steam does not have far to go before blowing up. These behaviors, then, do not necessarily indicate serious pathology when they occur in the teen years and must be measured against the intensity of the precipitating cause, the appropriateness of the reaction from the perception of the youth, and his or her usual level of functioning in other areas. Repetitive loss of self-control unexplainable by normal midteen frustrations and in excess of the provocation warrant particularly close examination for possible predisposing factors such as an impulse disorder (see next section).

EVALUATION AND MANAGEMENT

If called when an adolescent is out of control, the physician's first and most imperative step is to assess the degree of danger to self or others quickly and to act to contain the patient and prevent harm. The following procedures may be tried:

1. Remove any apparent precipitating cause immediately. This may be an individual such as parents or teachers in a confrontational rage situation, or, in the ill adolescent, misunderstood or overheard medical information of dire import or, in the face of a threatening piece of medical apparatus, even a needle and syringe.

2. Try to establish visual contact and act with quiet reassurance. Attempt to calm the patient with concerned and empathic words, "You are O.K. and I will see that you will not be harmed. What can I do to help?" Answers should be respected; if the patient asks to be left alone, it is appropriate to do so, provided he or she promises not to hurt himself or others.

3. If the patient is beyond such efforts, either initially or after a modest trial of "talking him down," forceful containment may be necessary. Although nonassaultive methods are always preferable, preventing serious injury is paramount.

4. Medication is indicated if the patient continues struggling after contained. Chlorpromazine or sodium amytal intramuscularly, either one in a dose of 25 mg for a Tanner V (mature) youth, will decrease excessive anxiety and help the patient regain self-control. Medication, however, should not be used in an extended manner or as a pharmacologic straight jacket.

Several words to the wise. Do not succumb to your own sense of panic. Do not be a hero; get help if possible, but try to avoid calling the police unless the youth is armed or there is no other resource. Uniforms frequently only escalate matters and bringing in the law puts the patient before the public eye as well. Keep talking to the patient in calm, reassuring tones at all times.

A careful history should be obtained after the crisis situation has passed and the patient is accessible, usually within half an hour. The patient should be questioned first, then parents and others who may be involved. The following points should be ascertained:

1. Appropriateness of response to precipitating cause.

2. Presence or absence of similar past episodes.

3. Any evidence of impulse disorder.

4. Psychosocial developmental status.

5. Cultural factors (for example, some cultural groups are more likely to respond to a crisis with heightened emotionalism than others).

6. Possible "mob" psychology factors (out-of-control behaviors evidenced by a group do not speak to the psychopathology of any single group member and comprise a unique phenomenon).

7. Possible implication of hallucinogenic drugs with panic being related to psychotogenic features.

When loss of control is the result of clear situational provocation, the patient quickly reorganizes himself or herself when the stress is removed and support provided. In the absence of similar events in the past or other significant historic data, reassurance coupled with one or two followup visits in support is all that is needed. When matters are complicated by other signs of dysfunctionality, further evaluation and treatment are indicated. In some instances the counseling approach (Chapter 23) is sufficient; in more confirmed or resistant cases psychiatric referral is required.

Impulse Disorders

Impulse disorders arise from failure in early childhood to internalize external controls over instinctive drives (superego development). Triggered by seemingly minimal stress, manifestations include rage responses to ordinary discipline, truancy, sporadic running away, petty thievery, and some forms of sexual promiscuity or excessive risk-taking behavior. Extreme examples of an impulse-ridden character structure are juvenile delinquents unable to perceive right from wrong, drug addicts, and rapists.

Most impulse disorders are of the lesser form and may be amenable to interventions such as peer "rap" groups, individual counseling, or therapeutic day programs. The selection of an approach is based on a knowledge of the patient and his or her family, the duration and seriousness of the problem, and the willingness of the adolescent to be involved in treatment. Many youngsters in this category are unable to perceive their own com-

plicity. There is a paranoid quality to their committed belief that their behavior is wholly justified by the unresponsiveness or provocativeness of others. Of course, these are not particularly lovable youths, and their behavior is trying at best. Negative perceptions of the outside world become a self-fulfilling prophecy and create an even more difficult situation with hostility all around.

Treatment is particularly difficult due to the well-entrenched, chronic nature of the psychopathology. Mild degrees may be responsive to counseling, but severer forms (or lesser symptoms resistant to change after 2–3 months' treatment) warrant referral for psychiatric help. Residential programs may be necessary when the adolescent is unable to use support systems while remaining at home. In some instances, however, resistance to change is insurmountable, and the patient will need support of one sort or another indefinitely. Impulse disorders also may lead the adolescent into trouble with the law. Regardless of the treatment plan, matters may be taken out of the therapist's hand if the patient has been involved and caught in an illegal act.

Psychoses

A psychotic individual is one whose mental capacity, affective response, ability to recognize reality, and/or ability to communicate and relate to others are so compromised as to impair effective environmental interaction. Three generic forms have been identified: organic, cyclical, and schizophrenic (Table 26-3).

ORGANIC PSYCHOSES

Organic psychoses result from chronic or acute central nervous system insults. In adolescents, organic psychoses are most commonly encountered with head trauma or drug ingestion. Indeed, drug toxicity should be the first diagnostic choice in any young person exhibiting unprecedented psychotic behavior. Some drugs closely mimic the schizophrenic state, particularly lysergic acid diethylamide (LSD), phencyclidine (PCP), and atropinic drugs. It also may be difficult to discriminate between the effects of central nervous system stimulants or atropinic drugs and manic states. Chapter 20 discusses differential features.

Signs and symptoms of an organic psychosis include disorientation, hallucinations, fluctuating states of consciousness, intellectual impairment, and fragmented thinking. Initial evaluation and ongoing monitoring rely heavily on serial mental status examinations (see Chapter 23), physical and neurologic

TABLE 26-3
CLASSIFICATION OF PSYCHOSES

Organic brain syndromes	Affective disorders	Schizophrenia
Alcoholic	Major	Acute
Drugs, poisons	a. Unipolar (depression or mania)	Hebephrenic
Central nervous system	b. Bipolar (manic-depressive)	Catatonic
a. Infections	Minor	Paranoid
b. Trauma	a. Hypomanic disorder	Undifferentiated
Endocrine and metabolic	b. Depressive neurosis	Residual
	c. Cyclothymia	Schizoaffective
	Primary and secondary	
	Exogenous vs endogenous	

assessment, and appropriate laboratory tests. Treatment focuses on the underlying organic cause. Whether long-term treatment will be required depends on the extent of residual symptoms after the acute stage is passed (or, in the case of drug toxicity, any underlying emotional problem). Management proceeds as for any chronic situation and depends on the nature of persistent symptoms.

CYCLICAL DISEASE

This group of disorders is characterized by cyclical exacerbations and remissions of inappropriate affect. They now are considered to have a biological origin, although environmental precipitants clearly contribute to decompensation. Three types have been described: manic-depressive, depressive-depressive, and manic-manic. They may appear at any time during the teen years, but more commonly are first seen in late adolescence and young adulthood. Depressive components are as previously described under constitutional depression. The manic stage is characterized by euphoria, insomnia, anorexia, general excitation, spending sprees, denial, hostility, and paranoid thinking. Differential diagnosis should not overlook intoxication from central nervous system stimulants. Hospitalization usually is indicated and psychiatric consultation mandatory.

SCHIZOPHRENIA

Schizophrenia can manifest in childhood but rises in incidence from midadolescence through age 30 and then declines. Genetic and neurobiologic factors are clearly implicated, but the precise etiology remains obscure. Several forms have been described (Table 26-3) according to the dominance of various characteristic symptoms. These include:

1. Autism: withdrawal, refusal to communicate, bizarre or impoverished communications, thought incoherence, thought insertion and/or broadcasting in which patients believe someone is putting thoughts in their heads or they are receiving radio messages.

2. Abnormal affect: blunt, flat, or inappropriate feeling, tone or mood, but to be distinguished from giggling as a cover-up of embarrassment, or reserve and shyness in a new situation or flatness due to depression.

3. Disordered associations: loose ideation, hallucinations (usually auditory), delusions (paranoid, phobic, somatic, grandiose, religious, nihilistic, of being controlled by another, etc.).

4. Emotional ambivalence: opposite extremes present at the same time in excess of ordinary mixed feelings.

5. Disorganized behavior: impairment in daily function, deterioration in dress and hygiene.

The most common early symptom in adolescence is acute hypochondriasis, often in association with bizarre fears and acute school phobia. Other frequent signs are insomnia, agitation, poor judgment, and concrete and/or paranoid thinking. Intelligence and orientation, however, are usually spared. Without intervention, the picture rather rapidly deteriorates over a period of days or several weeks into florid disorganization.

The primary care physician should be able to make a provisional diagnosis based on the history and a careful mental status examination (Chapter 23, Table 26-4). Psychiatric consultation is always indicated. Prompt management with psychotherapeutic agents, however, is an important step in preventing progressive disorganization. When a psychiatric consultation cannot be arranged immediately, the primary care physician should institute treatment with one of the phenothiazides; 50 mg of chlorpromazine p.o. four times a day (total daily dose, 200 mg) is a good starting dose for the average-size adolescent. Much larger doses in the range of two to three times the starting dose may ultimately be needed for

TABLE 26-4
SIGNS AND SYMPTOMS OF PSYCHOSIS IN ADOLESCENCE
(Some, but rarely all, features will be present in a given case)

Organic brain syndrome
Altered state of consciousness: coma, semicoma, confusion, disorientation
Altered thinking: toxic delirium, visual hallucinations (primarily)
Positive history for precipitant: illness, drug/poison ingestion, trauma
Physical or laboratory abnormalities: fever, toxic blood levels of drug/poison, meningitis or other infection, encephalitis, CNS trauma, neurologic findings of significance, endocrine or metabolic abnormalities

Affective disorders
Depressive features (differentiate from other types of depression):
Dysphoric mood
Psychomotor retardation
Impaired concentration
Agitation
Loss of interest
Thoughts of death or suicide
Self-reproach or guilty thoughts
Loss of weight or appetite
Insomnia, morning fatigue
Manic features (differentiate from CNS stimulant intoxication):
Euphoria or expansive mood
Irritability or aggressiveness
Grandiosity
Distractibility, short attention span
Sleep loss without morning fatigue
Hyperactivity, spending sprees

Hypersexuality, sexual heroics
Push of speech, garrulousness
Flight of ideas
Bizarre dress

Schizophrenia (differentiate from hallucinogen ingestion or toxic psychosis from CNS stimulant overdose):
Delusions: somatic, body image distortions, sexual, guilt, persecution, reference, religious, nihilistic, paranoid, grandiosity, bizarre
Hypochondriasis: marked, well beyond normal adolescent preoccupations
Hallucinations: auditory (primarily)
Formal thought disorder: illogical thinking, flight of ideas, thought insertion, others
Confusion: poor understanding, uncertainty as to time and place
Emotional lability/ambivalence: rapid extreme mood swings or extremes present simultaneously
Inappropriate affect: inappropriate laughter, blunt or flat affect (do not confuse with nervous giggling over embarrassing topic, natural reserve in new situation with guarding, or "down" tone seen in depression of any type)
Catatonia or repetitive mannerisms: do not confuse repetitive mannerisms with habit tics or Gilles de la Tourette syndrome
Disorganized behavior: impairment of daily function, deterioration in dress and hygiene
Regressive behavior: withdrawal and isolation, infantilism, nudity

optimal symptomatic control, but amounts of this magnitude should be introduced only through a gradual buildup.

A patient who presents with florid disorganization usually warrants hospitalization and should remain under the treatment of a psychiatrist for several years after discharge. In less advanced cases, stabilization and reorganization adequate for reasonable function usually is achieved in a fairly short time. In this instance, it may well be within the scope of the primary physician's skill to continue management through individual and family counseling, vocational planning for low-stress occupations, and appropriate drug therapy. Thioridazine (Mellaril), trifluoperazine (Stelazine), or haloperidol (Table 23-7) are better choices for chronic maintenance than chlorpromazine because they have less of a sedative effect. These drugs are not without complications, however, and the physician who plans to use one or another of these agents over any pro-

longed period of time should become familiar with their side effects in some detail.

Many schizophrenics are ambulatory and can be maintained with only simple, highly concrete support. Particular attention is needed at times of increased environmental stress or when significant decisions have to be made. These patients may have considerable difficulty in exercising judgment in making and implementing the best choice among several options.

Adolescent schizophrenics, in particular, often do well and improve significantly with time when the high-stress demands of meeting developmental tasks are passed. These young people can look forward to achieving reasonably stable and rewarding lives by their midtwenties. Nonetheless, some form of support will be necessary over an indefinite period of time and a full cure cannot be expected. The primary care physician will need to decide whether it is within the range of his or her comfort, skill, and willing commitment to manage such a patient.

Bibliography*

Baldessarini, R. J. 1977. Schizophrenia. *N. Engl. J. Med.* 297:988.

Brandes, N. S. 1971. A discussion of depression in children and adolescents. *Clin. Pediatr.* 10:470.

Carlson, G. A., and Strober, M. 1978. Manic-depressive illness in early adolescence. *J. Am. Acad. Child Psychiatr.* 17:138.

Flaherty, L., and Sarles, R. M. 1981. Psychosis during adolescence. *J. Adolescent Health Care* 1:301–307.

Friedman, S. B., and Sarles, R. M. 1980. Out of control behavior in adolescents. *Pediatr. Clin. North Am.* 27:97–108.

Glaser, K. 1967. Masked depression in children and adolescents. *Am. J. Psychother.* 21:565.

Groves, J. E. 1981. Borderline personality disorder. *N. Engl. J. Med.* 305:259–262.

Herzog, D. B., and Rathbun, J. M. 1982. Childhood depression: developmental considerations. *Am. J. Dis. Children* 136:115–120.

Hofmann, A. D. 1975. Adolescents in distress: suicide and out-of-control behaviors. *Med. Clin. North Am.* 56:1429.

Loeb, L. 1969. Adolescent schizophrenia. In *The schizophrenic syndrome*, editors L. Bell and L. Loeb. New York: Grune and Stratton.

Manschreck, T. C. 1981. Schizophrenic disorders. *N. Engl. J. Med.* 305:1628–1632.

Marks, A. 1979. Management of the suicidal adolescent on a nonpsychiatric adolescent unit. *J. Pediatr.* 95:305–308.

Mättsson, A. 1979. Depression and suicide in adolescence. In *The clinical practice of adolescent medicine*, editor J. T. Y. Shen. New York: Appleton-Century-Crofts.

McIntire, M. S., and Angle, C. R. 1975. Evaluation of suicide risk in adolescents. *J. Family Practice* 2:339.

McIntire, M. S., and Angle, C. R. 1980. *Suicide attempts in children and youth.* Hagerstown, Md.: Harper & Row.

Mitchell, J. 1975. *The adolescent predicament.* Toronto: Holt-Rhinehart.

Rinsley, D. B. 1972. A contribution to the nosology and dynamics of adolescent schizophrenia. *Psychiatr. Qtrly.* 46:159.

Rohn, R. D.; Sarles, R. M.; Kenny, T. J.; et al. 1977. Adolescents who attempt suicide. *J. Pediatr.* 90:636.

Slipp, S. 1973. The psychotic adolescent in the context of his family. In *The emotionally troubled adolescent and the family physician*, editor M. C. Kalogerakis. Springfield, Ill.: Charles C Thomas.

Toolan, J. M. 1973. Depression and suicide. In *The emotionally troubled adolescent and the family physician*, editor M. G. Kalogerakis. Springfield, Ill.: Charles C Thomas.

Weinberg, S. 1970. Suicidal intent in adolescence: a hypothesis about the role of physical illness. *J. Pediatr.* 77:579.

Winnecott, D. W. 1969. Adolescent process and the need for personal confrontation. *Pediatrics* 44:752.

*Note: Also see other bibliographies in Part IV.

Appendix I
Selected Tables

TABLE 1
HEIGHT PERCENTILES IN CENTIMETERS AND INCHES OF UNITED STATES YOUTHS AGED 12–17 YEARS BY AGE AND SEX

Sex and age	In centimeters Percentile							In inches Percentile						
	5th	10th	25th	50th	75th	90th	95th	5th	10th	25th	50th	75th	90th	95th
Male														
12 years	138.2	138.9	145.3	150.2	156.1	161.6	163.8	54.4	54.7	57.2	59.1	61.5	63.6	64.5
12½	139.2	141.4	146.3	152.2	156.4	161.1	163.7	54.8	55.7	57.6	59.9	61.6	63.4	64.4
13	141.6	145.5	149.9	155.7	161.1	166.6	170.3	55.8	57.3	59.0	61.3	63.4	65.6	67.1
13½	145.9	148.8	153.6	159.4	165.9	173.2	175.2	57.4	58.6	60.5	62.8	65.3	68.2	69.0
14	149.1	152.0	157.4	163.4	169.9	174.3	177.7	58.7	59.8	62.0	64.3	66.9	68.6	70.0
14½	152.2	155.0	159.7	167.9	173.2	177.2	179.7	59.9	61.0	62.9	66.1	68.2	69.8	70.8
15	155.5	158.9	163.8	169.8	175.0	179.2	181.8	61.4	62.6	64.5	66.8	68.9	70.6	71.6
15½	159.3	161.9	167.0	171.5	175.5	180.3	183.4	62.7	63.7	65.8	67.5	69.1	71.0	72.2
16	161.7	164.2	169.2	173.9	177.8	180.8	183.6	63.7	64.6	66.6	68.5	70.0	71.2	72.3
16½	164.3	166.6	171.1	174.8	178.6	182.8	185.2	64.7	65.6	67.4	68.8	70.3	72.0	72.9
17	163.3	166.3	170.1	175.8	179.9	183.9	186.5	64.3	65.5	67.0	69.2	70.8	72.4	73.4
17½	162.9	167.1	170.5	175.8	179.8	185.4	188.2	64.1	65.8	67.1	69.2	70.8	73.0	74.1
18	162.5	167.1	171.1	175.5	180.4	185.1	186.6	64.0	65.8	67.4	69.1	71.0	72.9	73.5
Female														
12 years	142.0	145.8	149.7	153.5	156.7	162.1	167.6	55.9	57.4	58.9	60.4	61.7	63.8	66.0
12½	141.3	144.9	150.9	155.5	160.5	164.3	166.7	55.6	57.1	59.4	61.2	63.2	64.7	65.6
13	144.8	147.8	152.4	15.72	161.7	166.5	169.0	57.0	58.2	60.0	61.9	63.7	65.6	66.5
13½	147.4	150.3	154.7	158.9	163.8	168.2	170.1	58.0	59.2	60.9	62.6	64.5	66.2	67.0
14	149.1	151.5	156.2	160.7	164.5	167.8	169.8	58.7	59.6	61.5	63.3	64.8	66.1	66.8
14½	150.6	153.6	157.3	161.3	165.3	169.8	171.3	59.3	60.5	61.9	63.5	65.1	66.8	67.4
15	152.1	154.3	157.4	161.8	166.6	169.7	171.8	59.9	60.8	62.0	63.7	65.6	66.8	67.6
15½	151.7	153.2	157.3	162.5	167.7	171.5	173.7	59.7	60.3	62.0	64.0	66.0	67.5	68.4
16	151.2	153.6	158.0	162.6	166.7	170.1	171.9	59.5	60.5	61.9	64.0	65.6	67.0	67.7
16½	151.6	153.7	158.1	163.1	166.6	170.7	172.7	59.7	60.5	62.2	64.2	65.6	67.2	68.0
17	151.6	155.0	158.8	163.6	166.9	171.6	174.1	59.7	61.0	62.5	64.4	65.7	67.6	68.5
17½	151.9	154.7	158.3	162.9	167.1	170.7	172.3	59.8	60.9	62.3	64.1	65.8	67.2	67.8
18	152.5	154.3	157.6	162.4	167.7	171.4	175.2	60.0	60.8	62.1	63.9	66.0	67.5	69.0

From National Center for Health Statistics. 1973. Series 11–No. 124, DHEW pub. no. (HSM) 73–1606. Washington, D.C.: U.S. Government Printing Office.

TABLE 2
WEIGHT PERCENTILES IN KILOGRAMS AND POUNDS OF UNITED STATES YOUTHS AGED 12-17 YEARS BY AGE AND SEX

Sex and age	In kilograms Percentile							In pounds Percentile						
	5th	10th	25th	50th	75th	90th	95th	5th	10th	25th	50th	75th	90th	95th
Male														
12 years	28.51	30.58	35.63	39.51	45.92	54.83	59.56	62.9	67.4	78.6	87.1	101.2	120.9	131.3
12½	31.20	32.79	36.03	40.65	46.94	55.28	58.86	68.8	72.3	79.4	89.6	103.5	121.9	129.8
13	31.38	34.37	38.81	44.37	50.80	59.25	62.36	69.2	75.8	85.6	97.8	112.0	130.6	137.5
13½	36.10	37.16	41.34	48.53	56.84	66.73	70.59	79.6	81.9	91.1	107.0	125.3	147.1	155.6
14	38.11	40.18	45.11	51.43	59.63	68.68	76.92	84.0	88.6	99.5	113.4	131.5	151.4	169.6
14½	38.90	41.25	49.37	55.59	62.57	71.24	79.19	85.8	90.9	108.8	122.6	137.9	157.1	174.6
15	42.90	46.17	51.06	58.33	66.43	74.01	76.54	94.6	101.8	112.6	128.6	146.5	163.2	163.7
15½	46.86	49.38	54.60	59.63	66.54	76.19	83.89	103.3	108.9	120.4	131.5	146.7	168.0	184.9
16	46.75	50.30	56.37	62.03	68.61	77.17	86.03	103.1	110.9	124.2	136.8	151.3	170.1	189.7
16½	50.21	52.60	57.24	62.83	69.90	78.21	81.74	110.7	116.0	126.2	138.5	154.1	172.4	180.2
17	50.14	52.97	59.32	64.79	72.84	80.55	85.78	110.5	116.8	130.8	142.8	160.6	177.5	189.1
17½	52.84	56.45	61.25	66.80	74.30	85.49	90.93	116.5	124.5	135.0	147.3	163.8	188.5	200.5
18	54.01	56.01	60.35	67.22	73.82	79.98	96.17	119.1	123.5	133.0	148.2	162.7	176.3	212.0
Female														
12 years	32.73	34.33	38.28	43.83	49.84	58.69	62.57	72.2	75.7	84.4	96.6	109.9	129.4	137.9
12½	31.82	34.78	39.14	45.46	52.53	59.41	63.65	70.2	76.7	86.3	100.2	115.8	131.0	140.3
13	34.91	37.18	41.64	47.14	53.50	62.36	67.47	77.0	82.0	91.8	103.9	117.9	137.5	148.7
13½	36.35	38.65	43.83	49.63	56.44	62.97	72.51	80.1	85.2	96.6	109.4	124.4	138.8	159.9
14	38.29	40.22	46.15	51.04	57.45	63.81	68.11	84.4	88.7	101.7	112.5	126.7	140.7	150.2
14½	41.03	43.19	47.00	52.35	59.86	68.20	72.05	90.5	95.2	103.6	115.4	132.0	150.4	158.8
15	41.38	44.13	48.07	54.01	59.82	65.92	71.25	91.2	97.3	106.0	119.1	131.9	145.3	157.1
15½	41.05	44.22	48.99	55.27	60.81	72.42	82.46	90.5	97.5	108.0	121.8	134.1	159.7	181.8
16	44.46	46.45	50.77	54.86	60.62	68.98	77.75	98.0	102.4	111.9	120.9	133.6	152.1	170.3
16½	45.42	46.66	50.51	55.25	62.83	71.67	83.62	100.1	102.9	111.4	121.8	138.5	158.0	184.4
17	44.42	47.04	50.21	56.79	62.04	72.61	79.14	97.9	103.7	110.7	125.2	136.8	160.1	174.5
17½	44.73	46.92	50.88	55.59	63.25	69.82	82.00	98.6	103.4	112.2	122.6	139.4	153.9	180.8
18	44.43	46.34	50.67	55.71	61.75	71.24	75.28	98.0	102.2	111.7	122.8	136.1	157.1	166.0

From National Center for Health Statistics. 1973. Series 11–No. 124, DHEW pub. no. (HSM) 73–1606. Washington, D.C.: U.S. Government Printing Office.

TABLE 3
TRICEPS SKINFOLD IN MILLIMETERS
OF YOUTHS AGED 12-17 YEARS BY RACE, SEX, AND AGE AT LAST BIRTHDAY

	Percentile				
Race, sex and age	5th	10th	50th	90th	95th
White					
Male					
12 years	5.2	5.7	9.7	19.8	23.2
13	4.8	5.4	9.4	19.7	22.6
14	4.3	5.0	8.2	17.4	21.2
15	4.3	4.8	7.8	16.4	21.3
16	4.2	5.0	7.6	16.5	20.5
17	4.1	4.5	7.7	15.8	20.7
Female					
12 years	6.1	7.1	12.0	22.1	25.1
13	6.6	7.6	12.7	22.7	25.4
14	7.3	8.5	14.2	23.5	26.8
15	7.5	8.8	15.1	25.4	29.9
16	8.1	9.7	16.0	25.5	29.1
17	8.5	10.1	16.3	25.3	29.5
Negro					
Male					
12 years	3.8	4.7	7.4	15.3	23.2
13	3.6	4.2	7.2	15.6	25.2
14	3.6	4.1	6.4	14.2	19.2
15	3.9	4.2	6.4	10.6	14.7
16	4.0	4.3	6.7	11.7	12.8
17	4.2	4.6	6.1	14.0	15.8
Female					
12 years	6.0	6.5	10.6	22.5	25.6
13	6.0	6.3	9.8	23.9	27.2
14	5.5	6.7	12.5	22.1	24.6
15	7.2	8.2	12.8	22.7	25.8
16	7.0	7.6	13.1	26.4	31.5
17	7.1	7.6	13.4	23.3	25.8

From National Center for Health Statistics. 1974 *Skinfold thickness of youths 12–17 years*, Series 11, No. 132, (DHEW pub. no. (HRA) 74–1614). Washington, D.C.: U.S. Government Printing Office.

TABLE 4
PARAMETERS OF THE ADOLESCENT GROWTH SPURT

	Males	Females
Linear growth (accounts for 16% of final adult height)		
Age of onset (range)	12–14 years	10–12 years
Average gain	9.1 cm/yr	8.2 cm/yr
Cessation of all growth	By 20 years	By 17–19 years
Weight gain (accounts for approximately 50% of final adult weight)		
Average gain	9 kg/yr	8.3 kg/yr
Duration of gain	Parallels linear growth spurt	Parallels linear growth spurt
Dominant composition	Muscle and bone	Fat

TABLE 5
STAGES OF SEXUAL MATURATION (TANNER STAGING) AND NORMAL AGE RANGES: MALES

Stage	Pubic hair	Age in years -2 SD +2 SD Mean		Penis and testes	Age in years -2 SD +2 SD Mean		Comments
I	None; prepubertal			Prepubertal; testes approximately 2–2.5 cm in length			
II	Long, lightly pigmented, downy; at base of penis	11.36 13.44	15.62	Testes definitely enlarged; pigmentation and thinning of scrotum; penis beginning to enlarge	9.50 11.64	13.76	Testicular enlargement is earliest sign of puberty and antecedes pubic hair appearance by about 1½ years
III	Increased in amount and pigmentation; curly; still limited to base of penis	11.86 13.90	15.98	Further enlargement of testes and penis, particularly in length	10.77 12.85	14.93	Height spurt initiates at about this time; 50% may have downy facial hair at corners, upper lip, and on cheeks in front of ears
IV	Adult in type; extends about halfway out to inguinal regions	12.10 14.36	16.52	Further enlargement of testes and penis, particularly in circumference	11.73 13.77	15.81	Axillary hair appears here or in stage III; facial hair only slightly increased but extends across lip; beginning deepening voice; deceleration of height spurt
V	Adult in type, quantity, and lateral distribution, extending out to thighs	13.04 15.18	17.32	Adult size, may appear disproportionately large in boys who have not yet attained full skeletal growth	12.72 14.92	17.12	Upper lip hair conspicuous; may have sparse chin hair; body hair continues developing well into 20s; growth in height may continue significantly past stage V in some

After Tanner, J. M. 1962. *Growth at adolescence*, 2nd ed. Oxford: Blackwell; Root, A. W. 1973. Endocrinology of puberty. *J. Pediatr.* 83:1–19; and Hofmann, A.; Becker, R.; and Gabriel, H. 1976. *The hospitalized adolescent.* New York: The Free Press.

TABLE 6
STAGES OF SEXUAL MATURATION (TANNER STAGING) AND NORMAL AGE RANGES: FEMALES

Stage	Pubic hair	Age in years -2 SD	+2 SD Mean	Breasts	Age in years -2 SD	+2 SD Mean	Comments
I	None; prepubertal			Prepubertal; elevation papilla only			
II	Long, lightly pigmented, downy; along labia	9.27	14.11 / 11.69	Breast bud stage; elevation of breast and papilla as small mound and enlargement of areolar diameter	8.95	13.25 / 11.15	Onset of breast and pubic hair development more or less simultaneous; initiation of height spurt will soon follow
III	Increased in amount and pigmentation; curly; still limited to labia	10.16	14.56 / 11.69	Breast and areola show further enlargement with no separation of contours	9.97	14.33 / 12.15	Menarche usually occurs about this time or 1½ years after onset of breast development; axillary hair first appears here or in stage IV
IV	Adult in type; covers mons and extends about halfway out to inguinal regions	10.83	15.07 / 12.95	Areola and papilla project to form a secondary mound above the level of the breast itself (variable; not always present)	10.81	15.31 / 13.11	Height spurt begins to decelerate
V	Adult in type, quantity, and lateral distribution; extending out to thighs	12.17	16.65 / 14.41	Mature with projection of papilla only due to recession of general contour of entire breast	11.85	18.81 / 15.33	Growth almost complete and most epiphyses closed; may grow 1–2 cm more

After Tanner, J. M. 1962. *Growth at adolescence*, 2nd ed. Oxford: Blackwell; Root, A. W. 1973. Endocrinology of puberty. *J. Pediatr.* 83:1–19; and Hofmann, A.; Becker, R.; and Gabriel, H. 1976. *The hospitalized adolescent.* New York: The Free Press.

TABLE 7
NORMAL BLOOD VALUES OF SELECTED TESTS BY AGE AND MATURATIONAL LEVEL*

Test		Age						Tanner stage				
		13	14	15	16	17	18	I	II	III	IV	V
Serum alkaline phosphatase† (International units)												
Male	Mean	100±45	102±36	103±39	75±28	64±46	42±14	74±21	89±29	116±41	103±43	70±39
	Range	49–240	36–192	41–195	32–142	21–228	23–63	43–130	42–204	46–240	32–228	21–228
Female	Mean	78±29	52±19	38±16	31±10	28±6	21±4	79±16	93±21	84±30	39±21	32±12
	Range	25–144	22–91	17–91	13–56	16–46	18–24	51–108	49–138	26–148	16–144	13–76
Hematocrit (%)‡,§												
Male	White	40	41	42	47	45	—	39.5	40	41	42	43.5
	Black	39	41	40	42	44	48	37.5	38.5	39.5	41	42.5
Female	White	40	40	39	40	41	40	39	39	39	39	39
	Black	38	40	38	38	39	39	37	39	38	38	39
Hemoglobin g/100 ml‡,∥												
Male	White	13.3	13.7	14.1	16.1	16.0	—	14.4	14.2	14.7	15.2	15.9
	Black	13.0	13.6	13.4	14.0	14.3	14.8					
Female	White	13.5	13.4	13.0	13.6	13.3	13.2	13.3	13.4	13.2	13.4	13.3
	Black	12.7	12.8	12.5	12.5	12.4	13.1					
Plasma cholesterol mg/ml¶ (fasting)												
Male	Mean	154	151	146	149	152	—	—	—	—	—	—
	Range	112–202	116–197	112–194	115–192	117–209	—	—	—	—	—	—
Female	Mean	154	156	155	152	155	—	—	—	—	—	—
	Range	119–195	117–195	119–187	119–196	118–196	—	—	—	—	—	—
Plasma triglycerides mg/ml¶ (fasting)												
Male	Mean	71	70	76	74	74	—	—	—	—	—	—
	Range	37–162	37–143	44–165	36–163	42–174	—	—	—	—	—	—
Female	Mean	80	75	76	74	74	—	—	—	—	—	—
	Range	48–142	44–141	44–154	39–114	41–108	—	—	—	—	—	—

*Other common tests have normal values in the adult range.

†Bennett, D.; Ward, M.; and Daniel, W. 1976. The relationship of serum alkaline phosphatase concentrations to sex maturity ratings in adolescence. *J. Pediatr.* 88:633.

‡Daniel, W.; and Rowland, A. 1969. Hemoglobin and hematocrit values of adolescents. *Clin. Pediatr.* 8:181.

§Young, H. B., et al. 1968. Evaluation of physical maturity at adolescence. *Dev. Med. Child Neurol.* 10:338.

∥Daniel, W. 1973. Hematocrit: maturity relationship in adolescence. *Pediatrics* 52:388.

¶deGroot, I.; Morrison, J.; Kelley, K.; et al. 1977. Lipids in school children 6–17 years of age: upper normal limits. *Pediatrics* 60:437 and U.S. Department of Health, Education, and Welfare, Vital and Health Statistics. 1980. *Serum cholesterol levels of persons 4–74 years of age*, DHEW Pub. No. (PHS) 80-1667. Hyattsville, Md.: National Center for Health Statistics.

Also see Friedman, I. M., and Goldberg, E. 1980. Reference materials for the practice of adolescent medicine. *Pediatr. Clin. North Am.* 27:193.

TABLE 8
HORMONE VALUES: THYROID HORMONE AND
GONADOTROPIN LEVELS BY AGE AND MATURATIONAL LEVEL

Test	Age	Mean	Range	Tanner stage	Males	Females
Thyroxine (RIA) (μg/dl)	10–15	8.1	5.6–11.7	I	10.7	10.1
	15	7.6	——	II	9.4	10.3
	——	——	——	III	8.9	10.2
	——	——	——	IV	8.5	8.9
	——	——	——	V	8.4	10.8
Triiodothyronine (RIA) (ng/dl)	10–15	133	83–213	I	139	140
	15	125	——	II	121	143
	——	——	——	III	134	139
	——	——	——	IV	146	137
	——	——	——	V	131	128
Thyroid-stimulating hormone (TSH) (RIA) (μU/ml)	10–15	1.9	0.6–6.3	I	8.5	10.5
	15	1.9	0.6–6.3	II	8.7	9.8
	——	——	——	III	10.8	7.4
	——	——	——	IV	12.5	8.3
	——	——	——	V	15.7	8.9
Basal serum LH (mIU/ml, IRP-2-hMG)	11–12	<1–12	<1–9	I	<1–5	<1–6
	13–14	3–15	3–10	II	<1–8	<1–9
	15–20	5–25	4–25	III	3–15	3–15
	——	——	——	IV	3–20	3–20
	——	——	——	V	5–25	4–25
Basal urine LH levels (IU, IRP-2-hMG/24 hrs)	11–12	3–13	1–15	I	<0.5–5	<0.5–3
	13–14	10–28	5–30	II	3–20	——
	——	——	——	III	5–25	2–20
	15–20	10–60	10–60	IV	10–35	——
	——	——	——	V	15–60	10–60
Basal serum FSH levels (mIU/ml, IRP-2-hMG)	11–12	2–12	3–11	I	<1–5	2–4
	13–14	3–15	3–15	II	<1–10	2–10
	15–20	5–10	4–20	III	3–15	3–15
	——	——	——	IV	3–20	3–20
	——	——	——	V	5–20	4–20
Basal urine FSH levels (IU, IRP-2-hMG/24 hrs)	11–12	1.5–5	1–8	I	<0.5–4.5	<0.5–3
	13–14	2–12	1–10	II	2–8	——
	15–20	2.5–20	1–12	III	2–13	1–8
	——	——	——	IV	3–25	——
	——	——	——	V	4–18	3–12

From Johnson, T.; Moore, W.; and Jeffries, J. 1978. *Children are different*, 2nd ed. Columbus, Ohio: Ross Laboratories, and Reiter, E. O., and Root, A. W. 1975. Hormonal changes of adolescence. *Med. Clin. North Am.* 59:1289.

TABLE 9
HORMONE VALUES: PLASMA SEX STEROIDS BY AGE AND SEXUAL MATURATION*

Age	E_1 (pg/ml)	E_2 (pg/ml)	T ng/dl)	A (ng/dl)	DHA ng/dl)	DHAS (μg/dl)	17-KS (mg/24 hr urine)
Females							
10–12	20–67	10–200	10–65	40–150	150–600	25–150	3.34
12–14	20–177	10–270	20–80	40–150	150–700	50–150	4.34
14–16	20–100	15–400	20–85	40–150	200–700	125–225	——
Tanner stage							
I	<20	<10	<20	10–100	——	——	1.18
II	10–53	5–62	<20–65	——	——	——	1.79
III	15–91	9–126	<20–80	——	——	——	——
IV	16–177	10–270	<20–85	40–150	——	——	3.31
V	29–77	15–400	<20–85	40–150	——	——	4.50
Males							
12–13	14–50	2–30	131–249	57–90	200–500	50–250	3.3–4.5
14–15	15–50	5–40	328–643	87–140	300–500	75–250	5.2
Tanner stage							
I	<20	2–6	17–25	60–62	——	——	1.8
II	15–36	2–10	25–85	60–62	——	——	1.8
III	21–51	8–16	52–328	——	——	——	2.2
IV	23–50	11–23	134–532	43	——	——	3.8
V	27–48	14–29	328–643	78	——	——	6.4

*Adapted from Johnson, T.; Moore, W.; Jeffries, J. 1978. *Children are different*, 2nd ed. Columbus, Ohio: Ross Laboratories; and Reiter, E., and Root, A. 1975. Hormonal changes of adolescence. *Med. Clin. North Am.* 59:1289.

Abbreviations: E_1, estrone; E_2, estradiol; T, testosterone; A, androstanedione; DHA, dehydroepiandrosterone; DHAS, dehydroepiandrosterone sulfate; 17-KS, 17-ketosteroids.

TABLE 10

PULMONARY FUNCTION TESTS: NORMAL VALUES IN YOUTHS AGED 12-17 YEARS

Age	Height 50th percentile (cm)		Vital capacity (ml)		Functional residual capacity (ml)		Total lung capacity (ml)		Peak expiratory flow rate (L/min)	
Age	Male	Female	Male	Female	Male	Female	Male	Female	Male	Female
12	150	152	2800	2620	1710	1660	3810	3625	375	360
13	155	157	3090	2890	1890	1790	4207	3957	400	375
14	163	160	3575	3040	2190	1880	4871	4160	459	400
15	168	161	3880	3090	2200	1900	5310	4217	475	409
16	172	162	4140	3150	2580	1950	5685	4312	510	415
17	172	163	4295	3190	2670	1980	5891	4372	520	420
Adult	176	165	4780	3320	2180	1670	5970	4160	525	425

From Johnson, T.; Moore, W.; and Jeffries, J. 1978. *Children are different*, 2nd ed. Columbus, Ohio: Ross Laboratories.

TABLE 11
BLOOD PRESSURE VALUES FOR WHITE AND BLACK ADOLESCENTS (mm Hg)

Age	White			Black		
	Mean	±2.5 SD	95th percentile	Mean	+2.5 SD	95th percentile
Females			*Systolic pressure*			
12	124.3	11.6	144.2	121.8	10.6	138.9
15	127.9	12.1	149.5	124.0	10.5	141.6
17	128.2	12.1	148.7	129.7	11.1	147.4
			Diastolic pressure			
12	71.7	7.5	82.5	72.9	7.9	85.5
15	75.3	7.6	87.0	72.9	7.8	89.7
17	76.4	7.4	87.9	77.5	7.8	90.3
Males			*Systolic pressure*			
12	120.1	10.9	138.2	117.5	9.7	132.9
15	133.8	11.9	151.9	129.1	11.7	148.8
17	138.1	12.7	162.0	133.5	11.7	152.3
			Diastolic pressure			
12	70.3	7.2	82.5	70.8	6.6	82.4
15	75.8	7.6	88.3	76.9	8.5	90.3
17	79.0	7.6	90.4	81.6	7.4	94.4

Adapted from the National Health Survey. 1980. Vital and health statistics, Series II, Nos. 135 and 136. In *Compendium of resource materials on adolescent health*, DHHS, PHS. Rockville, Md.: Bureau of Community Health Services.

Appendix II
Selected Resources for Professional and Lay Information

These resources variably provide patient education materials, professional guidelines, technical reports (particularly governmental clearinghouses), consultations, further referral resources, and/or advocacy and support in special problem areas. Notation as to subject areas of concern and services other than educational is made when relevant or not self-evident. Inquiry about full range of services, publication lists, and so on should be made directly to the organization in question. Organizations also are cross-referenced by title only when applicable with headings under which the address may be found given in parentheses.

General Health
MULTIPLE TOPICS
American Academy of Pediatrics
P. O. Box 1034
Evanston, IL 60204   (312) 869-4255

American College Health Association
152 Rollins Avenue, Suite 208
Rockville, MD 20852

American Medical Association
Department of Health Education/
Department of Publications
535 North Dearborn Street
Chicago, IL 60610

National Center for Health Statistics
3700 East-West Highway
Hyattsville, MD 20782   (301) 436-8500

Society for Adolescent Medicine
P. O. Box 3462
Granada Hills, CA 91344   (213) 368-5996
(Referral lists, fellowship information, speakers bureau, journal)

NUTRITION
General Mills, Inc.
Nutrition Department
Minneapolis, MN 55460

National Dairy Council
Rosemont, IL 60018

SPECIAL HEALTH ISSUES
American Cancer Society, Inc.
777 Third Avenue
New York, NY 10017
(Breast exam, smoking)

National Cancer Institute
Office of Cancer Communications
Bethesda, MD 20014
(Breast exam, smoking, DES)

American Diabetes Association
600 Fifth Avenue
New York, NY 10020

Juvenile Diabetes Foundation
2200 Benjamin Franklin Parkway
Philadelphia, PA 19130   (215) 567-4307

Epilepsy Foundation of America
1828 L Street NW
Washington, DC 20036

Mental Health
National Clearinghouse—Mental Health Information
Room 11 A-33, Parklawn Building
5600 Fishers Lane
Rockville, MD 20857   (301) 443-4273

Sexuality

Sex Education (broadly defined)

Also see *Sex Education for Adolescents; an Annotated Bibliography of Low Cost Publications*, available from the American Academy of Pediatrics or Planned Parenthood Federation of America (addresses given in other sections of this Appendix).

Ed-U-Press
P. O. Box 583
Fayetteville, NY 13066
(Publisher for Institute for Family Research and Education, University of Syracuse; also publications on sexually transmitted disease.)

Emory University-Grady Memorial Hospital Family Planning Program
80 Butler Street SE
Atlanta, GA 30303

National Clearinghouse–Family Planning Information
Box 2225
Rockville, MD 20852   (301) 443-4273

Ortho Pharmaceutical Corp.
Raritan, NJ 08869

Planned Parenthood, Alameda-San Francisco
1660 Bush Street
San Francisco, CA 94109

Planned Parenthood Federation of America
810 Seventh Avenue
New York, NY 10019   (212) 541-7800

Planned Parenthood Center of Syracuse
1120 East Genesee Street
Syracuse, NY 13210

Rocky Mountain Planned Parenthood
2030 East Twentieth Avenue
Denver, CO 80205

Sex Information and Education Council of the U.S. (SIECUS)
84 Fifth Avenue, Suite 407
New York, NY 10011   (212) 929-2300
(Professional guidelines, reference library, advocacy, newsletter, plus bibliography, patient education materials, and so on.)

Also see American College Health Association (general health); American College of Obstetricians and Gynecologists (pregnancy); American Medical Association (general health); Do-It-Now Foundation (substance abuse).

SEXUALLY TRANSMITTED DISEASE

(Also many of above.)
American Social Health Association
260 Sheridan Avenue
Palo Alto, CA 94306

(Also publications on general sex education, substance abuse; also see National Hot Lines under social services section.)

ADOLESCENT PREGNANCY/ PARENTHOOD

American College of Obstetricians and Gynecologists
1 East Wacker Drive
Chicago, IL 60601
(Also general sex education, task force on adolescent pregnancy, professional workshops)

Child Welfare League of America
67 Irving Place
New York, NY 10003   (212) 254-7410
(Advocacy, research, education, information on child welfare, adolescent parenthood initiative, and publications)

Department of Health and Human Services
Office of Adolescent Pregnancy Programs
Parklawn Building, Room 16A-17
5600 Fishers Lane
Rockville, MD 20857
(Granting agency for service programs, clearinghouse, newsletter.)

Family Service Association of America
44 East 23rd Street
New York, NY 10010   (212) 674-6100
(Technical and statistical publications concerning family life, including adolescent pregnancy.)

National Foundation–March of Dimes
1275 Mamaroneck Avenue
White Plains, NY 10605
(Wide range of educational material for individuals and schools.)

The Salvation Army
120 West 14th Street
New York, NY 10011
("Education for parenthood" curriculum designed for adolescents.)

HOMOSEXUALITY

Dignity International
1500 Massachusetts Avenue NW, No. 11
Washington, DC 20005
(Catholic support group.)

National Gay Health Coalition
26 North 35th Street
Philadelphia, PA 19104
(Advocacy group for improved health care and health services.)

National Gay Task Force
80 Fifth Avenue, Suite 1601
New York, NY 10011   (212) 741-5800
(Educational materials.)

The National Federation of
Parents and Friends of Gays
5715 Sixteenth Street NW
Washington, DC 10011   (202) 726-3223
(Support group with regional branches; pamphlet
with regional telephone numbers.)

Also see *Gay Yellow Pages* available in many book-
stores; gives local hot lines and other regional services.

Substance Abuse

Alcoholics Anonymous (also see telephone directory
for local branches)
Box 452
Grand Central Annex
New York, NY 10017

Alateen (Group program for teenagers of alcoholic
parents; see local listings for AA or Alateen.)

Alanon (Group program for spouses of alcoholic
partner)
Alanon Family Group Headquarters
115 East 23rd Street
New York, NY 10010
(Also see local directory listings.)

Do-It-Now Foundation
Box 5115
Phoenix, AR 85010
(Also publications on sex education, sexually trans-
mitted disease, others.)

National Association for the Prevention of Narcotics
Abuse
305 East 79th Street
New York, NY 10021

National Clearinghouse–Alcohol Information
Box 2345
Rockville, MD 20852   (301) 948-4450

National Clearinghouse–Drug Abuse Information
Parklawn Building, Room 10 A-56
5600 Fishers Lane
Rockville, MD 20852   (301) 443-4273

National Clearinghouse on Smoking and Health
Center for Disease Control, Building 14
1600 Cliften Road
Atlanta, GA 30333

National Poison Center Network
125 DeSoto Street
Pittsburgh, PA 15213
(Also see telephone directory for local poison control centers)

Narcotics Education
6830 Laurel Avenue
Washington, DC 20012

HANDICAPPED
(Also see Education and Social Services sections.)
CLOSER LOOK: National Information Center for
the Handicapped
Box 1492
Washington, DC 20013   (202) 833-4160
(Information concerning services and funding for
handicapped, including youth.)

SOCIAL SERVICES
Directory of Hot Lines
The Communication Company
1826 Fell Street
San Francisco, CA 94117

National Hot Lines:
Operation Venus (VD counseling and referral)
(800) 523-1885; in Pennsylvania, (800) 462-4966

National Runaway Switchboard (parent-runaway
contact service) (800) 621-4000;
in Illinois, (800) 972-6004
Also see local telephone directory.

National Clearinghouse on Child Abuse and Neglect
Information
400 Sixth Street SW
Washington, DC 20201   (202) 755-0587

National Directory of Children and Youth Services
Child Protection Report
1301 20th Street NW
Washington, DC 20009
(Directory of public and private agencies at city,
county, state, and federal levels; $39 postage paid.)

National Youth Work Alliance
1346 Connecticut Avenue NW
Washington, DC 20036   (202) 785-0764
                              or (800) 424-6740
(Workshops, newsletter, information concerning services for and issues relating to youth, particularly
runaways; employment; juvenile justice; substance
abuse; pregnancy.)

Office of Human Development (DHHS)
Administration for Children, Youth and Families
P. O. Box 1182
Washington, DC 20013   (202) 755-7724
(Administers Head Start, national runaway program,
and some delinquency diversion programs.)

Education

American School Counselors Association
1607 New Hampshire Avenue NW
Washington, DC 20009   (202) 483-4633

National Association of School Psychologists
1511 K Street NW
Washington, DC 20005   (202) 347-3956

National Education Association of the U.S.
1201 16th Street NW
Washington, DC 20036   (202) 833-4000

National Institute of Education
1200 19th Street NW
Washington, DC 20208   (202) 254-5800

U.S. Department of Education
400 Maryland Avenue SW
Washington, DC 20202   (202) 245-8564

U.S. Department of Education bureaus (use Maryland Avenue address)
  Bureau of Education for the Handicapped,
  (202) 245-9661
  Office for Gifted and Talented Education,
  (202) 245-2482
  National Right-to-Read Office, (202) 245-8537
  Educational Resources Information Center (ERIC),
  (202) 254-5555 (computer searches in 16 different subject areas)
  Bureau of Elementary and Secondary Education
  Division of Education for the Disadvantaged,
  (202) 245-2722
  National Center for Education Statistics
  Statistical Information Branch, (202) 245-8511

Juvenile Delinquency

National Council on Crime and Delinquency
Continental Plaza
411 Hackensack Avenue
Hackensack, NJ 07601   (202) 488-0400
(Information clearinghouse on community-based delinquency prevention programs.)

National Criminal Justice Reference Service
1015 20th Street NW
Washington, DC 20036   (202) 862-2900
                              or (800) 424-2856
(Juvenile justice clearinghouse, information on federal legislation and federal programs.)

Also see Children's Defense Fund (advocacy)
Coalition for Children and Youth (advocacy)

Advocacy

American Academy of Pediatrics
Office of Governmental Affairs
1800 North Kent Street
Arlington, VA 22209   (703) 525-9560

(Concerned with federal legislation concerning health and health services for children and youth; information on status of specific legislation; newsletter.)

Center for Early Adolescence
Suite 223, Carr Mill Mall
Carrboro, NC 27510
(Also professional education, workshops, newsletter, publications.)

Children's Defense Fund
1520 New Hampshire Avenue NW
Washington, DC 20036   (800) 424-9602
(Also information on problems and issues affecting children and youth via toll free line—no individual consultations; core issues: education, health care, child care and development, juvenile justice; publications.)

Coalition for Children and Youth
815 15th Street NW
Washington, DC 20005   (202) 347-9380
(1500 member groups; core issues: health, day care, juvenile justice; publications.)

Audiovisuals

B.F.A. (Division of CBS, Inc.)
2211 Michigan Avenue
P. O. Box 1795
Santa Monica, CA 90406
(Mental health, sexually transmitted disease, substance abuse.)

Churchill Films
662 North Robertson Boulevard
Los Angeles, CA 90069
(Nutrition, puberty, sexually transmitted disease, substance abuse.)

Lawren Productions, Inc.
P. O. Box 666
Mendocino, CA 95460
(Mental health, educational problems.)

Multi-Media Resource Center
1525 Franklin Street
San Francisco, CA 94109
(Sexuality, sex dysfunction, substance abuse.)

Perennial Education, Inc.
477 Roger Williams
P. O. Box 855
Highland Park, IL 60035
(Contraception, nutrition, pregnancy, sexuality, sexually transmitted disease, substance abuse.)

Picture Films Distribution Corp.
43 West 16th Street
New York, NY 10011
(Pregnancy, substance abuse.)

Sunburst Communications
41 Washington Avenue, Room 5
Pleasantville, NY 10570
(Mental health, nutrition, pregnancy, sexuality, sexually transmitted disease, substance abuse.)

Texture Films, Inc.
1600 Broadway
New York, NY 10019
(Sexuality.)

"Triggertapes"
Learning Corporation of America
1350 Avenue of the Americas
New York, NY 10019
(Decision making, sexuality, pregnancy.)

Professional Publications

Journal of Adolescent Health Care. Official Journal of the Society for Adolescent Medicine. Subscription, $30 individuals; $15 interns and residents. Elsevier North Holland, Inc., 52 Vanderbilt Avenue, New York, NY 10017.

Transitions. Professional courtesy publication. Syntex Laboratories, Inc., 3401 Hillview Avenue, Palo Alto, CA 94304.

Organizations Offering Useful Services, Information, and/or Educational Materials at the Local Level

(Check local telephone directory for address and telephone number.)

PEER GROUP AND ROLE MODEL PROGRAMS
Boys Clubs/Girls Clubs of America
Boy and Girl Scouts of America
Big Brothers/Big Sisters
Police Athletic League (PAL)

PRIVATE SOCIAL SERVICE AND MENTAL HEALTH AGENCIES
Catholic Charities
Jewish Family Services (or equivalent)
State and local organizations for the mentally handicapped, brain injured, retarded, etc. (for children and adults)
Community- and hospital-based mental hygiene clinics

SPECIAL HEALTH PROBLEMS
Adolescent medical clinics in local hospitals
Specific disease support groups (for example, diabetes, epilepsy, hemophilia)
Lighthouse for the Blind
Weight Watchers, TOPS, Overeaters Anonymous
Alcoholics Anonymous, Alanon, Alateen
Planned Parenthood

STATE AND LOCAL GOVERNMENT SERVICES*
Department of Health
  Preventive health services
  Acute health care services (for example, venereal disease treatment)
  School health
  Family planning services
  Services for the handicapped
Department of Mental Health
  Services for the brain injured, retarded
  Services for the emotionally disturbed
  Drug and alcohol abuse services (may be under separate department)
Department of Labor
  Youth employment services
Department of Education
  School guidance department
  School psychologist
  Bureau of special educational services or equivalent
Department of Social Service
  Medicaid administration
  Child and adolescent abuse
  Residential placement services
  Pregnancy programs
Department of Justice
  Family court
  Police; may have youth delinquency diversion programs
Office of Vocational Rehabilitation (or equivalent); services for disabled adults.

*Adolescents may qualify for either child or adult services depending on age. If under 18, eligible for child services; between 18 and 21 is variable; check local regulations.

Index